W9-BVX-563

CLINICAL

NUCLEAR

CARDIOLOGY

George A. Beller, M.D.
Chief, Cardiovascular Division
Department of Internal Medicine
University of Virginia Health Sciences Center
Charlottesville, Virginia

W.B. SAUNDERS COMPANY
A Division of Harcourt Brace & Company
Philadelphia • London • Toronto • Montreal • Sydney • Tokyo

W.B. SAUNDERS COMPANY
A Division of Harcourt Brace & Company

The Curtis Center
Independence Square West
Philadelphia, Pennsylvania 19106

Library of Congress Cataloging-in-Publication Data

Beller, George.
    Clinical nuclear cardiology/George A. Beller.

    p.   cm.

ISBN 0-7216-3332-3

1. Heart—Radionuclide imaging.   I. Title.

[DNLM: 1. Heart Diseases—radionuclide imaging.   WG 141.5.R3
1995]

RC683.5.R33B45   1995

616.1'207575—dc20

DNLM/DLC   94-25345

CLINICAL NUCLEAR CARDIOLOGY   ISBN 0-7216-3332-3

Copyright © 1995 by W.B. Saunders Company.

All rights reserved. No part of this publication may be reproduced or transmitted in any form or by any
means, electronic or mechanical, including photocopy, recording, or any information storage and retrieval
system, without permission in writing from the publisher.

Printed in the United States of America.

Last digit is the print number: 9   8   7   6   5   4   3   2   1

AV9573
Cummings, John

To my parents,
Irving and Joanna Beller,
for their sustained love and encouragement
through the years.

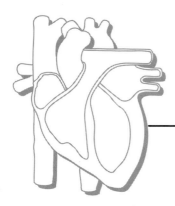

Preface

During the past 20 years, nuclear cardiology, as a subdiscipline of both cardiology and nuclear medicine specialties, has experienced a major expansion in the techniques offered and in associated clinical applications. Whereas for almost 15 years thallium-201 (Tl-201) was the dominant agent employed for myocardial perfusion imaging, today several new technetium-99m (Tc-99m)–labeled radionuclides have emerged as excellent alternatives to Tl-201 for the detection of coronary artery disease, prognostication, and even assessment of myocardial viability. Single-photon emission tomography (SPECT) has all but replaced planar imaging techniques for myocardial scintigraphy, and novel computer-derived quantitative analyses of regional tracer uptake have been introduced to enhance sensitivity and specificity for detection of abnormal myocardial blood flow in patients with coronary artery disease. Use of these new Tc-99m tracers has reduced the false-positive rate of scan interpretations. Pharmacologic stress imaging using either dipyridamole, adenosine, or dobutamine is a superb substitute for exercise stress in evaluation of patients with suspected or known coronary artery disease who are unable to exercise adequately. Distinguishing viable from irreversibly injured myocardium with SPECT or positron emission tomographic (PET) radionuclide methodologies has proved most valuable to clinicians by contributing important information regarding which patients with severe coronary artery disease and profound left ventricular dysfunction benefit most from revascularization. Such techniques also permit the noninvasive determination of the degree of myocardial salvage and the ability to distinguish stunned from necrotic myocardium after coronary reperfusion in the setting of acute myocardial infarction. Stress nuclear imaging approaches have aided in the noninvasive identification of coronary restenosis after angioplasty and bypass graft obstruction after revascularization surgery, thereby avoiding coronary angiography in many patients presenting with atypical symptoms following these procedures. These are just some of the clinical applications that have characterized the expansion of nuclear cardiology in recent years.

Clinical Nuclear Cardiology comprehensively presents the current and potential future uses of nuclear cardiology techniques in cardiovascular medicine by providing in-depth, state-of-the-art, and extensively referenced presentations of clinical applications of presently utilized techniques and critical discussion of the probable worth and potential limitations of new techniques now undergoing validation in experimental laboratories and studies in the clinical setting. The book took more than two years to complete and is different from most others in the field in that it does not merely emphasize the technical aspects of nuclear cardiology but focuses on clinical utility for a myriad of disease entities or syndromes. It is also written by a single author with 20 years of clinical research experience in the field of noninvasive cardiology and radionuclide imaging in particular. Chapters 1 and 2 review in detail the technical aspects of radionuclide imaging instrumentation for both SPECT and PET approaches and the biologic behavior of the array of radiopharmaceuticals employed, respectively. Many new agents such as Tc-99m sestamibi, iodine-123 IPPA, and carbon-11 hydroxyephedrine are discussed. The last is used with PET to assess cardiac sympathetic innervation. These early chapters contain introductory sections summarizing a vast amount of experimental laboratory data relevant to tracer kinetics, which form the basis for clinical imaging.

Subsequent chapters are organized by clinical applications or clinical syndromes, including detection of coronary artery disease (Chapter 3), assessment of prognosis (Chapter 4), evaluation of silent myocardial ischemia (Chapter 5), acute myocardial infarction (Chapter 6), unstable angina pectoris (Chapter 7), pharmacologic stress imaging (Chapter 8), assessment of myocardial viability (Chapter 9), evaluation of coronary bypass surgery and percutaneous transluminal coronary angioplasty (Chapter 10), extra-coronary and congenital heart disease (Chapter 11), and valvular heart disease (Chapter 12). In each chapter, the merits and drawbacks of a host of nuclear cardiology method-ologies are placed in perspective with other noninvasive and invasive diagnostic ap-proaches used in clinical practice. Comparisons are made, where pertinent, with exercise electrocardiographic stress testing, ambulatory electrocardiographic monitoring, and rest or stress echocardiography in the diagnostic and prognostic evaluation of patients with coronary artery disease and in assessment of myocardial viability. Also included are discussions related to clinical decision-making and outcomes analysis, with insertion of figures demonstrating decision-making algorithms based on literature reviews and current practice guidelines. Each chapter contains multiple graphic illustrations and representative nuclear scans from patients with a variety of cardiac abnormalities.

My hope is that this text will serve as a reference to clinical cardiologists seeking to better comprehend the value (or limitations) of nuclear cardiology tests to either solve a diagnostic problem (e.g., undiagnosed atypical chest pain) or assist in a patient manage-ment decision (e.g., coronary angioplasty versus medical therapy after acute myocardial infarction). I also hope that it will serve as a source book for nuclear medicine specialists and radiologists responsible for providing nuclear cardiology services. The style with which the text and illustrations are presented in the book should permit any physician or nonphysician interested in the field of nuclear cardiology to acquire the basic knowledge of instrumentation, properties of radiopharmaceuticals, and clinical indications for various tests presented with comparison to other invasive and noninvasive modalities.

GEORGE A. BELLER, M.D.

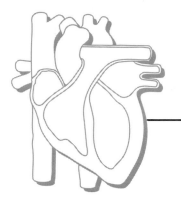

Acknowledgments

I would like to acknowledge the enormous contributions to the field of nuclear cardiology by my colleague of 17 years, Denny Watson, Ph.D., who provided critical input to the first chapter dealing with instrumentation, image generation, and image analysis. I am also grateful for the opportunity to have collaborated with so many talented individuals throughout the years, including Dr. William B. Hood, Jr., Dr. Thomas W. Smith, Dr. Edgar Haber, Dr. Sanjiv Kaul, Dr. Gerald M. Pohost, David Glover, Mirta Ruiz, and William H. Smith. I further want to recognize the immense contributions to our work by cardiology fellows and medical students who worked in my laboratory or participated in clinical research protocols. These individuals include Dr. Charles A. Boucher, Dr. Allen B. Nichols, Dr. Bruce C. Berger, Dr. Peter Ackell, Dr. Andrew M. Grunwald, Dr. Robert S. Gibson, Dr. Jerome E. Granato, Dr. Albert J. Sinusas, Dr. Nat C. Edwards, Dr. Allen Taylor, Dr. Michael Ragosta, Dr. Vedat Sansoy, and Bruce A. Koplan. I am grateful for the superb editorial assistance provided by Mr. Jerry Curtis in preparing the text of this book. The author gratefully acknowledges the American Heart Association, the American College of Cardiology, and the Society of Nuclear Medicine for allowing the reproduction of numerous figures and tables from Circulation, the Journal of the American College of Cardiology, and the Journal of Nuclear Medicine, respectively. Finally, I want to thank my wife, Emily Couric, whose patience during the two years it took to write this book was indeed heroic.

GEORGE A. BELLER, M.D.

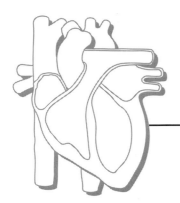

Contents

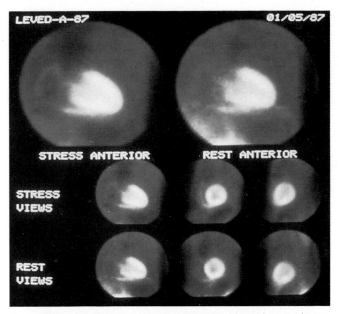

Color Figure 1–10. Stress and rest anterior planar images in top row with anterior 45-degree LAO and 70-degree LAO stress and rest images in bottom rows employing the green-to-white intensity scale. These normal images were acquired in a patient with chest pain and less than 5% likelihood of CAD.

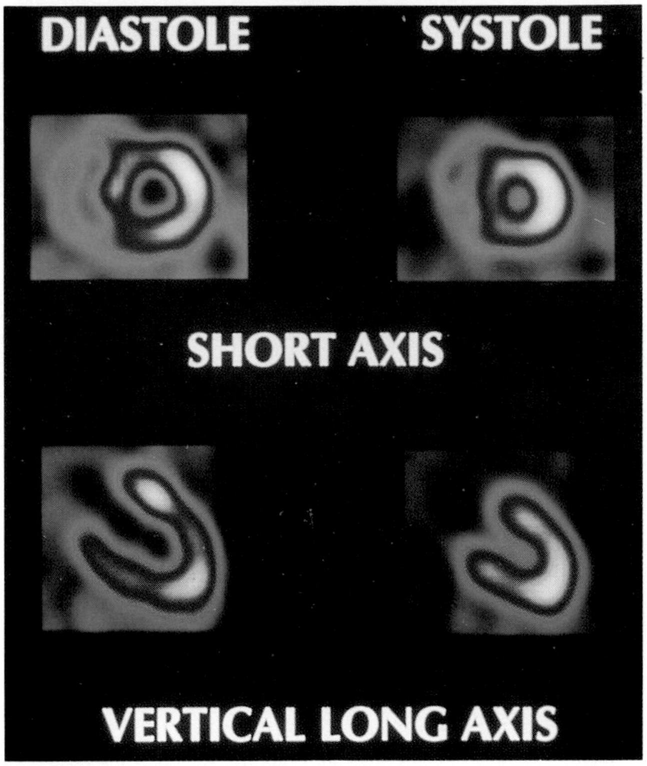

Color Figure 1–26. End-diastolic (diastole) and end-systolic (systole) short-axis and vertical long-axis SPECT images in a subject with slightly diminished septal activity.

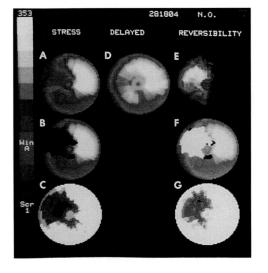

Color Figure 1–25. The stress bull's-eye images *(first column)* demonstrate a significant anteroseptal defect, which shows complete reversibility on the delayed image *(second column)*. Bull's-eye plot *B* in the first column shows a "blackout" area that exceeded 2.5 standard deviations from the mean of normal Tl-201 distribution. Bull's-eye plot *C* uses the color scale to depict the number of standard deviations any given area differs from the mean. Subtracting each point in a normalized stress image from the corresponding point in the normalized delay image yields a polar plot of "reversibility" as shown in *E*. Regions that were irreversible are depicted in black. The "whiteout" bull's-eye in *F* duplicates the results of the stress blackout bull's-eye, in which areas that fall below 2.5 standard deviations from the mean are blacked out. However, regions that have significantly reversed on delayed images are whited out. The bull's-eye plot in *G* is a reversibility plot that depicts the number of standard deviations from the mean of normal reversibility using a varying color scale. (Reprinted by permission of the Society of Nuclear Medicine from Klein JL, et al.: J Nucl Med 1990;31:1240–1246.)

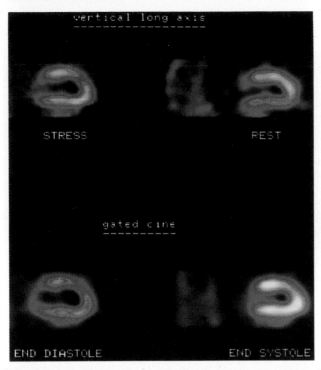

Color Figure 1–27. Comparison of ungated *(top panels)* and gated *(bottom panels)* vertical long-axis tomographic Tc-99m–sestamibi images. In the ungated study, an anterior defect is observed that normalizes on the resting study. On the gated study, the end-systolic image shows thickening depicted by increased brightness as compared with the defect observed in the end-diastolic image. (Garcia EV: J Nucl Cardiol 1994;1:83–93.)

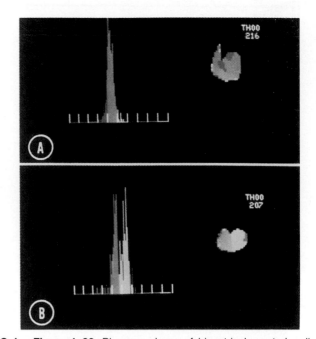

Color Figure 1–38. Phase analyses of biventricular gated radionuclide angiographic studies in a patient with normal conduction and normal contraction **(A)** and in a patient with left bundle branch block **(B). A.** In the upper right-hand corner, "THOO" signifies that the color scale is set so that each of eight colors covers a range of 10% of the cycle, or 36 degrees. The number "216" signifies color scale has been translated so that its center (between yellow and brown) was at 216 degrees. The eight colors, in order of increasing (later) phase, were light blue, dark green, light green, yellow, brown, red, purple, and white. The phase image shown below the color scale shows that the phase was relatively uniform across both ventricles. The histogram to the left of the phase image represents the "phase distribution," the number of pixels in the ventricles with each phase value. The X axis represents channels with a width of 3 degrees for phase angle, and the Y axis represents the number of pixels in each channel. In this patient with normal conduction, the histogram had a single, discrete peak. **B.** With left bundle branch block, there is demonstrated a later phase over the left ventricle (yellow and brown) relative to the right ventricle (green). The phased distribution histogram has now two distinct peaks. (Swiryn S, et al.: Am Heart J 1981;102:1000–1010.)

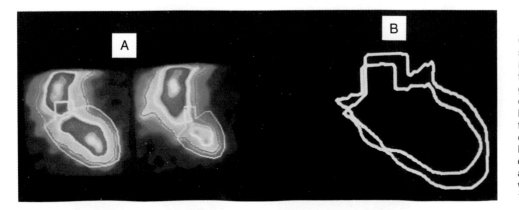

Color Figure 1–33. A. End-diastolic and end-systolic blood pool images of the left ventricle from a first-pass radionuclide angiographic study. Isocontour lines are drawn around the border of the left ventricle and through the aortic valve plane. **B.** Superimposed end-diastolic and end-systolic outlines are depicted. Homogeneous contraction can be seen in the anterior wall, apex, and inferior wall. (Jengo JA, et al.: Circulation 1978;57:326–332.)

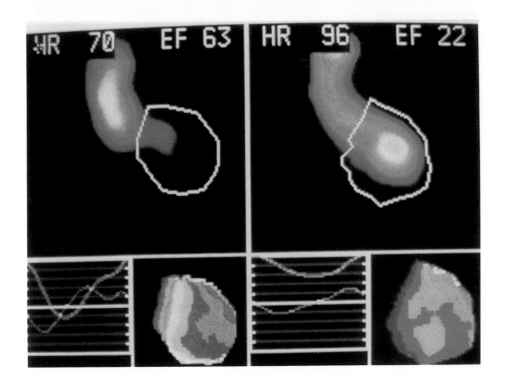

Color Figure 1–41. Example of a first-pass radionuclide angiogram utilizing a mobile multiwire gamma camera and tantalum-178 at baseline *(left)* and after left anterior descending coronary artery occlusion *(right)*. The end-diastolic frame is superimposed on the end-systolic silhouette shown as an outer white ring. Normal wall motion with an EF of 63% is shown on the baseline study. The EF was 22%, and a severe anterior and anterolateral wall motion abnormality is shown with a left anterior descending coronary occlusion. Below these images are the regional EF image showing diffuse LV deterioration. (Key: HR, heart rate.) (Reprinted with permission from the American College of Cardiology (Journal of the American College of Cardiology, 1992, Vol. 19, pp. 297–306).)

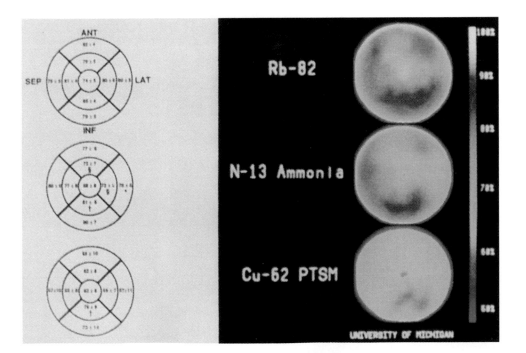

Color Figure 1–42. Polar maps from short-axis images of myocardial blood flow. The tracers shown include Rb-82, N-13 ammonia, and Cu-62-PTSM. (Reprinted by permission of the Society of Nuclear Medicine from Schwaiger M.: J Nucl Med 1994;35:693–698.)

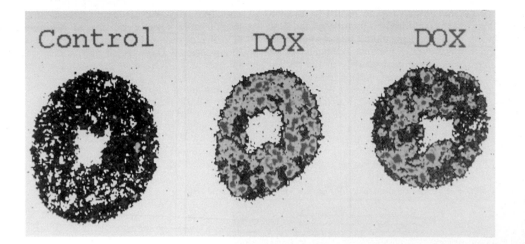

Color Figure 2–34. Audioradiographs of excised hearts in control rats and doxorubicin-treated ones *(middle* and *right)* after administration of indium 111 antimyosin antibody. A higher uptake of radioactivity in the heart is depicted by the red color, and a lower uptake by the blue color. (Hiro EM, et al.: Circulation 1992; 86:1965–1972.)

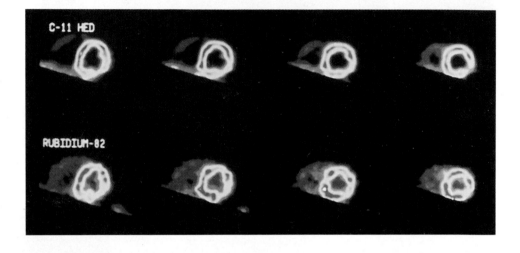

Color Figure 2–44. Cross-sectional PET images of the left ventricle of a normal volunteer after administration of Ru-82 and C-11 HED. The C-11 HED images were acquired 30 to 40 minutes after intravenous tracer injection. (Schwaiger M, et al.: Circulation 1990;82:457–464.)

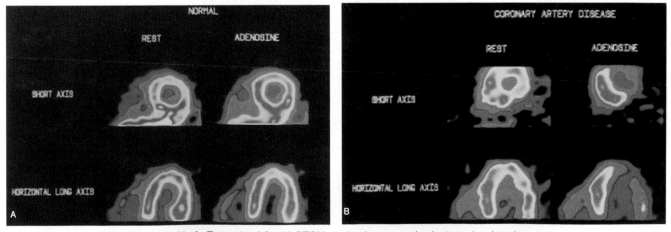

Color Figure 2–46. A. Example of Cu-62-PTSM studies in a normal volunteer showing short-axis and horizontal long-axis views at rest *(left)* and following adenosine-induced vasodilation *(right)* employing PET imaging. Note the good image quality. **B.** An example of Cu-62-PTSM tomographic studies in a patient with two-vessel coronary artery disease. Note that perfusion abnormalities in anterior, lateral, and apical walls are consistent with impaired flow reserve in these regions. (Reprinted by permission of the Society of Nuclear Medicine from Beanlands RSB: J Nucl Med 1992;33:684–690.)

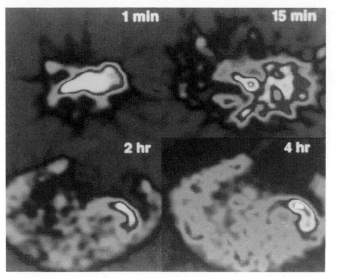

Color Figure 2–49. Serial PET images of F-18 fluoromisonidazole uptake in ischemic anterior wall myocardium in a dog with ischemia in the territory of the left anterior descending coronary artery. The images represent a cross section through the chest cavity that is roughly parallel to the long axis of the heart. The septum is on the left, whereas the apex of the left ventricle is to the right. One minute after injection, the tracer is concentrated in the blood pool. The 2- and 4-hour postinjection images show some enhancement of activity in the distal anterior wall and apex of the left ventricle. (Reprinted by permission of the Society of Nuclear Medicine from Martin GV, et al.: J Nucl Med 1992;33:2202–2208.)

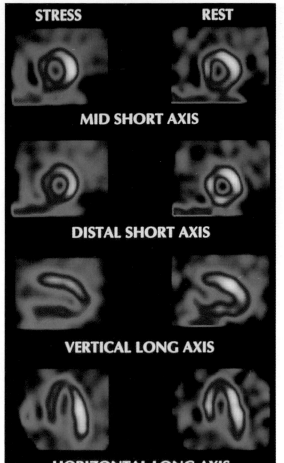

Color Figure 4–13. Example of a high-risk SPECT myocardial perfusion scan in a patient who underwent exercise sestamibi imaging for evaluation of chest pain. The exercise images are shown on the left and rest images on the right. Representative short-axis tomograms demonstrate reversible anteroseptal and inferior defects. The vertical long-axis tomogram reveals a partially reversible inferior defect and a persistent apical defect. Increased activity is also seen in the anterior wall when comparing rest and stress images. The horizontal long-axis image reveals a reversible septal defect and a persistent apical defect. These scintigraphic findings are consistent with LAD and right CAD.

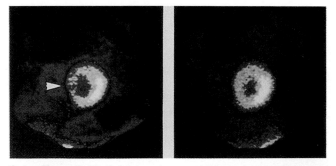

Color Figure 3–30. One-hour stress and 3-hour delayed 45-degree left anterior oblique Tc-99m–sestamibi images obtained in a patient with 95% left anterior descending coronary artery stenosis. The septal wall defect *(arrow)* observed 1 hour after Tc-99m–sestamibi injection at stress shows mild partial redistribution at 3 hours poststress. (Reprinted by permission of the Society of Nuclear Medicine from Taillefer R, et al.: J Nucl Med 1991;32:1961–1965.)

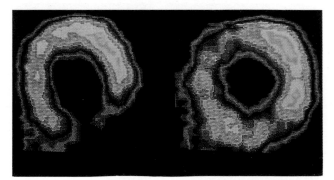

Color Figure 6–14. Tl-201 scintigram obtained in a patient before *(left)* and 24 hours after *(right)* successful coronary recanalization. Note the resolution of a large perfusion defect in the inferior segment of the left ventricle. (Schuler G, et al.: Circulation 1982;66:658–664.)

Tc-99m MIBI in Acute Myocardial Infarction: Thrombolysis Group

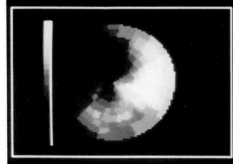

Admission

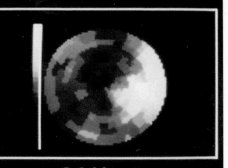

24 Hours

Color Figure 6–39. Bull's-eye SPECT images performed on admission before thrombolytic therapy and 24 hours later in a patient with an acute anteroseptal MI study at the Montreal Heart Institute. Note the marked improvement in Tc-99m–sestamibi uptake in the anteroseptal region, indicative of substantial salvage. (Kindly provided by Dr. Pierre Théroux, Montreal Heart Institute.)

Color Figure 7–5. Two-dimensional polar map display of a Tc-99m–sestamibi study obtained in a 48-year-old man admitted for atypical chest pain at rest. The study obtained during an episode of chest pain (left) shows a large perfusion defect involving anterior and septal walls. The polar map image in the absence of chest pain (right) shows almost complete recovery of the perfusion defect. A 70% left anterior descending stenosis was found in angiography. (Courtesy of Drs. J. Grégoire and P. Théroux.)

Tc-99m SESTAMIBI IN SPONTANEOUS CHEST PAIN

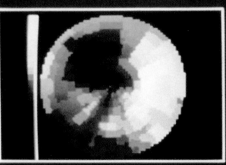

Onset of chest pain

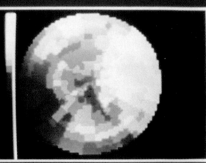

No chest pain

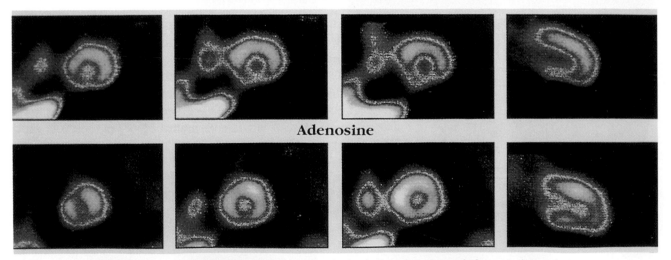

Adenosine

Color Figure 8–33. Teboroxime SPECT images obtained after adenosine and after rest, demonstrating a reversible inferior defect. (Reprinted with permission of the American College of Cardiology (Journal of the American College of Cardiology, 1992, Vol. 19, pp. 307–312).)

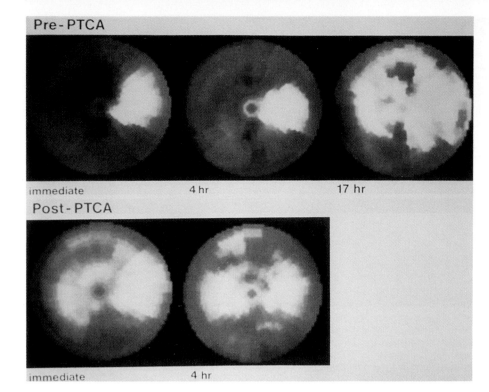

Pre-PTCA

immediate   4 hr   17 hr

Post-PTCA

immediate   4 hr

Color Figure 9–10. Bull's-eye maps from SPECT Tl-201 images obtained in a patient with angina pectoris before angioplasty (pre-PTCA) and 2 days after angioplasty (post-PTCA). Pre-PTCA images were obtained immediately (immediate) after stress and 4 and 17 hours later, and the post-PTCA scintigrams were obtained immediately and 4 hours after Tl-201 injection. Note the additional delayed redistribution at 17 hours compared to 4 hours in the pre-PTCA series of bull's-eye maps. After PTCA, Tl-201 activity is normal in both the stress and the 4-hour delayed images. (Reprinted with permission of the American College of Cardiology (Journal of the American College of Cardiology, 1988, Vol. 12, pp. 955–963).)

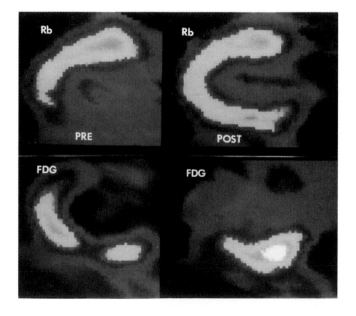

Rb   Rb
PRE   POST
FDG   FDG

Color Figure 9–39. Sagittal PET images with apex oriented to the left, which demonstrate improvement in Rb-82 uptake in the inferior wall after revascularization *(upper panels),* with persistent elevation of FDG activity in the inferior wall after surgery *(lower right panel).* (Marwick TH, et al.: Circulation 1992;85:1347–1353.)

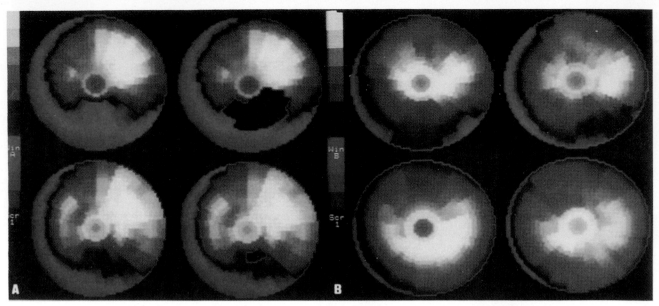

Color Figure 10–7. Bull's-eye polar maps from SPECT images obtained after exercise *(top row)* and 4 hours after tracer injection *(bottom row)*. The preangioplasty bull's-eye maps are shown in the left panel, **A,** and the postangioplasty bull's-eye maps are shown in the right panel, **B.** Note that, following successful right coronary artery angioplasty, both the immediate and 4-hour delayed bull's-eye plots are normal. In the preangioplasty study, a significant diminution in tracer uptake is seen in the inferior wall with partial redistribution at 4 hours. (DePuey E: Circulation 1991;84:I-59–I-65.)

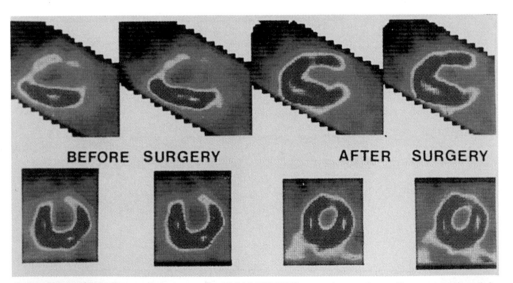

Color Figure 11–7. Pre- and postoperative Tl-201 SPECT images in a patient with an anomalous left coronary artery arising from the pulmonary trunk. The vertical long-axis slices *(upper row)* and the short-axis slices *(bottom row)* demonstrate reduced tracer uptake in the septum and the anterior wall before surgery. The postoperative images show resolution of these defects. (Reprinted by permission of the Society of Nuclear Medicine from Anguenot TJ, et al.: J Nucl Med 1991;32:1788–1790.)

Chapter 1

Instrumentation in Nuclear Cardiology

BASIC PHYSICS OF RADIOACTIVITY

Structure of the Atom

All nuclear cardiology techniques are based upon obtaining images of radioactivity emanating from radioactive tracers localized in heart muscle or the cardiac blood pool. To better comprehend the way in which nuclear cardiology images are obtained, a review of relevant physics of radioactivity may be useful. More detailed discussions of this subject can be found in recent books on the subject.[1-5] Figure 1–1 is a diagram of the components of an atom, which is the basic structure of any element. The atom is composed of a centrally positioned nucleus containing positively charged protons and electrically neutral neutrons. Protons and neutrons are often referred to as *nucleons*. Orbiting around the nucleus are electrons, which are negatively charged. The orbits are also called *energy shells*. Energy shells are designated by sequence, with the innermost shell identified as the K shell and proceeding outward sequentially to L, M, N shells, and so on. Energy shells can also be listed numerically, the number 1 shell being nearest to the nucleus (see Fig. 1–1). The first or K shell has a limit of two electrons; the second or L shell can have no more than eight electrons, and the third or M shell can have as many as 18 electrons. All electrons orbiting in a specific shell have the same energy state. Protons and neutrons both have approximately 1800 times the mass of the electron. An electron can jump from a higher orbit to a lower one. It conserves energy by emitting an x-ray of energy equal to the energy difference between the two orbits. The number of units of positive charge of the nucleus or number of electrons in orbit is equal to the atomic number of the atom

(Z) in the electrically neutral state. Figure 1–1 depicts the phosphorus atom, which has 15 protons and 15 electrons. The maximum number of electrons in each orbit is $2n^2$, where n is the quantum number of the energy shell. The atomic number provides the classification of an atom as one of the elements (e.g., atomic number 2 is helium).

Isotopes of a given element are atoms that have the same number of protons but different numbers of neutrons. Atoms with a stable neutron-proton ratio are called stable isotopes. These are not radioactive, and atoms in the first

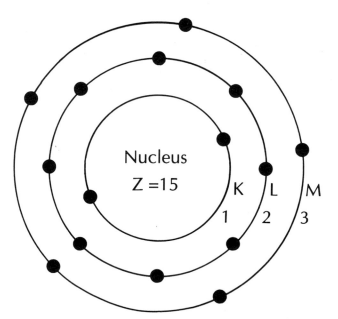

Figure 1–1. Diagram of the phosphorus atom demonstrating orbits of 15 electrons. Phosphorus has 15 protons and 16 neutrons in its nucleus. The nucleus is 10^5 times smaller than the atom.

two thirds of the Periodic Table have at least one form of the atom that has a stable neutron-proton ratio. There are other forms of these elements that do not have a stable neutron-proton ratio. These decay or disintegrate. In this process, the nucleus alters its components so that a neutron is changed to a proton, a proton is changed to a neutron, or an alpha particle is emitted so that the residual nucleus is stable. Such atoms are called *radionuclides*. Nuclear decay is usually accompanied by emissions of energy in the form of γ-rays (i.e., photons).

Some discussion of nuclear nomenclature is now warranted. Conventionally, the total number of nucleons (protons and neutrons) is put in the superscript position preceding the chemical symbol. This is the mass number, or A. The number of protons (i.e., atomic number Z) is placed in the subscript position preceding the chemical symbol. ^{131}I or ^{131}Xe indicates 131 nucleons in the nucleus. For ^{201}Tl the mass number, or *A,* indicates 201 protons. In this book, radionuclides are described with the atomic number following the chemical symbol (e.g., I-131, Tl-201, Rb-82).

Types of Radioactive Decay

Nuclei of radioactive atoms eject alpha, beta, beta-plus (β$^+$) particles, and the neutrino. Beta-plus decay is also known as *positron decay*. When protons change into neutrons, or neutrons into protons, another particle is created and ejected. The type of particle created with this change and ejected depends on the unstable conditions in the nucleus of the parent nuclide. With this unstable situation, the proton number either increases or decreases, and the remaining atom is, by necessity, a different element. The modes of decay include alpha, beta, positron, gamma, and electron capture (Table 1–1). With alpha decay, there is an emission of an alpha particle from a high–atomic weight

Table 1–1. **Types of Radioactive Decay**
Alpha decay
Emission of an alpha particle from a high–atomic weight radionuclide
Beta-minus decay
Emission of an electron from the nucleus
Positron decay
Emission of a positively-charged electron from the nucleus
Electron capture
Decay occurs when an electron is captured by the nucleus from an electron shell

radionuclide. An alpha particle is a helium nucleus, which consists of two neutrons and two protons bound together in a very stable condition. With beta-minus decay, there is emission of an electron from the nucleus. The particle comes from radionuclides that have excess neutrons in the nucleus. A neutron changes into a proton when the beta-minus particle is emitted. A neutrino is also emitted, which has no charge and carries off energy from the reaction. Phosphorus-32 (P-32) for example, is a pure beta emitter.

With positron decay there is emission of a β$^+$ particle, a positively-charged electron that is emitted from the nucleus. These particles are emitted from atoms that have excess protons in the nucleus. The proton is converted into a neutron upon emission of the positron. The positron attracts a negative electron and they annihilate each other, which results in emission of two γ-rays of 0.511 MeV (or 511 keV) each. The two γ-rays are emitted in precisely opposite directions from each other (Fig. 1–2). Decay by electron capture occurs when an electron in orbit is captured by a nucleus. The captured electron combines with a proton and forms a neutron with emission of a neutrino. This is accompanied by emission of a γ-ray and x-rays as the empty electron orbit is filled by an electron cascading from an energy shell more remote from the nucleus. Most electrons are captured from the K shell. Many nuclei decay by both

POSITRON EMISSION AND ANNIHILATION

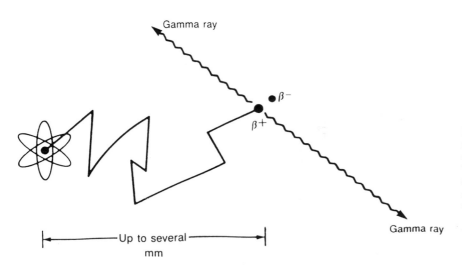

Gamma ray

β$^-$

β$^+$

Up to several mm

Gamma ray

Figure 1–2. Diagram of positron decay of a nucleus. See text for explanation. In this type of decay, the positron attracts a negative electron, resulting in annihilation, which produces an emission of two γ-rays 0.511 MeV each. As shown, the two γ-rays are emitted in exactly opposite directions from each other. (Bacharach SL: The physics of positron emission tomography. *In* Bergmann SR, Sobel BE (eds): *Positron Emission Tomography of the Heart.* Mt. Kisco, Futura, 1992, pp 13–44).

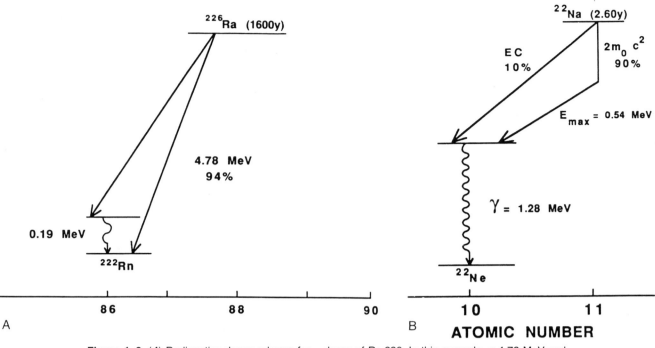

Figure 1–3. (*A*) Radioactive decay scheme for α-decay of Ra-226. In this example, a 4.78-MeV and α-particle is released during 94% of Ra-226 transitions. (*B*) Radioactive decay scheme for positron decay and electron capture of Na-22. In this example, 90% of all decays occur with an emission of a positron. The remaining 10% is by electron capture (EC). (Hendee WR, Ritenour R (eds): Medical Imaging Physics, ed 3. St. Louis, CV Mosby, 1992, pp 36–45.)

electron capture and positron emission (e.g., sodium-22). Figure 1–3 illustrates examples of the different types of radioactive decay.[5a]

The Compton effect, an important phenomenon with implications for nuclear imaging, occurs when a γ-ray or an x-ray strikes an outer-shell electron. The γ-ray or x-ray (photon) is changed in direction, and its energy is reduced. This is referred to as *Compton scatter*, which is a cause of image degradation.

Physical and Biologic Half-Lives

When a radionuclide is injected into a person, subsequently there is both physical decay of the radioactivity and elimination of the radioactive agent by biologic processes (e.g., urinary excretion). The activity of any radioactive material is expressed as the number of nuclear disintegrations per unit of time (dN/dt), and the fraction of the radioisotope that decays per unit of time is referred to as the *decay constant* (λ). The decay constant (λ) is defined as $0.693/T_p$, where T_p is the physical half-life. Also, the $T_{1/2}$ is equal to $0.693/\lambda$. The accepted unit of radioactivity is the curie (Ci), defined as 3.7×10^{10} nuclear disintegrations per second. The millicurie (mCi) and microcurie (μCi) are the subunits of the curie. Recently, the curie has been replaced with the becquerel (Bq) which is the accepted SI (*le Système international d'Unités*) unit of radioactivity. A bec-

querel is defined as one radioactivity disintegration per second, and 1 mCi is equivalent to 37 MBq (megabecquerels).

The *physical half-life* is defined as the time required for half of the original number of atoms in a given nuclide to decay. The *biologic half-life* ($T_{1/2}$ [bio]) is defined as the time required for the body to eliminate 50% of an administered radioactive dose. The *effective half-life* ($T_{1/2}$ [eff]) is the time required for the administered radioactive dose to decrease by half within the body. The effective half-life considers both radioactive decay and biologic elimination (e.g., excretion, metabolism) and, therefore, is most applicable for radiation dosimetry. The effective half-life is calculated thus:

$$\frac{1}{T_{1/2}} + \frac{1}{T_{1/2}\,(\text{bio})} = \frac{1}{T_{1/2}\,(\text{eff})}$$

DETECTION OF RADIATION

The high-energy photons of electromagnetic radiation (γ-rays and x-rays) emitted from an injected radionuclide are important for nuclear medicine. This radiation should not substantially interact with the patient but should be totally absorbed by a detector.

Certain characteristics of radiation detectors have significance for clinical nuclear cardiology techniques. Chandra summarizes these characteristics in the following manner:[5b] The *intrinsic efficiency* or *sensitivity* of a detector measures its capability to detect radiation and is defined as the ratio of the number of α-, β-, or γ-rays detected to the number of rays of a given radiation incident on the sensitive volume of the detector. An intrinsic efficiency of 50% implies that half of the rays incident on the sensitive volume of the detector are being detected. The higher the intrinsic efficiency, the better is its use for imaging. *Dead time* or *resolving time* is a measure of the capability of a radiation detector to detect rays at high count rates or radiation flux. With high count rates or high radiation flux (or intensity), the second ray arrives and interacts with the detector while it is still processing the first ray. Ideally, the detector should have as short a dead time as possible. For fast dynamic radionuclide imaging (e.g., first-pass radionuclide angiography), dead times for a detector system must be less than 5 μsec. *Energy resolution,* another important characteristic, is defined as the ability of a detector to distinguish between two radiations of different energies. Full width at half maximum (FWHM), a term used as a measure of energy resolution, represents the minimum difference necessary between the energies of two γ-rays if they are to be identified as possessing different energies. A lower value of FWHM indicates better energy discrimination capability. For example, an FWHM of 20 keV means that two γ-rays with an energy difference of 10 keV could not be distinguished from each other.

Certain materials have the property of absorbing γ-rays or x-ray photons and converting them to flashes of light called scintillations. The sodium iodide (NaI) crystal is one of these detectors. With the NaI crystal doped with small amounts of thallium (NaI [Tl]), the detection process begins when the γ-ray enters the crystal. The energy is absorbed inside the crystal when the photons interact with electrons in the crystal. When electrons absorb energy, light is produced. The intensity of the light is proportional to the amount of absorbed energy. The light is directed by photomultiplier tubes, which are the light-sensitive devices in the detector.

Photomultiplier tubes are composed of a photocathode facing the window through which light enters, a series of metallic electrodes called dynodes arranged in a geometric pattern, and an anode. The photomultiplier tube, which is optically linked with the scintillation crystal, converts the light from the crystal to electrical energy by the emission of electrons from the photocathode in proportion to the amount of light received. This process yields measurable electronic pulses. The original number of electrons released in proportion to photons striking the photocathode is amplified electronically by a factor of approximately 1 million. This amplification is accomplished by multiplication of electrons striking the dynodes. Finally, the electrons are collected by the anode and shaped by a preamplifier to generate an electrical pulse of a few microamperes in amplitude and about a microsecond in duration. The height of this pulse, or voltage, created by a single scintillation is directly proportional to the amount of light released within the crystal, which, in turn, is proportional to the energy of the γ-ray absorbed by the crystal. This pulse is delivered to a preamplifier, usually mounted on the photomultiplier tube. The output of the preamplifier is directed to a linear amplifier for amplification to several volts. Figure 1–4 depicts in diagrammatic form this process of converting γ-ray energy to an electrical pulse height after light is released.

A pulse height analyzer or selector is an electronic device used to select pulses from a range of available energies to be counted. An energy window is created in this manner, and pulses corresponding to γ-rays of energies outside this window are rejected and not recorded. The use of a pulse height analyzer for imaging of radiation is important in that energies below a certain threshold are rejected, and γ-rays that have lost their original energy and direction during a Compton scatter event in the patient but that continue to strike the crystal are eliminated. Simply stated, the pulse height analyzer rejects background and scattered radiation. The window for the energy range is usually set with an upper-level discriminator and a lower-level discriminator. With respect to technetium-99m (Tc-99m), a 20% window for the 140 keV would range from 126 keV to 154 keV. A

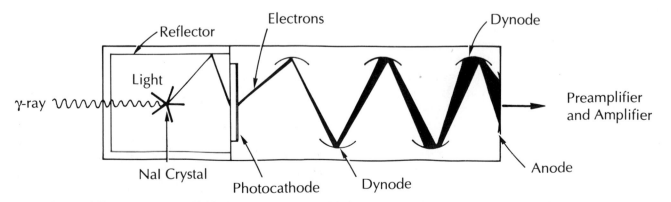

Figure 1–4. Schematic depiction of a sodium iodide (NaI) crystal and photo multiplier tube. See text for explanation.

Tl-201 Energy Spectrum

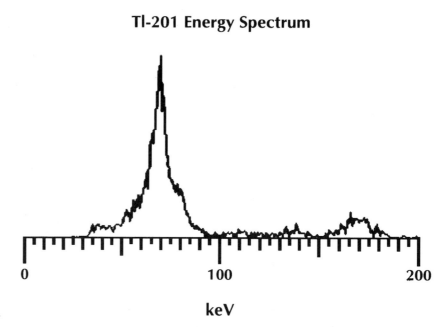

0   100   200

keV

Figure 1–5. Pulse height spectrum for Tl-201.

scaler is used to count and display the number of pulses by measuring the number of γ-rays absorbed by the crystal. Figure 1–5 shows the energy spectrum of Tl-201 around its photopeak.

IMAGING INSTRUMENTATION

Detection and Localizing Scintillation Events

The basic types of NaI (Tl) detectors to localize scintillation events are the single-crystal (Anger) camera and the multicrystal camera. There are also nonimaging probes, which can monitor radioactive counts but do not produce an image of the heart.

Single-Crystal Camera

The single-crystal gamma scintillation camera uses a large NaI (Tl) crystal with a set of photomultiplier tubes arranged in a hexagonal array. The crystal is usually 0.25- to 0.5-inch thick. The diameter of the crystal varies from 11 to 20 inches. The thinner the crystal, the better the intrinsic resolution. The trade-off for better resolution is a reduction in sensitivity. The γ-rays emanating from the heart, for example, are initially "collimated" to allow only γ-rays of a desired direction to strike the crystal. This is required so an accurate image of the distribution of radioactivity in a patient can be produced. The locations of absorption of γ-rays in the scintillation camera should be related to the origin of these rays within the patient. The γ-rays pass through the holes of the collimator and are absorbed by the crystal and give rise to scintillation. The photomultiplier tubes detect the light given off by the scin-

tillation and feed the output into a computer-directed analyzer. The circuitry of this analyzer permits the determination of the point at which each scintillation occurs and x- and y coordinates are assigned to the event. A z signal or pulse is also generated, which represents the summed output of all photomultiplier tubes. The x-y coordinate signals are normalized to the z pulse, yielding a size of an image that is independent of the energy of the γ-rays striking the crystal.

It is the z signal that is analyzed by the pulse height analyzer that has been programmed to accept only a certain range of energies. Only when this z-pulse has been accepted by the analyzer is the scintillation event counted. If the z-pulse is not within the selected range, it is not applied to the plates of the cathode ray tube (CRT). The x, y, and z signals can be recorded using a CRT in analog format. When the z pulse or signal enters the CRT, there is an emission of electrons from the electron gun. The x and y positional signals are applied to vertical and horizontal plates. This results in a deflection in the path of electrons which directly corresponds to the coordinates of the scintillation pulse. These electrons then strike the phosphor screen of the CRT, producing light recorded as a dot on photographic film. When a new γ-ray interacts in the crystal, a new set of x, y, and z signals is produced, which then places the light spot to a new location dictated by these signals. The image obtained from radionuclide distribution in an organ like the heart is a collection of these dots. The location of the dots is related directly to the radioactivity localized in the patient. The electronics placed in the single-crystal camera provide certain corrections by real-time signal processing to more precisely position the scintillation event in the body. These include tube drift correction, used to calibrate the photomultiplier tubes so that each generates the same pulse voltage when it accumulates the same light from the point light source. There is an energy correction circuit to normalize each photomultiplier tube so that it generates the same energy spectrum. Finally, there is a correction to achieve linearity, ensuring straight radioactive lines using phantom line sources.

Collimators

Collimators are lead disks containing multiple holes that block γ-rays that are not traveling in the desired pathway. Collimators have both a high-density and a high-attenuation coefficient for the γ-rays less than 500 keV, which are those of interest for nuclear medicine. The parallel-hole collimator, the one most commonly used in cardiac nuclear imaging, has a large number of parallel holes, which are aligned perpendicular to the face of the crystal. The larger the diameter of the holes or the shorter the length of the holes, the greater is the sensitivity of the detector but the lower the spatial resolution of the detector system. Spatial resolution is defined as the ability to distinguish two distinct radioactive objects in an image. A longer, narrower hole sees a smaller area, which is accompanied by better resolution but lower sensitivity. Figure 1–6 shows in diagrammatic form the components of a simple lead collimator from the text of Hendee and Ritenour.[5a]

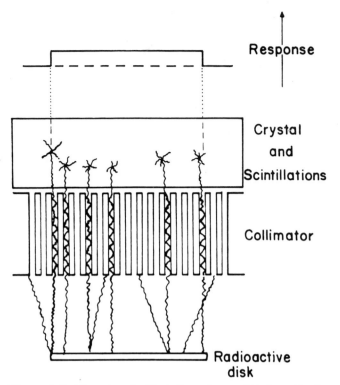

Figure 1–6. Diagrammatic illustration of a multi-hole collimator where γ-rays admitted in line with the collimator holes are transmitted to the crystal, whereas γ-rays emitted obliquely are absorbed by the collimator septa. (Hendee WR, Ritenour R (eds): Medical Imaging Physics, ed 3. St. Louis, CV Mosby, 1992, p 315.)

Multicrystal Camera

A multicrystal gamma camera consists of a detector comprising 294 (1 cm × 1 inch) NaI (Tl) crystals. These crystals are arranged in an array of 14 rows by 21 columns with 35 photomultiplier tubes. There is one photomultiplier tube for each row and each column. Each crystal is coupled to two photomultiplier tubes, one for the x axis and one for the y axis. The light from a scintillation emitted for each γ-ray absorbed by the crystal is detected by the corresponding horizontal and vertical photomultiplier tubes, which identify the position in the crystal. The multicrystal camera has a high count rate capability and is able more accurately to record the count rate from an intense radioactive source. In the multicrystal camera, the detection of an interaction does not include collection of position information, so much higher count rates can be processed without appreciable count rate loss or positioning errors. As will be discussed subsequently in this chapter, the multicrystal camera is the instrument used for first-pass imaging of a radionuclide through the central circulation. Since the collimator has holes more closely approximating the dimensions of the crystals, there is a higher γ-ray flux on the crystals. This high sensitivity results in the recording of more than 400,000 counts per second in the image. The downside of the multicrystal camera is the relatively poor spatial and energy resolution.

Nonimaging Probes

Several nonimaging devices are available for assessment of dynamic changes in radioactivity within the blood pool of the left and right ventricles.[5c, 6–8] One of the first devices was referred to as a *nuclear stethoscope,* which consisted of a sodium iodide crystal which was 2 inches in diameter and 1.5 inches thick.[6] It was interfaced with a photomultiplier and a single-bore, flat-field converging collimator. The stethoscope was mounted on an arm and interfaced to a microprocessor. The microprocessor records counts in real time originating from the field of view of the device and is linked to the electrocardiographic (ECG) signal from the patient. After accurate positioning of the probe to obtain the highest count rate, beat-to-beat left ventricular (LV) time-activity curves are recorded and displayed. The LV ejection fraction (LVEF) is then calculated. The radioactive counts from the LV blood pool are corrected for background activity using the probe and interfaced microprocessor.

Another nonimaging device has been referred to as the VEST.[7] With this device, the detector, electronics, and recorder are inserted in a vestlike jacket worn by the patient. The detector used is 5.5 cm in diameter and is equipped with a parallel-hole collimator. The detector weighs approximately 0.75 kg. The radioactive counts from the ventricular

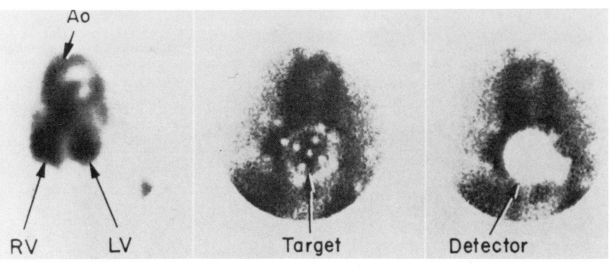

Figure 1–7. Static imaging of the LV and RV blood pools in the left anterior oblique position are required for accurate positioning of the VEST. In the middle panel, a positional target can be seen overlying the LV blood pool. The right panel shows the target removed and replaced with the detector. (Reprinted with permission from the American College of Cardiology (Journal of the American College of Cardiology, 1990, Vol. 15, p. 1500).)

blood pool are obtained at a rate of 32 times per second. ECG recordings are made simultaneously. In contrast to the nuclear stethoscope, positioning of the VEST is undertaken with the assistance of a gamma camera (Fig. 1–7). The VEST permits continuous, ambulatory monitoring of LVEF during ambulatory activities, similar to what is acquired by ambulatory ECG monitoring for arrhythmias or ischemic ST-segment depression.

A third device is a miniature nuclear probe system called the Cardioscint used for continuous on-line monitoring of cardiac function and ST-segment depression similar to the VEST.[8] The probe has a diameter of 0.48 cm. This device also allows for the measurement of EF, relative cardiac LV volumes, and ST-segment changes, which are displayed at the end of each acquisition, ranging from 10 to 300 seconds. As with VEST, the Cardioscint probe can be positioned with the assistance of a gamma camera. Or, as with the nuclear stethoscope, it can be positioned based on maximum stroke counts recorded.

Acquisition of Planar Scintigraphic Images

Most gamma scintillation cameras are interfaced to a computer. Digital computers are necessary to acquire, analyze, store, and display a great deal of complex information. The x, y, and z pulses, which are sent to the CRT in an analog camera, are also directed to the computer interface, which converts the pulses to digital information. The computer has an analog-to-digital converter (ADC), transforming the height of the pulses to an integer. The ADC commonly used for digitizing x and y signals of the scintillation camera are 6- or 7-bit, so that x and y ranges are divided into 2^6 (64) or 2^7 (128) equal divisions, respectively. Com-

puters in gamma cameras have direct memory access, hardware instrumentation that constantly updates the memory to free-up the computer for continued acquisition of imaging data.

Planar studies are acquired in what is called a *frame mode*. The computer memory is used to represent an image acquired for preset time or preset radioactive counts. The camera field of view is divided into a grid using a matrix of memory locations in the computer memory. Each memory location allocated to a frame represents a digital counter of how many scintillation pulses occurred at each single picture element (pixel) location during acquisition. A specific area on the crystal corresponds to a specific pixel. Matrix size for acquisition is typically 64 × 64 or 128 × 128. The analog image is, thus, divided into 4096 (64 × 64) or 16,384 (128 × 128) pixels. When time of acquisition for a frame has elapsed (as with preset time of acquisition or preset counts acquired), the frame is transferred to a disk for storage.

For planar imaging using Tl-201, images are obtained for a preset time of 8 to 10 minutes per view and typically are obtained in the anterior, 45-degree left anterior oblique (LAO), and a steep (70-degree) LAO view.[9] Since cardiac rotation can influence the configuration of myocardial scintigrams, some have advocated the "best septal" image as a substitute for a standard 45-degree LAO view projection image. For women, a lateral view may often be preferred to the steep 70-degree LAO view, to minimize attenuation from overlying breast tissue. Figure 1–8 shows normal anterior, 45-degree LAO, and 70-degree LAO Tl-201 images in a normal subject. Figure 1–9 shows that obtaining a left lateral image yielded a more normal looking anterior wall than a 70-degree LAO image, which showed a breast attenuation artifact. Several factors influence the diagnostic qual-

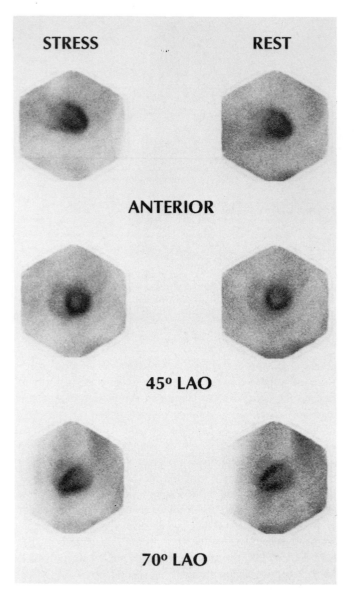

STRESS   **REST**

ANTERIOR

45° LAO

70° LAO

Figure 1–8. Example of a normal exercise (STRESS) and 2.5-hour redistribution (REST) anterior, 45-degree left anterior oblique (LAO) and 70-degree LAO planar Tl-201 images.

ity of planar Tl-201 images. The specifications of gamma cameras and collimators vary. Resolution, sensitivity, and field uniformity are all important in Tl-201 imaging. Unfortunately, these factors are interrelated: the improvement in one is frequently at the expense of another. The best system performance, thus, results from a good compromise between different system components, including the collimator and the imaging chain. Most cameras provide field-nonuniformity correction capability. Care must be taken in performing correction floods on cameras because errors can produce artifacts which are then impressed into all subsequent images.

Compton scattering is a major problem associated with the low-energy photons from Tl-201, since 80-keV photons can scatter through an angle greater than 90 degrees with

loss of only 10 keV. For example, an energy window of 25% centered on the photopeak accepts photons that have been scattered up to 90 degrees. Using a narrower window to limit the acceptance of scatter photons, would, however, reduce the detection efficiency to such a degree that a loss in image quality would result. A window width of 20% to 30% is an optimal compromise between loss of statistical definition from a narrow window and loss of image contrast from a wide window because of acceptance of excessive Compton scatter. Image contrast is adversely influenced by background activity and scattered radiation.

A medium-resolution (general all-purpose) collimator may be preferable to a high-resolution collimator for Tl-201 imaging, since it allows higher count rates and shorter imaging times, which are important for detecting transient perfusion defects that may fill in rapidly by redistribution. The general all-purpose collimator has nearly the same resolution as the high-resolution collimator but loses resolution more rapidly with increasing distance from the collimator face. This appears to be an acceptable compromise

70° LAO   **LLAT**

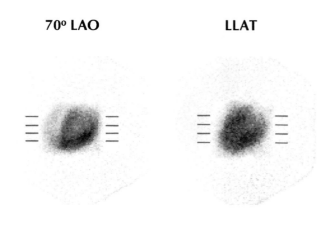

STRESS   **STRESS**

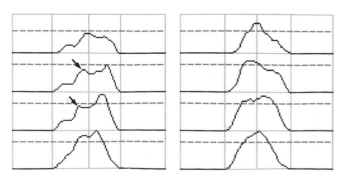

HORIZONTAL PROFILES

Figure 1–9. A 70-degree left anterior oblique (LAO) image in a woman showing breast attenuation. The quantitative count profiles are shown below the images and demonstrate *(arrows)* diminished septal counts on the 70° LAO view. This artifact can often be avoided by obtaining a steep left lateral (LLAT) projection image. The breast artifact is then displaced anterior to the heart. Note the increase in septal counts on the quantitative profiles shown below the LLAT image.

to reduce imaging time and achieve a more rapid image sequence. For Tc-99m sestamibi imaging, a high-resolution collimator may be preferable.

All Tl-201 imaging studies should be recorded on a computer for standardized image formation. Image contrast and density are standardized, allowing enhanced ability to differentiate clinically relevant defects from insignificant image variables. By varying levels of background suppression, artifactual defects can appear. Similarly, manually adjusting the gray scale is associated with arbitrary modification of defect size and severity. Smith and Watson have pointed out that standardization of video and hard copy images (e.g., transparency film) is considered necessary for reproducible image interpretation.[10] They recommend the use of the Society for Motion Picture and Television Engineers (SMPTE) test pattern to fix the video contrast and brightness levels and adjust the film imager to achieve recommended values of film density for the test pattern.[11] Smith and Watson[10] point out that no arbitrary manipulation of background cutoff, contrast, brightness, or film density should be permitted when displaying planar images for interpretation. All images are made employing standardized settings. Background levels are set for a film density of 0.05 to 0.1 density units, and maximum film density is set between 1.5 and 1.7. These density values are in accordance with the recommendations of the SMPTE.[12]

Watson et al.[13] recommend a standardized intensity scale designed to provide intuitively linear monochromatic conversion of count density and perceived brightness values. A standard "green scale" is used that ranges from dark green through light green, and finally to pure white. The standard green scale is designed so that image count density is re-

lated linearly to perceived brightness value. Green is the primary video color in the center of the spectrum of human visual sensitivity. The standard green scale runs from 20% to 100% CRT beam intensity rather than commencing at zero. Figure 1–10 shows an example of a set of planar images displayed using the green scale. Interpretation of images is often undertaken using multiple color scales. This allows for more dramatic image displays, but small gradations in tracer uptake are difficult to detect. Our laboratory does not employ such multiple color displays.

Quantitation of Planar Images

Since visual interpretation of analog Tl-201 images is subject to substantial variability, quantitation of initial distribution and subsequent washout of Tl-201 has been recommended.[9, 14–16] Quantitative evaluation of Tl-201 images cannot be accomplished without adequate background subtraction techniques. Background activity is variable and obviously has nonuniform distribution. Moreover, the distribution of background activity changes quite significantly over the interval between stress and delayed rest images. This is why methods that subtract a constant background are inappropriate. Background activity degrades the contrast of perfusion defects and prevents accurate measurement of regional Tl-201 activity from the myocardium.

The background subtraction used in our laboratory before quantitation of regional Tl-201 activity, which is a modification of the Goris method,[9, 10, 16] first entails placing a rectangular region of interest (ROI) around the heart. Each ROI is placed so that the box just touches the heart on all

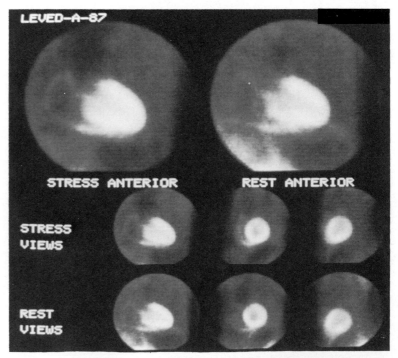

Figure 1–10. Stress and rest anterior planar images in top row with anterior 45-degree LAO and 70-degree LAO stress and rest images in bottom rows employing the green-to-white intensity scale. These normal images were acquired in a patient with chest pain and less than 5% likelihood of CAD. (See Color Figure 1–10.)

See Color Figure 1–10.

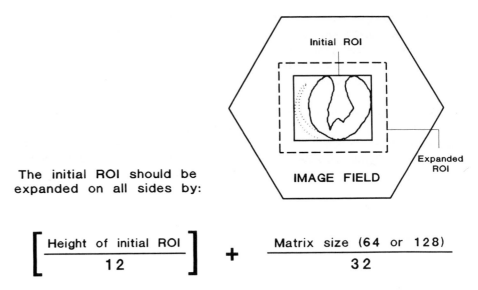

The initial ROI should be
expanded on all sides by:

Figure 1–11. For accomplishing the interpolative background subtraction, a placement of a region-of-interest (ROI) must be placed around the heart on all sides including the right ventricle. (Smith WH, Watson DD: Am J Cardiol 1990;66:16E–22E.)

$$\left[\frac{\text{Height of initial ROI}}{12}\right] + \frac{\text{Matrix size (64 or 128)}}{32}$$

sides and includes the right ventricle in the rectangle (Fig. 1–11). The portion of the right ventricle extending beyond the superior or inferior borders of the left ventricle is not included. The same size ROI is placed on both the exercise and rest images. The user is permitted to reposition the same box on the rest image but not to change the size. This yields less operator variability. The user can at any time rescale the image to the maximum counts in the heart to optimize placement of the ROI. Rescaling may be useful for unprocessed Tc-99m sestamibi images, since splanchnic activity may cause improper scaling. Once the ROI is placed, the computer program automatically rescales the

images to the hottest pixel inside the ROI. The ROI is also used for background subtraction and image registration.

As mentioned, with the interpolative background subtraction algorithm, a rectangular background boundary is set by the operator to touch the edges of the heart.[9] The computer program expands this boundary and generates a background reference plane according to the equations shown in Figure 1–12. The equations are written to be independent of matrix size. This background subtraction algorithm removes the "tissue cross-talk" from the raw image.[17] More complex weighting functions have been introduced as a modification of the original Goris method.[9] A further modification of the

INTERPOLATIVE
BACKGROUND SUBTRACTION

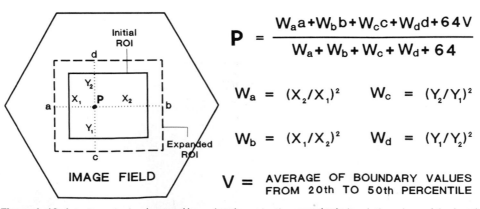

$$P = \frac{W_a a + W_b b + W_c c + W_d d + 64 V}{W_a + W_b + W_c + W_d + 64}$$

$$W_a = (X_2/X_1)^2 \qquad W_c = (Y_2/Y_1)^2$$

$$W_b = (X_1/X_2)^2 \qquad W_d = (Y_1/Y_2)^2$$

$$V = \text{AVERAGE OF BOUNDARY VALUES FROM 20th TO 50th PERCENTILE}$$

Figure 1–12. A rectangular background boundary is set by the operator to touch the edges of the heart as described for Figure 1–11. The computer program expands this boundary and generates a background reference plane according to the equation shown on the right. This equation is written to be independent of matrix size. The constant, 64, is unrelated to the matrix but actually controls the steepness of the rolloff from the boundary to background beneath the heart. Pixel counts on the expanded boundary are sorted from the lowest to the highest, and V is the average of all those values included from the 20th to the 50th percentile. (Smith WH, Watson DD: Am J Cardiol 1990;66:16E–22E.)

Watson interpolative background algorithm used for Tl-201 was developed for Tc-99m sestamibi.[18, 19] These weighting functions provide proximity weighting near the edges of the background-defining region, which also causes more rapid fall-off of the generated background because it is extrapolated beneath the myocardial rim in the proximity of intense background regions such as the liver and stomach.

For each planar sestamibi image, a background is generated automatically from the smoothed image using an expanded boundary for the ROI. With the smoothing technique, images are filtered to diminish statistical fluctuations. The background is subtracted from the unsmooth raw image, leaving myocardial activity in a random pattern of residual counts outside the heart (Poisson statistical noise).

To accurately compare rest and exercise images for detection of Tl-201 redistribution, images must be in "registration" with each other. Image registration is defined as the alignment of sequential images in a particular projection (e.g., 45-degree LAO). Image registration can be undertaken without operator interaction. For the Watson method,[9, 20] each background-corrected image is initially centered by finding the two-dimensional (2-D) centroid of the image inside the expanded ROI, and then shifting the image so that the centroid is in the center of the image matrix (Fig. 1–13). This procedure is applied for both the rest and exercise background-corrected images. After approximate centroid centering, a cross-correlation technique is performed that precisely aligns the rest and exercise images according to a 2-D least-squares criterion. This is accomplished by iteratively translating the position of the rest image to maximize the cross-correlation coefficient with the exercise image (Fig. 1–14). The x and y summed profiles are used instead of calculating a pixel-by-pixel correlation coefficient. This image registration procedure ensures that the same regions on the exercise and rest images are sampled by the count profiles. After subtraction of the

reference plane to compensate for tissue cross-talk and registration of the images is accomplished, quantification is undertaken by displaying horizontal count profiles across the heart (Fig. 1–15). For the Watson method,[9] four profiles will sample the myocardial count distribution adequately within the limitations of image resolution. Each profile represents an average of about a 1-cm wide slice across the heart.

An alternative to the horizontal count profile quantitative approach is the circumferential profile method. This method was pioneered by Garcia.[21–23] With this method, images are also compensated for tissue cross-talk by performing interpolative background subtraction followed by spatial smoothing using a nine-point weighted average. Circumferential profiles are then generated. Profiles are generated of the maximum counts per pixel along each of 60 radii spaced 6 degrees apart and plotted clockwise (Fig. 1–16). The profiles quantitate the segmental activity as an angular function reference from the visually located center of the LV cavity. The operator assigns the maximum and minimal radius to which the computer is to search, which prevents the algorithm from searching outside the heart. The profiles are aligned so that the apex in each view is assigned to 90 degrees, permitting correction for the variation in the position of the heart. With the ventricular apex oriented to 90 degrees in each projection, a profile of maximal counts at each successive clockwise 6-degree radius is plotted. The circumferential profile method provides a more compact and dense single-curve display of counts sampled around the myocardial rim and allows the simple plot of a second profile, which indicates normal limits. As shown in Figure 1–17, assignment of the center of the left ventricle with this technique is crucial to prevent image artifacts. If the center is erroneously placed too close to the apex, as in this example, an apical artifact will be seen, which results from "fanning" of the radii.

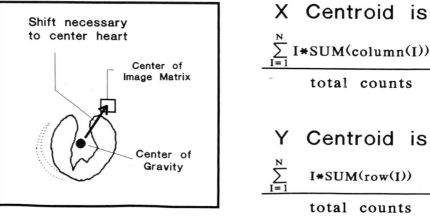

Figure 1–13. The background-corrected image is centered by computing the X- and Y-centroids, which define the center of gravity. Then, the image is shifted so the center of gravity now lies in the center of the image matrix. Any counts outside the expanded ROI (not shown) are not included in the computations. (Smith WH Watson DD, Am J Cardiol 1990;66: 16E–22E.)

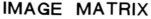

CROSS-CORRELATION CORRECTION

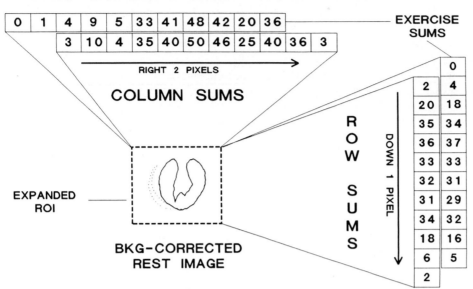

| 0 | 1 | 4 | 9 | 5 | 33 | 41 | 48 | 42 | 20 | 36 |

| 3 | 10 | 4 | 35 | 40 | 50 | 46 | 25 | 40 | 36 | 3 |

RIGHT 2 PIXELS →

COLUMN SUMS

EXERCISE SUMS

EXPANDED ROI

BKG-CORRECTED REST IMAGE

R O W   S U M S

DOWN 1 PIXEL ↓

	0
2	4
20	18
35	34
36	37
33	33
32	31
31	29
34	32
18	16
6	5
2	

Figure 1–14. The final adjustment is made to the positioning of the background-corrected rest image by maximizing the cross-correlation coefficient for the exercise image. The computation is performed using the X (columns) sums and the Y (row) sums inside the expanded ROI. This cross-correlation technique is performed after centering and comprises aligning the rest image with the exercise image according to a two-dimensional least-squares criterion. (Smith WH, Watson DD: Am J Cardiol 1990;66:16E–22E.)

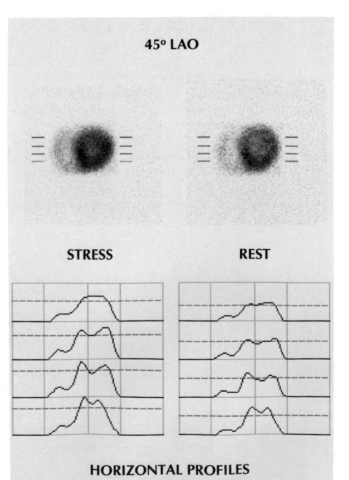

45° LAO

STRESS   **REST**

HORIZONTAL PROFILES

Figure 1–15. Stress and rest horizontal count profiles shown below background-subtracted 45-degree LAO images. The bottom of the four profiles are representative of inferoapical activity, whereas the top profiles are taken from the upper septum and upper posterolateral wall. Note that the rest profiles are lower than the stress profiles, reflecting uniform Tl-201 washout from all myocardial segments. The short horizontal lines adjacent to the images depict the location of the horizontal count profiles shown below the images.

ALGORITHM

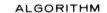

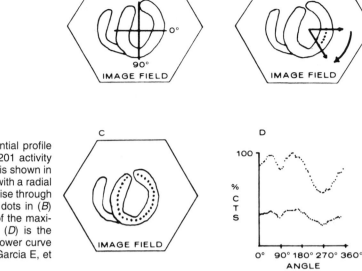

Figure 1–16. Diagrammatic representation of the circumferential profile quantitative approach to determining changes in regional Tl-201 activity from stress to rest conditions. Polar coordinate reference axis is shown in (*A*). Image pixels for circumferential profile analysis are found with a radial search for maximum value at 6-degree intervals plotted clockwise through 360 degrees as shown (*B*). Maximal values shown as black dots in (*B*) and (*C*) are replotted in (*D*) for each angle as a percentage of the maximum value for the circumferential profile. The top curve in (*D*) is the circumferential profile from the stress Tl-201 image, and the lower curve is the circumferential profile from the 4-hour delayed image. (Garcia E, et al.: J Nucl Med 1981;22:309–317.)

The Garcia program incorporates lower limits of normal circumferential profiles generated from patients with a less than 1% pretest likelihood of coronary artery disease (CAD). There is more operator interaction and variability with the circumferential profile method than with the linear profile approach. This is because there is a requirement for location of the center and edge of the myocardium and a computer search for a parameter, usually maximum counts along a radial profile from center to edge. The apex must also be located by an operator.

Other computer-assisted quantitative techniques for assessing planar myocardial perfusion images have been utilized.[24–26] Like the two methods described previously, these also are highly reproducible with good inter- and intraobserver variability. Figure 1–18 describes the method employed by Wackers et al.[26a] for quantitating defect size on planar Tl-201 images utilizing the circumferential profile analysis technique. The clinical utility of such quantitative techniques for detection of CAD is described in greater detail in Chapter 3.

Although no longer used clinically for routine image interpretation, the regional myocardial washout rate of Tl-201 can be quantitatively determined by calculating percentage of reduction in counts in a specific region between initial and delayed images. Normal washout rates have been derived for multiple myocardial regions from subjects with

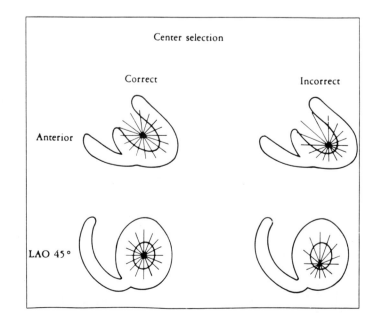

Figure 1–17. Diagram of the left ventricle in anterior and 45-degree LAO views showing correct (*left*) and incorrect (*right*) designation of the center of the left ventricle for subsequent generation of circumferential profiles. If the center of the left ventricular cavity is placed too close to the apex, "fanning" of the radii would result in an artifactual defect at the apex. (Maddahi J, et al.: Assessment of myocardial perfusion by single-photon agents. *In* Pohost GM, O'Rourke RA (eds): Principles and Practice of Cardiovascular Imaging. Boston, Little, Brown, 1991, pp 179–219.)

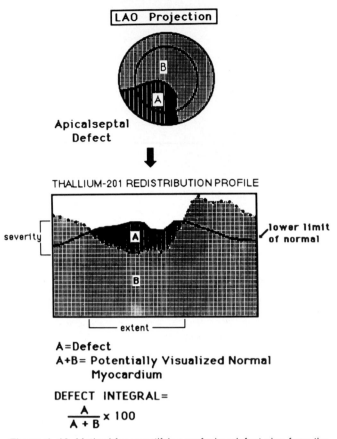

| LAO Projection |

Apicalseptal Defect

THALLIUM-201 REDISTRIBUTION PROFILE

severity

A

lower limit of normal

B

extent

A=Defect
A+B= Potentially Visualized Normal Myocardium

DEFECT INTEGRAL=
$$\frac{A}{A+B} \times 100$$

Figure 1–18. Method for quantifying perfusion defect size from the LAO projection with a hypothetical apical-septal defect. The Tl-201 distribution profile is shown below. The apical-septal defect is graphically shown as the portion of the profile that falls below the lower limit of normal (A). The defect can be described in terms of extent (the number of data points below the lower limit of normal) as well as severity (the nadir of the curve below the lower limit of normal). Defect size can be quantitated as the integral of the defect area (A) and the potentially visualized normal myocardium (A plus B). (Wackers FJT, et al.: J Am Coll Cardiol 1993;21:1064–1074.)

angiographically normal coronary arteries or less than 1% likelihood of CAD. The Garcia approach employs washout circumferential profiles that are calculated as percentage washout from the stress to the approximately 4-hour redistribution image. Figure 1–19 shows that the half-life for myocardial Tl-201 washout in normal myocardium is related to peak exercise heart rate. The higher the exercise heart rate, the faster the Tl-201 clearance rate.[15]

Single-Photon Emission Computed Tomography

Most nuclear imaging laboratories perform single-photon emission computed tomography (SPECT) imaging, which was introduced in the late 1970s.[26b] The SPECT imaging approach yields images of slices of the heart without interference of activity from noncardiac or overlapping myocardial regions and is similar in principle to x-ray computed tomography. It does this by collecting data about the heart from multiple views and using these data to construct tomograms through the heart. Tomographic images are "computed" from the registration of interactions of individual γ-rays in a crystal. The SPECT image represents an assignment of radioactivity concentration to pixels. SPECT imaging yields better contrast resolution, enhancing detection of small regions of hypoperfusion. Overlap of normal and abnormal segments on planar images makes detection and localization of small perfusion abnormalities difficult. Because SPECT images are free of background, lesion contrast is higher, and the size of lesions is made greater by tomographic reconstructed views than on planar projections obtained in anterior, 45-degree LAO, and 70-degree LAO projections. However, the cost of improvement in contrast resolution is a loss of spatial resolution.[21] Because reorientation is performed on all hearts, the views are more standardized with respect to cardiac orientation.

To perform SPECT imaging,[21, 27] a gamma camera mounted on a gantry is rotated around the patient up to a full 360 degrees' angular sampling. Table 1–2 summarizes the considerations for selecting SPECT imaging parameters as outlined by Garcia.[21, 21a] Tomographic acquisition for SPECT imaging is best accomplished with a large–field of view gamma camera equipped with a low-energy general-purpose collimator. Detector orbits can be elliptical or circular. Elliptical orbits are characterized by having the detector closer to the patient during rotation, preserving spatial resolution when the detector is far from the patient during image acquisition. Circular orbits may be associated with

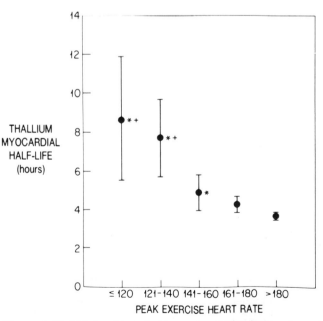

THALLIUM MYOCARDIAL HALF-LIFE (hours)

PEAK EXERCISE HEART RATE

Figure 1–19. Relationship between peak exercise heart rate and myocardial clearance of Tl-201 in 89 normal subjects. *$P < 0.05$ compared with heart rate >180; $P < 0.05$ compared with heart rate of range of 161–180. (Kaul S, et al.: Semin Nucl Med 1987;17:131–144.)

Table 1–2. **Considerations for Selecting SPECT Imaging Parameters**

Energy window: symmetric vs. asymmetric
Collimator: low-energy, general-purpose vs. high-resolution
Orbit: 180 degrees vs. 360 degrees; elliptical vs. circular
Step-and-shoot vs. continuous acquisition
Time per projection and number of projections
Single vs. multiple detector systems
ECG gated or nongated

(Adapted from Garcia EV: Physics and instrumentation of radionuclide imaging. *In* Marcus M, et al. (eds): Cardiac Imaging: A Companion to Braunwald's "Heart Disease." Philadelphia, WB Saunders, 1991, pp 977–1005.)

greater loss of spatial resolution than elliptical orbits. However, with elliptical orbits there is more regional nonuniformity, which can create image artifacts.[21a, 28] Figure 1–20 from Garcia[21a] depicts 180-degree circular and elliptical orbits. Presently, the most commonly employed mode of SPECT acquisition is called a *step-and-shoot method.* The detector halts at predetermined angles and acquires the γ-rays while it is stationary for a preselected period. When the time is up for collection of counts in each projection, the camera "steps" to the next angular position.

The 180-degree orbit is preferred to the 360-degree orbit, to provide adequate sampling angles but minimize highly attenuated and scattered photons resulting from imaging myocardium from the right posterior oblique projection. The 180-degree orbit is characterized by high spatial and contrast resolution, whereas the 360-degree orbit is associated with enhanced field uniformity. The 180-degree imaging protocol involves collecting data from the 45-degree right anterior oblique (RAO) to the 45-degree left posterior oblique projection. Typically, the camera makes 32 or 64 stops for 40 seconds each for the 180-degree acquisition. Each of the projections is corrected for field nonuniformity and for misalignment of the mechanical center of rotation with respect to the reconstruction matrix.

After the orbit is complete, the series of planar images taken at different angles around the patient are back-projected into the transverse axial images, which are slices that are oriented perpendicular to the axis of rotation. Back-projection is undertaken to reconstruct transverse tomograms encompassing the heart from apex to base. Thus, these transaxial images correspond to the long axis of the patient. The transaxial images are then reoriented to produce horizontal long-axis and vertical long-axis images. The final images are displayed in a slice-by-slice format for visual analysis. Figure 1–21 shows how short-axis, vertical long-axis, and horizontal long-axis SPECT tomograms are displayed in a left-to-right or top-to-bottom format, per the recommendation of the American College of Cardiology, American Heart Association, and Society of Nuclear Medicine.[28a] Figure 1–22 shows a normal SPECT scintigram.

The standard filtered back-projection method has a disadvantage in that it causes blurring, producing loss of spatial resolution. Using such a filtered back-projection approach, a blur-corrected tomogram from processed planar projections can be derived by using a Ramp filter. This high-pass filter corrects for the blurring from unfiltered back-projection. Garcia states that filtered back-projection may be thought of as, first, extracting the edges of a three-dimensional (3-D) radioactive source from different angles and, second, back-projecting the edges from the different angles to generate the count distribution in a transaxial tomogram.[21] As a result of enhancing higher frequencies, the Ramp filter may propagate high-frequency noise when there are low-count statistics. To compensate for this high-

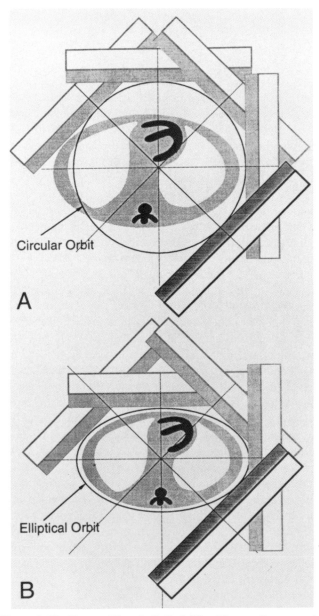

Figure 1–20. Circular (**A**) and elliptical (**B**) orbits are diagrammatically depicted. With the circular orbit rotating 180 degrees around the thorax, the detector is closer to the apex and anterior wall in the 45-degree LAO projection compared with 45 degrees right anterior oblique or left posterior oblique projections. For the 180-degree elliptical orbit around the thorax, the detector is closer to the heart than with the circular orbit. (Garcia EV: J Nucl Cardiol 1994;1:83–93.)

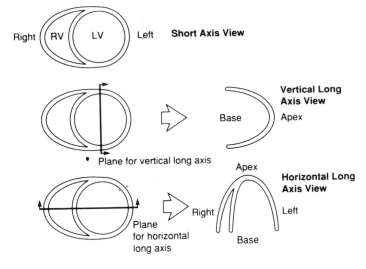

Figure 1–21. Display for SPECT images per the recommendation of the American Heart Association, American College of Cardiology, and Society of Nuclear Medicine. (J Nucl Cardiol 1994;1:117–119.)

frequency noise, the Ramp filter is usually combined with a low-pass (smoothing) filter. The Hanning and the Butterworth filters are two examples of low-pass filters that can be combined with a Ramp filter to produce different degrees of tradeoff between reduction of noise and degradation of spatial and contrast resolution.

There are SPECT systems with two detector heads mounted in 90-degree or in 180-degree opposition and SPECT machines with three detector heads mounted at 120-degree intervals.[28b] Garcia states that, for 180-degree tomographic acquisition of the heart, the best detector configuration is two heads separated by 90 degrees.[21a] That way, the full 180-degree orbit can be acquired in half the time with only 90 degrees of motion. This increases throughput by cutting acquisition time in half. The three-head system has some advantages, including extremely high resolution, and by using fan-beam or cone-beam collimators, both spatial resolution and sensitivity can be enhanced. Fan-beam or cone collimation should permit simultaneous attenuation correction. Bateman et al.[28c] found that acquisition using a three-detector camera provides more data than can serve to minimize, but not correct, for the effects of localized attenuation if incorporated into the final reconstruction set.

Acquisition parameters for gated SPECT Tc-99m sestamibi imaging have been formulated.[28, 28d] Acquisition usually involves using a high-resolution, parallel-hole collimator with a step-and-shoot circular, patient-centered orbit with a 180-degree imaging arc with no zoom and eight frames per cardiac cycle. Summed frames are prefiltered with a Ramp filter and then filtered with the 2-D Butterworth filter (critical frequency, 0.52; power, 5.0). Frames are typically reconstructed 1 pixel thick. Slice display is as single slices of 6.4 mm thickness or in staggered pairs with a thickness of 12.8 mm.

Quantitation of SPECT Images

There are several computer quantitation approaches to enhance the detection of abnormalities in myocardial per-

fusion on SPECT reconstructed images.[21, 27, 29–38a] One of the most common techniques for quantitating myocardial perfusion is 2-D polar maps.[35] The polar maps are constructed by mapping sequential maximal-count circumferential profiles, ranging from apex to the base of the heart, into successive rings on the polar map (Fig. 1–23). The apex is placed in the center of the map, and the base is displayed at the periphery. A display of the three coronary artery territories on the polar map is shown in Figure 1–24. Conventionally, only the short-axis slices are quantified in this manner. Klein et al.[36] described the quantification process with this technique. It consists of extracting maximal-count circumferential profiles on each of the short-axis slices in 9-degree arcs ranging from apex to base, yielding 40 data points for each slice. The data are then interpolated to the equivalent of 15 slices and stored in two 15 by 40 arrays, one for the stress data and one for the resting data. The data are then transformed into the polar plot referred to as the *bull's-eye plot*. The bull's-eye plot consists of a series of 15 concentric circles made from the 15 profiles interpolated from the 12 slices from apex to base. In these series of 15 concentric circles, the apex is at the center and the base at the periphery. Bull's-eyes are constructed for the stress and delayed images, as well as for percentage of washout.

Normalization of bull's-eyes is usually accomplished by comparison with normal files obtained from subjects with a low probability of CAD. Mean values and standard deviations are derived from the normal population for each of the angular locations in each of the 15 profiles. Normal files have to be generated separately for each radionuclide perfusion agent, and a normal Tl-201 database cannot be used for quantitating Tc-99m sestamibi SPECT images. Comparing each patient's bull's-eye to a gender-matched normal file results in the conversion of the bull's-eye into a standard deviation map displaying pixels color-coded to the number of standard deviations away from normal. Figure 1–25 from Klein et al.[36] shows a Tl-201 bull's-eye polar map display of a patient with disease of the left anterior

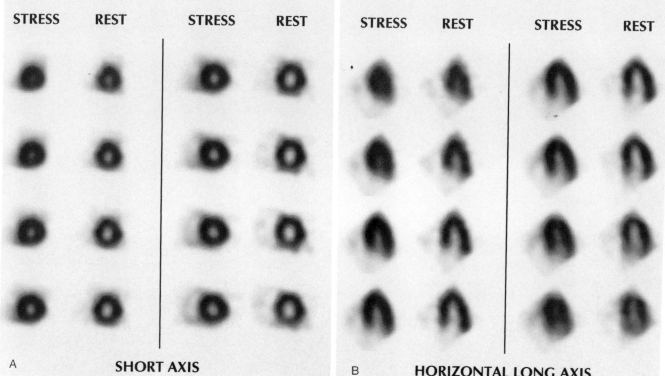

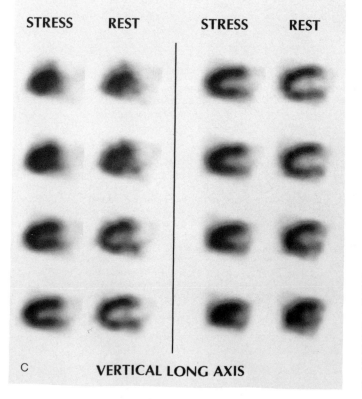

Figure 1–22. Normal stress and rest Tc-99m–sestamibi SPECT images obtained in a 45-year-old man with a normal resting electrocardiogram, who achieved 12.9 METS and a peak heart rate of 152/bpm during exercise. **A,** Short-axis tomograms with apex at upper left and basilar slices at lower right; **B,** horizontal long-axis tomograms with superior slices at upper left and inferior slices at lower right; **C,** vertical long-axis tomograms with right ventricular and septal slices at upper left and lateral wall slices at lower right. The tomograms are shown with the apex pointing to the left rather than to the right as recommended in Figure 1–21.

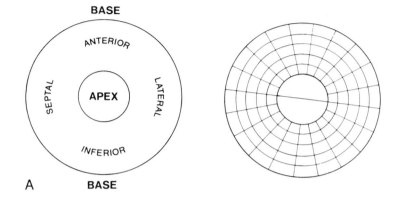

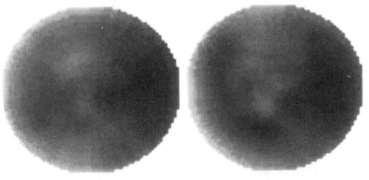

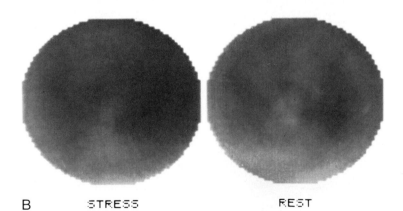

Figure 1–23. (*A*) Polar map display in diagrammatic form of the various regions of the left ventricle with these regions divided into 102 sections (*right*). (Reprinted with permission from the American College of Cardiology (Journal of the American College of Cardiology, 1989, Vol. 14, pp. 1689–1699).) (*B*) Normal Tc-99m sestamibi bull's-eye maps at stress and rest in a normal male *(bottom)* and a normal female *(top)*. The normal male bull's-eye map shows some diminished activity in the inferior region secondary to attenuation, whereas the bull's-eye map from the normal female patient shows some diminished activity in the anterior wall due to breast attenuation.

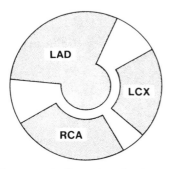

Figure 1–24. Diagrammatic illustration of polar map display of the three coronary artery territories. (Key: LAD, left anterior descending coronary artery; LCX, left circumflex coronary artery; RCA, right coronary artery.) (Reprinted with permission from the American College of Cardiology (Journal of the American College of Cardiology, 1989, Vol. 14, pp. 1689–1699).)

descending coronary artery (LAD). For profile points that fall below 2.5 standard deviations of the normal value, a blackout area within the bull's-eye plot defines the extent of hypoperfusion (Fig. 1–25). The Emory group has also shown that washout and reversibility bull's-eyes can be generated.[36] Reversibility bull's-eyes are generated by subtracting the stress profiles from the corresponding delayed

profiles after normalizing to a 5 by 5 pixel maximal-count reference area in the exercise Tl-201 study. Figure 1–25 shows a reversibility bull's-eye plot in the patient with a stenosis of the LAD.

Botvinick et al.[38b] emphasize the importance of recognizing patient motion during acquisition as artifacts on quantitative SPECT imaging. Others have also provided ways to better detect motion artifacts and correct for them.[38c–38f] The clinical application and limitations of both qualitative and quantitative SPECT perfusion imaging are reviewed in Chapter 3.

As mentioned previously, Tc-99m sestamibi stress images can be gated so that the perfusion pattern during exercise can be compared with resting regional function at the time images are acquired 30 to 60 minutes after tracer injection. This assists in viability detection. Figure 1–26 shows end-diastolic and end-systolic short-axis and vertical long-axis SPECT images in a normal subject. Note the smaller LV cavity in the end-systolic images with greater activity in the myocardial walls indicated by increased "brightness." Figure 1–27 compares ungated and gated vertical long-axis tomograms in a patient with an anterior perfusion abnormality.

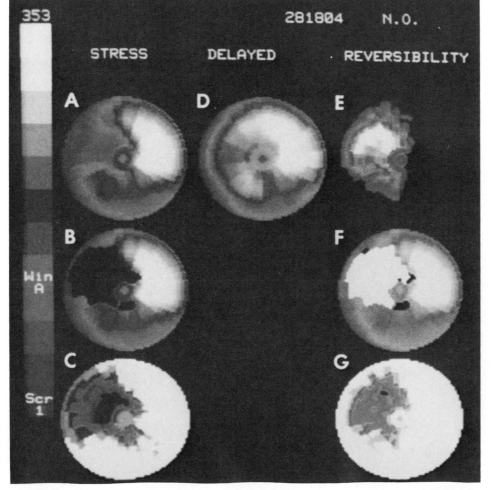

Figure 1–25. The stress bull's-eye images (*first column*) demonstrate a significant anteroseptal defect, which shows complete reversibility on the delayed image (*second column*). Bull's-eye plot B in the first column shows a "blackout" area that exceeded 2.5 standard deviations from the mean of normal Tl-201 distribution. Bull's-eye plot C uses the color scale to depict the number of standard deviations any given area differs from the mean. By subtracting each point in a normalized stress image from the corresponding point in the normalized delay image yields a polar plot of "reversibility" as shown in E. Regions that were irreversible are depicted in black. The "white-out" bull's-eye in F duplicates the results of the stress blackout bull's-eye, in which areas falling below 2.5 standard deviations from the mean are blacked out. However, regions that have significantly reversed on delayed images are whited out. The bull's-eye plot in G is a reversibility plot that depicts the number of standard deviations from the mean of normal reversibility using a varying color scale. (See Color Figure 1–25.) (Reprinted by permission of the Society of Nuclear Medicine from: Klein JL, et al.: J Nucl Med 1990;31: 1240–1246.)

See Color Figure 1–25.

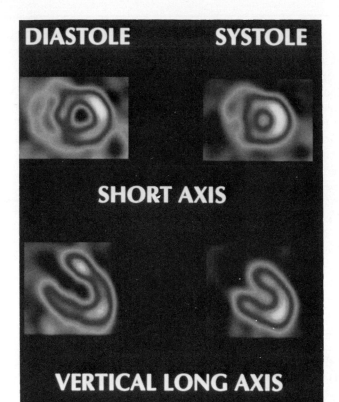

See Color Figure 1–26.

Figure 1–26. End-diastolic (diastole) and end-systole (systole) short-axis and vertical long-axis SPECT images in a normal subject. (See Color Figure 1–26.)

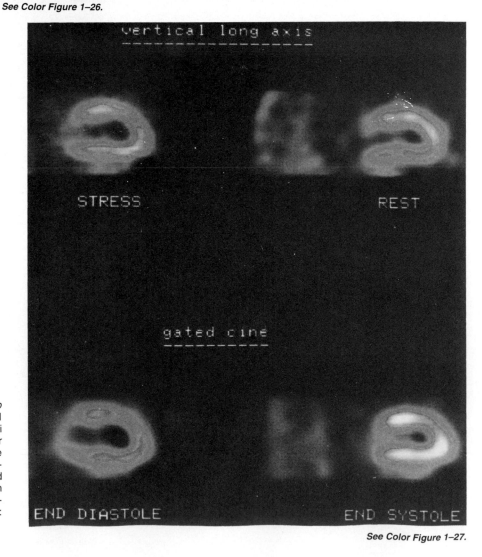

See Color Figure 1–27.

Figure 1–27. Comparison of ungated (*top panels*) and gated (*bottom panels*) vertical long-axis tomographic Tc-99m–sestamibi images. In the ungated study, an anterior defect is observed that normalizes on the resting study. On the gated study, the end-systolic image shows thickening depicted by increased brightness as compared with the defect observed in the end-diastolic image. (See Color Figure 1–27.) (Garcia EV: J Nucl Cardiol 1994;1:83–93.)

RADIONUCLIDE ANGIOGRAPHY

Radionuclide angiography implies the dynamic imaging of the LV and right ventricular (RV) blood pools employing ECG gating. This noninvasive technique is referred to in this text as *radionuclide angiography* (RNA). For the most part, RNA is undertaken employing a single-crystal gamma scintillation camera. Two approaches to gated RNA have emerged: the *first-pass* and the *equilibrium* method.[39, 40]

Equilibrium-Gated Method

The equilibrium radionuclide angiographic method is also referred to as a MUGA nuclear scan study. This is because there is *multiple-gated acquisition* in which there is repetitive sampling of blood pool counts from equal subdivisions of the R-R interval (Fig. 1–28). Generally, a framing interval of 30 to 50 msec is employed in the resting state, and 20 to 30 msec for exercise. Imaging is performed for as many as 200 successive cardiac cycles, until images of good photon density are acquired. The R wave of the ECG is used as the marker to initiate acquisition of count data with each cardiac cycle. From these "resultant" images, both regional wall motion and global ventricular function are evaluated. From the series of images, changes in radioactivity that occur within the cardiac chambers during the cardiac cycle can be digitized and displayed in the form of a relative volume curve (see Fig. 1–28). The images that are acquired have approximately 200,000 counts per frame. Figure 1–29 shows selected frames from MUGA studies in a normal individual and a patient with abnormal LV function from the paper of Burow et al.[41] To obtain a volume curve with the highest resolution, a standard–field of view camera is used, and the images are acquired in approximately 5 minutes.

The volume curve is based on the principle that a change in radioactivity is proportional to the change in blood volume, and when background corrections have been performed, the LV time-activity curve represents the average change in blood volume when all the cardiac cycles have been integrated to form a composite cycle (Fig. 1–30). This equilibrium-gated radionuclide angiogram can be displayed in an endless-loop cineformat in which frames are displayed in a movie mode. This average cardiac cycle is displayed over and over again and simulates the beating heart, as compared with what is observed with a contrast ventriculogram. Chamber size and segmental wall motion are subjectively assessed from the cineangiogram or computer-assisted quantitation of regional EF and ventricular volumes.

To adequately assess regional wall motion, multiple imaging views are obtained. They include the best "septal" projection corresponding normally to a 45-degree LAO view, an anterior view projection, a steep 70-degree LAO view, and, at times, a left lateral view. This latter view provides an elongated display of the inferior wall, permitting improved assessment of wall motion of the posterobasal segment. Figure 1–31 shows examples of normal end-systolic and end-diastolic frames of a radionuclide angiogram in these three projections.

ECG gating may be performed by using either frame mode or list mode acquisitions. In the frame mode acquisition, the imaging data are sorted into the appropriate location of the picture file or added to the previous data in that memory and then eliminated. Most computer systems with limited memory capability employ this approach. Using the list mode, count data are stored consecutively, word by word, in one of two buffer memories. The imaging data are acquired with timing marks as well as ECG signals. The list mode acquisition requires expanded computer memory. An advantage of list mode acquisition is that it permits reformatting of data. Data from ectopic beats or those with significant variation in R-R interval can be readily excluded. Some have proposed that the diastolic portion of

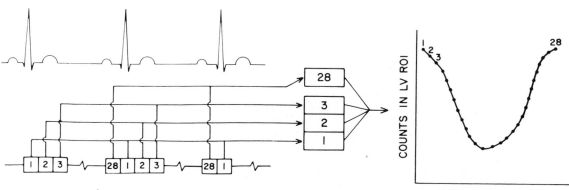

Figure 1–28. Diagram of the multiple-gated cardiac blood pool imaging (MUGA) technique for equilibrium radionuclide angiography. In this example, each R-R interval is subdivided into 28 equal frames. Data from consecutive beats are summed, resulting in a single representative cardiac cycle. Each of the 28 frames becomes a corresponding image, and counts in the left ventricle can be quantitated using a region of interest (ROI) yielding a left ventricular volume curve (*right*). (Zaret B, Berger H: Progress in Cardiology. Philadelphia, Lea & Febiger, 1983, pp 33–58.)

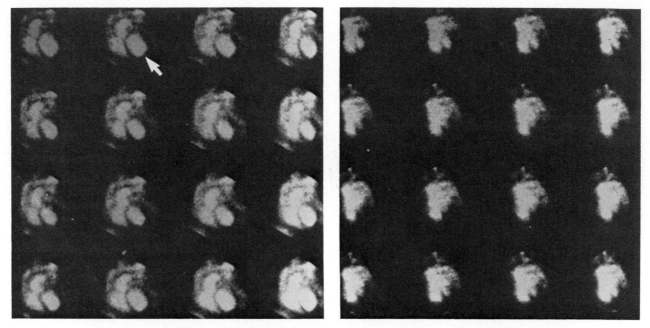

Figure 1–29. Selected frames from an equilibrium-gated cardiac blood pool study (MUGA) performed in the left anterior oblique position in a patient with diminished left ventricular function (*left*) and in a patient with normal left ventricular function (*right*). Note that throughout the cardiac cycle, the left ventricular blood pool (*arrow*) is enlarged in the patient with cardiac disease with minimal change from diastole through systole. In contrast, the left ventricular chamber is considerably smaller in the normal patient with virtual cavity obliteration during systole (*second and third rows*). (Burow RD, et al.: Circulation 1977;56:1024–1028.)

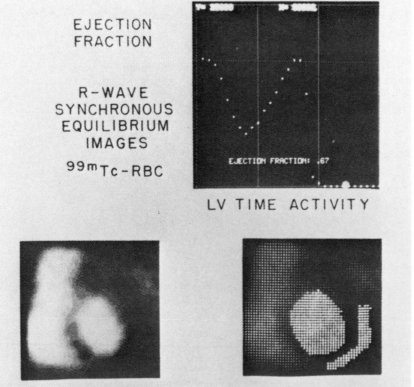

Figure 1–30. Illustration of the gated equilibrium blood-pool method for generating left ventricular (LV) time-activity curves reflecting changes in LV volume over time. The 45-degree LAO image of the heart at end-diastole is depicted in the lower left frame. In the lower right frame, the LV and background (BK) regions of interest have been outlined by a light pen. The frame in the upper right-hand corner shows the synchronized composite time-activity curve generated during several hundred cardiac cycles from the background-subtracted LV region of interest. (Reprinted by permission of the Society of Nuclear Medicine from: Folland ED, et al.: J Nucl Med 1977;18:1159–1166.)

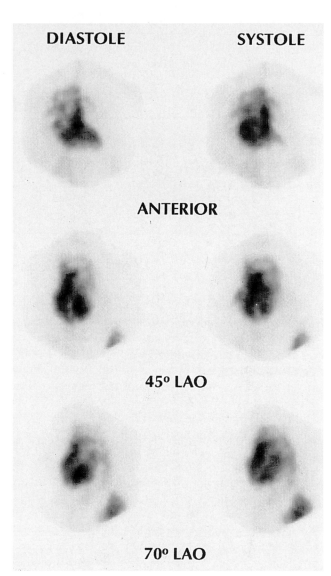

DIASTOLE   SYSTOLE

ANTERIOR

45º LAO

70º LAO

Figure 1–31. Normal end-systolic (SYSTOLE) and end-diastolic frames (DIASTOLE) in anterior, 45-degree left anterior oblique (LAO) and 70-degree LAO projections.

the volume curve is improved since the LV time-activity curve can be constructed using forward-backward framing.

The LVEF is calculated from the LV volume curve after appropriate background subtraction using a "counts-based" method.[41–43] To optimally calculate EF, the measurement of count rate changes must be confined solely to the LV blood pool. Thus, the 45-degree LAO or a "best septal" oblique projection must be employed. The LV region of interest is manually or automatically derived. A background region of interest is also outlined manually or by computer. The method used for calculation of the EF is called the *area-counts technique.* The premise utilized for this technique is that there is proportionality between Tc-99m counts in the cardiac blood pool and actual blood volume. The end-diastolic counts are proportional to end-diastolic volume, and the end-systolic counts are propor-

tional to the end-systolic volume. The changes in radioactivity in the LV blood pool between end-diastole and end-systole are proportional to stroke volume and are called the stroke counts.

Background correction is intended to correct for radioactivity in the LV region of interest that does not originate from the LV blood pool itself. Most often, a background region of interest is placed immediately adjacent to the posterolateral wall segment of the left ventricle (see Fig. 1–30). The EF is computed as the end-diastolic counts minus the end-systolic counts (stroke counts) divided by the end-diastolic counts. This, of course, is undertaken after background subtraction has been accomplished. The area-counts technique for calculation of LVEF correlates very well with EF assessed from contrast ventriculography.[41, 44] Studies in the literature have reported excellent reproducibility and

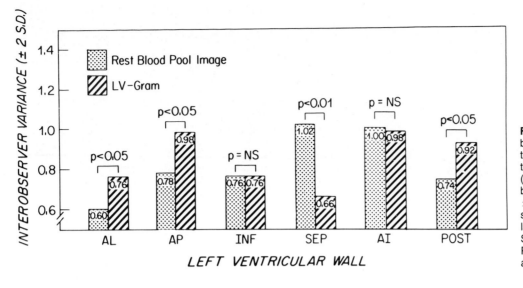

Figure 1–32. Intraobserver variability in the evaluation of left ventricular regional wall motion using the contrast left ventriculogram (LV gram) and the rest multigated blood-pool image, expressed as ±2 SD employing a five-point scoring system. (Key: AL, anterolaterals; AP, apical; INF, inferior; SEP, septal; AI, apical-inferior; POST, posterior.) (Okada RD, et al.: Circulation 1980;61:128–136.)

intraobserver variability by measuring the EF in this manner. Okada et al. in this study[45] found an intraobserver variance for EF determination of ±5.8% and interobserver variance of ±6.0%. Figure 1–32 shows the interobserver variance in the evaluation of LV regional wall motion using the contrast ventriculogram and the resting gated equilibrium radionuclide angiogram in this study.

When sufficient temporal resolution is employed in the acquisition of the radioisotope data, other hemodynamic parameters, such as peak systolic ejection rate, ejection time, and early systolic EF, can be measured from the ejection portion of the curve, and they reflect the speed of systolic emptying. Other indices that can be obtained from the radionuclide angiogram include RVEF, relative or absolute end-diastolic and end-systolic volumes, cardiac output, and regurgitant fraction. The accurate quantitative measurement of ventricular volume and cardiac output is dependent on the attenuation correction used.[46] To provide time-activity volume curves with sufficient temporal resolution for use in generating the systolic ejection rate, data should be acquired using a rapid framing rate.

First-Pass Method

With the first-pass method, a single bolus is injected rapidly via the intravenous route, and analysis is limited to the initial transit of radioactivity through the central circulation.[47–49c] Since there is both temporal and anatomic separation of radioactivity within each cardiac chamber, both RV and LV performance can be evaluated from the same study employing indicator-dilution techniques for functional analysis. In the first-pass method, Tc-99m radiopharmaceuticals with a high specific activity are used. Since serial studies require separate injections of the radiotracer, Tc-99m–labeled agents other than sodium pertechnetate are preferable. When serial studies are undertaken during rest

and under exercise, the first injection can be made either with Tc-99m sulfur colloid, which is extracted from the blood pool by the reticuloendothelial system, or with Tc-99m pertechnetate, which is cleared by the kidneys.

For first-pass studies, a scintillation camera and computer are required, which provide adequate temporal and spatial resolution with good counting statistics. This is because data are derived from only a few cardiac cycles during the initial passage of the radioactive bolus. Multicrystal scintillation cameras are preferable to the single-crystal Anger camera for first-pass RNA because high count rates of up to 400,000 counts per second are obtainable with the multicrystal device. The initial phase of evaluation of a first-pass study involves the visual evaluation of images derived at 1-sec intervals. The mean transit time that correlates with cardiac output can be calculated from the interval of the appearance of the bolus in the right and left sides of the circulation. Figure 1–33 shows end-diastolic and end-systolic images of the LV blood pool using first-pass RNA from the paper by Jengo et al.[48]

Ejection fractions of the right and left ventricles can be measured with the first-pass method by identifying the regions of the blood pool of both chambers on the computer display and determining the time-activity curve as the bolus of radioactivity traverses the heart (Fig. 1–34). The LVEF is determined by averaging several individual beats or from a summed cardiac cycle by adding several beats. The ejection rates of both ventricles can also be determined. The peaks and valleys of the time-activity curves correspond to end-diastole and end-systole, respectively (see Fig. 1–34). As with the equilibrium method, the EF for the first-pass method is calculated by subtracting the end-systolic from the end-diastolic radioactive counts and dividing by the end-diastolic counts. The method of EF measurement is independent of ventricular geometry and is ideally suited for evaluating the ventricle with regional dysfunction. Ventricular volumes can be evaluated using a geometric or

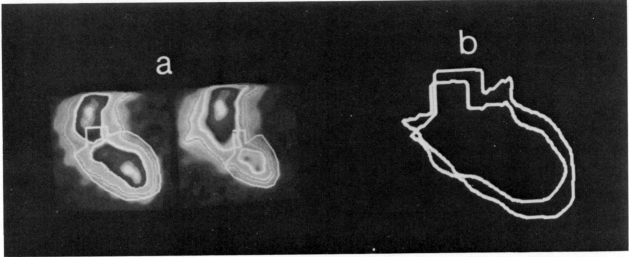

See Color Figure 1–33.

Figure 1–33. (*A*) End-diastolic and end-systolic blood pool images of the left ventricle from a first-pass radionuclide angiographic study. Isocontour lines are drawn around the border of the left ventricle and through the aortic valve plane. (*B*) Superimposed end-diastolic and end-systolic outlines are depicted. Homogeneous contraction can be seen in the anterior wall, apex and inferior wall. (See Color Figure 1–33.) (Jengo JA, et al.: Circulation 1978;57:326–332.)

count-based analysis of the LV blood pool. Regional wall motion can be assessed by viewing the display of multiple images obtained during the cardiac cycle in a cine format or by computer superimposition of end-diastolic and end-systolic images.[49c]

Comparison of Equilibrium and First-Pass Methods

There are advantages and disadvantages to first-pass and equilibrium-gated techniques for assessment of cardiac dynamics. The first-pass approach has certain advantages over the equilibrium approach for evaluating ventricular performance during rest or with exercise stress. One is that it can be repeated rapidly. A resting study can usually be finished in less than 30 seconds. Also, with the first-pass approach, body motion is not much of a problem and, therefore, upright exercise can be employed. In an equilibrium study, exercise is usually performed in the supine position because of the adverse effect of such body motion. RV function is probably best evaluated with the first-pass technique (Fig. 1–35), as is the assessment of intracardiac shunts.[49b] Wall-motion evaluation may also be superior using the first-pass approach, since imaging of the left ventricle can be carried out with virtually any view without

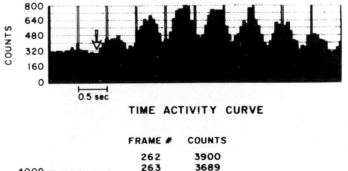

TIME ACTIVITY CURVE

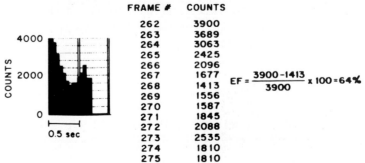

FRAME #	COUNTS
262	3900
263	3689
264	3063
265	2425
266	2096
267	1677
268	1413
269	1556
270	1587
271	1845
272	2088
273	2535
274	1810
275	1810

$$EF = \frac{3900 - 1413}{3900} \times 100 = 64\%$$

Figure 1–34. Time-activity curve and representative cycle used to calculate EF in a normal patient using the first-pass technique. Actual time-activity curve is shown in the upper panel, with summed representative cycle and EF calculation in the lower panel. The arrow in the time-activity curve indicates the region of background selection. Counts for each summed 0.05-sec frame of the representative cycle are shown along with EF calculation. In this example, end-diastolic counts were 3900; end-systolic counts were 1413, and the calculated EF was 64%. (Marshall RC, et al.: Circulation 1977;56:820–829.)

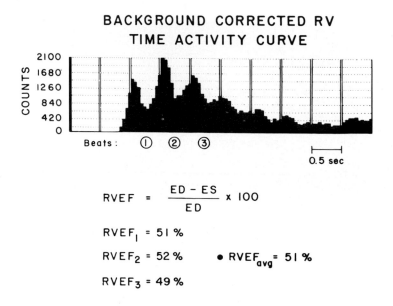

BACKGROUND CORRECTED RV TIME ACTIVITY CURVE

$$RVEF = \frac{ED - ES}{ED} \times 100$$

$RVEF_1 = 51\%$

$RVEF_2 = 52\%$ ● $RVEF_{avg} = 51\%$

$RVEF_3 = 49\%$

Figure 1–35. Calculation of the RVEF for three beats taken from the background-corrected RV time-activity curve from a first-pass radionuclide angiogram. The RVEF is measured from counts at end-diastole (ED) minus counts at end-systole (ES), divided by counts at end-diastole. (Berger HJ, et al.: Am J Cardiol 1978;41:897–905.)

interference by overlying left atrial or RV activity. In contrast, a single-crystal camera usually employed for equilibrium-gated RNA has an advantage over the multicrystal detector used in first-pass imaging in that it provides relatively better spatial resolution. Although first-pass RNA can be acquired in any oblique position relative to the imaging camera, the anterior projection is preferred for assessment of both RV and LV function. Even though the relative background correction for first-pass studies is substantially lower than that for gated-equilibrium RNA, the background activity must still be taken into account. Using the first-pass approach, a fixed region of interest corresponding to the end-diastolic image is most often utilized. Exclusion of the proximal aorta from the LV region of interest is most critical.

Disadvantages of the first-pass method include a lower photon concentration, and therefore a lower resolution in gated studies, the technical difficulty of performing serial evaluations owing to the confounding effect of residual Tc-99m activity and the need for a multicrystal camera for optimal data acquisition.[47]

Using the first-pass method, the end-diastolic boundary can be used to derive an end-diastolic volume. The geometric area-length method is used when the diastolic image is considered to resemble an ellipsoid. Using the end-diastolic volume measurement as well as the EF derived from a count-based calculation, end-systolic volume, stroke volume, and cardiac output can be derived. The major pitfalls of this approach are the inaccurate determination of the LV edges (edge detection) and delineation of the aortic valve plane. Gal et al. developed a count-based method that requires only the area of pixel, the total counts in the LV, and the maximum pixel count to calculate LV volume.[50]

The high-count photon yield of equilibrium-gated RNA is an advantage to the first-pass technique for evaluation of regional wall motion. In addition, the equilibrium approach permits assessment of all cardiac structures simultaneously.

The bolus injection technique is of great importance in attaining an optimal first-pass study. When the bolus injection is poor or when there is delayed radionuclide clearance from the right heart, as in marked pulmonary hypertension, assessment of LV function is compromised.

Visual Evaluation of Radionuclide Angiograms

A systematic approach should be employed when interpreting either first-pass or equilibrium-gated radionuclide angiograms. Structures outside the heart and great vessels should be examined for abnormalities. An area of deficient photon flux surrounding the right and left ventricles appearing as a halo is consistent with a pericardial effusion. LV hypertrophy can be identified by observing increased thickness of both the septum and lateral free wall of the left ventricle. In many instances, total cavity obliteration will be seen during systole in such patients. The right atrium should be evaluated in every study, since enlargement of this chamber seen in the anterior view might provide a clue that the patient has a left-to-right shunt (e.g., atrial septal defect or increased pulmonary vascular resistance). Tricuspid regurgitation may be identified visually by reflux of radioactive counts into the inferior vena cava as detected on the first-pass transit of the radionuclide through the chambers of the heart.

RV function should always be assessed, and it often demonstrates abnormal systolic function after inferior myocardial infarction (Fig. 1–36). As will be discussed in Chapter 11, primary or secondary abnormalities of RV function due to pressure or volume overload can easily be identified. Patients with an atrial septal defect or cor pulmonale show increased RV volume.

LV size should then be assessed, followed by a description of global and regional LV systolic function. Regional wall motion abnormalities should be visually assessed by

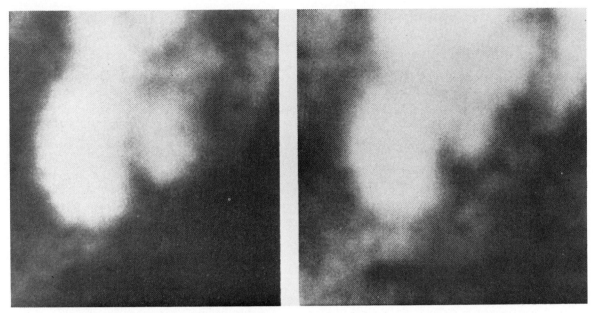

Figure 1–36. Severe global right ventricular dysfunction as assessed from end-diastolic (*left*) and end-systolic (*right*) 45-degree left anterior oblique gated blood pool images. Note that the left ventricle contracts normally. (Bateman TM, et al.: Circulation 1985;71:1153–1161.)

viewing the anterior and three oblique projections simultaneously on one screen. Images are best interpreted after spatial and temporal smoothing. The images should be adjusted on the computer display to maximize visualization of the LV borders. In the anterior projection, the enlarged right ventricle may obscure inferior wall movement, which should therefore be assessed in the 70-degree LAO or lateral projection. With respect to the septum, visualization of thickening, or lack thereof, is the best visual approach to identifying septal asynergy.

With respect to exercise radionuclide ventriculography, new stress-induced wall motion abnormalities are best assessed by viewing the exercise and rest projections simultaneously side by side (see Chap. 3). When the left ventricle is dilated because of severe valvular regurgitation, diffuse hypokinesis is seen, although more asynergy may be evident at the apex. The left lateral or left posterior oblique position provides optimal visualization of the posterobasal and inferior segments as well as viewing the anterior and apical portions of the left ventricle. Various quantitative scoring systems have been utilized in the visual assessment of regional wall motion. A system employed at Yale University involves dividing the left ventricle into 11 segments as seen on three or four views.[51] Each segment is graded on a five-point scale, with 3 as normal, 2 as mildly hypokinetic, 1 as severely hypokinetic, 0 as akinetic, and −1 as dyskinetic. A total LV wall motion score is then derived, with normal being 33.

A 10-degree caudal tilt with the detector pointed toward the patient's feet is often employed to minimize left atrial contributions within the LV region of interest. This also improves the assessment of regional wall motion in LV segments.

Detection of Left-to-Right Shunts and Estimation of Valvular Regurgitation

Left or right intracardiac shunts can be quantitated using radionuclide angiographic methods (see Chap. 11). Maltz and Treves were the first to describe and validate this noninvasive approach to quantitating shunt fraction.[52] In their method, the ratio of pulmonary-to-systemic blood flow (QP/QS) is calculated from A_1 divided by $(A_1 - A_2)$. A_1 is the integral of a γ-variate function fitted to the first-pass portion of the lung time-activity curve, and A_2 is the integral of a γ variate fitted to the early recirculation peak. The recirculation peak is identified by subtracting the γ-variate fit from the observed lung time-activity curve. This method has been modified by Madsen et al.,[53] in which the γ variate, which is fitted to the first-pass portion of the lung time-activity curve, is used to generate a curve that simulates the response of a normal lung curve with systemic recirculation. The shunted activity is then calculated as the difference between the estimated curve and the actual observed lung curve. This modification is not subject to the bias of the operator performing the analysis with respect to having to select the appropriate portion of the recirculation curve for the second fitting. In addition, this modification avoids the possibility of not distinguishing between normal systemic recirculation of the tracer and shunted activity.

Semiquantitative assessment of valvular regurgitation can be assessed by equilibrium radionuclide angiographic techniques by measuring the ratio of the LV stroke volume to the RV stroke volume.[54, 55] In the absence of valvular regurgitation, the stroke counts from the RV and LV should be nearly comparable. In patients with no valvular regurgitation in a study by Rigo et al.,[54] the LV-RV stroke counts ratio was approximately 1.15, whereas in patients with aortic or mitral regurgitation it averaged 1.36. Studies using this technique have shown significant overlap between patients who have mild regurgitation and those who have none. It can be utilized to distinguish between significant regurgitation and none at all. Overlap of atrial activity may alter the measurement of ventricular stroke counts. Right atrial activity can be excluded by using caudal tilt of the collimator or by subtracting right atrial activity.[55] This radionuclide method for quantitating left-sided valvular regurgitation is invalid if there is combined left- and right-sided valvular regurgitation or intracardiac shunting. With first-pass RNA, tricuspid regurgitation is manifested by reflux of Tc-99m activity into the inferior vena cava.[56] This noninvasive radionuclide method is not widely utilized in current practice for detection of mild to moderate regurgitation. Doppler echocardiography, particularly with color-flow technology, is more sensitive and more accurate for quantitating left-sided regurgitation than the radionuclide stroke counts ratio method.

Absolute Ventricular Volume Determination

Absolute determination of LV volume from gated RNA has been attempted utilizing geometric techniques or nongeometric counts-based methods. The geometric technique has not yielded accurate measurements, particularly when there is coexisting regional myocardial asynergy. One approach employing a nongeometric technique involved converting the count rate from the LV cavity to volume units using activity measured from a small sample of the patient's blood. This method is based on the assumption that because of the proportionality of the Tc-99m counts in the blood sample and blood volume, the LV cavity counts should be proportional to the LV volume. However, this assumption does not take into account the photon attenuation occurring through the chest wall. Thus, an absolute measurement of LV volume using the imaging of the peripheral blood sample cannot be accurately determined. Correction for tissue attenuation is required to convert this volume index into an actual volume measurement. In the absence of attenuation correction, background-corrected LV counts determined from the "best septal" LAO view are divided by the counts per millimeter of peripheral blood, yielding an index that is somewhat related to the LV blood volume.

There are other pitfalls to nongeometric radionuclide imaging approaches to determine LV volumes. Separation of the LV chamber from the atria and aorta is incomplete, even using the "best septal" LAO projection. Defining the borders (edge detection) of the LV cavity by manually drawing a region of interest around the ventricle is somewhat subjective and is associated with unavoidable intraobserver variability. No highly reproducible automatic edge detection algorithm is available that can be applied accu-

rately for this purpose. There may be an incorrect estimate of the background activity that has to be subtracted. When the background is oversubtracted because it is overestimated, the result is underestimation of the LV volume. Scatter of radioactivity from the heart and adjacent tissues may contribute to this overestimation of background. As mentioned previously, there is significant chest-wall attenuation of radiation emanating from the left ventricle, as well as self-attenuation within the LV blood pool that has to be corrected when measuring absolute cardiac volumes.

Despite these multiple factors that have the potential to introduce errors into the ventricular volume measurements, reported validation studies[46, 57–59] demonstrate surprisingly good correlation of radionuclide-derived stroke volumes with contrast ventriculographic and Fick-determined stroke volumes. A major advance in this area occurred when an appropriate attenuation-correction technique was introduced by Links et al.[46] Attenuation correction is accomplished successfully by counting a venous sample of known volume under the collimator of the gamma camera and determining the depth of the center of the left ventricle. LV volume, in milliliters, is then calculated from the following equation:

$$LV \text{ volume (ml)} = \frac{\text{Tc-99m counts in LV-background}}{\text{Blood sample counts/ml-background}} \times e^{-ud}$$

where e^{-ud} is the attenuation corrector factor; u is 0.15 cm^{-1}, which is the linear attenuation coefficient of water; and d is the depth of the center of the left ventricle. Figure 1–37 shows the relationship between angiographic volumes derived from cardiac catheterization and radionuclide volumes quantitated from the method of Links et al.[46]

Phase Analysis

Phase analysis of the radionuclide ventriculogram has been employed as an adjunctive method for assessment of regional wall motion.[60–64] Each point in the phase image is coded to indicate its time course of contraction with respect to a reference point. The phase image is a computer-derived functional image, based on the analysis of time-activity curves in each pixel location of the gated cardiac blood pool scan. Within the ventricular regions of interest, the phase angle is roughly equivalent to the time of onset of counts diminution or to the time of onset of systolic contraction, and is expressed in degrees from 0 to 360. A gray-scale or color-coded image of such a regional phase angle, the *phase image,* can be interpreted as a map of sequential systolic contraction. Contraction in a normal left ventricle is relatively homogeneous, and thus, the phase analysis of each of the segments within the left ventricle is quite uniform (Fig. 1–38). In patients with ischemic heart disease and subtle contraction abnormalities in regional myocardial

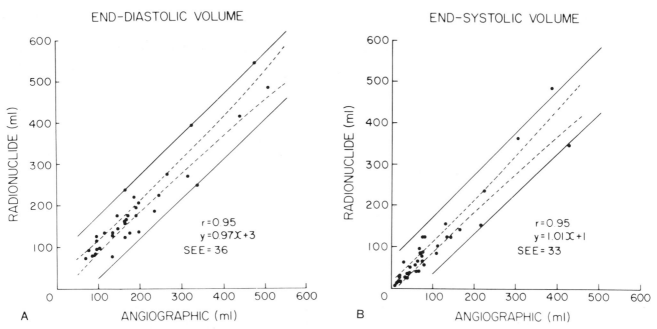

END-DIASTOLIC VOLUME

END-SYSTOLIC VOLUME

r=0.95
y=0.97X+3
SEE=36

r=0.95
y=1.01X+1
SEE=33

A   ANGIOGRAPHIC (ml)

B   ANGIOGRAPHIC (ml)

Figure 1–37. A. Relationship between angiographic volume and radionuclide end-diastolic volume. The radionuclide volume was derived from equilibrium-gated blood pool studies utilizing attenuation correction (see text). **B.** Relationship between angiographic volume and radionuclide end-systolic volume utilizing attenuation correction. (Links JM, et al.: Circulation 1982;65:82–91.)

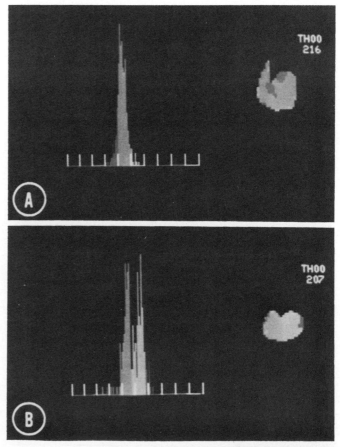

Figure 1–38. Phase analyses of biventricular gated radionuclide angiographic studies in a patient with normal conduction and normal contraction (**A**) and in a patient with left bundle branch block (**B**). **A,** In the upper right-hand corner, "THOO" signifies that the color scale is set so that each of eight colors covers a range of 10% of the cycle, or 36 degrees. The number "216" signifies color scale has been translated so that its center (between yellow and brown) was at 216 degrees. The eight colors, in order of increasing (later) phase, were light blue, dark green, light green, yellow, brown, red, purple, and white. The phase image shown below the color scale shows that the phase was relatively uniform across both ventricles. The histogram to the left of the phase image represents the "phase distribution," the number of pixels in the ventricles with each phase value. The x axis represents channels with a width of 3 degrees for phase angle, and the y axis represents the number of pixels in each channel. In this patient with normal conduction, the histogram had a single, discrete peak. **B,** With left bundle branch block, there is demonstrated a later phase over the left ventricle (yellow and brown) relative to the right ventricle (green). The phased distribution histogram has now two distinct peaks. (See Color Figure 1–38.) (Swiryn S, et al.: Am Heart J 1981;102:1000–1010.)

See Color Figure 1–38.

wall motion, there is greater dispersion of the phase angles within the ventricle. Myocardial regions with a normal but delayed onset of ventricular ejection (asynchrony) can be detected with these images in areas of dyskinesia, which are displayed as being out of phase with the other normal areas of the ventricle.

The phase analysis is usually displayed as a functional image of the left ventricle on a pixel-by-pixel method. The individual regional phase measurement is derived from the first harmonic of the Fourier expansion of the regional ventricular volume. The volume-time curve from each pixel, since it resembles a sinusoidal wave, can be estimated with a single cosine component with the frequency of the heart rate. That is, the regional volume curve is fitted to the cosine function, and the phase angle determined as a degree shift in the peak of the cosine function relative to zero degrees.

Although regional phase angle is affected by contraction abnormalities, it may also be altered by intraventricular conduction abnormalities (see Fig. 1–38). The sequence of activation and pattern of contraction can be described by these phase maps in patients with bundle branch blocks[64] and Wolff-Parkinson-White syndrome[65, 66] and in patients with pacemakers. In patients with Wolff-Parkinson-White syndrome, the site of earliest ventricular phase angle corresponds to the site of the bypass tract as determined by endocardial mapping.[66]

Regional Ejection Fraction

To acquire a more objective, operator-independent approach to assessing regional myocardial function, a more quantitative approach that permits measurement of regional EF in the left ventricle has been proposed.[67–69] This more quantitative assessment of regional LV function is accomplished by dividing the LV region of interest in the LAO view into multiple sectors (Fig. 1–39). Time-activity curves are generated from each of the sectors, yielding a regional EF for each of them. No study has been published to date that demonstrates the superiority of the regional EF method over visual assessment of wall motion for detection of localized myocardial asynergy.

Assessment of Ventricular Diastolic Function

Ventricular diastolic function can also be evaluated by radionuclide angiographic techniques.[70–78] Using the gated-equilibrium technique, the rate of ventricular filling or peak filling rate and time-to-peak filling have been obtained from the high–temporal resolution volume curve of the left ventricle (Fig. 1–40). These parameters are indices of the compliance, or stiffness of LV myocardium. LV diastolic filling at rest can be determined by analysis of the time-activity curves acquired at 20 msec per frame. Diastolic filling pa-

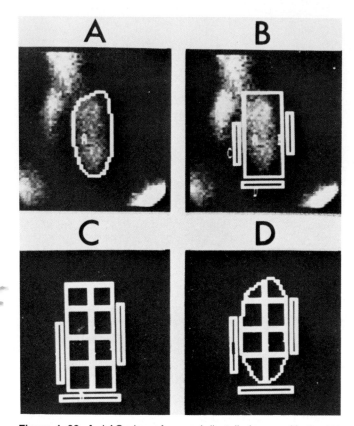

Figure 1–39. A. LAO view of an end-diastolic image with the LV perimeter shown by the white line around the chamber. **B.** LV perimeter with three background correction regions indicated by the small rectangles. **C.** Exscribed rectangle derived from the LV perimeter with eight subdivisions. **D.** Final regions of interest with LV perimeter and the eight subdivisions. (Maddox DE, et al.: Circulation 1979;59:1001–1009.)

rameters are influenced by heart rate and LV systolic function. Correction for age is necessary, since the rate and extent of rapid diastolic filling are diminished in the elderly age groups.[79] The peak filling rate is measured as the peak slope of a third-order polynomial fit to the rapid-filling phase of diastole. Peak filling rate is measured in counts per second, normalized for the number of counts at end diastole and expressed as end-diastolic volume per second (EDV/s). Time to peak filling rate (TPFR) is measured from end systole (minimal volume on the time-activity curve) to the time of peak LV filling rate. The contribution of rapid filling to total LV filling volume is measured by determining the end of the rapid-filling phase on the time-activity curve by visual inspection and computing the ventricular filling volume during rapid filling as a percentage of total LV stroke volume.

The National Institutes of Health (NIH) group[70–73] has identified the normal limits for some of these variables. The normal limit for peak filling rate is at least 2.5 EDV/s; the normal limit of TPFR is 180 msec, and the relative contribution of rapid filling to total filling volume is at least 69%. Regional systolic asynchrony in patients with CAD affects the relaxation and filling phases of diastole and contributes

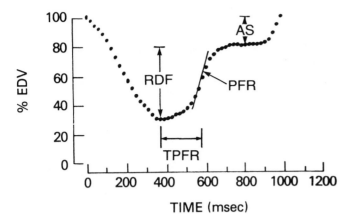

Figure 1–40. An example of a high temporal resolution time-activity curve obtained from radionuclide angiography for assessment of diastolic function. Each point represents 20 msec. Variables utilized to evaluate LV rapid filling and include peak filling rate (PFR), time to PFR (TPFR), and atrial systole (AS). The vertical axis represents percentage of end-diastolic volume (EDV). (Key: RDF, rapid diastolic filling.) (Bonow RO: Circulation 1991;84:I-208–I-215.)

to diastolic dysfunction in this patient population.[77] Clinically, this technique for evaluating diastolic function is not commonly employed, and 2-D echocardiography with Doppler is the noninvasive technique used most frequently for this purpose.

Tomographic Radionuclide Ventriculograms

Gated tomographic radionuclide ventriculography has been advanced by the work of Corbett and coworkers.[80] This approach is the 3-D analog to standard planar RNA. The advantage over the planar approach is the ability to completely interrogate the cardiac blood pool in three dimensions and to slide the resulting volume in any plane while maintaining complete separation of the cardiac chambers. The imaging systems used to obtain tomographic blood pool scintigrams are similar to those used for SPECT myocardial perfusion scintigraphy. Endocardial motion quantification in the tomograms can be accomplished utilizing computer-processing. Corbett's method involves using a three-headed rotating gamma camera equipped with a low-energy general-purpose collimator. One hundred and twenty gated projections are acquired over 360 degrees using the closest elliptical orbit. A total of 16 equally spaced time frames over the cardiac cycle are created. Each projection is acquired for a present time of 25 seconds into a 64 × 64 matrix with a pixel size of 5 mm × 5 mm. The total imaging time is estimated at 17 minutes. The projections are reconstructed into transverse image sets using filtered-back projection. Only those projections from 45 degrees RAO to 45 degrees left posterior oblique are reconstructed. Cerqueira et al.[81] used a floating axis system in which the geometric center of the left ventricle was individually determined for end-diastole and end-systole, to more

accurately measure regional EF using quantitative gated blood pool tomography.

Pulmonary Blood Volume Ratio

Okada et al.[82] proposed that assessing the ratio of pulmonary blood volume at exercise and at rest on RNA would provide important information on the changes in pulmonary capillary wedge pressure consequent to stress. The concept proposed was that patients with significant CAD would demonstrate a rise in left atrial pressure and an increase in pulmonary blood volume secondary to exercise-induced diastolic dysfunction due to ischemia. In this method, a region of interest is drawn on the LAO image just posterior to the aorta, and counts per pixel are measured. The ratio of Tc-99m activity on the exercise image to the activity on the rest image is then calculated. A ratio of 1.06 or less was observed in normal patients. In a variety of patients with cardiac disease, the directional changes in the pulmonary blood volume ratio corresponded with directional changes in the wedge pressure. This variable is somewhat helpful in separating patients with abnormal and normal LV function.

Multiwire Gamma Camera and Tantalum-178 First-Pass Radionuclide Angiography

An alternative to first-pass RNA with the multicrystal camera employs a multiwire camera used in combination with tantalum-178 (Ta-178),[83] a radionuclide with a 9.3-minute half-life. This system can acquire images of high count statistics and improved resolution, permitting quantitative assessment of global and regional ventricular function. The instrumentation has been compacted into a mobile unit. Tantalum-178 dosages are obtained from a Tungsten-178 (W-178) *N* Ta-178 generator by elution. The detector on the multiwire camera can be rotated 180 degrees horizontally and vertically. The dimensions of the detector are 25 × 25 cm^2. First-pass RNA with this instrumentation has been acquired in the anterior view using a 32 × 32-pixel, a 16-bit matrix and a time resolution of 25 msec/frame. Figure 1–41 shows an example of a radionuclide angiogram at baseline and after occlusion of the LAD in a patient from the study of Verani et al.[83] using the multiwire gamma camera and Ta-178.

POSITRON EMISSION TOMOGRAPHY

Instrumentation

Positron emission tomography (PET) affords quantitative noninvasive imaging of regional concentration of positron-emitting tracers.[5, 84–86] The capability for quantitation exists because photon attenuation can be measured and appropri-

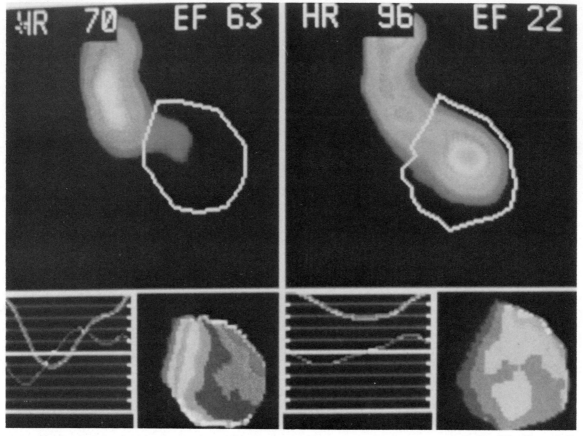

See Color Figure 1–41.

Figure 1–41. Example of a first-pass radionuclide angiogram utilizing a mobile multiwire gamma camera and tantalum-178 at baseline (*left*) and after left anterior descending coronary artery occlusion (*right*). The end-systolic frame is superimposed on the end-diastolic silhouette shown as an outer white ring. Normal wall motion with an EF of 63% is shown on the baseline study. The EF was 22%, and a severe anterior and anterolateral wall motion abnormality is shown with left anterior descending coronary occlusion. Below these images are the regional EF image showing diffuse LV deterioration. (Key: HR, heart rate.) (See Color Figure 1–41.) (Reprinted with permission from the American College of Cardiology (Journal of the American College of Cardiology, 1992, Vol. 19, pp. 297–306).)

ately corrected for and because of in-depth independent spatial resolution. A review of the radioactive tracers employed with PET imaging is found in Chapter 2. PET is undertaken with various short-lived positron-emitting isotopes such as carbon-11, nitrogen-13, oxygen-15, fluorine-18, and rubidium-82. Positrons are particles that are positively charged whose mass is equal to that of electrons. When combined with an electron, they "annihilate," which means that the combined mass of the positron and electron is converted into energy and pairs of 511-keV photons leaving the site of annihilation in diametrically opposite directions. These 511-keV photons are detected by a pair of radiation detectors positioned 180 degrees from each other and connected by coincidence circuitry. When both photons simultaneously strike two scintillation detectors connected by this circuitry, the decay is recorded. That is, if both detectors are activated simultaneously by the pairs of 511-keV photons, the annihilation event is recorded. If their radioactive decay occurs outside the sample volume between the detectors, they are excluded from the accumu-

lation of count data. An unpaired photon that strikes only one of the detectors is not counted or recorded. Since the two photons were emitted at an angle of 180 degrees, the site of the annihilation event can be located within the field between the scintillation detectors.

Generation of Images

Multiple detector pairs arranged in circular arrays allow localization of the site of annihilation events. Collimation which excludes the stray radiation is accomplished electronically. Most positron cameras contain 1000 to 1500 detectors in three to eight banks of rings, which are attached to photomultiplier tubes (PMT) in ratios ranging from one to eight detectors for each PMT. Back-projection techniques and reconstruction algorithms locate the distribution of positron-emitting radionuclides in space and form images of their concentrations in tissue. A transmission image for attenuation correction is obtained by placing a ring of activity around the patient for imaging of the heart before injection of a positron-emitting radionuclide. An emission image is then obtained, using the back-projection technique after intravenous administration of a positron radionuclide. This emission image is corrected for attenuation as well as for random coincidences and scattered radiation.

Static or dynamic transaxial tomographic images of the uptake, retention, and clearance of positron-emitting tracers in the myocardium can be obtained with the positron camera. The transaxial images can be reoriented into short-axis and long-axis sections of the LV myocardium. The static images display the relative uptake and retention of positron radionuclides in the myocardium. The spatial distribution of a radionuclide in the myocardium can be displayed in the form of polar maps, as described previously for SPECT Tl-201 images. Figure 1–42 shows normal PET images of myocardial blood flow to the heart from the review by Schwaiger.[87]

Dynamic image acquisition allows measurement of the arterial input function of a radiotracer and what happens in the myocardium after tracer delivery. Quantitative imaging implies that the true distribution of activity in the heart uninfluenced by tissue attenuation (corrected by the transmission scan) can be acquired. Most positron cameras can simultaneously acquire 15 to 22 planes with a 7-mm inter-plane distance and an axial field of view of 10 to 15 cm. Spatial resolution is usually 5 to 6 mm (FWHM). Schelbert[84] states that the physical size of individual detectors or the density of detector packing predominantly determines the spatial resolution characteristics and counting efficiency and sensitivity of the PET device. Also, the smaller the detector, the higher the spatial resolution. Image acquisition can be gated with the patient's ECG, and 16 to 32 frames for a single cardiac cycle can be collected. This allows assessment of regional wall motion.

Certain errors can influence the quality of the PET scintigrams. They include positional changes between transmission and emission images, low count statistics, partial volume effect, and activity spillover. Corrections for the partial-volume effect leading to underestimation of true tracer tissue concentrations can be made with knowledge of regional wall thickness. Thickness of the myocardial wall can be quantitated by echocardiography or derived from the positron images themselves. When radioactivity is extremely high in the LV blood pool relative to the myocardial wall, myocardial activity will be misinterpreted because of spillover activity from the LV blood pool. Under these conditions, regional myocardial tissue tracer concentration will be falsely high. Correction for this spillover can be accomplished utilizing measurements of activity with a

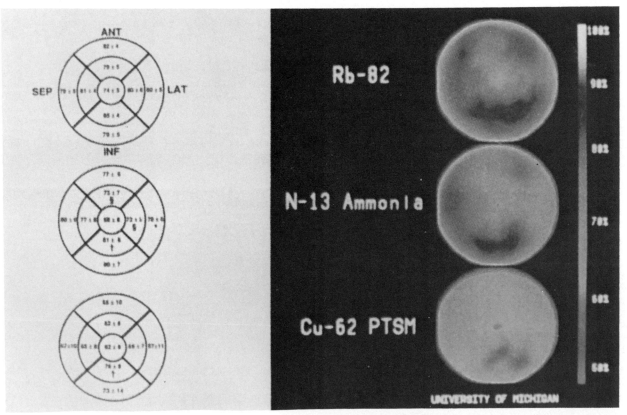

See Color Figure 1–42.

Figure 1–42. Polar maps from short-axis images of myocardial blood flow. The tracers shown include Rb-82, N-13 ammonia, and Cu-62-PTSM. (See Color Figure 1–42.) (Reprinted by permission of the Society of Nuclear Medicine from Schwaiger M.: J Nucl Med 1994;35:693–698.)

region of interest in the blood pool adjacent to the myocardium and assessing activity in a region of interest on the myocardium. A spillover fraction is derived and used to correct for the observed myocardial tissue activity. There can also be some spillover from the myocardial blood volume (particularly with hyperemia and an increased intravascular volume).

The quantitation of positron-emitting radionuclides is accomplished in a manner not too dissimilar from that described for quantitating SPECT Tl-201 images. A circumferential profile analysis is performed by generating radii from the center of the LV cavity at 6-degree intervals. Relative regional radioactivity is exhibited as a function of the angle along the circumference of the curve. Circumferential profiles obtained from patients or subjects are compared with profiles obtained from a normal data base to define regional abnormality of tracer uptake. Bull's-eye plots can also be generated to quantitatively display regional activity of PET tracers. The clinical applications of PET imaging are discussed in further detail in subsequent chapters.

REFERENCES

1. Iskandrian AS: Nuclear Cardiac Imaging: Principles and Applications. Philadelphia, FA Davis, 1987.
2. Pohost GM, O'Rourke RA (eds): Principles and Practice of Cardiovascular Imaging. Boston, Little, Brown, 1991.
3. Marcus ML, Schelbert HR, Skorton DJ, Wolf GL (eds): Cardiac Imaging: A Companion to Braunwald's "Heart Disease." Philadelphia, WB Saunders, 1991.
4. Zaret BL, Beller GA (eds): Nuclear Cardiology: State of the Art and Future Directions. St. Louis, CV Mosby, 1993.
5. Bergmann SR, Sobel BE: Positron Emission Tomography. Mount Kisco, Futura, 1992.
5a. Hendee WR, Ritenour R: Medical Imaging Physics, ed 3. St. Louis, CV Mosby, 1992, pp 36–45.
5b. Chandra R: Detection of high-energy radiation. *In* Chandra R (ed): Introductory Physics of Nuclear Medicine. Philadelphia, Lea & Febiger, 1992, pp 99–119.
5c. Zaret BL, Jain D: Continuous monitoring of left ventricular function with miniaturized nonimaging detectors. *In* Zaret BL, Beller GA (eds): Nuclear Cardiology: State of the Art and Future Directions. St. Louis, CV Mosby, 1993, pp 111–145.
6. Bacharach SL, Green MV, Borer JS, Ostrow HG, Redwood DR, Johnston GS: ECG-gated scintillation probe measurement of left ventricular function. J Nucl Med 1977;18:1176–1183.
7. Wilson RA, Sullivan PJ, Moore RH, Zielonka JS, Alpert NM, Boucher CA, McKusick KA, Strauss HW: An ambulatory ventricular function monitor: Validation and preliminary clinical results. Am J Cardiol 1983;52:601–606.
8. Broadhurst P, Cashman P, Crawley J, Raftery E, Lahiri A: Clinical validation of a miniature nuclear probe system for continuous on-line monitoring of cardiac function and ST-segment. J Nucl Med 1991;32:37–43.
9. Watson DD, Campbell NP, Read EK, Gibson RS, Teates CD, Beller GA: Spatial and temporal quantitation of plane thallium myocardial images. J Nucl Med 1981;22:577–584.
10. Smith WH, Watson DD: Technical aspects of myocardial planar imaging with technetium-99m sestamibi. Am J Cardiol 1990;66:16E–22E.
11. Gray JE, Lisk KG, Haddick DH, Harshbarger JH, Oosterhof A, Schwenker R: Test pattern for video displays and hard-copy cameras. Radiology 1985;154:519–527.
12. Gray JE, Lisk KG, Haddick DH, Harshbarger JH, Oosterhof A, Schwenker R, Members of the SMPTE Subcommittee on Recom-

mended Practices for Medical Diagnostic Display Devices. Test pattern for video displays and hard-copy cameras. Radiology 1985;154:519–527.
13. Watson DD, Leidholtz E, Beller GA, Teates CD: Defect perception in myocardial perfusion images (Abstract). J Nucl Med 1980;21:p61–p62.
14. Watson DD: Methods for detection of myocardial viability and ischemia. *In* Zaret BL, Beller GA (eds): Nuclear Cardiology: State of the Art and Future Directions. St. Louis, Mosby, 1993, pp 111–145.
15. Kaul S, Chesler DA, Boucher CA, Okada RD: Quantitative aspects of myocardial perfusion imaging. Semin Nucl Med 1987;17:131–144.
16. Berger BC, Watson DD, Taylor GJ, Craddock GB, Martin RP, Teates CD, Beller GA: Quantitative thallium-201 exercise scintigraphy for detection of coronary artery disease. J Nucl Med 1981;22:585–593.
17. Watson DD, Smith WH: Sestamibi and the issue of tissue crosstalk (Editorial; comment). J Nucl Med 1990;31:1409–1411.
18. Sinusas AJ, Beller GA, Smith WH, Vinson EL, Brookeman V, Watson DD: Quantitative planar imaging with technetium-99m methoxyisobutyl isonitrile: Comparison of uptake patterns with thallium-201. J Nucl Med 1989;30:1456–1463.
19. Koster K, Wackers FJ, Mattera JA, Fetterman RC: Quantitative analysis of planar technetium-99m-sestamibi myocardial perfusion images using modified background subtraction. J Nucl Med 1990;31:1400–1408.
20. Read ME, Watson DD, Read EK, Leidholtz E: A method for automatic overlapping of sequestered images (Abstract). J Nucl Med 1980;21:61.
21. Garcia EV: Physics and instrumentation of radionuclide imaging. *In* Marcus M, Schelbert H, Skorton D, Wolf G (eds): Cardiac Imaging: A Companion to Braunwald's "Heart Disease." Philadelphia, WB Saunders, 1991, pp 977–1005.
21a. Garcia EV: Quantitative myocardial perfusion single-photon emission computed tomographic imaging: quo vadis (where do we go from here)? J Nucl Cardiol 1994;1:83–93.
22. Garcia EV, Van Train K, Maddahi J, Prigent F, Friedman J, Areeda J, Waxman A, Berman DS: Quantification of rotational thallium-201 myocardial tomography. J Nucl Med 1985;26:17–26.
23. Garcia E, Maddahi J, Berman D, Waxman A: Space/time quantitation of thallium-201 myocardial scintigraphy. J Nucl Med 1981;22:309–317.
24. Kaul S, Chesler DA, Okada RD, Boucher CA: Computer versus visual analysis of exercise thallium-201 images: A critical appraisal in 325 patients with chest pain. Am Heart J 1987;114:1129–1137.
25. Sigal SL, Soufer R, Fetterman RC, Mattera JA, Wackers FJ: Reproducibility of quantitative planar thallium-201 scintigraphy: quantitative criteria for reversibility of myocardial perfusion defects. J Nucl Med 1991;32:759–765.
26. Wackers FJ, Fetterman RC, Mattera JA, Clements JP: Quantitative planar thallium-201 stress scintigraphy: A critical evaluation of the method. Semin Nucl Med 1985;15:46–66.
26a. Wackers FJ, Bodenheimer M, Fleiss JL, Brown M and the Multicenter Study on Silent Myocardial Ischemia (MSSMI) Thallium-201 Investigators: Factors affecting uniformity in interpretation of planar thallium-201 imaging in a multicenter trial. J Am Coll Cardiol 1993;21:1064–1074.
26b. Garvin AA, Cullum J, Garcia EV: Myocardial perfusion imaging using single-photon emission computed tomography. Am J Card Imag 1994;8:189–198.
27. Garcia EV, Cooke CD, Van Train KF, Folks R, Peifer J, DePuey EG, Maddahi J, Alazraki N, Galt J, Ezquerra N, et al.: Technical aspects of myocardial SPECT imaging with technetium-99m sestamibi. Am J Cardiol 1990;66:23E–31E.
28. Maniawski PJ, Morgan HT, Wackers FJ: Orbit-related variation in spatial resolution as a source of artifactual defects in thallium-201 SPECT. J Nucl Med 1991;32:871–875.
28a. ACC/AHA/SNM policy statement: Standardization of cardiac tomographic imaging. J Nucl Cardiol 1994;1:117–119.
28b. Faber TL: Multiheaded rotating gamma cameras in cardiac single-photon emission computed tomography. J Nucl Cardiol 1994;1:292–303.
28c. Bateman TM, Kolobrodov VV, Vasin AP, O'Keefe JH Jr: Extended acquisition for minimizing attenuation artifact in SPECT cardiac perfusion imaging. J Nucl Med 1994;35:625–627.
28d. Cooke CD, Garcia EV, Cullom J, Faber TL, Pettigrew RI: Deter-

mining the accuracy of calculating systolic wall thickening using a fast Fourier transform approximation: A simulation study based on canine and patient data. J Nucl Med 1994;35:1185–1192.

29. Garcia EV, Van Train K, Prigent F, Friedman J, Areeda J, Waxman A, Berman DS: Quantification of rotational thallium-201 myocardial tomography. J Nucl Med 1985;26:17–26.
30. Prigent F, Maddahi J, Garcia E, Van Train K, Friedman J, Berman D: Noninvasive quantification of the extent of jeopardized myocardium in patients with single-vessel coronary disease by stress thallium-201 single-photon emission computerized rotational tomography. Am Heart J 1986;111:578–586.
31. Van Train KF, Maddahi J, Berman DS, Kiat H, Areeda J, Prigent F, Friedman J: Quantitative analysis of tomographic stress thallium-201 myocardial scintigrams: A multicenter trial. J Nucl Med 1990;31:1168–1179.
32. Maddahi J, Van Train KF, Prigent F, Wong C, Gurewitz J, Friedman J, Waxman A, Berman D: Quantitation of Tl-201 myocardial single-photon emission computed rotational tomography: Developments, validation, and prospective application of an optimized computerized method (Abstract). J Nucl Med 1986;27:899.
33. Mahmarian JJ, Boyce TM, Goldberg RK, Cocanougher MK, Roberts R, Verani MS: Quantitative exercise thallium-201 single photon emission computed tomography for the enhanced diagnosis of ischemic heart disease. J Am Coll Cardiol 1990;15:318–329.
34. Kiat H, Van Train KF, Friedman JD, Germano G, Silagan G, Wang FP, Maddahi J, Prigent F, Berman DS: Quantitative stress-redistribution thallium-201 SPECT using prone imaging: Methodologic development and validation. J Nucl Med 1992;33:1509–1515.
35. Garcia EV, DePuey EG, Sonnemaker RE, Neely HR, DePasquale EE, Robbins WL, Moore WH, Heo J, Iskandrian AS, Campbell J: Quantification of the reversibility of stress-induced thallium-201 myocardial perfusion defects: A multicenter trial using bull's-eye polar maps and standard normal limits. J Nucl Med 1990;31:1761–1765.
36. Klein JL, Garcia EV, DePuey EG, Campbell J, Taylor AT, Pettigrew RI, D'Amato P, Folks R, Alazraki N: Reversibility bull's-eye: A new polar bull's-eye map to quantify reversibility of stress-induced SPECT thallium-201 myocardial perfusion defects. J Nucl Med 1990;31:1240–1246.
37. Maddahi J, Van Train K, Prigent F, Garcia EV, Friedman J, Ostrzega E, Berman D: Quantitative single photon emission computed thallium-201 tomography for detection and localization of coronary artery disease: optimization and prospective validation of a new technique. J Am Coll Cardiol 1989;14:1689–1699.
37a. Maddahi J, Rodrigues E, Berman DS: Assessment of myocardial perfusion by single-photon agents. In GM Pohost and RA O'Rourke (eds): Principles and Practice of Cardiovascular Imaging. Boston, Little, Brown, 1991, pp 179–219.
38. DePasquale EE, Nody AC, DePuey EG, Garcia EV, Pilcher G, Bredlau C, Roubin G, Gober A, Gruentzig A, D'Amato P, et al.: Quantitative rotational thallium-201 tomography for identifying and localizing coronary artery disease. Circulation 1988;77:316–327.
38a. Germano G, Van Train KF, Garcia EV, et al.: Quantitation of myocardial perfusion with SPECT: current issues and future trends. In Zaret BL, Beller GA (eds): Nuclear Cardiology: State of the Art and Future Directions. St. Louis, CV Mosby, 1993, pp 77–88.
38b. Botvinick EH, Zhu YY, O'Connell WJ, Dae MW: A quantitative assessment of patient motion and its effect on myocardial perfusion SPECT images. J Nucl Med 1993;34:303–310.
38c. Cooper JA: Detection of patient motion during tomographic myocardial perfusion imaging. J Nucl Med 1993;34:1341–1348.
38d. Germano G, Chua T, Kavanaugh P, Kiat H, Berman D: Detection and correction of patient motion in dynamic and static myocardial SPECT using a multi-media detector camera. J Nucl Med 1993;34:1349–1355.
38e. DePuey EG: How to detect and avoid myocardial perfusion SPECT artifacts. J Nucl Med 1994;35:699–702.
38f. Germano G, Kavanagh PB, Kiat H, Van Train K, Berman DS: Temporal image fractionation: Rejection of motion artifacts in myocardial SPECT. J Nucl Med 1994;35:1193–1197.
39. Rozanski A, Rodriguez E, Nichols K, Berman S: Equilibrium and first-pass radionuclide angiography. In Pohost GM, O'Rourke RA (eds): Principles and Practice of Cardiovascular Imaging. Boston, Little, Brown, 1991, pp 221–260.
40. Bonow R: Gated equilibrium blood pool imaging: Current role for

diagnosis and prognosis in coronary artery disease. In Zaret BL, Beller GA (eds): Nuclear Cardiology: State of the Art and Future Directions. St. Louis, CV Mosby, 1993, pp 123–136.
41. Burow RD, Strauss HW, Singleton R, Pond M, Rehn T, Bailey IK, Griffith LC, Nickoloff E, Pitt B: Analysis of left ventricular function from multiple gated acquisition cardiac blood pool imaging. Comparison to contrast angiography. Circulation 1977;56:1024–1028.
42. Green MV, Ostrow HG, Douglas MA, Myers RW, Scott RN, Bailey JJ, Johnston GS: High temporal resolution ECG-gated scintigraphic angiocardiography. J Nucl Med 1975;16:95–98.
43. Bacharach SL, Green MV, Borer JS, Douglas MA, Ostrow HG, Johnston GS: A real-time system for multi-image gated cardiac studies. J Nucl Med 1977;18:79–84.
44. Schelbert HR, Verba JW, Johnson AD, Brock GW, Alazraki NP, Rose FJ, Ashburn WL: Nontraumatic determination of left ventricular ejection fraction by radionuclide angiocardiography. Circulation 1975;51:902–909.
45. Okada RD, Kirshenbaum HD, Kushner FG, Strauss HW, Dinsmore RE, Newell JB, Boucher CA, Block PC, Pohost GM: Observer variance in the qualitative evaluation of left ventricular wall motion and the quantitation of left ventricular ejection fraction using rest and exercise multigated blood pool imaging. Circulation 1980;61:128–136.
46. Links JM, Becker LC, Shindledecker JG, Guzman P, Burow RD, Nickoloff EL, Alderson PO, Wagner HN: Measurement of absolute left ventricular volume from gated blood pool studies. Circulation 1982;65:82–91.
47. Adelstein SJ: Optimal resources for radioactive tracer studies of the heart and circulation. Circulation 1984;70:525A–536A.
48. Jengo JA, Mena I, Blaufuss A, Criley JM: Evaluation of left ventricular function (ejection fraction and segmental wall motion) by single pass radioisotope angiography. Circulation 1978;57:326–332.
49. Hecht HS, Mirell SG, Rolett EL, Blahd WH: Left-ventricular ejection fraction and segmental wall motion by peripheral first-pass radionuclide angiography. J Nucl Med 1978;19:17–23.
49a. Marshall RC, Berger HJ, Costin JC, et al: Assessment of cardiac performance with quantitative radionuclide angiography: Sequential left ventricular ejection fraction, normalized left ventricular ejection rate and regional wall motion. Circulation 1977;56:820–829.
49b. Berger HJ, Matthay RA, Loke J, Marshall RC, Gottschalk A, Zaret BL: Assessment of cardiac performance with quantitative radionuclide angiocardiography: Right ventricular ejection fraction with reference to findings in chronic obstructive pulmonary disease. Am J Cardiol 1978;41:897–905.
49c. DePuey EG, Salensky H, Melancon S, Nichols KJ: Simultaneous biplane first-pass radionuclide angiocardiography using a scintillation camera with two perpendicular detectors. J Nucl Cardiol 1994;35:1593–1601.
50. Gal RA, Grenier RP, Port SC, Dymond DS, Schmidt DH: Left ventricular volume calculation using a count-based ratio method applied to first-pass radionuclide angiography. J Nucl Med 1992;33:2124–2132.
51. Zaret B, Berger H: Radionuclide studies of ventricular performance in coronary artery disease. In Yu PN, Goodwin JF (eds): Progress in Cardiology, vol 12. Philadelphia, Lea & Febiger, 1983, pp 33–58.
52. Maltz DL, Treves S: Quantitative radionuclide angiocardiography: Determination of Qp: Qs in children. Circulation 1973;47:1049–1056.
53. Madsen MT, Argenyi E, Preslar J, Grover-McKay M, Kirchner PT: An improved method for the quantification of left-to-right cardiac shunts. J Nucl Med 1991;32:1808–1812.
54. Rigo P, Alderson PO, Robertson RM, Becker LC, Wagner HN Jr: Measurement of aortic and mitral regurgitation by gated cardiac blood pool scans. Circulation 1979;60:306–312.
55. Henze E, Schelbert HR, Wisenberg G, Ratib O, Schon H: Assessment of regurgitant fraction and right and left ventricular function at rest and during exercise: A new technique for determination of right ventricular stroke counts from gated equilibrium blood pool studies. Am Heart J 1982;104:953–962.
56. Handler B, Pavel DG, Lam W, Byrom E, Swiryn S, Pietras R, Rosen KM: Tricuspid insufficiency detected by equilibrium gated radionuclide study. Clin Nucl Med 1981;6:485–488.
57. Melin JA, Wijns W, Robert A, Nannan M, De Coster P, Beckers C, Detry JM: Validation of radionuclide cardiac output measurements during exercise [published erratum appears in J Nucl Med 1987 28:401–402]. J Nucl Med 1985;26:1386–1393.

58. Verani MS, Gaeta J, LeBlanc AD, Poliner LR, Phillips L, Lacy JL, Thornby JI, Roberts R: Validation of left ventricular volume measurements by radionuclide angiography [published erratum appears in J Nucl Med 1987 Mar;28(3):401–402]. J Nucl Med 1985;26:1394–1401.

59. Kronenberg MW, Parrish MD, Jenkins DW, Jr., Sandler MP, Friesinger GC: Accuracy of radionuclide ventriculography for estimation of left ventricular volume changes and end-systolic pressure-volume relations. J Am Coll Cardiol 1985;6:1064–1072.

60. Frais M, Botvinick E, Shosa D, O'Connell W, Pacheco Alvarez J, Dae M, Hattner R, Faulkner D: Phase image characterization of localized and generalized left ventricular contraction abnormalities. J Am Coll Cardiol 1984;4:987–998.

61. Frais MA, Botvinick EH, Shosa DW, O'Connell WJ, Scheinman MM, Hattner RS, Morady F: Phase image characterization of ventricular contraction in left and right bundle branch block. Am J Cardiol 1982;50:95–105.

62. Henze E, Tymiec A, Delagardelle C, Adam WE, Bitter F, Stauch M: Specification of regional wall motion abnormalities by phase analysis of radionuclide angiograms in coronary artery disease and non-coronary artery disease patients. J Nucl Med 1986;27:781–787.

63. Johnson LL, Seldin DW, Yeh HL, Spotnitz HM, Reiffel JA: Phase analysis of gated blood pool scintigraphic images to localize bypass tracts in Wolff-Parkinson-White syndrome. J Am Coll Cardiol 1986;8:67–75.

64. Swiryn S, Pavel D, Byrom E, Witham D, Meyer-Pavel C, Wyndham CR, Handler B, Rosen KM: Sequential regional phase mapping of radionuclide gated biventriculograms in patients with left bundle branch block. Am Heart J 1981;102:1000–1010.

65. Botvinick EH, Frais MA, Shosa DW, O'Connell JW, Pacheco-Alvarez JA, Scheinman M, Hattner RS, Morady F, Faulkner DB: An accurate means of detecting and characterizing abnormal patterns of ventricular activation by phase image analysis. Am J Cardiol 1982;50:289–298.

66. Johnson LL, Seldin DW, Yeh HL, Spotnitz HM, Reiffel JA: Phase analysis of gated blood pool scintigraphic images to localize bypass tracts in Wolff-Parkinson-White syndrome. J Am Coll Cardiol 1986;8:67–75.

67. Gibbons RJ, Morris KG, Lee K, Coleman RE, Cobb FR: Assessment of regional left ventricular function using gated radionuclide angiography. Am J Cardiol 1984;54:294–300.

68. Maddox DE, Wynne J, Uren R, Parker JA, Idoine J, Siegel LC, Neill JM, Cohn PF, Holman BL: Regional ejection fraction: a quantitative radionuclide index of regional left ventricular performance. Circulation 1979;59:1001–1009.

69. Papapietro SE, Yester MV, Logic JR, Tauxe WN, Mantle JA, Rogers WJ, Russell RO Jr, Rackley CE: Method for quantitative analysis of regional left ventricular function with first pass and gated blood pool scintigraphy. Am J Cardiol 1981;47:618–625.

70. Bonow RO: Radionuclide angiographic evaluation of left ventricular diastolic function. Circulation 1991;84:I208–I215.

71. Bonow RO, Bacharach SL, Green MV, Kent KM, Rosing DR, Lipson LC, Leon MB, Epstein SE: Impaired left ventricular diastolic filling in patients with coronary artery disease: Assessment with radionuclide angiography. Circulation 1981;64:315–323.

72. Bonow RO, Vitale DF, Bacharach SL, Frederick TM, Kent KM, Green MV: Asynchronous left ventricular regional function and impaired global diastolic filling in patients with coronary artery disease: Reversal after coronary angioplasty. Circulation 1985;71:297–307.

73. Bonow RO, Ostrow HG, Rosing DR, Cannon RO, Lipson LC, Maron BJ, Kent KM, Bacharach SL, Green MV: Effects of verapamil on left ventricular systolic and diastolic function in patients with hypertrophic cardiomyopathy: Pressure-volume analysis with a nonimaging scintillation probe. Circulation 1983;68:1062–1073.

74. Bonow RO, Frederick TM, Bacharach SL, Green MV, Goose PW, Maron BJ, Rosing DR: Atrial systole and left ventricular filling in hypertrophic cardiomyopathy: Effect of verapamil. Am J Cardiol 1983;51:1386–1391.

75. Iskandrian AS, Heo J, Segal BL, Askenase A: Left ventricular diastolic function: Evaluation by radionuclide angiography. Am Heart J 1988;115:924–929.

76. Friedman BJ, Drinkovic N, Miles H, Shih WJ, Mazzoleni A, DeMaria AN: Assessment of left ventricular diastolic function: comparison of Doppler echocardiography and gated blood pool scintigraphy [published erratum appears in J Am Coll Cardiol 1987;9:1199]. J Am Coll Cardiol 1986;8:1348–1354.

77. Perrone-Filardi P, Bacharach SL, Dilsizian V, Bonow RO: Effects of regional systolic asynchrony on left ventricular global diastolic function in patients with coronary artery disease. J Am Coll Cardiol 1992;19:739–744.

78. Spirito P, Maron BJ, Bonow RO: Noninvasive assessment of left ventricular diastolic function: Comparative analysis of Doppler echocardiographic and radionuclide angiographic techniques. J Am Coll Cardiol 1986;7:518–526.

79. Lakatta EG, Yin FC: Myocardial aging: Functional alterations and related cellular mechanisms. Am J Physiol 1982;242:H927–H941.

80. Corbett JR, Jansen DE, Lewis SE, Gabliani GI, Nicod P, Filipchuk NG, Redish GA, Akers MS, Wolfe CL, Rellas JS, et al.: Tomographic gated blood pool radionuclide ventriculography: analysis of wall motion and left ventricular volumes in patients with coronary artery disease. J Am Coll Cardiol 1985;6:349–358.

81. Cerqueira MD, Harp GD, Ritchie JL: Quantitative gated blood pool tomographic assessment of regional ejection fraction: Definition of normal limits. J Am Coll Cardiol 1992;20:934–941.

82. Okada RD, Osbakken MD, Boucher CA, Strauss HW, Block PC, Pohost GM: Pulmonary blood volume ratio response to exercise; a noninvasive determination of exercise-induced changes in pulmonary capillary wedge pressure. Circulation 1982;65:126–133.

83. Verani MS, Lacy JL, Guidry GW, Nishimura S, Mahmarian JJ, Athanasoulis T, Roberts R: Quantification of left ventricular performance during transient coronary occlusion at various anatomic sites in humans: A study using tantalum-178 and a multiwire gamma camera. J Am Coll Cardiol 1992;19:297–306.

84. Schelbert HR: Principles of positron emission tomography. In Marcus MM, Schelbert HR, Skorton DJ, Wolf G (eds): Cardiac Imaging: A Companion to Braunwald's "Heart Disease." Philadelphia, WB Saunders, 1991, pp 1140–1168.

85. Schelbert HR, Czernin J: PET studies of myocardial blood flow and metabolism in patients with acute myocardial infarction. In Zaret BL, Beller GA (eds): Nuclear Cardiology: State of the Art and Future Directions. St. Louis, CV Mosby, 1993, pp 294–302.

86. Schelbert HR, Mody FV: Positron emission tomography. In Pohost GM, O'Rourke RA (eds): Principles and Practice of Cardiovascular Imaging. Boston, Little, Brown, 1991, pp 293–316.

87. Schwaiger M: Myocardial perfusion imaging with PET. J Nucl Med 1994;35:693–698.

Chapter 2

Radiopharmaceuticals in Nuclear Cardiology

Basic knowledge of active and passive transport mechanisms for concentrating monovalent cations in myocardial tissue first led to the investigation of the use of radioisotopes of potassium, rubidium, ammonia, and thallium for evaluation of regional myocardial perfusion and viability employing radionuclide imaging technology. The uptake of these cations in myocardial cells is proportional to blood flow, myocyte integrity, and the size of the regional potassium pool. When administered intravenously, their uptake by the myocardium approximates the fraction of the cardiac output perfusing the heart. Before equilibrating intracellularly, these cations must first traverse the capillary wall, interstitial space, and cell membrane. Both passive and active transport mechanisms are operative for this intracellular uptake. The active transport system involves the adenosine triphosphate (ATP)–dependent sodium-potassium exchange mechanism. An abnormal reduction in regional myocardial blood flow, a functional or anatomic alteration in cell membrane Na^+, K^+-ATPase activity, a lack of adequate energy production, or an abnormality in cellular energy utilization results in diminished uptake of these radionuclide monovalent cations. The active transport system requires availability of ATP, which is supplied by either aerobic or anaerobic intermediary pathways of the myocardial cell.

The first potassium analogs available for human use, potassium-42 (K-42) and rubidium-86 (Rb-86), were not ideal for imaging with gamma scintillation detectors because the excessively high-energy gamma radiation was difficult to detect and the presence of beta radiation caused an excessive radiation dose for the patient. K-43 was one of the first radionuclides to be utilized successfully for imaging in humans but was limited by its rather high-energy photons (373 keV peak), which made imaging with

the gamma scintillation camera quite difficult. There is also a significant photon peak at 619 keV that caused substantial degradation of the image due to scatter. The significant beta emission results in a high absorbed radiation dose for the patient. Despite these limitations, K-43 scintigraphy was able to accurately localize zones of myocardial infarction and stress-induced ischemia.[1] The successful application of K-43 imaging encouraged further exploration to identify a more appropriate radioactive monovalent cation for imaging and heralded a new era in cardiac diagnostic medicine.

The next radionuclide monovalent cation to be tested was Rb-81, a potassium analog with myocardial uptake and clearance characteristics similar to those of K-43. Myocardial perfusion imaging with Rb-81 was accomplished with a scintillation camera equipped with a special collimator that prevented penetration of the high-energy emission of both Rb-81 and Rb-82m, the latter being a contaminant in commercially available Rb-81. High sensitivity and specificity values were reported for detection of coronary artery disease (CAD) with Rb-81 using exercise stress.[2, 3] Although the clinical studies cited above yielded satisfactory results, several limitations of Rb-81 scintigraphy soon became apparent. Image interpretation using a pinhole collimator is difficult if the heart is not well centered within the camera's field of view. Camera sensitivity is not uniform across a flood field; peak activity occurs in the center. Thus, patient positioning becomes critical, since small shifts within the field have the potential to create differences in image intensity, making analysis of regional tracer uptake patterns quite difficult.

At about the time that further investigation was being planned to improve image quality with Rb-81, radioactive thallium was shown to have biologic properties similar to those of other potassium analogs but with superior physical properties for imaging with a scintillation camera.[4] Today, thallium-201 (Tl-201) is still the most clinically used radiopharmaceutical for myocardial perfusion imaging with a conventional gamma scintillation camera.

Throughout the decade of the 1980s, intense basic research was conducted to develop technetium-99m (Tc-99m)–labeled myocardial perfusion agents that would have physical characteristics superior to those of Tl-201 for imaging with a gamma scintillation camera. From this laboratory research effort, several new compounds emerged that proved clinically useful. These were the Tc-99m–labeled isonitrile compounds, of which Tc-99m methoxyisobutyl isonitrile (sestamibi) is the most applicable for clinical use, and Tc-99m teboroxime, which belongs to a class of neutral lipophilic, technetium-containing complexes known as boronic acid adducts of technetium dioxime (BATO) complexes. Another Tc-99m–labeled agent, Tc-99m tetrofosmin, was developed for myocardial imaging in the early 1990s. This agent is a lipophilic, cationic diphosphine agent that in early clinical trials has shown promise for detection of CAD.

Short-lived positron emitters have been developed for myocardial perfusion imaging and myocardial metabolic imaging utilizing positron-emission tomography (PET) scintigraphy. Perhaps the most widely used agents are nitrogen-13 (N-13)–labeled ammonia (N-13 ammonia) and Rb-82. The latter is an ultrashort-lived positron-emitting radiopharmaceutical that most often is injected intravenously with dipyridamole or adenosine. Table 2–1 lists all the radionuclides that have been utilized for assessment of regional myocardial perfusion.

Other radiopharmaceuticals used for imaging myocardial necrosis, cardiac sympathetic nerves, intravascular thrombosis, and cellular hypoxia have been introduced for potential clinical applicability in patients with cardiovascular disease.

THALLIUM-201 KINETICS

Physical Properties

Thallium is a metallic element in group III-A of the Periodic Table. Tl-201 decays by electron capture (half-life 73 hours). Its principal photo peaks are at 135 and 167 keV, and it emits mercury x-rays of 69 to 83 keV with 98% abundance. The 80-keV mercury x-ray is at the lower end of the energy spectrum for resolution with a gamma scintillation camera. The 69- to 80-keV x-rays emitted by Tl-201 allow imaging with high-resolution, low-energy collimators, which were not practical for imaging of radioactive potassium or rubidium in the myocardium.

A 1.0 mCi dose of Tl-201 administered intravenously delivers to the whole body a radiation dose of 0.21 rad/mCi. The dose to the testes is 0.59 rad/mCi, and the dose

Table 2–1. Radionuclides Utilized for Noninvasive Assessment of Regional Myocardial Perfusion

Single-photon agents
  Potassium-43
  Rubidium-81
  Thallium-201
  Technetium-99m sestamibi
  Technetium-99m tetrofosmin
  Technetium-99m teboroxime
  Technetium-99m Q12
  Technetium-99m albumin
    microspheres
Positron-emitting agents
  Nitrogen-13 ammonia
  Rubidium-82
  Potassium-38
  Oxygen-15 water
  Copper-62 PTSM

to the kidneys and the dose to the thyroid gland are 1.17 and 1.03 rad/mCi, respectively.

Thallium is biologically similar to potassium. Lebowitz provides the physicochemical explanation for the biologic similarity of thallium and potassium, observing that the hydrated ionic radius of thallium[+] is between those of potassium and rubidium,[4] and this radius has been suggested as the property that determines passive penetration through a membrane.[5]

Several other properties of Tl-201 made it a very attractive radionuclide for imaging the myocardium. In comparison with K-43 and Rb-81, the percentage of the total dose of Tl-201 that concentrates in the myocardium is greater (2.08% at 10 minutes, compared with 1.25% for K-43 and 1.15% for Rb-81).[6] Hepatic and gastric uptake of Tl-201 are also relatively less avid than that of the other two tracers.[6]

Initial Myocardial Uptake

Thallium-201 Extraction

The initial myocardial uptake of Tl-201, after intravenous administration, depends on both myocardial blood and the myocardial extraction fraction for thallium.[6, 7, 7a] Strauss et al.[6] showed in dogs with an occluded left anterior descending coronary artery (LAD) that the uptake of Tl-201 was comparable to the uptake of K-43 (Fig. 2–1). Weich et al.[7] assessed the extraction of Tl-201 in a canine model and found that, under basal conditions, the extraction fraction measured 88% ±2.1%. The extraction fraction measurement evaluates only the ability to extract the tracer from the blood in the first pass through the coronary circulation. Weich et al.[7] showed that, following pacing to a rate of 195 bpm, the extraction fraction remained unchanged at 88.5%. Similarly, the extraction fraction for thallium was not significantly altered by changes in pH or by propranolol, insulin, or digitalis. Hypoxia caused a slight but significant

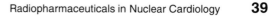

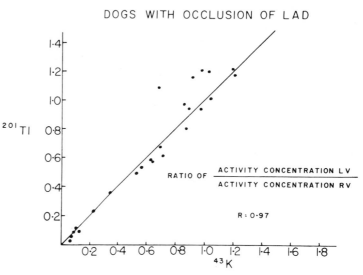

DOGS WITH OCCLUSION OF LAD

RATIO OF $\dfrac{\text{ACTIVITY CONCENTRATION LV}}{\text{ACTIVITY CONCENTRATION RV}}$

R : 0·97

Figure 2–1. Regional myocardial distribution of Tl-201 and K-43 in dogs whose left anterior descending coronary artery (LAD) is ligated. Data points depict the ratio of activity in the section of the left ventricle (LV) to that of the right ventricle (RV). (Strauss HW, et al.: Circulation 1975;51:641–645.)

decrease in extraction fraction, to 77.9%. As would be expected for any diffusible indicator, the extraction fraction fell with increasing coronary blood flow to hyperemic values. Leppo et al.[8] also examined the effect of cellular hypoxia on extraction of Tl-201 by the myocardium. They found that first-pass extraction and the permeability surface area product (PS) for Tl-201 were not affected by hypoxia that caused severe cardiac hemodynamic dysfunction. In another study by Leppo and coworkers,[9] myocardial uptake of Tl-201 during a constant infusion into an isolated rabbit heart was unaffected by hypoxia when coronary flow was held constant. Friedman et al. reported a small (14%) decrease in Tl-201 uptake during hypoxia in cultured chick ventricular cells.[10]

McCall et al.[11] investigated the kinetics of thallium exchange in cultured rat myocardial cells. Uptake of Tl-204 was best described by a single exponential with a half-time ($T_{1/2}$) of exchange that was approximately half that of potassium and that was largely independent of the extracellular thallium concentration. Some 60% of thallium uptake occurred via an "active" or ouabain-inhibitable mechanism. Figure 2–2 shows the effect of increasing doses of ouabain on thallium uptake in this experimental preparation. Increasing extracellular potassium caused significant, concentration-dependent decreases in both the total and the active component of thallium influx. Overall, the studies by McCall et al. showed that active membrane transport accounted for the greater portion of the influx of thallium and that the transport occurred via a mechanism common with potassium. Melin and Becker[12] examined the quantitative relationship between fractional myocardial Tl-201 uptake and ouabain-induced inhibition of Na+, K+-ATPase. Six dogs received an intravenous injection of ouabain, 0.030 mg/kg, followed 30 minutes later by a second injection of 0.010 mg/kg. This dose was sufficient to provoke arrhythmias in all dogs, to decrease heart rate by 3%, and to increase arterial blood pressure by 16%. This dose of oua-

bain did not affect early Tl-201 uptake in their canine model. Krivokapich and Shine[13] also reported that the influx of Tl-201 was not inhibited by a digitalis analog, acetylstrophanthin, in the isolated perfused rabbit septum. Thus, physiologic doses of digitalis do not appear to affect Tl-201 uptake substantially.

Okada et al.[14] used implantable, miniature cadmium telluride radiation detectors positioned against the endocardium for defining myocardial uptake and clearance kinetics

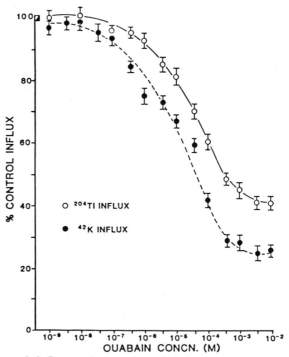

Figure 2–2. Dose-response curve of ouabain on K-42 and Tl-204 influx in myocardial cells at 37° C. Cultured rat myocardial cells were utilized in these experiments. Some 60% of thallium uptake occurred via the active transport mechanism. (McCall D, et al.: Circ Res 1985;56:370–376.)

for Tl-201 in canine myocardium. Using this technique for constantly monitoring Tl-201 activity in vivo, they found that such activity reached 80% of peak uptake within 1 minute after intravenous injection and peaked in a mean time of 24 ± 18 minutes, after which Tl-201 activity decreased monoexponentially. This rapid myocardial uptake is associated with rapid clearance of the tracer from the blood pool. Figure 2–3 shows the plot of Tl-201 activity versus time after injection for both myocardium and blood on a semilogarithmic scale. The decay constants for myocardium and blood were comparable.

Extraction Versus Perfusion Pressure

When the coronary perfusion pressure is transiently lowered, as with a focal coronary occlusion with an experimental constrictor, the extraction fraction for Tl-201 is not significantly altered as long as infarction has not occurred. Grunwald et al.[15] found that the average extraction fraction at normal blood flows was 82% ± 6% in anesthetized dogs. The extraction fraction remained unchanged at 85% ± 7%

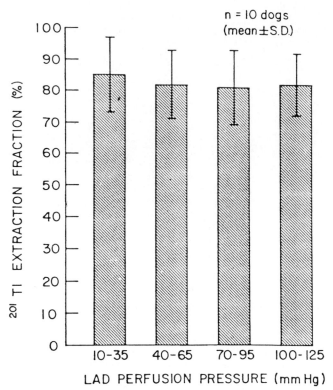

Figure 2–4. First-pass Tl-201 as a function of LAD coronary artery perfusion pressure in 10 dogs. Extraction fractions were determined 10 minutes after each stabilization period with progressive LAD narrowing. (Grunwald AM, et al.: Circulation 1981;64:610–618.)

at coronary perfusion pressures of 10 to 35 mm Hg. Figure 2–4 shows the first-pass Tl-201 extraction fractions as a function of LAD perfusion pressure in this canine model. First-pass extraction of Tl-201 is normal in stunned myocardium characterized by postischemic dysfunction following repetitive, brief periods of flow reduction[16] (see Chap. 9). With a chronic low-flow state (short-term hibernation), myocardial Tl-201 uptake is not impaired out of proportion to the flow diminution, despite severe systolic dysfunction.[17] The overall conclusion of these experimental findings is that intracellular extraction of Tl-201 via transport across the sarcolemmal membrane is not appreciably affected by transient alterations in hemodynamics or metabolic alterations such as hypoxia, so long as irreversible membrane injury is avoided. Tl-201 extraction is high, permitting an adequate heart-background ratio for external imaging of tracer distribution.

Thallium-201 Uptake and Regional Blood Flow

Several studies have investigated the relationship of initial myocardial Tl-201 concentration to regional blood flow as determined by the radioactive microsphere technique. Over a wide range of physiologic blood flows, the uptake of thallium in the canine heart is proportional to flow.[6, 15–19] Similarly, relative Tl-201 uptake in the LAD perfusion zone is comparable with Tl-201 uptake in circumflex artery–

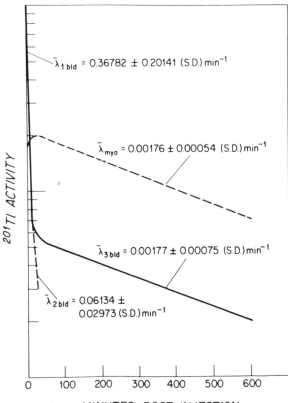

Figure 2–3. Tl-201 activity versus time after intravenous (i.v.) administration of the tracer. Values represent mean ± SD for nonlinear least-squares estimation of Tl-201 decay constants for myocardium (λmyo) and blood (λbld). Tl-201 activity is depicted on a semilogarithmic scale. Continuous on-line monitoring of myocardial thallium activity was undertaken with an implantable miniature cadmium telluride radiation detection device inserted through the left ventricular apex and positioned against the endocardium. (Okada RD, et al.: Circulation 1982;65:70–77.)

perfused myocardium in patients and proportional to absolute flow values as determined by the intracoronary xenon washout method.[20] Figure 2–5 shows a linear correlation between regional myocardial blood flow measured in the LAD and left circumflex (LCx) distributions during rapid atrial pacing in patients with significant lesions in the left coronary system. Figure 2–5 also shows a linear correlation between Tl-201 activity recorded in the LAD and the LCx distributions from exercise images in the same patients. Nielsen et al.[19] compared the myocardial distribution of Tl-201 and regional myocardial blood flow during ischemia and the physiologic stress of exercise in conscious dogs. The maximum increase in blood flow at peak exercise in these animals ranged from 3.3 to 7.2 times resting control values. In each dog, there was a close linear relationship between Tl-201 distribution and direct measurements of regional myocardial blood flow. Linear regression analyses demonstrated a correlation coefficient of 0.98 or greater in each dog (Fig. 2–6). Pohost et al.[21] investigated the relationship between Tl-201 uptake and relative regional myocardial blood flow determined by radioactive microspheres in dogs undergoing coronary occlusion for 2 hours. In areas of low flow, myocardial Tl-201 uptake exceeded flow in this region. This observation suggests that there is increased intracellular extraction of Tl-201 in areas of marked flow diminution and suggests that the absolute flow decrement would be underestimated by the magnitude of the decrease in Tl-201 activity relative to nonischemic zone activity.

Thallium-201 Uptake and Irreversible Myocardial Injury

Damaged myocardial tissue cannot concentrate Tl-201 intracellularly (see Chap. 9). In a model where myocardial accumulation of Tl-201 in response to ischemia-like myocardial injury was assessed in a cultured mouse heart prep-

aration, Tl-201 accumulation within injured hearts, as compared with that for controls, was related in a monotonically decreasing fashion to the loss of lactic dehydrogenase.[22] Ingwall et al.[23] evaluated the effect of ischemia-like insults on net Tl-201 uptake. Anoxia, deprivation of oxidizable substrate, and introduction of lactic acid were employed to create a model of ischemia. In these experiments, net Tl-201 uptake was determined as a function of time over a 5-hour period for control hearts exposed to 95% oxygen and normal substrate and injured hearts. By 2 hours' exposure to Tl-201, hearts deprived of oxidizable substrate accumulated significant levels of Tl-201, but the extent of accumulation was reduced compared with that of controls. The percentage of reduction in Tl-201 uptake was equal to the percentage of cells that ultimately became necrotic as measured by lactic dehydrogenase depletion. The investigators concluded that extraction of Tl-201 from the medium was depressed only when irreversible cell damage was present. In their model, an ischemic insult that did not produce cell necrosis did not appear to depress Tl-201 uptake.

Redistribution Kinetics

Tl-201 does not remain fixed in myocardial cells after the initial extraction phase. Rather, data from many studies support the concept that it is continually exchanged with new Tl-201 from systemic recirculation. This process of continuous exchange explains why perfusion defects, noted early after Tl-201 administration and resulting from transient hypoperfusion or a chronic reduction in regional blood flow, are demonstrated to resolve on delayed images obtained 2½ to 4 hours later.[14, 15, 21, 24–37]

In experimental studies, when Tl-201 was injected during a period of temporary coronary occlusion, initial intracellular Tl-201 concentration was markedly decreased. Subse-

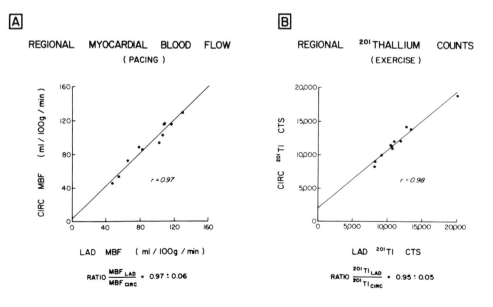

Figure 2–5. A. Linear correlation between regional myocardial blood flow (MBF) measured in the LAD and left circumflex (CIRC) distributions during rapid atrial pacing in patients without significant coronary stenoses. **B.** Linear correlation between Tl-201 activity (counts) recorded in CIRC and LAD distributions from exercise scintigrams in the same patients as in **A.** (Nichols AB, et al.: Circulation 1983;68:310–320.)

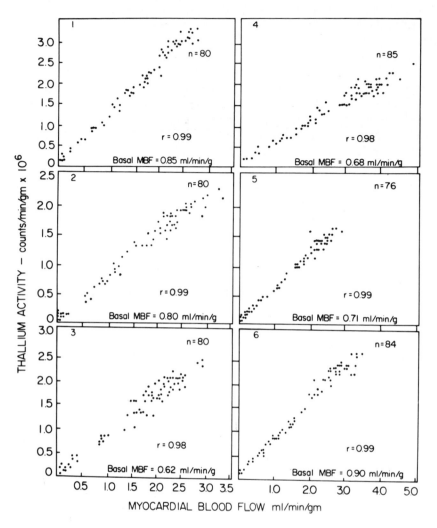

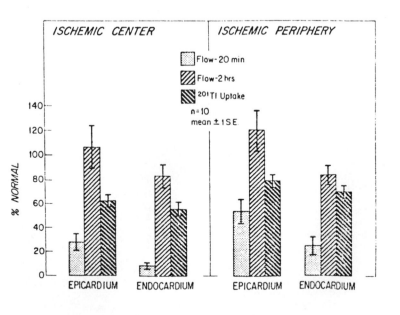

Figure 2–6. Relationship between Tl-201 activity and myocardial blood flow (ml/min/g) in six dogs during exercise-induced ischemia (n, number of samples analyzed). Each dog was exercised on a treadmill at speeds of 5 to 9 mph at a 5-degree incline. After 1 minute of exercise, the circumflex coronary artery was occluded and Tl-201 and microspheres were injected. (Nielsen AP, et al.: Circulation 1980;61:797–801.)

Figure 2–7. Regional myocardial blood flow (% normal) and Tl-201 uptake (% normal) in epicardial and endocardial samples from central and peripheral ischemic zones in 10 dogs undergoing 20 minutes of coronary occlusion and 100 minutes of reperfusion. Tl-201 was administered after 10 minutes' occlusion. Tl-201 uptake in ischemic zones is significantly higher than the flow *(stippled bars)* at the time of Tl-201 administration, reflecting redistribution of the tracer during the 100-minute reperfusion. However, Tl-201 activity at 2 hours' redistribution is still less than reperfusion flow *(cross-hatched bars* in middle of each group of bars). (Pohost GM, et al.: Circulation 1977;55:294–302.)

quently, however, with restoration of perfusion, myocardial cellular Tl-201 concentration increased over time.[21] Figure 2–7 shows regional blood flow and Tl-201 activity values expressed as a percentage of nonischemic values in epicardial and endocardial samples from the ischemic zone in dogs undergoing 20 minutes' LAD occlusion and 100 minutes' reperfusion. Tl-201 was administered after 10 minutes of occlusion. Tl-201 uptake at 100 minutes of reflow is significantly higher than occlusion flow at the time of Tl-201 administration, reflecting delayed redistribution. The time course of this delayed normalization of myocardial Tl-201 concentration after transient occlusion of the LAD was ascertained.[24] In this set of experiments, Tl-201 activity was reduced by 80% compared with normal myocardial activity during LAD occlusion when the tracer was injected. With flow restoration by removal of the ligature after only 20 minutes of occlusion, near normalization of activity between nonischemic and ischemic zones (redistribution) occurred by 4 hours (Fig. 2–8). Significant filling in of the defect was observed, however, as early as 20 minutes after flow restoration. This was one of the first studies to show that Tl-201 redistribution after transient myocardial ischemia is related to both delayed accumulation of Tl-201 into ischemic myocardial segments and to more rapid washout of the tracer from normal segments. The mechanism for these disparate clearance rates will be discussed later.

In a canine model characterized by permanent fixed stenosis with chronic reduction of coronary blood flow, Tl-201 defects observed soon after tracer administration also showed delayed resolution.[31] Figure 2–9 shows the relationship between Tl-201 activity 4 hours after Tl-201 administration and regional microsphere flow at the time of Tl-201 administration in dogs with chronic reduction in blood flow. The plots show Tl-201 "excess" relative to flow, indicating the degree of rest redistribution. The investigators found that the resolution of defects at rest was significantly related to both release of Tl-201 from the nonischemic zone and accumulation of Tl-201 in the hypoperfused zone distal to the persistent severe coronary artery stenosis. These conclusions are drawn from these studies: (1) The distribution of Tl-201 in delayed images is not equivalent to the distribution obtained initially after a resting injection. (2) Tl-201 "redistribution" can occur even when there is no change in coronary blood flow between the initial and delayed images. Continuous extraction of Tl-201 from systemic recirculation accounts for disappearance of initial Tl-201 defects. The clinical application of Tl-201 redistribution kinetics for differentiating ischemic from scarred myocardium for determination of myocardial viability is discussed in Chapter 9.

Thallium-201 Washout Rate

The rate at which Tl-201 is exchanged between myocardium and the systemic pool is determined by the *intrinsic* myocardial washout rate. This reflects only the rate of Tl-201 efflux from the myocardium and must be determined in a manner that excludes continuous reintroduction of Tl-201 to the myocardium from the systemic pool. In contrast, the *net* myocardial Tl-201 washout rate reflects only the net

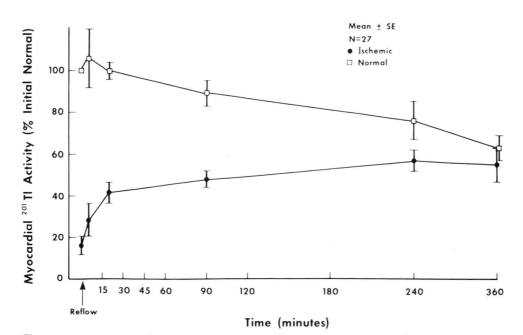

Figure 2–8. Serial determination of myocardial Tl-201 activity, expressed as a percentage of initial (before reflow) normal Tl-201 activity in five groups of dogs occluded for 20 minutes and reperfused for 5, 20, 90, 240, and 360 minutes. The initial value of Tl-201 activity in the ischemic region (●) was obtained before reperfusion and represents the mean ±SE for all 27 dogs. Near-equalization of Tl-201 concentration in normal and previously ischemic myocardial regions appears by 4 hours. (Beller GA, et al.: Circulation 1980;61:791–797.)

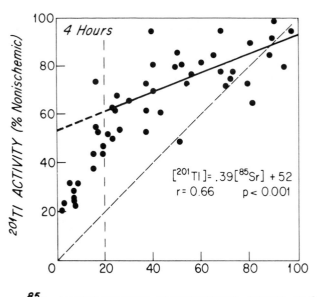

Figure 2–9. Relationship between Tl-201 activity (% nonischemic) and initial Sr-85 microsphere–determined blood flow (% nonischemic) in the zone of chronic low flow from dogs killed 4 hours after administration of Tl-201. The light dashed line represents line of identity. The regression line *(solid line)* is depicted for ischemic flows of 20% to 100% of nonischemic flow and has been extrapolated to zero flow *(dashed portion)*. The increase above the line of identity reflects degree of "rest redistribution." (Pohost GM, et al.: Circ Res 1981;48:439–446.)

difference between rates of input and output. The two washout rates must be considered independently. The intrinsic washout rate depends solely on factors intrinsic to the myocardium. The net clearance rate, however, depends on how rapidly the tracer is being recirculated back to the heart from all body organs and, therefore, depends on factors extrinsic to the myocardium, including the blood pool concentration. The $T_{1/2}$ for net Tl-201 clearance from the myocardium is 7 to 8 hours after a resting injection.

The intrinsic washout rate has been determined experimentally by serial measurement of myocardial Tl-201 activity after direct intracoronary injection of the tracer in closed-chest anesthetized dogs.[15] Under these conditions, a negligible amount of Tl-201 is being recirculated back to the heart from systemic compartments. With intracoronary administration, approximately 85% of the injected dose is initially distributed to the heart, as compared with 2% to 4% in the instance of an intravenous injection. Figure 2–10 shows the intrinsic myocardial Tl-201 washout curve in a representative experimental animal. Note that, in this example, the intrinsic washout rate after intracoronary injection of Tl-201 is significantly more rapid than the net clearance of Tl-201 from the myocardium measured after intravenous injection. The $T_{1/2}$ for intrinsic Tl-201 washout in normal dogs with normal coronary perfusion pressures averaged 54 ±7 minutes.[15] The intrinsic washout curve is monoexponential over the time range of 5 minutes to 2

hours after injection. This finding implies that the intrinsic Tl-201 washout rate is proportional to the myocardial Tl-201 concentration. That is,

$$dC(t)/dt = kC(t)$$

This relationship is directly implied from experimental data indicating that $C(t)$ equals $C_o e^{-kt}$, where $C(t)$ is the myocardial Tl-201 concentration at time t and k is the intrinsic clearance coefficient ($0.693/T_{1/2}$). Two distinct components of the intrinsic Tl-201 washout curve are observed after intracoronary tracer injection. The first, a rapid component with a $T_{1/2}$ of about 2.5 minutes, is observed immediately after intracoronary injection and represents the myocardial clearance of unextracted Tl-201 from the interstitial space (Fig. 2–11A). Between approximately 5 minutes and 2 hours after intracoronary Tl-201 administration, the intrinsic washout curve is monoexponential (Fig. 2–11B).

As the coronary perfusion pressure is reduced in a graded manner below normal, the $T_{1/2}$ for intrinsic washout becomes markedly prolonged, approaching 300 minutes when the vessel is obstructed to a degree that approaches its critical closing pressure (Fig. 2–12). The reason for the

MYOCARDIAL THALLIUM ACTIVITY vs TIME

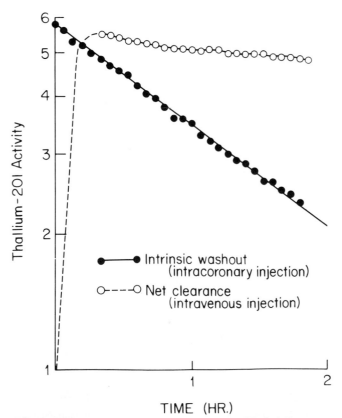

Figure 2–10. Intrinsic Tl-201 washout rate *(solid circles)* and net thallium clearance rate *(open circles)* in a representative dog. The intrinsic washout rate is determined after intracoronary injection of the radionuclide and is significantly more rapid than the net clearance of thallium from the myocardium measured after intravenous injection. (Grunwald AM, et al.: Circulation 1981;64:610–618.)

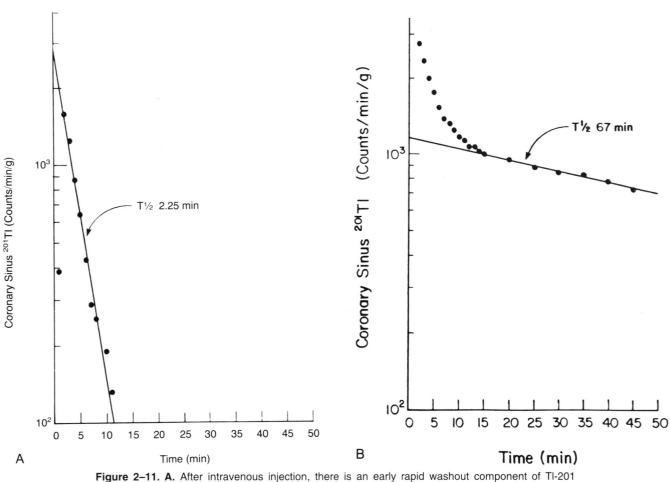

Figure 2–11. A. After intravenous injection, there is an early rapid washout component of Tl-201 clearance. This rapid component is apparent between 0 and 10 minutes after tracer injection. Coronary sinus Tl-201 counts versus time for this early component is shown and is attributed to the rapid washout of the tracer from the interstitial compartment. **B.** Coronary sinus Tl-201 counts versus time after intracoronary injection in the same dog. The $T_{1/2}$ for the intrinsic Tl-201 washout was 67 minutes. This washout rate was calculated from the slower washout component depicted by the solid line. (Grunwald AM, et al.: Circulation 1981;64:610–618.)

slowing of Tl-201 efflux with reduction in coronary perfusion pressure is not entirely clear, but it may reflect either reduced flow, altered membrane metabolic activity, alterations in Tl-201 diffusion kinetics between the plasma compartment and the myocardial cells in low-flow regions, or undetermined causes.

Okada et al.[36] also examined the intrinsic Tl-201 washout rate after intracoronary administration of the tracer in anesthetized dogs. Using the miniature cadmium telluride detection device, they showed that myocardial Tl-201 activity after intracoronary injection peaked in a mean time of 2.0 ± 0.8 minutes, then decreased monoexponentially with a $T_{1/2}$ of 84 ± 12 minutes. They also showed that Tl-201 clearance from the myocardium after intracoronary administration was significantly greater than after intravenous injection. In a subsequent study, these investigators showed reduced clearance of Tl-201 in a zone perfused by a coronary vessel involved by stenosis in dogs that received norepinephrine infusion to simulate exercise stress.[37]

A reduction in the intracellular efflux rate of Tl-201 with chronic ischemia provides a plausible explanation for Tl-201 redistribution (delayed defect resolution) in the situation of a chronic reduction in regional blood flow (rest redistribution). An initial defect in Tl-201 uptake is observed because of relative hypoperfusion of myocardium distal to the subtotal occlusion. With serial monitoring of Tl-201 activity in this region, however, delayed relative accumulation of Tl-201 in the hypoperfused zone is observed in conjunction with a net decrease in Tl-201 activity in normally perfused myocardium, as discussed previously. The disparate net clearance rates—higher in normally perfused myocardium and lower in the region of hypoperfusion—subsequently result in equalization of Tl-201 activity in normal and hypoperfused zones, despite no significant change in regional blood flow. Thus, rest redistribution occurs because in the region of myocardial hypoperfusion the intrinsic washout rate is slower than normal.

As mentioned previously, the net rate of clearance of Tl-201 from the myocardium determined after intravenous in-

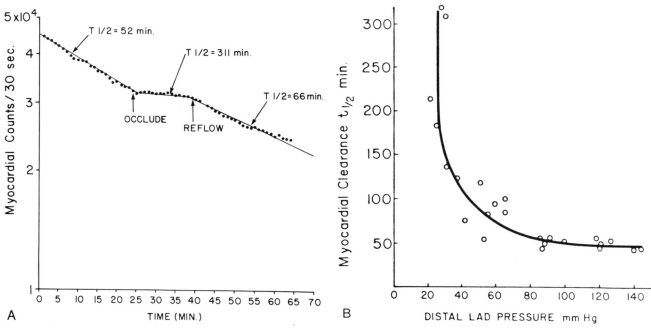

Figure 2–12. A. Intrinsic myocardial Tl-201 washout ($T_{1/2}$) during controlled conditions, after coronary occlusion (Occlude), and after reflow (Reflow). Myocardial Tl-201 counts per 30 seconds are plotted over time. The $T_{1/2}$ of intrinsic Tl-201 washout markedly increased after occlusion of the left anterior descending coronary artery and returned toward normal after flow restoration. **B.** Intrinsic Tl-201 washout ($T_{1/2}$) plotted as a function of the mean perfusion pressure in the distal left anterior descending coronary artery (LAD). The $T_{1/2}$ increases markedly, approaching 300 minutes at the lowest perfusion pressures. (Grunwald AM, et al.: Circulation 1981;64:610–618.)

jection of Tl-201 is slower than the intrinsic washout rate. The explanation for the slower net rate is that, as Tl-201 leaves the myocardium after intravenous injection, it is continuously replaced by new Tl-201 recirculating from the systemic blood pool at almost the same rate. Thus, there is only a slow reduction in myocardial Tl-201 concentration over time after injection.

Compartmental Model for Thallium-201 Redistribution

Understanding Tl-201 uptake and washout kinetics permits optimal use of this radionuclide for detecting CAD and distinguishing ischemia from scar.[35] *Redistribution* is defined as the total or partial resolution of initial defects over time after Tl-201 administration. The process of continuous exchange of Tl-201 between the myocardium and the extracellular compartment defines the process of Tl-201 redistribution observed after transient regional myocardial hypoperfusion or with a chronic reduction in blood flow. If Tl-201 is injected during a hyperemic phase following resolution of spontaneous ischemia, a perfusion defect may not be demonstrated.[38] For example, if Tl-201 is injected during a period of coronary vasospasm but relief of spasm occurs immediately after Tl-201 administration, an actual "hot spot" of Tl-201 activity may be observed. Rapid Tl-

201 clearance from this hyperemic zone would ensue. For a given degree of reversible myocardial ischemia at the time of Tl-201 injection, the perfusion defect observed on the initial scintigram is influenced by both the duration of the ischemic state after injection and the magnitude of postischemic reactive hyperemia.[26]

Redistribution begins immediately and proceeds continuously until an equilibrium distribution is reached, which is determined by a net balance between myocardial Tl-201 input and output. Redistribution results from a continuous exchange of Tl-201 between myocardium and all other extracardiac compartments.

To better understand the mechanism of Tl-201 redistribution, a simplified compartmental model described by Dr. Denny Watson from the University of Virginia is useful.[35] In this model, Tl-201 is distributed within three major compartments: blood, myocardium, and all other extracardiac organs. The latter contain all of the extravascular Tl-201 except that in the myocardium. Figure 2–13 depicts this model to help the reader visualize the compartmental exchange of Tl-201. In Figure 2–13A, the dark-shaded region indicates the concentration of Tl-201 just after injection into the blood. Tl-201 is extracted avidly by most organs in the body, and within a few minutes is distributed roughly in proportion to the distribution of cardiac output (Fig. 2–13B). The light-shaded region of the heart is presumed to have diminished blood flow in comparison with the dark-shaded region of the heart, and consequently to have taken up proportionally less Tl-201. The actual concentration of Tl-201 at this time would be proportional to the product of perfusion and extraction fraction. Approximately 4% of the Tl-201 that was injected is now in the heart, and more than 90% is in other body organs. Thus, there is a very large systemic reservoir of Tl-201 outside the heart. Tl-201 is in equilibrium with the systemic pool and the cardiac blood pool, while the blood acts as the transport vehicle. A portion of Tl-201 from this exchangeable pool enters the myocardium. This is referred to as Tl-201's being *imported*. On the other hand, Tl-201 may wash out of the myocardium, as described in the previous section, and be sequestered in the systemic pool. This washout can be thought of as Tl-201 being *exported* from the myocardium.

In the type of exchange process just described, in which Tl-201 is both entering and leaving a myocardial region, the net concentration of Tl-201 in that region may change if there is an imbalance between the rate of import and the rate of export. For example, in Figure 2–13B, the area of myocardium where initially the concentration was high might be exporting Tl-201 to the systemic pool more rapidly than it can import it from the same pool, resulting in a decrease in net Tl-201 concentration. In contrast, the area of myocardium with initially low concentration might tend to import more Tl-201 than it exports and consequently increases net concentration over time. Thus, the local concentration of Tl-201 continues to change until a static equilibrium condition is achieved, so that import of Tl-201 is equal to export. Ultimately, the total amount of Tl-201 extracted is related to the ability of the cell to maintain the electrochemical Tl-201 gradient. Under the condition of static equilibrium, no further net change in concentration occurs. At this point, this redistribution process has yielded normalization of initial defects caused by the flow heterogeneity between myocardial regions. The delayed equilibrium phase is depicted in Figure 2–13C.

Redistribution is not a true equilibrium, since there is continued net loss of Tl-201 owing to systemic excretion as blood pool activity falls; however, total body loss of Tl-201 is quite slow compared to the rate of systemic exchange.

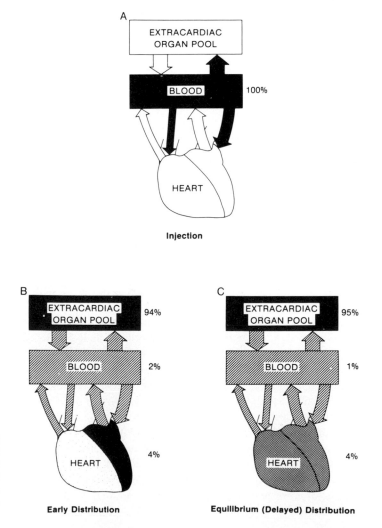

Figure 2–13. Compartmental model demonstrating different phases of Tl-201 uptake and delayed redistribution (see text for discussion). The light area of the heart in panel **B** represents a region of abnormal perfusion. The percentages represent the amount of Tl-201 in each compartment during the phases shown. (Beller GA, et al.: Cardiovascular Nuclear Medicine. St. Louis, CV Mosby, 1979.)

Thus, the exchange and the equilibrium are unaffected by systemic excretion, except that there is a gradual net loss of total circulating Tl-201.

Factors That Affect Thallium-201 Kinetics

The clearance of Tl-201 from the myocardium is influenced not only by myocardial ischemia but also by certain other factors. Kaul et al.[39] showed by linear regression analysis that a decrease in peak heart rate of 1 bpm was associated with a slower Tl-201 clearance (longer half-life) of 0.05 hour. Nordrehaug et al.[40] found a linear relationship between heart rate and Tl-201 clearance ($r = 0.80$). Clearance was altered by 0.024 heart rate/heart beat. The slower Tl-201 clearance at slower heart rates has clinical significance for patient imaging. Regional washout abnormalities are more likely to represent ischemia when they are observed at high exercise heart rates, whereas a downsloping washout pattern is seen in normally perfused myocardium.

Tl-201 redistribution can be influenced by a metabolic intervention such as intravenous ribose infusion. Angello et al.[41] found significant enhancement of Tl-201 redistribution in ribose-treated pigs with experimental ischemia as compared with ribose-untreated animals. These investigators proposed that ribose administration during the redistribution phase may permit earlier and better recognition of redistribution after transient ischemia.

Persistent Thallium-201 Defects and Partial Redistribution

When Tl-201 is administered intravenously under conditions of total occlusion of a coronary vessel or in the presence of a myocardial scar, a "persistent" defect is observed in the coronary supply region of the irreversibly damaged area. In the presence of infarction or scar, a defect is noted soon after Tl-201 administration and several hours later when repeat imaging is performed. In this situation, no delayed redistribution can be detected. Partial redistribution is observed if there is physiologically significant collateral flow to viable myocardium in the distribution of an occluded artery or if some antegrade flow is preserved. Partial redistribution indicates the presence of some viable myocardium in the distribution of a stenotic or occluded coronary artery. In a canine infarct model, Khaw et al. showed that persistent Tl-201 defects correlated with irreversibly damaged myocardium as assessed by radiolabeled antimyosin antibody uptake.[42] An inverse relationship between the amount of Tl-201 redistribution and the magnitude of radiolabeled antibody uptake was seen. As discussed in greater detail in Chapter 9, some persistent Tl-201 defects do not represent irreversibly injured myocardium and can show improved Tl-201 uptake after coronary revascularization with corresponding improvement in regional wall motion. Several new Tl-201 imaging protocols have emerged that have been shown to enhance detection of defect revers-

ibility on serial Tl-201 images. These protocols are discussed in detail in Chapter 9.

Reverse Thallium-201 Redistribution

Reverse redistribution is defined as the appearance of a defect for the first time on images obtained 2 to 3 hours after Tl-201 injection. The early initial images appear to be normal, or nearly so, having no significant focal defects. Reverse redistribution has been observed when serial imaging was performed in patients who have undergone reperfusion therapy after myocardial infarction (MI). When Tl-201 is injected during exercise, or even in the resting state, in a patient who previously underwent successful reperfusion with a thrombolytic agent or angioplasty, there may be significant exercise-induced hyperemia in the subepicardial but viable regions of the infarct zone. The enhanced Tl-201 uptake in these hyperemic subepicardial layers prevents detection of the zone of necrosis, which may be confined to the subendocardium. Thus, early images do not demonstrate relative defect when compared to the contralateral, presumably normal, myocardial region. Subsequently Tl-201 is cleared faster from this hyperemic region that was reperfused than from the normal zone, and a significant defect is seen for the first time on delayed scintigrams.

A second mechanism for reverse redistribution is delayed accumulation of Tl-201 uptake in a zone of ischemia coupled with enhanced Tl-201 washout from another area that is a mixture of scar and viable myocardium. The images obtained soon after Tl-201 administration might show "balanced" Tl-201 uptake in the ischemic zone and the partially scarred zone. The delayed images show the appearance of a new defect because the ischemic zone accumulates Tl-201 over time and the partially infarcted zone demonstrates a net washout pattern. Reverse redistribution is seen because the area composed of a mixture of normal myocardium and scar is perceived as a significant defect only in the delayed image, owing to uneven regional Tl-201 clearance. This mechanism of reverse redistribution signifies multivessel CAD.

A third mechanism for reverse redistribution relates to an artifact that can be produced by oversubtraction of background activity by computer processing.[43] Lear et al.[43] noted that reverse redistribution is more prevalent as an artifact on single-photon emission computed tomography (SPECT) than on planar Tl-201 images. If reverse redistribution is seen in a patient with a low pretest likelihood of CAD and no other evidence of exercise-induced ischemia, the finding is most likely artifactual.

TECHNETIUM-99M SESTAMIBI KINETICS

In recent years, several technetium-99m (Tc-99m)–labeled myocardial perfusion agents have been under investigation to determine their efficacy in assessing regional myocardial blood flow and cellular viability.[44–49c] These Tc-99m agents prove superior to Tl-201 for myocardial perfusion imaging because of better physical characteristics. The 140-keV photon energy peak of Tc-99m is optimal for gamma camera imaging and can produce higher quality images than those produced by Tl-201. The relatively short half-life (6 hours) of Tc-99m provides favorable patient dosimetry and makes it possible to administer a dose of the radiopharmaceutical 10 to 15 times larger than that of Tl-201, yielding better images in a shorter time.

Initial efforts were directed at developing cationic Tc-99m complexes, and although preliminary animal experiments were promising, these agents demonstrated an unfavorable heart–background activity ratio in humans.[50, 51] Recent work has been directed at a new class of cationic technetium compounds, the hexakis alkylisonitrile technetium (I) complexes. The Tc-99m–labeled isonitrile complexes have the general formula $[Tc(CNR_6)]^-$, where R is an alkyl group.

In 1986, Holman et al.[52] presented the first human Tc-99m perfusion imaging studies, done with Tc-99m tertiary butylisonitrile (TBI). The clinical usefulness of this agent was hampered by persistently high hepatic and lung activity. The higher background activity resulted in failure to identify a significant number of hypoperfused myocardial regions demonstrated on Tl-201 scintigrams in the same patients, thus diminishing sensitivity. Later studies with the less lipophilic Tc-99m–labeled carbomethoxyisopropyl isonitrile (CPI) yielded images of higher quality with less lung and hepatic uptake than was seen with TBI[53]; however, heart-background ratios were not ideal. The next agent in the isonitrile compound class to be evaluated was Tc-99m methoxyisobutyl isonitrile (sestamibi). This compound showed the most favorable myocardial-background ratio for myocardial imaging of any of the isonitriles. The kinetics of this myocardial perfusion agent have been investigated in a number of experimental models.[7a, 45, 49] Tc-99m sestamibi has emerged as the most clinically applicable of the various isonitrile compounds.

Myocardial Uptake of Technetium-99m Sestamibi

There is convincing experimental evidence that Tc-99m sestamibi is a suitable agent for evaluating regional myocardial blood flow and cellular viability. Piwnica-Worms et al.[54] investigated the fundamental cellular uptake mechanism of Tc-99m sestamibi and found that its transport involves passive distribution across plasma and mitochondrial membranes. At equilibrium it is sequestered largely within mitochondria by the large negative transmembrane potentials. When plasma or mitochondrial membrane potentials are depolarized, net uptake of Tc-99m sestamibi is inhibited and the radionuclide is retained. When mitochondrial and plasma membrane potentials are hyperpolarized, cellular uptake and retention of Tc-99m sestamibi are increased. Mitochondrial membrane depolarization is a feature of irreversible myocyte injury.

Cellular Uptake and Retention Related to Viability

Metabolic derangements simulating ischemia or hypoxia can result in diminished Tc-99m sestamibi uptake independent of flow. This can occur with metabolism-induced membrane polarization changes. Tc-99m–sestamibi depletion has been observed in heart cells with carbonyl cyanide *m*-chlorophenylhydrazone (CCCP) and 2,4-dinitrophenol, both of which depolarize mitochondrial membrane potentials. Other agents, such as rotenone, nigericin, and dimethylsulfoxide, have no significant effect on Tc-99m–sestamibi retention since these latter metabolic inhibitors have no detrimental effects on the negative potential across the inner mitochondrial membrane. Figure 2–14 from the work of Piwnica-Worms[54] shows a plot of the effect of these metabolic inhibitors on Tc-99m–sestamibi retention in cultured heart cells. Subsequent studies by this group of investigators further demonstrated dependence of Tc-99m–sestamibi uptake on viability of myocardial mitochondrial and plasma membranes.[54a, 54b] Beanlands et al. investigated Tc-99m–sestamibi kinetics in isolated rat heart preparations.[55] Under constant flow conditions, sodium cyanide, a cytochrome C oxidase inhibitor, and Triton X-100, a sarcolemmal membrane detergent, reduced peak accumulation of Tc-99m ses-

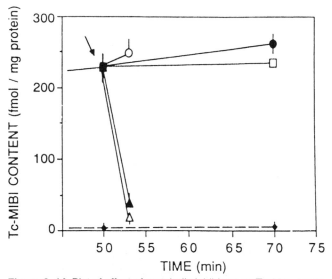

Figure 2–14. Plot of effect of metabolic inhibitors on Tc-99m–sestamibi (Tc-MIBI) retention in heart cells. Preparations were incubated in control buffer containing 1.26 nM Tc-MIBI for 50 minutes, at which point various drugs were added. (Key: solid square, control net uptake; solid triangles, CCCP administration; open triangles, dinitrophenol administration; solid circles, rotenone administration; open circles, nigericin; open squares, dimethyl sulfoxide administration; solid diamond, freeze-thawed preparations incubated in loading buffer [see text for mechanism of action of these metabolic inhibitors].) (Piwnica-Worms D, et al.: Circulation 1990;82:1826–1838.)

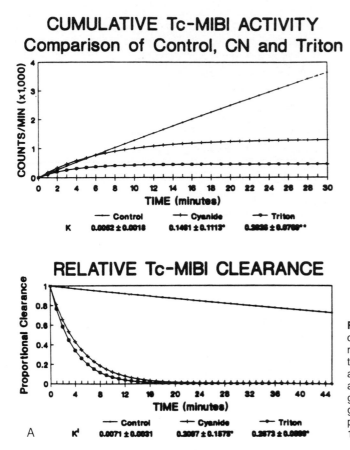

CUMULATIVE Tc-MIBI ACTIVITY
Comparison of Control, CN and Triton

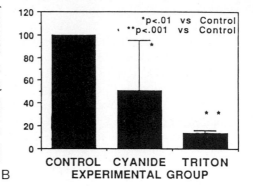

MEAN PERCENT UPTAKE OF Tc-MIBI

B

RELATIVE Tc-MIBI CLEARANCE

A

Figure 2–15. A. Time-activity curves for accumulation *(top)* and clearance *(bottom)* of Tc-99m–sestamibi (Tc-MIBI) activity. Cyanide- and Triton X-100–induced injury alters accumulation of the tracer. Triton- and cyanide-induced injury also lead to rapid clearance *(bottom)* of technetium-99m sestamibi. For clearance, the y axis is the proportion of peak activity, where the peak activity is given a value of 1.0. Clearance constant (K′) is shown for each group. **B.** Bar graph of mean uptake activity for each group as a percentage of control. (Beanlands RSB, et al.: Circulation 1990;82:1802–1814.)

tamibi and resulted in loss of cellular retention of the radionuclide. Figure 2–15A shows time-activity curves for accumulation and clearance of Tc-99m sestamibi in isolated rat hearts from this study with introduction of cyanide and triton. Note that cellular injury induced by these agents results in impaired uptake and rapid clearance. Figure 2–15B shows a bar graph of mean percentage of uptake of Tc-99m sestamibi for control, cyanide, and triton experimental groups. Thus, adverse metabolic conditions induced by chemical agents simulating ischemia or hypoxia result

in inhibition of cellular Tc-99m–sestamibi uptake and failure of Tc-99m–sestamibi retention.

Beller et al.[56] showed in intact dogs that Tc-99m–sestamibi retention was dependent on myocardial viability. Tc-99m sestamibi was administered intravenously to dogs at baseline under normal conditions, after which the LAD was occluded for 3 hours and then reperfused for another 3 hours. Animals were killed 4 minutes, 30 minutes, or 180 minutes into reperfusion. In dogs that were preloaded with Tc-99m sestamibi, 3 hours' LAD occlusion and 3 hours'

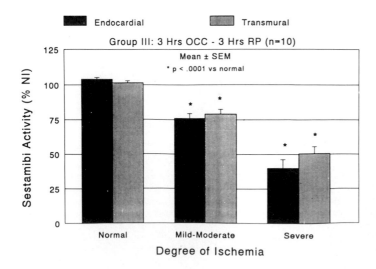

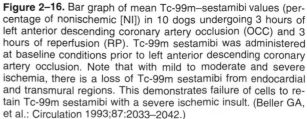

Figure 2–16. Bar graph of mean Tc-99m–sestamibi values (percentage of nonischemic [NI]) in 10 dogs undergoing 3 hours of left anterior descending coronary artery occlusion (OCC) and 3 hours of reperfusion (RP). Tc-99m sestamibi was administered at baseline conditions prior to left anterior descending coronary artery occlusion. Note that with mild to moderate and severe ischemia, there is a loss of Tc-99m sestamibi from endocardial and transmural regions. This demonstrates failure of cells to retain Tc-99m sestamibi with a severe ischemic insult. (Beller GA, et al.: Circulation 1993;87:2033–2042.)

reflow resulted in a loss of Tc-99m sestamibi in the endo-cardial zone of the ischemic region to 40% ±6% of the nonischemic level (Fig. 2–16). This loss corresponded to sustained elevation of coronary sinus activity throughout the reflow period. The loss was also greater than that observed in dogs killed after 4 or 30 minutes' reflow. Thus, an ischemic insult can cause cells to "dump" Tc-99m sestamibi into the coronary venous effluent, presumably secondary to mitochondrial and sarcolemmal membrane injury.

Ouabain infusion has little effect on peak myocardial extraction or the permeability surface area product of Tc-99m sestamibi.[57] Maublant et al.,[58] using a preparation of cultured rat myocytes, also showed that ouabain did not affect Tc-99m–sestamibi uptake whereas Tl-201 uptake was inhibited. These observations suggest that active membrane transport mechanism plays a small role, if any, in intracellular transport of Tc-99m sestamibi.

Further evidence that myocardial Tc-99m–sestamibi uptake depends on cellular viability is that such uptake is not significantly affected by myocardial stunning. Sinusas et al.[17] reported that administration of Tc-99m sestamibi during reperfusion preceded by 15 minutes of coronary occlusion resulted in unaltered Tc-99m–sestamibi uptake in the region of "stunned" myocardium, which exhibited severe postischemic systolic dysfunction (Fig. 2–17). In this model of transient occlusion and reperfusion, Tc-99m–sestamibi uptake was comparable to Tl-201 uptake and proportional to regional flow. Myocardial Tc-99m–sestamibi uptake also was not adversely affected in a canine model of "short-term" hibernation.[17] There was preserved Tc-99m–sesta-

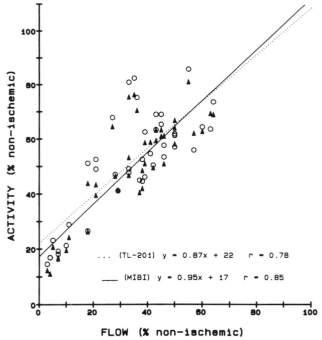

Figure 2–18. Central ischemic endocardial Tc-99m and Tl-201 activity versus flow in dogs with a chronic stenosis in which flow to the endocardium was reduced to not more than 60% of baseline flow. (Key: open circles, values for Tl-201; closed triangles, Tc-99m–sestamibi values.) (Reprinted with permission from the American College of Cardiology (Journal of the American College of Cardiology, 1989, Vol. 14, pp. 1785–1793).)

mibi uptake in anesthetized dogs with a partial coronary stenosis that reduced flow to 60% of the control level. Despite severe systolic dysfunction, Tc-99m–sestamibi uptake was still proportional to the residual flow in the ischemic zone and comparable to Tl-201 uptake in the same dogs (Fig. 2–18). Sansoy et al.[58a] showed greater Tl-201 uptake than Tc-99m–sestamibi uptake 2 hours after tracer injections in dogs with a 50% reduction in regional flow. In this study, greater Tl-201 than Tc-99m–sestamibi redistribution was noted. However, the difference in uptake only averaged 5% and significant Tc-99m–sestamibi uptake was observed in asynergic myocardium. Results from these experiments suggest that postischemic dysfunction or sustained low-flow ischemia producing a profound reduction in systolic thickening does not affect Tc-99m–sestamibi uptake as long as myocardial cells remain viable. A discussion of myocardial Tc-99m–sestamibi kinetics for evaluation of viability is also presented in Chapter 9.

Regional Blood Flow and Technetium-99m–Sestamibi Uptake

Uptake of Tc-99m sestamibi in viable myocardium is proportional to regional blood flow.[59–64] Okada et al.[59] demonstrated a good correlation ($r = 0.92$) between myocardial blood flow as measured by radioactive microspheres and Tc-99m–sestamibi uptake in anesthetized dogs subjected to partial occlusion of a coronary vessel (Fig. 2–19A). In a similar model, Glover and Okada[60] demonstrated a linear

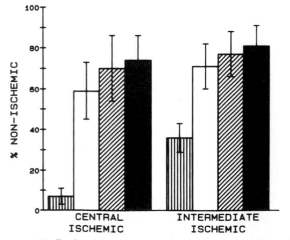

Figure 2–17. Regional blood flow and myocardial activity in dogs undergoing myocardial stunning with 15 minutes of coronary occlusion followed by reperfusion. Illustrated are occlusion *(vertically hatched bars)* and reperfusion flows *(open bars)* and Tl-201 *(diagonally hatched bars)* and Tc-99m–sestamibi *(solid bars)* activity for central ischemic ($N=29$) and intermediate ischemic ($N=21$) endocardial segments expressed as a percent of nonischemic values. Both Tl-201 and Tc-99m–sestamibi activity levels were comparable to reperfusion flow and central and intermediate ischemic segments. (Reprinted with permission from the American College of Cardiology (Journal of the American College of Cardiology, 1989, Vol. 14, pp. 1785–1793).)

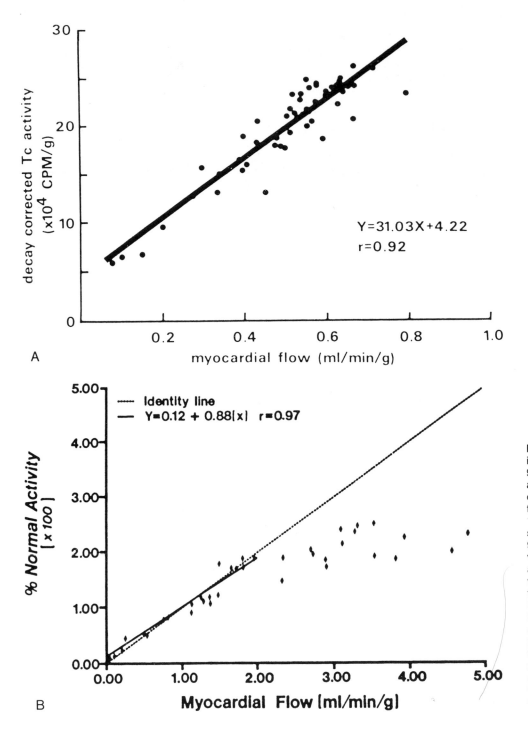

A.

B.

Figure 2–19. **A.** Relationship of initial myocardial blood flow to Tc-99m–sestamibi activity (vertical axis) in 12 dogs with a partially occluded circumflex coronary artery. (Okada RD, et al.: Circulation 1988;77:491–498.) **B.** Scatter plot showing percentage of normal Tc-99m–sestamibi activity distribution versus microsphere blood flow after dipyridamole infusion in dogs with mild to moderate left circumflex coronary stenoses. Line of identity is shown as the dashed line, and the regression line is shown as solid. Tc-99m–sestamibi distribution is linearly related to flow, up to approximately 2.0 ml/min/g. A plateau is then reached for flows above this value. (Glover DK, Okada RD: Circulation 1990;81:628–636.)

relation ($r = 0.97$) between initial myocardial uptake of Tc-99m sestamibi and regional myocardial blood flow at flow rates up to 2.0 ml/min/g when the radionuclide was injected after dipyridamole infusion (Fig. 2–19B). Like other diffusible indicators such as Tl-201, Tc-99m sestamibi underestimates myocardial blood flow at high flow rates. In low-flow regions, uptake of Tc-99m sestamibi is higher relative to nonischemic uptake than is the microsphere-determined regional blood flow. This may be attributed to increased extraction of the tracer at slow flow rates. Melon et al.[61] compared the myocardial retention of Tc-99m sestamibi and Tl-201 over a wide range of blood flow values induced by dipyridamole in a canine coronary occlusion model. Tl-201 demonstrated greater absolute tissue retention than did Tc-99m sestamibi. Retention of both tracers underestimated myocardial blood flow at high flow rates. This finding again points out that, with hyperemic flow, the peak extraction of a radionuclide perfusion agent decreases, thus underestimating the true increase in blood flow. Glover et al.[62] confirmed these findings using intravenous adenosine infusion in anesthetized dogs that had either critical or mild LAD stenosis. Figure 2–20 shows the

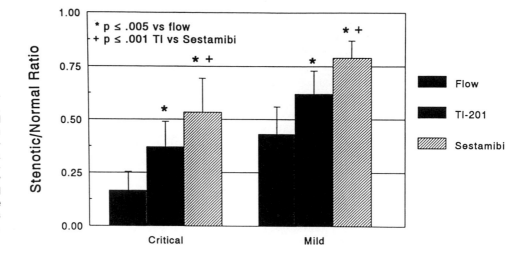

Figure 2–20. Stenotic:normal uptake ratios of blood flow (first bar), Tl-201 activity (second bar), and sestamibi activity (third bar) in dogs receiving intravenous adenosine with either critical *(left)* or a mild *(right)* stenosis of the left anterior descending coronary artery (LAD). Note that both Tl-201 and sestamibi values underestimate flow, but the underestimation was greater for sestamibi. (Glover DK, et al.: Circulation 1994, in press.)

ischemic-normal ratios of flow, Tl-201 uptake, and Tc-99mm–sestamibi uptake in these experiments. Note that in dogs with either a critical stenosis or a mild stenosis, Tl-201 and Tc-99m–sestamibi uptake underestimated the actual microsphere-determined flow ratio. As reported by Melon et al.,[61] the degree of this underestimation was greater for Tc-99m sestamibi than for Tl-201. Nevertheless, the gamma-camera images of myocardial slices from these dogs showed that Tc-99m–sestamibi defects could be resolved, although they were less severe than the Tl-201 defect magnitudes. Finally, Leon et al.[63] compared myocardial SPECT images of Tc-99m–sestamibi and Tl-201 distribution in the same dog undergoing partial coronary occlusion or pharmacologic vasodilatation with adenosine. Tc-99m–sestamibi SPECT imaging underestimated the area of the defect as compared with Tl-201 and with the pathologic estimation of the underperfused myocardial region.

Canby et al.[64] also showed a close positive linear corre-lation between Tc-99m–sestamibi uptake and regional flow when the radionuclide was administered before reperfusion after 2 hours of coronary occlusion. As expected, Tc-99m–sestamibi extraction was enhanced in zones where flow was reduced by approximately 10% to 40% of control flow, indicating increased extraction of this radionuclide by myocardial tissue in that region.

Leppo and Meerdink[65] investigated myocardial transmicrovascular transport of Tc-99m sestamibi in a blood-perfused, isolated rabbit heart model. They showed an inverse relationship between coronary flow and fractional extraction (E_{max}) of Tc-99m sestamibi and Tl-201 (Fig. 2–21). The mean E_{max} value for Tc-99m sestamibi (39% $\pm 9\%$) was significantly less than that for Tl-201 (73% $\pm 10\%$). The net myocardial extraction (E_{net}), an estimate of myocardial retention of a diffusible tracer measured over 2 to 5 minutes, also was significantly less for Tc-99m sestamibi (41% $\pm 15\%$) than for Tl-201 (57% $\pm 13\%$). Tl-201 was

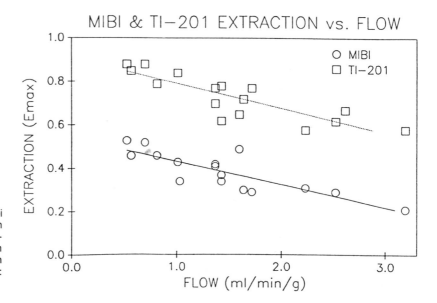

Figure 2–21. Comparison of Tc-99m–sestamibi (MIBI, lower line) and Tl-201 (upper line) extraction values versus coronary blood flow. Note that the extraction (E_{max}) is higher for Tl-201 than for Tc-99m sestamibi, though both tracers show a reduction in extraction at higher flows. (Leppo JA, Meerdink DJ: Circ Res 1989;65:632–639.)

shown to have a higher transcapillary exchange rate than Tc-99m sestamibi. The mean capillary permeability surface area product (PS) for Tc-99m sestamibi was approximately 33% of the value for Tl-201, but Tc-99m sestamibi had a significantly higher parenchymal cell permeability and higher volume of distribution in Tl-201. This would yield a longer residence time for Tc-99m sestamibi.

The net result of these differences in kinetics between Tc-99m sestamibi and Tl-201 is that little difference would be observed in the myocardial uptake of the two agents when imaged in vivo. This is because capillary permeability for Tl-201 is higher than for Tc-99m sestamibi, but the reverse is true at the parenchymal cell wall. With myocardial ischemia followed by reperfusion, the extraction (net) of Tc-99m sestamibi increases, whereas under the same experimental conditions, Tl-201 extraction diminishes (Fig. 2–22).[65a] These experiments were undertaken employing no-flow ischemia and reperfusion in the isolated, blood-perfused rabbit heart.

Marshall and his collaborators also investigated the myocardial extraction and retention of Tc-99m sestamibi as compared with Tl-201 in an isolated rabbit heart model.[66] Mean Tc-99m–sestamibi peak instantaneous extraction was lower (55% $\pm$ 10%) and more influenced by the flow rate than the peak instantaneous extraction of Tl-201 (83% $\pm$ 6%). As expected, the rate of Tl-201 washout was significantly faster and more dependent on perfusion than was Tc-99m–sestamibi washout. The initial myocardial retention of Tl-201 was higher than that of Tc-99m sestamibi, confirming the findings of the other investigators.[61, 62, 64] Owing to its faster washout rate, however, the superiority of Tl-201 over Tc-99m sestamibi as a myocardial perfusion agent was lost within 10 minutes of tracer injection with the single-pass experimental conditions used. Thus, net retention of Tc-99m sestamibi and of Tl-201 is comparable,

since back-diffusion of Tl-201 is relatively faster than that of Tc-99m sestamibi.

Clearance and Redistribution

After initial myocardial uptake subsequent clearance of Tc-99m sestamibi is slow. Okada et al.[59] reported that the 4-hour fractional Tc-99m sestamibi clearance values from normal and ischemic zones in their canine model were minimal and equivalent. Li et al.[67] investigated whether Tc-99m sestamibi redistribution after transient myocardial ischemia is comparable to what is observed with Tl-201. Both tracers were injected after 1 minute of experimental coronary occlusion in anesthetized dogs, and after 6 minutes, reflow was accomplished. Serial tomographic imaging in these animals showed a perfusion defect with some slight filling in after 2 hours, indicative of redistribution. The degree of redistribution was significantly less than that seen with Tl-201. Sinusas et al.[68] determined whether Tc-99m sestamibi would be redistributed when administered in the presence of a critical stenosis and a sustained diminution in coronary blood flow. In these experiments, the early myocardial distribution of Tc-99m sestamibi and of Tl-201 was comparable and correlated with the flow deficit. The late myocardial Tc-99m sestamibi concentration in the ischemic region was greater than the flow deficit, reflecting some redistribution. The magnitude of redistribution was less than that observed with Tl-201 in the same animals. Figure 2–23 compares early and late Tc-99m sestamibi uptake in dogs killed either 20 minutes or 3 hours after tracer administration. Flow values during administration of Tc-99m sestamibi are also shown. Note that some Tc-99m sestamibi redistribution is observed, which is reflected by higher values of Tc-99m sestamibi uptake in dogs killed 3 hours after tracer injection. Sansoy et al.[58a] confirmed the presence of some Tc-99m–sestamibi redistribution at rest when the tracer was administered to dogs with a 50% reduction in coronary flow. This redistribution was detected by quantitative planar gamma camera imaging. Glover and Okada[64a] could not visually detect Tc-99m–sestamibi redistribution in reperfused viable myocardium in a dog model but found evidence for delayed redistribution by gamma well counting after animals were killed. Thus, under conditions of sustained low flow there is some redistribution of Tc-99m sestamibi, though to a lesser extent than for Tl-201.

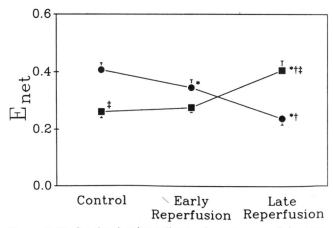

Figure 2–22. Graphs showing estimates for net myocardial extraction (E_{net}) for Tc-99m sestamibi *(solid squares)* and Tl-201 *(closed circles)*. Compared with paired Tl-201 values, the E_{net} for Tc-99m sestamibi was significantly lower at control, similar to Tl-201 at early reperfusion and significantly higher than Tl-201 at late reperfusion. (Meerdink DJ, Leppo JA: Circ Res 1990;66:1738–1746.)

Risk Area and Infarct Size

Several experimental studies have been performed to assess whether Tc-99m sestamibi can be employed to assess the risk area during coronary artery occlusion or the amount of salvaged myocardium after reperfusion. Verani et al.[69] found that the perfusion defect size on either planar or SPECT Tc-99m–sestamibi images correlated with the

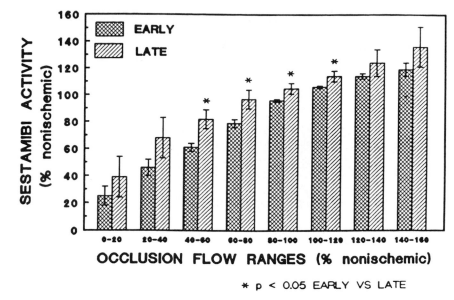

Figure 2–23. Tc-99m sestamibi activity for dogs killed at either 20 minutes (early) or 3 hours (late) after Tc-99m–sestamibi injection in dogs with a chronic low-flow state. Note that, in the dogs killed late, sestamibi activity (% nonischemic) is higher than values for the dogs killed early, for multiple ranges of occlusion flows. This difference reflects the degree of Tc-99m sestamibi from 20 minutes to 3 hours after tracer injection. (Sinusas AJ, et al.: Circulation 1994;89:2332–2341.)

pathologic infarct size in dogs subjected to 2 hours' coronary occlusion. After 48 hours of reperfusion, scintigraphic defect size was markedly reduced, and it correlated with the final infarct size. With reperfusion, myocardial uptake of Tc-99m sestamibi in the ischemic region increased significantly and correlated with the enhanced flow as determined by radioactive microspheres. Sinusas et al.[70] defined Tc-99m–sestamibi uptake before and after reperfusion in 17 open-chest dogs after 3 hours of LAD occlusion and 3 hours of reflow. When Tc-99m sestamibi was injected during occlusion, uptake of the radionuclide correlated well with the anatomic risk area as determined at postmortem examination. When Tc-99m sestamibi was injected after 90 minutes of reperfusion, uptake of the tracer correlated well with the final infarct area postmortem ($r = 0.98$). Among these dogs injected with Tc-99m sestamibi after 90 minutes of reperfusion, myocardial Tc-99m–sestamibi uptake did not correlate with reperfusion flow in either endocardial (Fig. 2–24) or transmural segments. In this group of animals, myocardial Tc-99m–sestamibi activity was significantly less than reperfusion flow at the time of tracer injection in the severely ischemic region (25% ±5% vs. 74% ±24% nonischemic). These findings indicate that Tc-99m sestamibi does not behave as a microsphere does and that it requires viable myocytes for intracellular concentration following reperfusion. This is why uptake of the tracer during reflow correlated with histologic infarct area rather than merely tracking reperfusion flow.

These findings from the experiments of Verani et al.[69] and Sinusas et al.[70] indicate that myocardial uptake of Tc-99m sestamibi during coronary occlusion correlates with occlusion flow and reflects the "area at risk." When Tc-99m sestamibi is given at 90 minutes of reperfusion, uptake reflects myocardial viability more than the degree of reperfusion. If Tc-99m sestamibi is administered intravenously immediately after reperfusion, myocardial infarct size is

underestimated[56] because early uptake of this tracer following reperfusion during the hyperemic state of reflow reflects reperfusion more than viability. If this agent is going to be utilized for assessing salvage after reperfusion therapy in the clinical setting, the tracer must be administered at least 60 minutes after flow restoration, to more accurately determine degree of salvage and residual viable myocardium in the perinecrotic regions. Also, the size of the Tc-99m defect

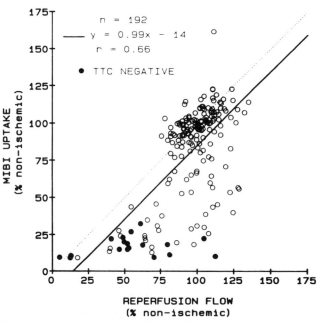

Figure 2–24. Myocardial Tc-99m–sestamibi (MIBI) activity expressed as a percentage of nonischemic activity versus reperfusion flow in dogs that received Tc-99m sestamibi during reperfusion. The solid circles represent values for nonviable endocardial segments unstained with triphenyltetrazolium chloride (TTC negative). Note that there is substantial impairment of Tc-99m–sestamibi uptake despite significant increases in reperfusion flow in necrotic regions. (Sinusas AJ, et al.: Circulation 1990;82:1424–1437.)

during ischemia and reperfusion is affected by alteration of left ventricular geometry.[70a] Coronary occlusion produces regional systolic thinning, which can create artifactual perfusion defects on Tc-99m–sestamibi images. This thinning causes partial volume effects that contribute to the defect size. The clinical application of serial Tc-99m sestamibi for evaluating patients receiving thrombolytic therapy in the setting of acute myocardial infarction is discussed in detail in Chapter 6. Also, Sinusas and Wackers recently reviewed the subject.[70b]

TECHNETIUM-99m TEBOROXIME

Tc-99m teboroxime is a neutral lipophilic agent which is in the class of compounds designated as boronic acid adducts of technetium oximes (BATO). Tc-99m–teboroxime uptake is not dependent upon an enzymatic mechanism. It has a very short half-life, approximately 12 minutes, which mandates a speedy imaging protocol (see Chap. 3).

Myocardial Uptake

Leppo and Meerdink compared the myocardial uptake kinetics of several Tc-99m–labeled BATO compounds with Tl-201 during varying levels of coronary flow in the isolated blood-perfused rabbit heart model.[71] As expected, there was an inverse relation between E_{max} and coronary blood flow for Tc-99m teboroxime. The E_{max} for Tc-99m teboroxime was higher than the Tl-201 value determined simultaneously. In these experiments, mean Tc-99m teboroxime extraction was 71%, a value 25% greater than the mean Tl-201 E_{max} of 0.57. The mean E_{net} for Tc-99m teboroxime was 55% $\pm$ 19%, which was 20% higher than the average Tl-201 values. Cellular retention of Tc-99m teboroxime was less than that of Tl-201 and Tc-99m sestamibi because of the high volume of back-diffusion of the tracer. Di Rocco et al.[72] showed that, soon after injection in a single-pass model in rats, Tl-201 and Tc-99m teboroxime values approximated true myocardial blood flow better than Tc-99m sestamibi. In multiple-pass experiments in dogs, Tl-201 approximated true flow changes with adenosine better than Tc-99m teboroxime.

Tc-99m–teboroxime uptake in the myocardium is substantial if activity is measured immediately after tracer administration, and this value can provide excellent contrast between normal and low flow regions as compared with Tl-201[72a]; however, myocardial retention diminishes rapidly over several minutes after injection of Tc-99m teboroxime. Beanlands et al.[73] examined the relationship between myocardial retention of Tc-99m teboroxime and myocardial blood flow at 1, 2, and 5 minutes after injection of tracer in a canine experimental model. At 1 minute after injection the relationship of retention to flow for Tc-99m teboroxime was linear over a wide range, becoming nonlinear at vol-

umes greater than 4.5 ml/min/g. After 5 minutes, myocardial uptake of tracer versus flow was linear only to 2.5 ml/min/g. Thus, only 5 minutes after Tc-99m–teboroxime administration, the myocardial uptake pattern underestimates flow increase in the moderate and high ranges. Figure 2–25 shows the decrease in myocardial teboroxime retention at flows of 1, 2, 3, and 4 ml/min/g versus time after injection. The decrease in retention is most rapid at the high flow rates. Glover et al.[74] reported similar findings in anesthetized dogs and showed that rapid clearance of Tc-99m teboroxime resulted in loss of defect contrast from 2 minutes to 4 minutes after tracer injection on gamma camera images of myocardial slices. By 2 minutes after injection, Tl-201 defect magnitude reflected the flow decrement better than Tc-99m–teboroxime defect magnitude in the same animals, which received both radionuclides after adenosine infusion in the presence of an LAD stenosis. These studies indicate that ultrarapid acquisition methods are required to adequately employ Tc-99m sestamibi for imaging of regional myocardial blood flow. *error*

Stewart et al.[75] injected Tc-99m teboroxime via the intracoronary route in open-chest dogs under baseline conditions and after intravenous dipyridamole administration. The first-pass myocardial retention fraction averaged 0.9 $\pm$ 0.04 in this model. There was, however, rapid clearance of the radionuclide soon after uptake was complete. Sixty-seven percent of retained activity cleared, with a $T_{1/2}$ of 2.3 $\pm$ 0.6 minutes. Thus, Tc-99m teboroxime exhibits high initial myocardial extraction but rapid tissue clearance. This rapid intrinsic clearance is the mechanism for loss of tissue retention over the first 5 minutes after initial uptake.

It may be possible to exploit the rapid myocardial washout of Tc-99m teboroxime for detection of significant CAD

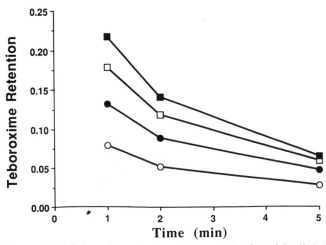

Figure 2–25. Teboroxime retention at flows of 1, 2, 3, and 4 ml/min/g derived from the retention–myocardial blood flow relationships versus time after injection in a canine model. A wide range of myocardial blood flows was induced in each experiment by coronary occlusion and dipyridamole infusion. Note the rapid decrease in retention over time at high flow rates. (Key: open circles, 1 ml/min/g; closed circles, 2 ml/min/g; open squares, 3 ml/min/g; solid squares, 4 ml/min/g.) (Beanlands R, et al.: J Am Coll Cardiol 1992;20:712–719.)

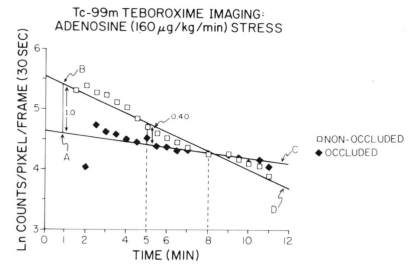

Figure 2–26. Log transform myocardial teboroxime clearance data from a dog with severe partial stenosis receiving adenosine. The clearance curves from the normal nonoccluded zone *(open squares)* and the occluded zone *(solid triangles)* intersect at 8 minutes postinjection. These quantitative "redistribution" curves correlated with fill-in of an anteroseptal perfusion defect. The myocardial clearance $T_{1/2}$ in the nonoccluded zone was 4.9 minutes; that in the occluded zone, 10.5 minutes. (Stewart RE, et al.: J Nucl Med 1991;32:2000–2008.)

(see Chap. 3). Stewart et al.[76] showed that myocardial Tc-99m–teboroxime washout is flow dependent. In regions of myocardium shown to have reduced flow, Tc-99m–teboroxime clearance is delayed as compared with regions of enhanced myocardial perfusion, where it is faster. In their studies, Tc-99m–teboroxime clearance in normal myocardium was accelerated by adenosine and by dipyridamole as compared with the rate in control subjects. Poststenotic Tc-99m–teboroxime clearance half-time was significantly longer than in the nonoccluded contralateral perfusion zone, as measured by adenosine stress (11.2 ±3.7 vs. 6.3 ±1.5 minutes) and by total coronary occlusion (12.1 ±3.3 vs 6.6 ±1.2 minutes). This differential tracer clearance from poststenotic and normal zones produced quantitative evidence of relative defect "redistribution." Figure 2–26 shows clearance data from a dog with a partial coronary stenosis that received adenosine before Tc-99m–teboroxime injection in this study.

Using time-activity curves generated over ischemic and normal zones on serial images in dogs after stress and rest injections, Gray and Gewirtz[77] observed delayed tracer clearance from the ischemic area. In their experiments, ischemic zone activity at 7 minutes fell to 78% ±6% of peak on the 30-second scan following the stress injection, as compared with 61% ±7% of peak activity in the normal zone. Since following stress injection Tc-99m–teboroxime washout was slower from the ischemic zone than from the normal zone, the ischemic-normal zone count ratio, reflecting defect magnitude, increased significantly between 30-second (0.50 ±0.14) and 7-minute scans (0.61 ±0.11). Figure 2–27 shows the ischemic-normal zone count ratios for stress and rest injections in this study and demonstrates an increase in this ratio between the 30-second and 7-minute scans. This change would give the scintigraphic correlate of "redistribution" as observed on serial Tl-201 scintigrams but over a much shorter interval (7 minutes vs.

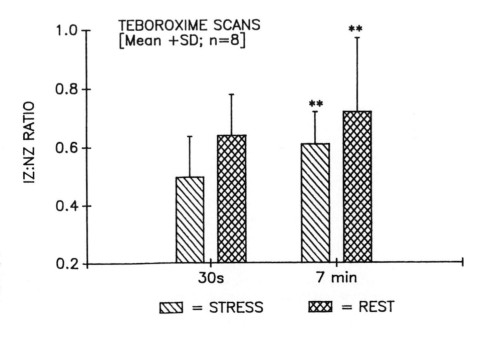

Figure 2–27. Ischemic-normal (Iz:Nz) count ratios for stress and rest teboroxime injections. The ratio increased significantly (** = P < 0.01) between 30-second and 7-minute scans following both stress and rest injections. (Gray WA, Gewirtz H: Circulation 1991;84:1796–1807.)

3.4 hours). Several groups[77a, 77b] have successfully utilized fast dynamic SPECT imaging for measuring myocardial blood flow employing kinetic modeling of Tc-99m teboroxine or compartmental analysis of teboroxine kinetics. Myocardial teboroxine extraction diminishes when the tracer is mixed with human red blood cells, and prolonged exposure with red blood cells significantly reduces extraction.[78a] In this study, teboroxine in saline solution showed an extraction of 0.89 in the isolated perfused rabbit heart. Extraction fell to 0.43 after prolonged incubation with human red blood cells, whereas a brief exposure reduced extraction to 0.60. When isolated rat hearts were perfused with Krebs-Hanseleit buffer, single-pass extraction rate for Tc-99m teboroxime was 96%.[78] When arterial blood was injected into the perfused heart, Tc-99m–teboroxime extraction decreased progressively over time. The authors concluded that, although much Tc-99m teboroxime is extracted on the first pass, extraction on subsequent recirculations may be affected by the binding of Tc-99m teboroxime to red blood cells and plasma proteins.

OTHER TECHNETIUM-99m MYOCARDIAL PERFUSION AGENTS

Technetium-99m Tetrofosmin

Tc-99m tetrofosmin is a cationic complex [^{99m}Tc-(tetrofosmin)$_2$O$_2$]$^+$ that has been synthesized and evaluated for possible use as a myocardial perfusion agent.[79] Tetrofosmin is the ether-functionalized diphosphine ligand 1,2 bis(2-ethoxyethyl)-phosphinol ethane. The complex shows good myocardial uptake with rapid clearance from blood and liver and little uptake in pulmonary tissue. Preliminary studies by Dahlberg et al.[79a] show that uptake of tetrofosmin is related linearly to coronary blood flow in the isolated blood-perfused rabbit heart. Sinusas et al.[79b] showed that myocardial Tc-99m–tetrofosmin uptake correlated linearly with microsphere-determined flow in a canine model of ischemia. As with other flow tracers, relative Tc-99m–tetrofosmin activity underestimated flow at high flow ranges above 2.0 ml/min/g. The heart:lung ratio of Tc-99m tetrofosmin was 3.57 ± 1.01 at 10 minutes post injection. Figure 2–28 depicts the relationship between myocardial Tc-99m–tetrofosmin activity and regional flow in 6 dogs in this study. Serial myocardium-lung and myocardium-liver ratios determined by planar Tc-99m–tetrofosmin dynamic studies reported by Nakajima et al.[79c] are summarized in Table 2–2. The myocardium-lung ratio was high, even 5 minutes postinjection, and the myocardium-liver ratio was 0.49.

Technetium-99m Q12

Like the other Tc-99m tracers described above, Tc-99m Q12 is taken up in the myocardium in proportion to blood

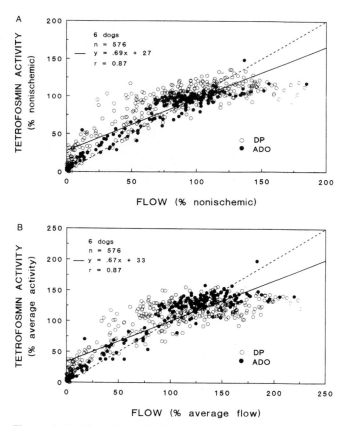

Figure 2–28. Normalized Tc-99m–tetrofosmin activity and microsphere flow in dogs with a coronary occlusion subjected to dipyridamole (DP) or adenosine (ADO) stress. **A.** Values normalized to nonischemic myocardial activity and flow. **B.** Mean values for each dog. A total of 576 segments were analyzed among the 6 dogs. (Reprinted by permission of the Society of Nuclear Medicine: from Sinusas AJ, et al: J Nucl Med 1994;35:664–671.)

flow. Gerson et al.[80] quantitated myocardial uptake of Tc-99m Q12 over 240 minutes after injection in open-chest dogs with Lcx coronary stenosis. The defect ratio (LCx:LAD) was 0.51 at 30 minutes and 0.48 at 240 minutes in this model. This implies no significant "redistribution" over time, similar to what has been reported for the other Tc-99m–labeled perfusion agents. Further investigation by this group[80a] showed that Tc-99m–Q12 myocardial activity is proportional to actual myocardial blood flow from 0 to 2 ml/min/g. Figure 2–29 shows the plateau in myocardial Tc-99m–Q12 uptake at flow values above 2.0 ml/min/g in dogs

Table 2–2. **Time Course of Technetium-99m Tetrofosmin***

Time	Heart-to-Lung Ratio	Heart-to-Liver Ratio
5	2.36 ± 0.72	0.49 ± 0.05
10	2.49 ± 0.85	0.41 ± 0.08
15	2.67 ± 1.11	0.41 ± 0.12
45†	2.74 ± 0.33	1.14 ± 0.51
180†	2.80 ± 0.43	2.33 ± 0.54

*n = 5, mean and SD.
†Measured with a static image after the first study. (Nakajima K, et al.: J Nucl Med 1993; 34:1478–1484.)

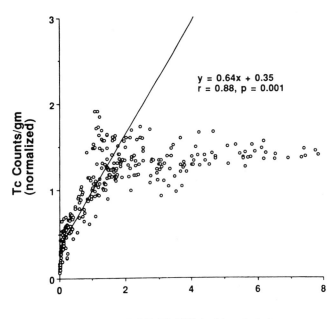

$$y = 0.64x + 0.35$$
$$r = 0.88, p = 0.001$$

Figure 2–29. Plot of myocardial microsphere-determined flow versus myocardial Tc-99m–Q12 activity in dogs with a left circumflex coronary artery occlusion that received intravenous dipyridamole prior to Q12 administration. Note the plateau in uptake at flows above 2.0 ml/min/g. (Gerson MC, et al: Circulation 1994;89:1291–1300.)

with a left circumflex coronary artery occlusion that received intravenous dipyridamole prior to Q12 injection.

TECHNETIUM-99m RED BLOOD CELLS

For gated cardiac blood pool imaging, the optimal blood pool label is one that is specific for the patient's own red blood cells.[81] Red blood cells can be labeled—in vivo or in vitro—with Tc-99m. For the in vivo technique for labeling red blood cells, unlabeled stannous pyrophosphate, reconstituted in normal saline, is injected intravenously 15 to 20 minutes before injection of 15 to 30 mCi of Tc-99m pertechnetate. With the in vitro technique, which is not often utilized, the labeling is achieved in a sterile vial, similar to other radiopharmaceutical kits. The patient's own blood is withdrawn and mixed with the stannous pyrophosphate. The dose of technetium pertechnetate is added 20 minutes later, and mixing is undertaken for approximately 10 minutes. The patient's own labeled red cells are reinjected. The technique for imaging the cardiac blood pools with Tc-99m–labeled red blood cells is discussed in detail in Chapter 1.

TECHNETIUM-99m PYROPHOSPHATE

Tc-99m pyrophosphate concentrates in zones of irreversible myocardial cell injury, providing a radionuclide imaging approach to detecting and sizing acute myocardial infarcts.[82] With irreversible cellular injury there is considerable calcification of mitochondria, particularly in zones of some residual blood flow. It is assumed that technetium pyrophosphate deposition occurs in necrotic areas of calcium overload.[83] With experimental infarction, the area of maximal Tc-99m–pyrophosphate uptake is the periphery of the infarct, where some collateral blood flow is preserved; uptake is less avid in the central infarct zones, where blood flow is markedly reduced.[84] Myocardial zones with flow reductions of 10% to 40% of control values are the areas of greatest Tc-99m–pyrophosphate uptake.[84, 85] This observation is consistent with the fact that, early after myocardial infarction, the peripheral zone of infarction with some residual flow to damaged tissue shows the greatest degree of calcium deposition. Uptake of this radionuclide in regions of necrosis is 10 to 50 times that noted in normal muscle. Uptake of technetium pyrophosphate is even greater after reperfusion following sustained coronary occlusion.[86]

In animal models, myocardial Tc-99m–pyrophosphate scintigrams demonstrate abnormalities 12 to 24 hours after ligation of a coronary vessel. From 24 to 72 hours, the scintigrams become more abnormal with greater tracer uptake in the zone of infarction. Following reperfusion, scintigrams can be positive within 2 hours after reflow. The Tc-99m–pyrophosphate scintigrams can remain abnormal for as long as a week after myocardial infarction.

INDIUM-111 ANTIMYOSIN ANTIBODIES

Cardiac myosin is an intracellular contractile protein consisting of two identical heavy chains and two pairs of light chains that comprise a molecule of 500 kd. Myosin molecules remain as insoluble myofibrils even after ischemic injury to the sarcolemmal membrane. The heavy chains do not wash out of damaged myocardium. This forms the rationale for use of radiolabeled antibodies specific for myosin for myocardial imaging of irreversible cell injury. Myosin-specific antibodies bind to the antigen only in necrotic myocardial tissue, whereas normal cell membranes prevent entry of the antibody into the cell.[87] With radiolabeling of the antibody, the extent of myocardial necrosis can be imaged with a conventional gamma scintillation camera.[88, 88a, 88b]

Fab fragments of antimyosin antibodies are labeled with indium-111 (In-111), which has two energy emission peaks, at 174 and 246 keV. In-111 imaging requires the use of a medium-energy collimator for optimal imaging of the myocardium. These Fab fragments of antimyosin antibodies have also been labeled with Tc-99m, which has a peak energy emission of 140 keV and is more suitable for imaging with a gamma camera and an all-purpose collimator. Fab fragments of antimyosin antibodies are cleared from the blood by 24 hours. At 48 hours after intravenous administration of the fragments, approximately 4% of the injected dose is present in the circulation.

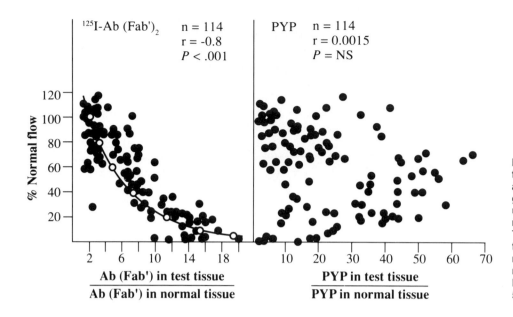

^{125}I-Ab (Fab')$_2$ n = 114
                            r = -0.8
                            P < .001

PYP   n = 114
        r = 0.0015
        P = NS

% Normal flow

Ab (Fab') in test tissue
Ab (Fab') in normal tissue

PYP in test tissue
PYP in normal tissue

Figure 2–30. Inverse relationship between Fab fragments of iodine 125 antimyosin antibody uptake and regional myocardial blood flow in dogs undergoing experimental myocardial necrosis. The relationship between Tc-99m–pyrophosphate (PYP) uptake and flow is quite different, maximum uptake being in regions of intermediate myocardial injury. (From Beller GA, et al.: Circulation 1977; 55:74–78.)

A number of experimental myocardial infarction studies in canine models have confirmed the high specificity of radiolabeled antimyosin antibody for identifying necrotic myocardium.[87, 89–91] Myocardial images of transverse slices in dogs with experimental infarction after intravenous administration of ^{131}I-labeled antimyosin (Fab')$_2$ showed good correlation with infarct size, as determined histochemically using triphenyltetrazolium chloride (TTC) staining.[92] There is an inverse exponential relationship between uptake of radiolabeled antimyosin and regional blood flow in ischemic myocardium.[89] Antimyosin uptake is maximal in the central region of necrosis as determined by microsphere–blood flow values (Fig. 2–30). In contrast, Tc-99m pyrophosphate shows no such direct inverse relationship to blood flow (see Fig. 2–30). Tc-99m–pyrophosphate uptake is greatest in zones of intermediate flow diminution; uptake decreases in the area of maximal flow reduction.

Infarct size determined by In-111 antimyosin was more accurate relative to histologic infarct size when compared with the Tc-99m–pyrophosphate infarct size, when measured simultaneously in the same dogs.[91] Tc-99m–pyrophosphate infarct size was significantly larger than the TTC infarct size, whereas antimyosin infarct size was not significantly different from the TTC infarct size. Perhaps the overestimation of infarct size with Tc-99m pyrophosphate relates to uptake in reversibly injured myocytes that accumulated calcium but survived without undergoing necrosis. Figure 2–31 shows in vivo gamma camera scintigraphic comparison of an experimental myocardial infarct delineated by In-111 antimyosin and by Tc-99m pyrophosphate 5 hours after injection of a mixture of both tracers.[91] In this example, the Tc-99m–pyrophosphate area of increased tracer uptake is larger than that delineated by In-111 antimyosin uptake. Alternatively, the larger scintigraphic estimate of infarct size with Tc-99m pyrophosphate may be due to greater uptake of the radionuclide in necrotic myocytes located at the boundary of the infarct, rather than to uptake in injured but viable tissue.[93] The clinical application of In-111–antimyosin imaging in patients with acute infarction is discussed in Chapter 6.

There is an inverse relation between antimyosin antibody uptake and final Tl-201 uptake as quantitated during the

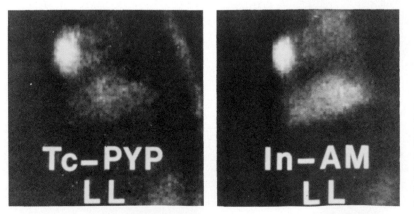

Figure 2–31. In vivo gamma camera images of Tc-99m pyrophosphate (Tc-PYP, *left*) and In-111 antimyosin antibody (In-AM, *right*). These are in vivo left lateral images of a dog injected intravenously with a mixture of Tc-99m pyrophosphate and In-111 antimyosin antibody following experimental myocardial infarction and reperfusion. (Reprinted by permission of the Society of Nuclear Medicine from: Khaw BA, et al.: J Nucl Med 1987;28:76–82.)

redistribution phase.[94] Areas showing no Tl-201 redistribution show the greatest uptake of radiolabeled antimyosin antibody. In-111 antimyosin antibody was also shown to be maximal in regions showing decreased Tc-99m–sestamibi activity in pigs undergoing LAD occlusion.[94a]

Radiolabeled antimyosin antibody is also taken up in myocardium that exhibits acute and chronic allograft rejection.[95, 95a] Experimental animals with allograft rejection show localization of radiolabeled antimyosin in areas of myocyte necrosis and white blood cell infiltration.[95a] In-111–antimyosin localization in transplanted hearts of animals treated with cyclosporin showed no increased uptake.[96] In those animals, pathologic inspection showed no evidence of myocyte necrosis. Figure 2–32 shows the relationship between degree of In-111–antimyosin uptake and the histologic degree of rejection in this study.

Antimyosin uptake has been found in animal models of Coxsackie virus–induced myocarditis in mice.[97, 98] In this animal model, specific localization of antimyosin was seen in necrotic myocardial tissue, and depression in cardiac function correlates with intensity of tracer uptake. Figure 2–33 depicts myocardial uptake of In-111 antimyosin Fab at various pathologic grades in virus-infected mice and infected mice from the study of Yamada et al.[98] Thus, it appears that imaging with radiolabeled antimyosin antibody can visualize the patchy myocardial necrosis found with heterotopic heart transplant rejection and acute myocarditis in experimental models. The clinical utility of this technique for detection of allograft rejection and diagnosing myocarditis is discussed in Chapter 11. In-111 antimyosin antibody shows promise for detecting cardiac damage in-

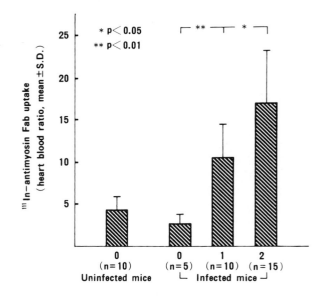

Figure 2–33. Myocardial uptake of In-111 antimyosin (Fab) expressed as a ratio of percent dose per gram of heart to percent dose per milliliter of blood. The bars represent antimyosin uptake according to pathologic grade (from 0 to 2) in virus-infected mice and uninfected mice. Data are represented as mean values ± SD. (Reprinted with permission from the American College of Cardiology (Journal of the American College of Cardiology, 1990, Vol. 16, pp. 1280–1286).)

duced by doxorubicin, a highly cardiotoxic agent.[99] Hiroe et al.[99] reported higher heart-blood and heart-lung uptake ratios in rats treated with doxorubicin than in control animals. Figure 2–34 shows examples of color autoradiographs from doxorubicin-treated rats in this study. In-111–antimyosin imaging can detect doxorubicin toxicity before the left ventricular ejection fraction deteriorates.[100]

POSITRON-EMITTING RADIONUCLIDES

Positron-emitting radionuclides can be employed to noninvasively assess persons who have any of a variety of disease states and pathophysiologic alterations for regional perfusion, metabolism, and the status of myocardial sympathetic and parasympathetic innervation. The principles of PET imaging were previously summarized in Chapter 1. The description of the radiopharmaceuticals employed for PET imaging is provided in the following paragraphs in this chapter.

Myocardial Blood Flow Radiotracers

Rubidium-82

Several positron-emitting radionuclides have been demonstrated to be useful for assessing regional myocardial blood flow.[101] Rb-82 is a monovalent cation that is generator produced and has an ultrashort half-life of 75 seconds.[102]

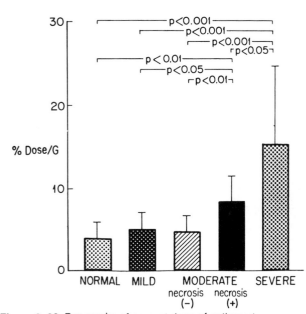

Figure 2–32. Bar graphs of percent dose of antimyosin per gram of grafted heart compared with histologic degree of rejection. Mice with moderate rejection were divided into groups according to absence (−) or presence (+) of myocyte necrosis. Mice with severe rejection showed a greater percent dose per gram than any other group. (Isobe M, et al.: Circulation 1991;84:1246–1255.)

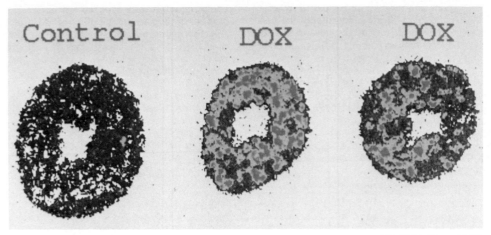

Figure 2–34. Audioradiographs of excised hearts in control rats and doxorubicin-treated rats *(middle* and *right)* after administration of indium-111 antimyosin antibody. A higher uptake of radioactivity in the heart is depicted by the red color, and a lower uptake by the blue color. (See Color Figure 2–34.) (Hiro EM, et al.: Circulation 1992;86:1965–1972.)

See Color Figure 2–34.

Sr-82 is the parent isotope in the generator system producing Rb-82. This generator has almost no breakthrough of strontium and is eluted with normal saline. Because of the short half-life of Rb-82, serial evaluations of regional myocardial perfusion can be made at intervals as short as 5 minutes. After intravenous injection, it takes the tracer between 60 and 90 seconds to clear from the blood, after which myocardial images are acquired. Because of the short physical half-life, doses as large as 50 to 60 mCi are required to achieve good count statistics. The first-pass extraction of Rb-82 at rest is approximately 50% to 60%, and extraction decreases at hyperemic blood flow rates.[103] The first-pass myocardial extraction is lower than that of N-13 ammonia and Tl-201, yet myocardial uptake is proportional to flow in the physiologic range. Rb-82 perfusion imaging is usually performed before and after vasodilator stress rather than with exercise. Infarcted myocardium does not retain intravenously administered Rb-82. After administration, it washes out rapidly from damaged myocardial cells following the initial uptake phase.[104] A mixture of reversi-

ble and irreversible myocardial tissue in the field of view results in an intermediate level of Rb-82 washout that is proportional to the percentage of viable or infarcted tissue. Comparison of Rb-82 activity in a late Rb-82 image and an early one reveals the extent of washout. A new defect or worsening of a defect on late Rb-82 images (120 to 360 seconds) as compared with early ones (15 to 110 seconds) reflects inability of damaged cells to retain Rb-82 and indicates necrosis. Figure 2–35 is a schematic of the protocol used by Gould et al.[104] for imaging the kinetic changes in myocardial Rb-82 activity to assess viability after infarction.

Tomographic data from Rb-82 images can be displayed using polar maps utilizing the bull's-eye approach with the apex located at the center and the base at the rim. Both relative and absolute flow reserve can be depicted on quantitative polar maps of Rb-82 activity.[101] In this manner, the rest and stress images are functionally interrelated. Three-dimensional (3-D) topographic displays of Rb-82 cardiac activity are more quantitative with respect to the polar

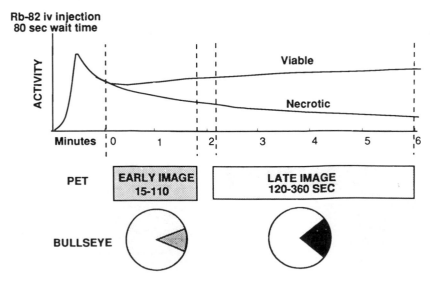

Figure 2–35. Schematic of the clinical protocol utilizing the kinetic changes of rubidium-82 after intravenous injection for assessing myocardial viability. (Reprinted by permission of the Society of Nuclear Medicine from: Gould KL, et al.: J Nucl Med 1991;32:1–9.)

maps. The 3-D topographic maps of cardiac positron emission tomographic (PET) images are derived from the short-axis data. The clinical use of Rb-82 imaging for detecting CAD and determining its extent is discussed in Chapter 8.

N-13 Ammonia

N-13 ammonia has also been utilized as an indicator of regional myocardial blood flow.[105–111] It has a half-life of 10 minutes and is produced by a cyclotron. The first-pass extraction fraction of N-13 ammonia is approximately 0.82 at normal resting flow values. As with other diffusible flow tracers, first-pass extraction diminishes with higher flows. N-13 ammonia is in the ionic form in the blood pool ($^{13}NH_4^+$) and crosses the myocardial cell membrane by passive diffusion. It then becomes metabolically trapped in the myocardium by the glutamate-glutamine reaction. First-pass extraction fraction of N-13 ammonia is slightly lower with experimental ischemia and acidosis.[110] The metabolic trapping phenomenon is not much influenced by alterations in myocardial metabolism.

For clinical imaging studies, approximately 20 mCi of N-13 ammonia is administered intravenously. As with Tl-201 and Rb-82, N-13 ammonia uptake is proportional to microsphere-determined flow but not in a linear fashion because of the roll-off at high flow rates. Figure 2–36 shows the relationship between myocardial blood flow as measured with N-13 ammonia and PET with microsphere-determined flow in dogs from the study of Shah et al.[111] Nienaber et al.[109] have described a method for quantitation of regional myocardial blood flow after intravenous injection of N-13 ammonia and rapid sequential imaging by dynamic PET. The quantitative technique has as its main feature tracer kinetic principles. The quantitative determination of flow is accomplished using an arterial sample to obtain an input function that is then combined with data from high temporal myocardial sampling to compute the index of myocardial blood flow. Concentrations of N-13–ammonia activity in blood are derived from a small region of interest located in the center of the left ventricular blood pool. The use of a two-compartment tracer kinetic model then corrects for the flow dependency of the extraction fraction, yielding an estimate of blood flow derived in vivo that correlates linearly with blood flow determined simultaneously by the microsphere approach. This model predicts progressively lower tracer extraction across a capillary membrane as the flow velocity through the capillary becomes greater. The regression equation inherent in the model permits direct conversion of observed net extraction of N-13 ammonia to blood flow, which compensates for the flow-dependent decrease in net extraction.

Kuhle et al.[110] improved on this technique of quantitating flow by using serially acquired and reoriented short-axis N-13–ammonia images rather than transaxially acquired images that limit the accuracy of regional partial volume corrections and precise localization of quantified regional flow values. Figure 2–37 shows serial short-axis images at a mid–left ventricular level, beginning with intravenous injection of N-13 ammonia from this study. Figure 2–38 depicts the comparison of calculated flow by the short-axis N-13–ammonia technique and microsphere flows from four dogs in this study that received an intravenous infusion of dipyridamole.

Muzik et al.[110a] developed a method for quantification of regional myocardial blood flow for clinical imaging with N-13 ammonia. The algorithm corrects for patient motion, provides automated definition of multiple regions, and displays absolute blood flows in polar map format. The automated region definition algorithm correlated well with the manually derived regions of interest. N-13-ammonia activity in the posterolateral wall is lower than in the septum.[110c] In this study the septum:posterolateral wall activity ratio

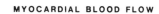

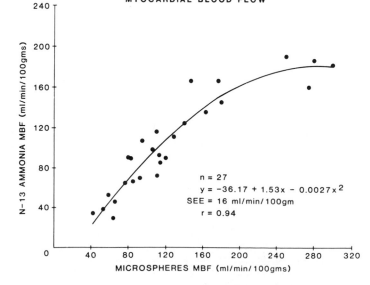

Figure 2–36. Relation between regional myocardial blood flow (MBF) determined by the microsphere technique and N-13 ammonia with PET in chronically instrumented dogs. (Reprinted with permission from the American College of Cardiology (Journal of the American College of Cardiology, 1985, Vol. 5, pp. 92–100).)

MYOCARDIAL BLOOD FLOW

N-13 AMMONIA MBF (ml/min/100gms)

MICROSPHERES MBF (ml/min/100gms)

n = 27
$y = -36.17 + 1.53x - 0.0027x^2$
SEE = 16 ml/min/100gm
r = 0.94

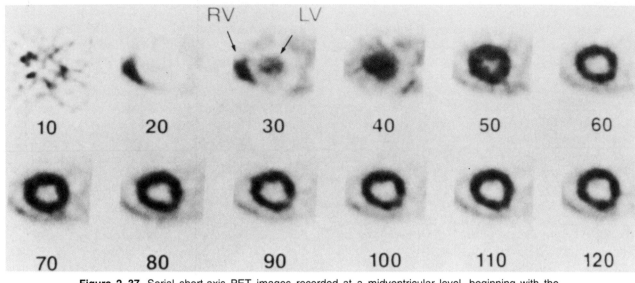

Figure 2–37. Serial short-axis PET images recorded at a midventricular level, beginning with the intravenous injection of N-13 ammonia. The number under each image indicates the elapsed time in seconds after tracer injection. The 30-second image illustrates the transit of the tracer through the right and left ventricles (RV, LV). (Reprinted by permission of the American College of Cardiology (Journal of the American College of Cardiology, 1992, Vol. 86, pp. 1007–1017).)

was 1.15 ± 0.07 in 28 normal volunteers. The percent maximal activity for N-13–ammonia in the inferior wall was greater than in the anterior and lateral walls. It was postulated that this increased inferior wall activity was due to cross-contamination of activity from the liver.

Oxygen-15 Water

Oxygen-15–labeled water (O-15 water) can be used quantitatively with PET for assessment of myocardial blood flow.[112–118c] O-15–labeled water is a positron-emitting flow tracer that is independent of metabolism with respect to

myocardial uptake. Its first-pass extraction fraction approaches 100%. It has an ultrashort half-life of 2 minutes, which requires that large doses of activity be administered. O-15 water is not only concentrated in the myocardium but is distributed into the blood pool, so blood pool activity must be accurately subtracted to assess myocardial O-15–water uptake. The blood pool subtraction utilizing O-15–carbon monoxide blood pool imaging is required (Fig. 2–39).

The intravenous method of O-15–water imaging has been well described.[116] After collection of attenuation data, 0.5 mCi/kg of O-15 water is injected as a bolus through a large-bore catheter inserted into an antecubital vein. Data

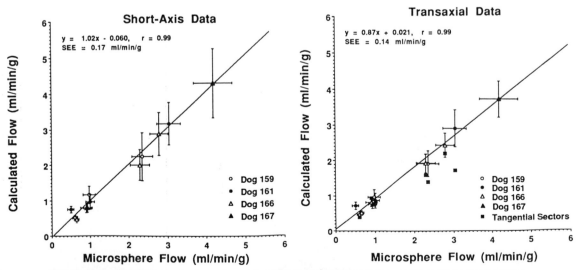

Figure 2–38. Comparison of microsphere blood flows and calculated flow using N-13 ammonia tomographic imaging utilizing reorientation and short-axis data. Plots of 12 flow points derived from the short-axis images are shown, one point for each experiment, each point being an average of 20 to 24 sectors. (Reprinted by permission of the American College of Cardiology (Journal of the American College of Cardiology, 1992, Vol. 86, pp. 1007–1017).)

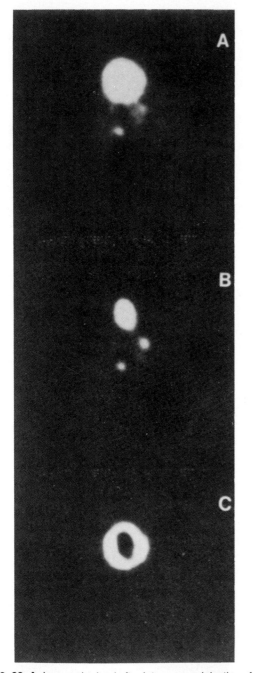

Figure 2–39. A. Image obtained after intravenous injection of O-15–labeled water in a dog experiment. The image depicts activity in myocardium, left ventricular blood pool, and lungs. **B.** Image recorded after inhalation of O-15–labeled carbon monoxide, which labels to red blood cells and depicts the left ventricular blood pool, aorta, and inferior vena cava. **C.** The blood pool activity has been subtracted from the myocardial activity, yielding an image outlining the O-15 activity in the left ventricular myocardium. (Schelbert HR: Semin Nucl Med 1987;17:145–181.)

collection is instituted at the start of infusion for 150 seconds in list mode, and with time-of-flight correction. After a 5-minute interval to allow decay of the tracer to baseline level, the subject inhales 40 to 50 mCi of O-15–labeled carbon monoxide to label the blood pool. The procedure can be repeated with intravenous infusion of dipyridamole.

For flow quantitation in experimental animals, a one-compartment mathematical model was used and the arterial input function and tissue radioactivity were directly measured.[112] Bergmann et al. have refined this technique to accurately measure absolute blood flow in humans by correcting for partial volume, spillover, and motion effects.[113] Figure 2–40 shows myocardial blood flow at rest and after administration of dipyridamole in 11 human volunteers from this study.

Shelton et al.[118a] assessed myocardial nutrient perfusion with PET and O-15 water before and after intravenous injection of dipyridamole and compared results with measurements of flow velocity reserve assessed in coronary conductance vessels determined at the time of catheterization using intracoronary Doppler probes. Perfusion reserve (ratio of absolute values of flow after dipyridamole to resting basal flow) estimated by PET correlated closely with flow velocity reserve using the Doppler wire (Fig. 2–41). Bol et al.[118b] compared N-13–ammonia uptake and O-15–water uptake with microsphere-determined flow values in the same experimental animals. Estimates of flow in absolute terms obtained noninvasively with PET tracers correlated closely over a wide range of flows. This good agreement was found in areas of high and low flows as well as in zones of infarction.

Myocardial blood flow with O-15–labeled water can also

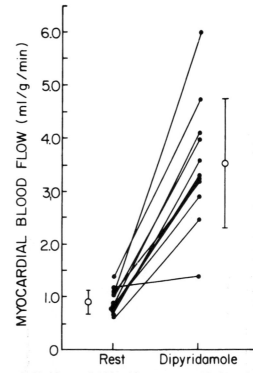

Figure 2–40. Myocardial blood flow, at rest and after administration of dipyridamole, in 11 human volunteers. Flow was measured with O-15–labeled water. After dipyridamole, the flow response was variable but increased to an average of 3.55 ± 1.15 ml/g/min. The resting flow averaged 0.90 ± 0.22 ml/g/min. (Reprinted by permission of the American College of Cardiology (Journal of the American College of Cardiology, 1989, Vol. 14, pp. 639–652).)

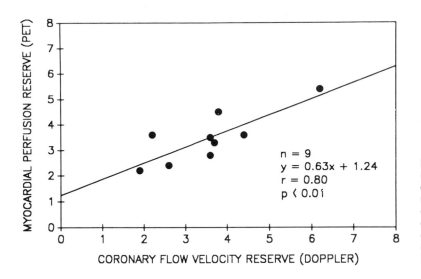

Figure 2–41. Correlation between myocardial perfusion reserve estimated by PET imaging with O-15–water under conditions of rest and after administration of intravenous dipyridamole and coronary flow velocity reserve estimated with an intracoronary Doppler flow probe under conditions of rest and after administration of intracoronary adenosine. (Reprinted by permission of the Society of Nuclear Medicine from: Shelton ME, et al: J Nucl Med 1993;34:717–722.)

be undertaken following inhalation of O-15–labeled carbon dioxide and rapid dynamic scanning. This technique involves continuous inhalation of O-15–labeled carbon dioxide, which is transformed into O-15–labeled water by the lung's carbonic anhydrase. In experimental studies, there was a good correlation between regional blood flow measured with O-15 water and radioactive microspheres using this inhalation administration technique.[115] The dynamic scanning protocol employs ungated acquisition, which is initiated 30 seconds before the start of O-15–carbon dioxide inhalation, enabling measurement of background activity. Approximately 24 time frames of varying length, ranging from 5 to 30 seconds, are then obtained.

Potassium-38

Potassium-38 (K-38) is another cyclotron-produced flow tracer employed with PET imaging. Melon et al. showed that high-quality myocardial images could be obtained with K-38.[115a] It has a 7.6-minute half-life, permitting rest and stress images to be acquired in a short time period. As with other extractable flow tracers, a plateau in myocardial uptake occurs at flows 1.6 times normal.[115a]

Positron-Emitting Tracers of Myocardial Metabolism

A major contribution of PET imaging is the ability to noninvasively evaluate regional myocardial metabolism with short-lived positron-emitting tracers. This has permitted radionuclide assessment of myocardial viability in patients with depressed myocardial function. Fatty acid and glucose metabolism can be evaluated separately, often in conjunction with assessing perfusion using blood flow tracers. The use of these tracers for clinical imaging of myocardial viability is discussed in Chapter 9.

Carbon-11–Labeled Palmitate

The uptake and tissue metabolism of carbon-11 (C-11) palmitate yields quantitative data on myocardial fatty acid metabolism in both normal and ischemic myocardium.[119–124] The C-11 label is in the 1 position of the 16-carbon fatty acid chain of palmitate. The initial myocardial uptake after intravenous injection reflects regional myocardial blood flow. The first-pass extraction fraction is approximately 0.67 at normal flow rates. After entering the cell by passive diffusion transport, C-11 palmitate is esterified to C-11 acyl-co enzyme A. This esterification competes with back-diffusion of nonmetabolized C-11 palmitate in the vascular pool. After intracellular sequestration, a portion of esterified C-11 palmitate undergoes beta oxidation in the mitochondria, a process that cleaves two carbon fragments from the long carbon chain, which then enters the tricarboxylic acid cycle and is oxided to carbon dioxide and water. Another fraction of the esterified C-11 palmitate is deposited as triglycerides and phospholipids in the lipid pool of the myocardium.

After intravenous injection, rapid dynamic images are recorded, which identify the initial bolus of C-11 palmitate in transit through the central circulation, followed by radiotracer uptake in the myocardium and then imaging the clearance of regional activity over time. Studies have shown that the clearance pattern from the myocardium is biexponential and the shape of the clearance curve corresponds to the metabolic disposition of C-11 palmitate in myocardial tissue, which in turn reflects the status of myocardial fatty acid metabolism.[119] There is a rapid-clearance component of the curve, which is thought to correspond to oxidation of the C-11 palmitate. A decrease in the size and slope of this rapid-clearance component occurs when there is a shift of fatty acid oxidation to an increase in glucose oxidation. The rapid-clearance curve also is altered in response to physiologic phenomena such as an increase in cardiac work and, thus, oxygen consumption. The slope of the clearance phase, often designated k_2, is representative of the deposition of C-11 palmitate in the endogenous lipid pool.

As expected, myocardial ischemia and hypoxia affect the clearance curve, which is characterized by a decrease in the slope and the relative size of the early washout component. This is indicative of impairment of fatty acid oxidation and the enhanced fatty acid deposition in the lipid pool associated with such insults.

Fluorine-18 2-Deoxyglucose

Fluorine-18 (F-18) 2-fluoro 2-deoxyglucose (FDG) is a glucose analog that is employed to assess glucose metabolism in the myocardium.[123, 125–128a] This radiotracer initially is taken up in myocardial cells and is trapped by conversion to FDG 6-phosphate. Unlike glucose 6-phosphate, FDG is not a substrate for glycolysis and is not used in glycogen synthesis. FDG 6-phosphate is impermeable to the cell membrane and remains within the cells at high concentrations for more than 40 to 60 minutes. Thus, it does not enter the pentose shunt. The transmembrane exchange in the initial metabolic step of FDG uptake in the myocardium has been well described. It diffuses across the capillary membrane and sarcolemmal membrane in proportion to the glucose concentration. In the cell, it competes with glucose for hexokinase and is phosphorylated to F-18 2-fluoro 2-deoxyglucose-6-phosphate. The phosphorylated form of FDG dwells in intracellular spaces in proportion to glucose concentration, so enough time is available for myocardial imaging. The magnitude of FDG activity on positron images is indicative of the rate of myocardial glucose consumption. PET images of the relative distribution of FDG uptake are obtained about 40 to 50 minutes after tracer injection, when the plateau phase of trapping is usually attained. Under conditions of ischemia, there is increased FDG uptake, presumably reflecting the substrate utilization

in the glycolytic pathway.[129–134] A tracer kinetic model can be employed for quantifying the regional rate of exogenous myocardial glucose use in animals and humans employing PET FDG imaging.[126] The clinical utility of FDG imaging for determining myocardial viability is reviewed in detail in Chapter 9.

Carbon-11 Acetate

Carbon-11 (C-11) acetate and dynamic PET imaging have been utilized for the noninvasive evaluation of regional myocardial oxidative metabolism.[135–147] The first-pass myocardial extraction fraction for C-11 acetate is high (64%), indicating that the initial distribution in the myocardium is proportional to myocardial blood flow.[139] After being extracted intracellularly, C-11 acetate is converted to acetyl-CoA, enters the tricarboxylic acid cycle, and is then oxidized to carbon dioxide and water. After the initial rapid accumulation phase in the myocardium, the tracer clears from the heart in a biexponential fashion, chiefly in the form of C-11–labeled carbon dioxide. The slope of the rapid-clearance curve component correlates well with myocardial oxygen consumption. Armbrecht et al.[139] found that C-11 acetate clearance is homogeneous in the left ventricular myocardium. The rate constants, K_1, which is obtained from biexponential fitting, and k_{mono}, which is obtained by monoexponential fitting of the initial linear portion of the time activity curves, correlate well with the rate-pressure product. Figure 2–42 shows regression plots of correlation between rate constants for the rapid C-11–acetate clearance phase (k_1) and myocardial oxygen consumption (MVO$_2$) from the study of Armbrecht et al.[139] Most investigators have suggested using monoexponential fitting of the short linear portion of the first exponential to assess regional myocardial oxygen consumption rather than using biexponential curve fitting. Figure 2–43 shows sequential cross-sectional images of myocardial C-11 activity after intrave-

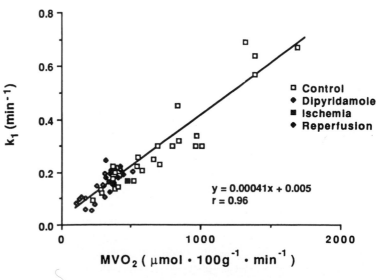

Figure 2–42. Regression plot of correlation between rate constants for the rapid C-11–acetate clearance phase (k_1) and myocardial oxygen consumption (MVO$_2$) in open-chest dogs under various conditions depicted by the symbols. C-11 acetate was injected directly into the left anterior descending coronary artery, and myocardial tissue–time activity curves were recorded with a gamma probe. As shown, the rate constant (k_1) for the rapid-clearance phase correlated closely with myocardial oxygen consumption in control, ischemia, reperfusion, and dipyridamole-induced hyperemia groups. (Armbrecht JJ, et al.: Circulation 1990;81:1594–1605.)

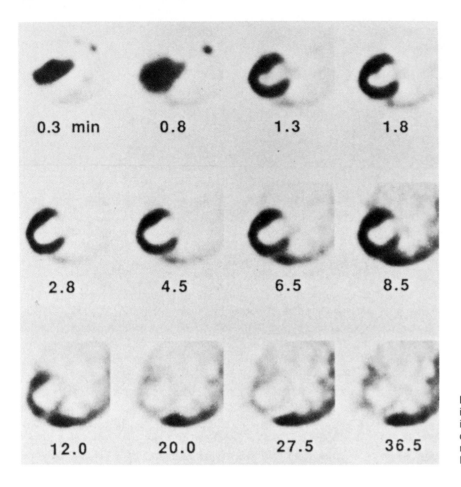

Figure 2–43. Sequential cross-sectional PET images of myocardial carbon-11 activity after intravenous injection of C-11 acetate in a closed-chest dog. Times under images are midacquisition times. (Buxton DB, et al.: Circulation 1989;79:134–142.)

nous administration of C-11 acetate in a closed-chest dog in the study of Buxton et al.[136] The 30-second image shows C-11 activity mostly in the left ventricular blood pool. Maximal myocardial activity was observed at 60 to 90 seconds after injection of the tracer. Washout is then rapid, so the myocardium is only faintly visible at 30 minutes postinjection.

In summary, PET imaging of C-11–acetate uptake and clearance provides a technique that combines evaluation of regional myocardial blood flow and regional rates of oxidative metabolism with just a single injection of a radiotracer. Clinical studies employing this tracer to evaluate regional myocardial viability are reviewed in Chapter 9.

Tracers for Assessment of Cardiac Sympathetic Nerves

Certain radiolabeled catecholamine analogs have been evaluated for the imaging of sympathetic nerve endings employing various radionuclide technologies. PET imaging of F-18 metaraminol (FMR) is an investigative approach for sympathetic nervous system imaging.[148] The retention of FMR in an open-chest canine model was determined by Schwaiger et al.[148] by assessing regional myocardial F-18-FMR concentrations after coronary occlusion and reperfu-sion. Myocardial F-18 activity reduction after reperfusion paralleled the reduction in tissue norepinephrine concentration. This agent is impractical for use in humans because of its relatively low specific activity, and the high concentration of metaraminol required for imaging may exert an unwanted pharmacologic effect.

Carbon-11 hydroxyephedrine (C-11 HED) is another physiologic tracer of norepinephrine activity that may be capable of functionally evaluating the cardiac sympathetic nervous system.[149] Uptake of C-11 HED by the heart is high, yielding a satisfactory heart-background ratio providing good image quality. Schwaiger et al.[149–151] found a heart-to-blood rate of 6:1 at 30 minutes after tracer injection. Figure 2–44 shows cross-sectional PET images in a normal volunteer after infusion of 20 mCi of C-11 HED and 60 mCi of Rb-82. One study by Wolpers et al.[150] showed that C-11 HED uptake was reduced in ischemic myocardial regions with no pathologic evidence of necrosis. This may reflect sympathetic nerve dysfunction in reversibly injured myocardium, which may be a potential mechanism of arrhythmias. Allman et al.[150a] performed PET imaging with C-11 HED in patients who had experienced a first acute MI and found that C-11 HED defects were larger than the flow deficit (assessed by N-13 ammonia) in cases of non–Q-wave infarction. In Q-wave infarct patients, ex-

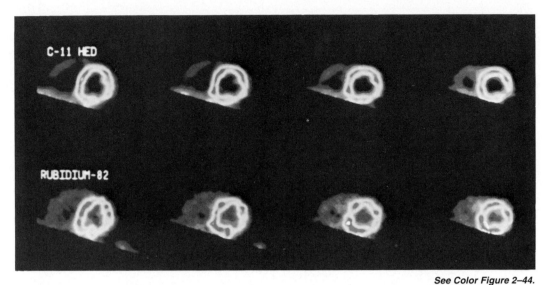

Figure 2–44. Cross-sectional PET images of the left ventricle of a normal volunteer after administration of rubidium-82 and C-11 HED. The C-11 HED images were acquired 30 to 40 minutes after intravenous tracer injection. (See Color Figure 2–44.) (Schwaiger M, et al.: Circulation 1990;82:457–464.)

tent of flow and C-11 HED abnormalities were comparable (Fig. 2–45). Melon et al.[150c] found markedly reduced myocardial retention of C-11 HED in dogs receiving intravenous cocaine. Calkins et al.[151] utilized C-11 HED imaging to assess cardiac sympathetic innervation in patients with the familial long QT syndrome. They found that patients with the long QT syndrome had normal cardiac sympathetic innervation. The authors concluded that if a decrease in right sympathetic activity is present in patients with familial long QT syndrome, it is unlikely to be attributed to an abnormal distribution of cardiac sympathetic nerves.

Merlet et al.[152] reported that C-11 CGP-12177 (CGP) has the potential to noninvasively assess β-adrenergic receptor density in the heart. Using this technique a 53% decrease in left ventricular concentration of β receptors was seen in patients with heart failure and idiopathic cardiomyopathy.

Goldstein and coworkers evaluated the utility of another catecholamine analog, F-18 fluorodopamine, for assessing cardiac sympathetic innervation and function.[153] After intravenous injection of this agent in normal animals, there was intense positron emission from the heart, as well as from the kidneys, liver, spleen, and salivary glands. With desipramine pretreatment, F-18 fluorodopamine uptake was significantly decreased. The experimental data from this study suggest that the sympathetic nerve terminals were labeled with this tracer. The agent successfully visualized left ventricular myocardium in humans without hemodynamic effects. Bromine-76 metabromobenzylguanidine (Br-76 MBBG) is another tracer shown to be capable of mapping sympathetic nerves of the heart.[153a] In both rats and dogs, myocardial uptake of this agent was avid. In rats, uptake was inhibited by desipramine. In summary, imaging of car-

diac sympathetic innervation is an exciting and innovative noninvasive approach to assessing the sympathetic nervous system in the heart, and it holds promise for having clinical utility.

Nitrogen-13 L-Glutamate

Certain abnormalities of myocardial amino acid metabolism occur in patients with CAD, particularly during episodes of ischemia. Glutamate is the only amino acid that has a positive arterial-venous difference in the human coronary circulation. This arterial-venous difference is greater in patients with CAD than in normal controls.[154] N-13 L-glutamate rapidly accumulates in myocardium after intravenous injection.[155] In areas of previous infarction, there is diminution of N-13–glutamate uptake, which correlates well with persistent Tl-201 defects in these regions. In patients with stress-induced ischemia, an inverse relationship between N-13–glutamate uptake and Tl-201 uptake has been observed.[156] Augmented accumulation of N-13 glutamate was seen in viable but reversibly injured myocardium. These authors have suggested that PET imaging of N-13 glutamate uptake may be useful for differentiating between viable and metabolically active myocardium from irreversibly damaged tissue.

Copper-62 Pyruvaldehyde bis (N-4 Methylthiosemicarbazone) Copper (II)

Copper-62 pyruvaldehyde bis (N-4 methylthiosemicarbazone) copper (II) (Cu-62 PTSM) (half-life 9.7 minutes)

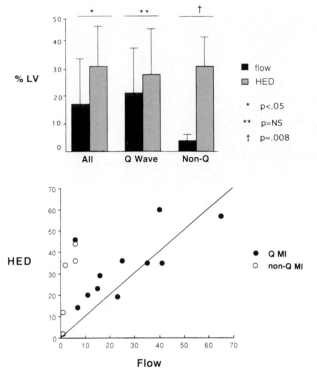

Figure 2–45. Extent of neuronal and flow abnormalities for imaging studies performed early after myocardial infarction in 16 patients. C-11 HED defects were larger, overall, than myocardial infarct size defined from N-13 ammonia flow images. In lower panel B is the scatter plot for individual patients, showing that non–Q-wave myocardial infarction patients showed C-11 HED abnormalities that were more extensive than that for flow. (Reprinted with permission of the American College of Cardiology (Journal of the American College of Cardiology, 1993, Vol. 22, pp. 368–375).)

is a generator-produced lipophilic compound that clears rapidly from the blood, yielding a high heart-lung ratio. This radionuclide is obtained from a zinc (Zn)-62–copper (Cu)-62 generator, eliminating the need for a cyclotron for flow assessment using PET. In isolated, perfused hearts, this agent is extracted by the myocardium with an extraction fraction of 0.45 throughout a wide range of conditions such as normal physiologic flow, ischemia, and hypoxia.[157] Interestingly, in the isolated heart, the extraction of Cu-62 PTSM was unaltered despite flows rising to the hyperemic range at 200% of normal. Shelton et al.[158] showed that good quality tomographic images could be obtained after intravenous administration of Cu-62 PTSM in dogs. The regional uptake of this agent in their studies corresponded closely with myocardial perfusion delineated by O-15–labeled water. Beanlands et al.[159] showed that good Cu-62 PTSM images could be obtained in humans at rest and after adenosine; however, there was only a 1.97-fold increase in activity between rest and adenosine (Fig. 2–46). The clearance half-time was 105 ±49 minutes at rest and 101 ±65 minutes following adenosine. Herrero et al.[160] estimated perfusion with Cu-62 PTSM using a two-compartment kinetic model from dynamic blood and tissue time-activity curves, along with the model parameter k_1 and the PET

parameter F_{BM} (the fraction of blood pool activity observed in tissue). Arterial blood activity was corrected for red blood cell–associated Cu-62. In a canine model, perfusion by Cu-62 PTSM correlated well ($r = 0.94$) with microsphere flow over a flow range of 0.23 to 6.14 ml/g/min (Fig. 2–47).

Fluorine-18 Fluoromisonidazole

F-18 fluoromisonidazole may have potential as an imaging agent for labeling hypoxic myocardium.[161–166] The agent accumulates in myocardium in inverse proportion to myocardial blood flow.[157] The ratios of binding to that of nonischemic tissue was 1.8:2.4 in myocardium where regional flow was reduced to 10% to 60% of normal. The compound binds covalently in viable myocardial cells inversely proportional to the partial pressure of oxygen (PO_2).[161] Cerqueira et al.[165] found increased binding of tritiated fluoromisonidazole in isolated rat myocytes exposed to anoxic conditions. They reported that binding of this agent was increased more than 10-fold by 180 minutes. Shelton et al.[162] reported that the biologic half-life of F-18 fluoromisonidazole was 40 hours in isolated perfused rabbit hearts rendered ischemic by lowering flow to 10% of control value, suggesting virtually irreversible binding. These authors found that F-18 fluoromisonidazole accumulates in myocardium in relation to diminished tissue oxygen content and not merely in relation to a reduction in flow. Figure 2–48 shows the residual fraction of F-18 activity in rabbit hearts subjected to ischemia or hypoxia as compared with control dogs from this study.[162] Further studies by Shelton et al.[163] in intact dogs demonstrated marked enhancement of extraction of F-18 fluoromisonidazole early after onset of acute ischemia (within 3 hours of occlusion) compared to 24 hours after coronary occlusion. Martin et al.[164] also found increased tissue uptake of F-18 fluoromisonidazole in dogs subjected to acute ischemia with pathologic confirmation that the enhanced uptake was not in the zone of necrosis. The agent also was taken up in myocardium perfused by a severely stenotic artery in another group of animals studied. Figure 2–49 shows serial PET images in one of the animals rendered ischemic in this study. Residual F-18–fluoromisonidazole activity can be seen in the 2-hour and 4-hour images in the anterior wall and apex.

An iodinated analog of misonidazole, iodovinylmisonidazole (IVM), labeled with I-131 showed regional deposition in ischemic myocardium that was inversely related to blood flow in dogs with an LAD stenosis receiving a catecholamine infusion to cause demand-type ischemia.[166a] The maximum tissue:blood ratio was 3.2, suggesting that this agent is also a potential marker for myocardial hypoxia. Similarly, Tc-99m–nitroimidazole (BMS181321) is trapped in zones of ischemia and hypoxia but is washed out rapidly from stunned myocardium.[166b]

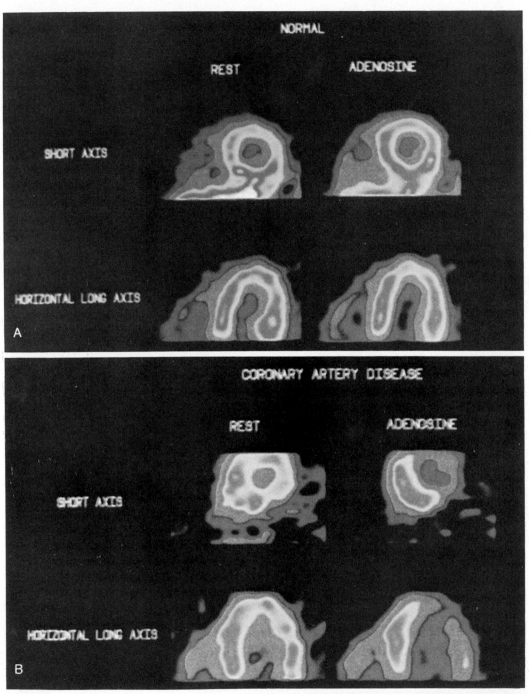

See Color Figure 2–46.

Figure 2–46. A. Example of Cu-62-PTSM studies in a normal volunteer showing short-axis and horizontal long-axis views at rest *(left)* and following adenosine-induced vasodilation *(right)* employing PET imaging. Note the good image quality. **B.** An example of Cu-62-PTSM tomographic studies in a patient with two-vessel coronary artery disease. Note that perfusion abnormalities in anterior, lateral, and apical walls are consistent with impaired flow reserve in these regions. (See Color Figure 2–46.) (Reprinted by permission of the Society of Nuclear Medicine from: Beanlands RSB: J Nucl Med 1992;33:684–690.)

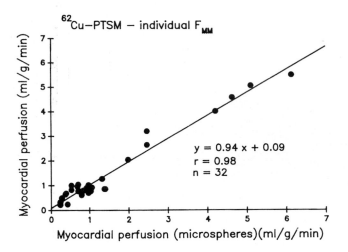

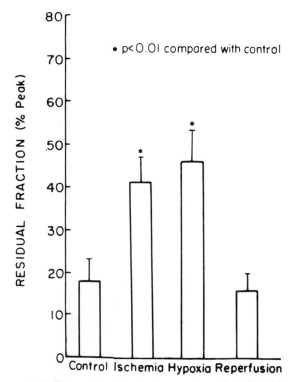

Figure 2–47. Plot showing relationship between myocardial blood flow by Cu-62 PTSM and microsphere-determined blood flow in intact dogs evaluated over a wide range of myocardial blood flow values. Note the excellent correlation between flow derived from Cu-62 PTSM and microsphere-derived flows. (Herrero P, et al.: Circulation 1993;87:173–183.)

INDIUM-111 PLATELET SCINTIGRAPHY

Autologous platelets can be labeled successfully with indium-111 and used for imaging left ventricular thrombi.[167] Most patients are imaged at least 48 hours after labeled platelet injection. The 173- and 247-keV gamma-photon peaks of indium-111 are counted for this imaging procedure. A study is defined as positive when a discrete area of intracardiac activity is clearly greater than that in the background blood pool in at least two planar views. The technique has also been used to detect coronary artery thrombi[168] and platelet deposition in saphenous vein bypass grafts.[169] A positive In-111 left ventricular platelet scan predicts increased risk of systemic embolism and is more specific than echocardiography for predicting future embolic events.[170]

IODINE-123 METAIODOBENZYLGUANIDINE SCINTIGRAPHY

Radiolabeled metaiodobenzylguanidine (MIBG), an analog of norepinephrine, concentrates in adrenergic neurons and has been used for scintigraphic assessment of regional cardiac adrenergic innervation.[171–183b] I-123 MIBG resides predominantly in the adrenergic neurons of the heart, and changes in concentrations of this agent reflect integrity of the nerves or their function. MIBG, although it shares with norepinephrine the same uptake, storage, and release mechanisms in adrenergic nerve terminals, does not get metabolized by catechol-*o*-methyltransferase and monoamine oxidase and, thus, it has great potential as a noninvasive tool for assessment of adrenergic nerve activity in pathologic cardiovascular states in vivo. Sisson et al.[172] reported that the uptake of I-123 MIBG is inhibited by the tricyclic drug, imipramine, which has also been shown to accelerate the loss of MIBG.

I-123 MIBG scintigraphy can identify the presence of denervation and subsequent reinnervation of sympathetic nerves in the myocardium. Maximum uptake of the tracer reflects the neuron density in the heart. Minardo et al.[173] showed that denervation occurring after phenol application or after transmural myocardial infarction produced defects on I-123 MIBG scans. Henderson et al.[174] found that I-123 MIBG activity was reduced in hearts of patients with

Figure 2–48. The residual fraction (percentage of peak activity retained in the myocardium) for control hearts, hearts subjected to ischemia, hearts subjected to hypoxia, and hearts subjected to reperfusion. Residual fraction of fluorine-18 fluoromisonidazole was higher in ischemic and hypoxic hearts than in control hearts and hearts subjected to ischemia followed by reperfusion. (Reprinted by permission of the Society of Nuclear Medicine from: Shelton ME, et al.: J Nucl Med 1989;30:351–358.)

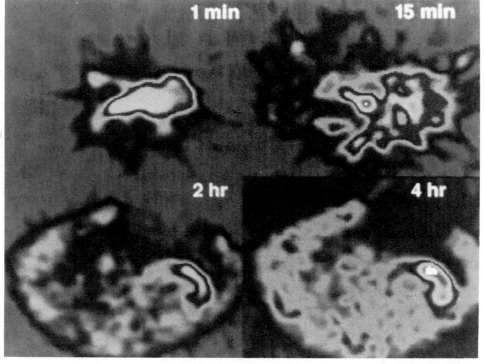

Figure 2–49. Serial PET images of fluorine-18 fluoromisonidazole uptake in ischemic anterior wall myocardium in a dog with ischemia in the territory of the left anterior descending coronary artery. The images represent a cross section through the chest cavity that is roughly parallel to the long axis of the heart. The septum is on the left, whereas the apex of the left ventricle is to the right. One minute after injection, the tracer is concentrated in the blood pool. The 2- and 4-hour postinjection images show some enhancement of activity in the distal anterior wall and apex of the left ventricle. (See Color Figure 2–49.) (Reprinted by permission of the Society of Nuclear Medicine from: Martin GV, et al.: J Nucl Med 1992;33:2202–2208.)

See Color Figure 2–49.

congestive cardiomyopathy, a finding consistent with the known alteration in sympathetic innervation in this patient population. Figure 2–50 depicts short-axis tomograms from a control patient and a patient with cardiomyopathy in this study. The control patient's images show a higher intensity of MIBG uptake. Similarly, I-123 MIBG accumulation is decreased in adriamycin-induced cardiomyopathy.[180] Cardiac MIBG heart-mediastinum ratio was shown to have prognostic value in patients with congestive heart failure. Merlet et al.[179] found that by multivariate stepwise regression analysis, cardiac MIBG uptake was a more potent predictor of survival than other indices. Cardiac sympathetic denervation, as assessed by I-123–MIBG imaging, was observed in 67% of 18 patients with ventricular tachycardia in absence of CAD, as compared with 8% in 12 patients without ventricular tachycardia.[181] In this study, regional cardiac sympathetic denervation was identified in 55% of patients whose heart was structurally normal. Similarly, Wichter et al.[182] reported localized sympathetic denervation in patients with arrhythmogenic right ventricular cardiomyopathy.

IODINE-LABELED FATTY ACID IMAGING

Of all of the radioactive iodine–labeled fatty acids evaluated for myocardial imaging, iodine-123 (I-123) phenylpentadecanoic acid (IPPA) has proven the most clinically applicable for patient imaging with SPECT.[184–189] I-123

IPPA is a synthetic long-chain fatty acid with myocardial kinetics similar to those of palmitate. The metabolism of I-123 IPPA does not result in liberation of free iodine, as occurred with hexadecanoic and heptadecanoic acids labeled with I-123. The metabolism of I-123 IPPA follows a biexponential clearance curve that is similar to what is described for palmitate.[184] Studies at the University of Texas, Southwestern have shown that IPPA is reduced in regions of infarction, whereas clearance of the tracer is prolonged relative to normal in peri-infarction zones.[185, 186] For human imaging, approximately 6 to 8 mCi of IPPA is injected 1 minute before termination of maximal symptom-limited exercise testing. Imaging commences approximately 9 minutes after tracer injection and is repeated 40 minutes later. Diminished initial uptake of I-123 IPPA is seen in zones of prior myocardial infarction and in areas perfused by severely stenotic coronary arteries. Delayed IPPA washout is seen in areas of myocardial ischemia. The explanation for the decreased washout is reduced beta oxidation with an increased percentage of fatty acids being incorporated as intracellular triglycerides. Reduced beta oxidation occurs because of shunting toward glucose metabolism with ischemia.

Murray et al.[187] assessed the utility of I-123 IPPA for determining myocardial viability in patients with a depressed left ventricular ejection fraction. They found that 73% of akinetic or dyskinetic segments exhibited preserved uptake of I-123 IPPA. Of these, 80% showed improved regional systolic function after revascularization. I-123

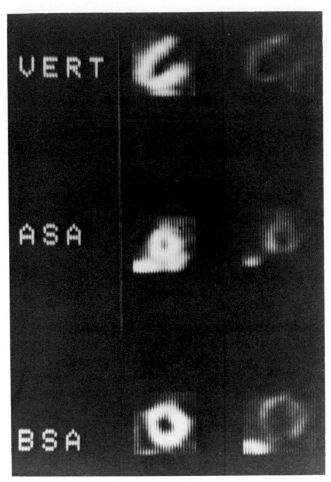

Figure 2–50. SPECT tomograms obtained after 85 minutes from a control subject *(left)* and a patient with cardiomyopathy *(right)* after administration of MIBG. The control subject exhibited more intense MIBG uptake than the patient with cardiomyopathy. (Key: VERT, vertical long axis; ASA, apical short axis; BSA, basal short axis.) (Henderson EB, et al.: Circulation 1988;78:1192–1199.)

IPPA imaging at 4, 12, 20, 28, and 36 minutes after a resting injection can be utilized to identify abnormal myocardial metabolic activity in patients with CAD, and resting left ventricular function.[188] Asynergic regions that demonstrated improved systolic function after revascularization had delayed washout of the tracer as determined from quantitation of activity over time on the SPECT images. A further discussion of clinical studies employing I-123 IPPA can be found in Chapter 9.

Iodine-123-iodophenyl-9-methyl-pentadecanoic acid (I-123 MPDA) is a modified long-chain fatty acid with 15 carbons that differs from I-123 IPPA by having a methyl branch on its 9-carbon location. In a study by Chouraqui et al.,[189] uptake and clearance kinetics of this radionuclide were similar to those described for I-123 IPPA. Initial myocardial uptake of this agent parallels segmental Tl-201 uptake, reflecting the dependency on regional blood flow distribution. The slower than normal clearance rate of this tracer from defect zones is similar to what was described

for I-123 IPPA, and it is thought to be secondary to reduced beta oxidation consequent to ischemia. I-123 15-(p-iodophenyl)3R, S-methylpentadecanoic acid (BMIPP) has also been proposed as a fatty acid probe for myocardial fatty acid utilization.[189a] This methyl-branched fatty acid does not enter the beta-oxidation pathway. Matsunari et al.[189a] reported accelerated clearance of BMIPP in myocardial segments corresponding to reversible stress-induced Tl-201 defects in patients with CAO. These authors postulated that this relatively increased clearance could be explained by back diffusion.

TECHNETIUM-99m–LABELED FRAGMENT E₁

Tc-99m–labeled fragment E₁ is a degradation product of human cross-linked fibrin that binds specifically to fibrin polymers.[190] Previously, I-123–labeled fragment E₁ was shown to be capable of imaging thrombi in patients.[191] More recently, this agent was successfully labeled with Tc-99m and shown to produce images of venous thrombi.[192] Figure 2–51 is a scintigram of a thrombus induced in a dog's femoral vein imaged 2 hours and 4 hours after injections of Tc-99m fragment E₁.

TECHNETIUM-99m–LABELED MONOCLONAL ANTIPLATELET ANTIBODY

The hybridoma-produced Fab′ fragment of the monoclonal antibody (S12) specific for the platelet membrane glycoprotein (GMP-140) was labeled with Tc-99m and tested as an in vivo marker of local platelet activation after peripheral balloon angioplasty in patients with CAD.[193] The ratio of activity in the local angioplasty site to activity in a

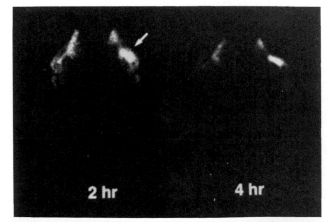

Figure 2–51. Gamma camera images of a dog with a thrombus induced in a femoral vein *(arrow)* at 2 hours and 4 hours following injection of Tc-99m fragment E₁. (Reprinted by permission of the Society of Nuclear Medicine from: Knight LC, et al.: J Nucl Med 1992;33:710–715.)

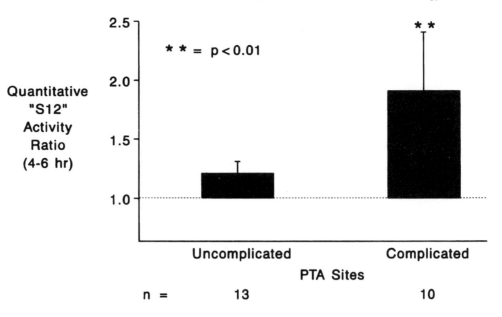

Figure 2–52. Bar graph shows Tc-99m-labeled platelet glyco-protein antibody S12 activity at complicated (*N*=10) and uncomplicated (*N*=13) percutaneous peripheral transluminal angioplasty sites at 4 and 6 hours after injection. A significant increase in quantitative S12 activity was noted in procedurally complicated sites (1.9 ±0.5 vs 1.2 ±0.1; *P*<0.01). (Miller DD, et al.: Circulation 1992;85:1354–1363.)

contralateral nonangioplasty arterial segment was 1.6 ±0.5. Vascular Tc-99m–S12 antibody activity was visually apparent in 78% of angioplasty sites at 4 to 6 hours after injection. Activity was greater in segments deemed "procedurally complicated" (ratio 1.9) than in uncomplicated segments (ratio 1.2). A summary of these results is depicted in Figure 2–52. A review of scintigraphic methods for detecting vascular thrombus by Knight is recommended.[194]

TECHNETIUM-99m-LABELED ANTI–NCA-95 ANTIGRANULOCYTE ANTIBODIES

The imaging of inflammatory valvular lesions with radiolabeled white blood cells holds promise for enhancing the diagnostic accuracy for detecting subacute infective endocarditis. Morguet et al.[195] labeled a murine monoclonal Ig G_1 antigranulocyte antibody with Tc-99m and administered a dose of 0.27 mCi/kg of body weight of the antibody to 72 consecutive patients with endocarditis. Sensitivity and specificity for endocarditis detection were 79% and 82%, respectively. The combination of scintigraphy and echocardiography yielded a sensitivity of 100% and specificity of 82%. Scintigraphy became negative on serial imaging in patients manifesting clinical improvement.

REFERENCES

1. Zaret BL, Strauss HW, Martin ND, Wells HP Jr, Flamm MD Jr: Noninvasive regional myocardial perfusion with radioactive potassium. Study of patients at rest, with exercise and during angina pectoris. N Engl J Med 1973;288:809–812.
2. Berman DS, Salel AF, DeNardo GL, Mason DT: Noninvasive detection of regional myocardial ischemia using rubidium-81 and the scintillation camera: Comparison with stress electrocardiography in patients with arteriographically documented coronary stenosis. Circulation 1975;52:619–626.
3. Mueller SP, Polak JF, Kijewski MF, Holman BL: Collimator selection for SPECT brain imaging: The advantage of high resolution. J Nucl Med 1986;27:1729–1738.
4. Lebowitz E, Greene MW, Fairchild R, Bradley-Moore PR, Atkins HL, Ansari AN, Richards P, Belgrave E: Thallium-201 for medical use. J Nucl Med 1975;16:151–155.
5. Kortüm F, Bockris J: *In* Textbook of Electrochemistry. Amsterdam, Elsevier, 1951, p 701.
6. Strauss HW, Harrison K, Langan JK, Lebowitz E, Pitt B: Thallium-201 for myocardial imaging. Relation of thallium-201 to regional myocardial perfusion. Circulation 1975;51:641–645.
7. Weich HF, Strauss HW, Pitt B: The extraction of thallium-201 by the myocardium. Circulation 1977;56:188–191.
7a. Dahlberg ST, Leppo JA: Myocardial kinetics of radiolabeled perfusion agents: Basis for perfusion imaging. J Nucl Cardiol 1994;1:189–197.
8. Leppo JA: Myocardial uptake of thallium and rubidium during alterations in perfusion and oxygenation in isolated rabbit hearts. J Nucl Med 1987;28:878–885.
9. Leppo JA, Macneil PB, Moring AF, Apstein CS: Separate effects of ischemia, hypoxia, and contractility on thallium-201 kinetics in rabbit myocardium. J Nucl Med 1986;27:66–74.
10. Friedman BJ, Beihn R, Friedman JP: The effect of hypoxia on thallium kinetics in cultured chick myocardial cells. J Nucl Med 1987;28:1453–1460.
11. McCall D, Zimmer LJ, Katz AM: Kinetics of thallium exchange in cultured rat myocardial cells. Circ Res 1985;56:370–376.
12. Melin JA, Becker LC: Quantitative relationship between global left ventricular thallium uptake and blood flow: Effects of propranolol, ouabain, dipyridamole, and coronary artery occlusion. J Nucl Med 1986;27:641–652.
13. Krivokapich J, Shine KI: Effects of hyperkalemia and glycoside on thallium exchange in rabbit ventricle. Am J Physiol 1981;240:H612–H619.
14. Okada RD, Jacobs ML, Daggett WM, Leppo J, Strauss HW, Newell JB, Moore R, Boucher CA, O'Keefe D, Pohost GM: Thallium-201 kinetics in nonischemic canine myocardium. Circulation 1982;65:70–77.
15. Grunwald AM, Watson DD, Holzgrefe HH Jr, Irving JF, Beller GA: Myocardial thallium-201 kinetics in normal and ischemic myocardium. Circulation 1981;64:610–618.
16. Moore CA, Cannon J, Watson DD, Kaul S, Beller GA: Thallium-201 kinetics in stunned myocardium characterized by severe postischemic systolic dysfunction. Circulation 1990;81:1622–1632.
17. Sinusas AJ, Watson DD, Cannon JM Jr, Beller GA: Effect of ischemia and postischemic dysfunction on myocardial uptake of technetium-99m–labeled methoxyisobutyl isonitrile and thallium-201. J Am Coll Cardiol 1989;14:1785–1793.

18. Mays AE Jr, Cobb FR: Relationship between regional myocardial blood flow and thallium-201 distribution in the presence of coronary artery stenosis and dipyridamole-induced vasodilation. J Clin Invest 1984;73:1359–1366.

19. Nielsen AP, Morris KG, Murdock R, Bruno FP, Cobb FR: Linear relationship between the distribution of thallium-201 and blood flow in ischemic and nonischemic myocardium during exercise. Circulation 1980;61:797–801.

20. Nichols AB, Weiss MB, Sciacca RR, Cannon PJ, Blood DK: Relationship between segmental thallium-201 uptake and regional myocardial blood flow in patients with coronary artery disease. Circulation 1983;68:310–320.

21. Pohost GM, Zir LM, Moore RH, McKusick KA, Guiney TE, Beller GA: Differentiation of transiently ischemic from infarcted myocardium by serial imaging after a single dose of thallium-201. Circulation 1977;55:294–302.

22. Goldhaber SZ, Newell JB, Alpert NM, Andrews E, Pohost GM, Ingwall JS: Effects of ischemic-like insult on myocardial thallium-201 accumulation. Circulation 1983;67:778–786.

23. Ingwall J, Kramer M, Klover N, et al.: Tl accumulation: Differentiation between reversible and irreversible myocardial injury (Abstract). Circulation 1979;60:678–678.

24. Beller GA, Watson DD, Ackell P, Pohost GM: Time course of thallium-201 redistribution after transient myocardial ischemia. Circulation 1980;61:791–779.

25. Shapiro W, Narahara KA, Park J: The effects of lidoflazine on exercise performance and thallium stress scintigraphy in patients with stable angina pectoris. Circulation 1982;65:I43–I50.

26. Wharton TP Jr, Neill WA, Oxendine JM, Painter LN: Effect of duration of regional myocardial ischemia and degree of reactive hyperemia on the magnitude of the initial thallium-201 defect. Circulation 1980;62:516–521.

27. Gerry JL Jr, Becker LC, Flaherty JT, Weisfeldt ML: Evidence for a flow-independent contribution to the phenomenon of thallium redistribution. Am J Cardiol 1980;45:58–61.

28. Bergmann SR, Hack SN, Sobel BE: ''Redistribution'' of myocardial thallium-201 without reperfusion: Implications regarding absolute quantification of perfusion. Am J Cardiol 1982;49:1691–1698.

29. Nishiyama H, Adolph RJ, Gabel M, Lukes SJ, Franklin D, Williams CC: Effect of coronary blood flow on thallium-201 uptake and washout. Circulation 1982;65:534–542.

30. Schelbert HR, Schuler G, Ashburn WL, Covell JW: Time-course of ''redistribution'' of thallium-201 administered during transient ischemia. Eur J Nucl Med 1979;4:351–358.

31. Pohost GM, Okada RD, O'Keefe DD, Gewirtz H, Beller G, Strauss HW, Chaffin JS, Leppo J, Daggett WM: Thallium redistribution in dogs with severe coronary artery stenosis of fixed caliber. Circ Res 1981;48:439–446.

32. Leppo J, Rosenkrantz J, Rosenthal R, Bontemps R, Yipintsoi T: Quantitative thallium-201 redistribution with a fixed coronary stenosis in dogs. Circulation 1981;63:632–639.

33. Okada RD, Leppo JA, Strauss HW, Boucher CA, Pohost GM: Mechanisms and time course for the disappearance of thallium-201 defects at rest in dogs. Relation of time to peak activity to myocardial blood flow. Am J Cardiol 1982;49:699–706.

34. Steingart RM, Bontemps R, Scheuer J, Yipintsoi T: Gamma camera quantitation of thallium-210 redistribution at rest in a dog model. Circulation 1982;65:542–550.

35. Beller GA, Watson DD, Pohost GM: Kinetics of thallium distribution and redistribution: Clinical applications in sequential myocardial imaging. In Strauss HW, Pitt B, eds. Cardiovascular Nuclear Medicine, ed 2. St. Louis, CV Mosby, 1979, pp 225–242.

36. Okada RD, Pohost GM: Effect of decreased blood flow and ischemia on myocardial thallium clearance. J Am Coll Cardiol 1984;3:744–750.

37. Okada RD: Myocardial kinetics of thallium-201 after stress in normal and perfusion-reduced canine myocardium. Am J Cardiol 1985;56:969–973.

38. Kronenberg MW, Robertson RM, Born ML, Steckley RA, Robertson D, Friesinger GC: Thallium-201 uptake in variant angina: Probable demonstration of myocardial reactive hyperemia in man. Circulation 1982;66:1332–1338.

39. Kaul S, Chesler DA, Pohost GM, Strauss HW, Okada RD, Boucher CA: Influence of peak exercise heart rate on normal thallium-201 myocardial clearance. J Nucl Med 1986;27:26–30.

40. Nordrehaug JE, Danielsen R, Vik-Mo H: Effects of heart rate on myocardial thallium-201 uptake and clearance. J Nucl Med 1989;30:1972–1976.

41. Angello DA, Wilson RA, Gee D: Effect of ribose on thallium-201 myocardial redistribution. J Nucl Med 1988;29:1943–1950.

42. Khaw BA, Strauss HW, Pohost GM, Fallon JT, Katus HA, Haber E: Relation of immediate and delayed thallium-201 distribution to localization of iodine-125 antimyosin antibody in acute experimental myocardial infarction. Am J Cardiol 1983;51:1428–1432.

43. Lear JL, Raff U, Jain R: Reverse and pseudoredistribution of thallium-201 in healed myocardial infarction and normal and negative thallium-201 washout in ischemia due to background oversubtraction. Am J Cardiol 1988;62:543–550.

44. Berman DS, Kiat H, Van Train K, Garcia E, Friedman J, Maddahi J: Technetium-99m sestamibi in the assessment of chronic coronary artery disease. Semin Nucl Med 1991;21:190–212.

45. Beller GA, Watson DD: Physiological basis of myocardial perfusion imaging with the technetium 99m agents. Semin Nucl Med 1991;21:173–181.

46. Sinusas AJ, Beller GA, Watson DD: Cardiac imaging with technetium 99m-labeled isonitriles. J Thorac Imaging 1990;5:20–30.

47. Leppo JA, DePuey EG, Johnson LL: A review of cardiac imaging with sestamibi and teboroxime. J Nucl Med 1991;32:2012–2022.

48. Liu P: New technetium 99m imaging agents: Promising windows for myocardial perfusion and viability. Am J Cardiac Imaging 1992;6:28–41.

49. Beller GA, Sinusas AJ: Experimental studies of the physiologic properties of technetium-99m isonitriles. Am J Cardiol 1990;66:5E–8E.

49a. Blackburn T, Beller G: Scintigraphic assessment of myocardial perfusion using thallium-201 and technetium-99m imaging. Coronary Artery Disease 1992;3:274–280.

49b. Maddahi J, Kiat H, Friedman JD, Berman DS, Van Train KF, Garcia EV: Technetium-99m–sestamibi myocardial perfusion imaging for evaluation of coronary artery disease. In Zaret BL, Beller GA (eds): Nuclear Cardiology: State of the Art and Future Directions. St. Louis, CV Mosby, 1993, pp 191–200.

49c. Berman DS, Kiat HS, Van Train KF, Germano G, Maddahi J, Friedman JD: Myocardial perfusion imaging with technetium-99m-sestamibi: Comparative analysis of available imaging protocols. J Nucl Med 1994;35:681–688.

50. Dudczak R, Angelberger P, Homan R, Kletter K, Schmoliner R, Frischauf H: Evaluation of ^{99m}Tc-dichloro bis (1,2-dimethylphosphino) ethane (^{99m}Tc-DMPE) for myocardial scintigraphy in man. Eur J Nucl Med 1983;8:513–515.

51. Gerundini P, Savi A, Gilardi MC, Margonato A, Vicedomini G, Zecca L, Hirth W, Libson K, Bhatia JC, Fazio F, et al.: Evaluation in dogs and humans of three potential technetium-99m myocardial perfusion agents. J Nucl Med 1986;27:409–416.

52. Holman BL, Campbell CA, Lister-James J, Jones AG, Davison A, Kloner RA: Effect of reperfusion and hyperemia on the myocardial distribution of technetium-99m t-butylisonitrile. J Nucl Med 1986;27:1172–1177.

53. Sia ST, Holman BL, McKusick K, Rigo P, Gillis F, Sporn V, Perez-Balino N, Mitta A, Vosberg H, Szabo Z, et al.: The utilization of Tc-99m-TBI as a myocardial perfusion agent in exercise studies: Comparison with Tl-201 thallous chloride and examination of its biodistribution in humans. Eur J Nucl Med 1986;12:333–336.

54. Piwnica-Worms D, Kronauge JF, Chiu ML: Uptake and retention of hexakis (2-methoxyisobutyl isonitrile) technetium(I) in cultured chick myocardial cells. Mitochondrial and plasma membrane potential dependence. Circulation 1990;82:1826–1838.

54a. Piwnica-Worms D, Chiu ML, Kronauge JF: Divergent kinetics of ^{201}Tl and ^{99m}Tc-sestamibi in cultured chick ventricular myocytes during ATP depletion. Circulation 1992;85:1531–1541.

54b. Carvalho PA, Chiu ML, Kronauge JF, Kawamura M, Jones AG, Holman BL, Piwnica-Worms D: Subcellular distribution and analysis of technetium-99m-MIBI in isolated perfused rat hearts. J Nucl Med 1992;33:1516–1521.

55. Beanlands RS, Dawood F, Wen WH, McLaughlin PR, Butany J, D'Amati G, Liu PP: Are the kinetics of technetium-99m methoxyisobutyl isonitrile affected by cell metabolism and viability? Circulation 1990;82:1802–1814.

56. Beller GA, Glover DK, Edwards NC, Ruiz M, Simanis, JP, Watson

DD: Technetium-99 sestamibi uptake and retention during myocardial ischemia and reperfusion. Circulation 1993;87:2033–2042.

57. Meerdink DJ, Leppo JA: Comparison of hypoxia and ouabain effects on the myocardial uptake kinetics of technetium-99m hexakis 2-methoxyisobutyl isonitrile and thallium-201. J Nucl Med 1989; 30:1500–1506.

58. Maublant JC, Gachon P, Moins N: Hexakis (2-methoxy isobutylisonitrile) technetium-99m and thallium-201 chloride: Uptake and release in cultured myocardial cells. J Nucl Med 1988;29:48–54.

58a. Sansoy V, Glover DK, Watson DD, Ruiz M, Smith WH, Simanis JP, Beller GA: Comparison of thallium-201 rest redistribution with technetium-99m sestamibi uptake and functional response to dobutamine for assessment of myocardial viability. Submitted to Circulation.

59. Okada RD, Glover D, Gaffney T, Williams S: Myocardial kinetics of technetium-99m-hexakis-2-methoxy-2-methylpropyl-isonitrile. Circulation 1988;77:491–498.

60. Glover DK, Okada RD: Myocardial kinetics of Tc-MIBI in canine myocardium after dipyridamole. Circulation 1990;81:628–637.

61. Melon PG, Beanlands RS, DeGrado TR, Nguyen N, Petry NA, Schwaiger M: Comparison of technetium-99m sestamibi and thallium-201 retention characteristics in canine myocardium. J Am Coll Cardiol 1992;20:1277–1283.

62. Glover DK, Ruiz M, Cunningham M, Edwards NC, Simanis JP, Smith W, Watson DD, Beller GA: Comparison between thallium-201 and Tc-99m sestamibi uptake during adenosine-induced vasodilation as a function of coronary stenosis severity. Circulation 1994 (in press).

63. Leon AR, Eisner RL, Martin SE, Schmarkey LS, Aaron AM, Boyers AS, Burnham KM, Oh DJ, Patterson RE: Comparison of single-photon emission computed tomographic (SPECT) myocardial perfusion imaging with thallium-201 and technetium-99m sestamibi in dogs. J Am Coll Cardiol 1992;20:1612–1625.

64. Canby RC, Silber S, Pohost GM: Relations of the myocardial imaging agents 99mTc-MIBI and 201Tl to myocardial blood flow in a canine model of myocardial ischemic insult. Circulation 1990;81:289–296.

64a. Glover DK, Okada RD: Myocardial technetium 99m sestamibi kinetics after reperfusion in a canine model. Am Heart J 1993;125:657–666.

65. Leppo JA, Meerdink DJ: Comparison of the myocardial uptake of a technetium-labeled isonitrile analogue and thallium. Circ Res 1989;65:632–639.

65a. Meerdink DJ, Leppo JA: Myocardial transport of hexakis (2-methoxyisobutylisonitrile) and thallium before and after coronary reperfusion. Circ Res 1990;66:1738–1746.

66. Marshall RC, Leidholdt EM Jr, Zhang DY, Barnett CA: Technetium-99m hexakis 2-methoxy-2-isobutyl isonitrile and thallium-201 extraction, washout, and retention at varying coronary flow rates in rabbit heart. Circulation 1990;82:998–1007.

67. Li QS, Solot G, Frank TL, Wagner HN Jr, Becker LC: Myocardial redistribution of technetium-99m methoxyisobutyl isonitrile (sestamibi). J Nucl Med 1990;31:1069–1076.

68. Sinusas A, Bergin JD, Edwards N, Watson DD, Ruiz M, Makuch RW, Smith WH, Beller GA: Redistribution of 99mTc-sestamibi and 201Tl in the presence of a severe coronary stenosis. Circulation 1994;89:2332–2341.

69. Verani MS, Jeroudi MO, Mahmarian JJ, Boyce TM, Borges-Neto S, Patel B, Bolli R: Quantification of myocardial infarction during coronary occlusion and myocardial salvage after reperfusion using cardiac imaging with technetium-99m hexakis 2-methoxyisobutyl isonitrile. J Am Coll Cardiol 1988;12:1573–1581.

70. Sinusas AJ, Trautman KA, Bergin JD, Watson DD, Ruiz M, Smith WH, Beller GA: Quantification of area at risk during coronary occlusion and degree of myocardial salvage after reperfusion with technetium-99m methoxyisobutyl isonitrile. Circulation 1990;82:1424–1437.

70a. Sinusas AJ, Shi Q-X, Vitols PJ, Fetterman RS, Maniawski P, Zaret BL, Wackers FJT: Impact of regional ventricular function, geometry and dobutamine stress on quantitative 99mTc-sestamibi defect size. Circulation 1993;88:2224–2234.

70b. Sinusas AJ, Wackers FJ Th: Assessing myocardial reperfusion with technecium-99m–labeled myocardial perfusion agents: Basic concepts and clinical applications. Am J Cardiac Imag 1993;7:24–38.

71. Leppo JA, Meerdink DJ: Comparative myocardial extraction of two technetium-labeled BATO derivatives (SQ30217, SQ32014) and thallium. J Nucl Med 1990;31:67–74.

72. Di Rocco RJ, Rumsey WL, Kuczynski BL, Linder KE, Pirro JP, Narra RK, Nunn AD: Measurement of myocardial blood flow using a co-injection technique for technetium-99m-teboroxime, technetium-96-sestamibi and thallium-201. J Nucl Med 1992;33:1152–1159.

72a. Weinstein H, Reinhardt CP, Leppo JA: Teboroxime, sestamibi and thallium-201 as markers of myocardial hypoperfusion: Comparison by quantitative dual-isotope autoradiography in rabbits. J Nucl Med 1993;34:1510–1517.

72b. Dahlberg ST. Gilmore MP, Leppo JA: Interaction of technetium-99m–labeled teboroxime with red blood cells reduces the compound's extraction and increases apparent cardiac washout. J Nucl Cardiol 1994;1:270–279.

73. Beanlands R, Muzik O, Nguyen N, Petry N, Schwaiger M: The relationship between myocardial retention of technetium-99m teboroxime and myocardial blood flow. J Am Coll Cardiol 1992;20:712–719.

74. Glover D, Ruiz M, Simanis J, Smith W, Watson D, Beller G: Comparison between Tl-201 and Tc-99m teboroxime uptake in a canine model of a coronary stenosis during pharmacologic vasodilation with adenosine (Abstract). J Nucl Med 1992;33:864–865.

75. Stewart RE, Schwaiger M, Hutchins GD, Chiao PC, Gallagher KP, Nguyen N, Petry NA, Rogers WL: Myocardial clearance kinetics of technetium-99m-SQ30217: A marker of regional myocardial blood flow. J Nucl Med 1990;31:1183–1190.

76. Stewart RE, Heyl B, O'Rourke RA, Blumhardt R, Miller DD: Demonstration of differential post-stenotic myocardial technetium-99m-teboroxime clearance kinetics after experimental ischemia and hyperemic stress. J Nucl Med 1991;32:2000–2008.

77. Gray WA, Gewirtz H: Comparison of 99mTc-teboroxime with thallium for myocardial imaging in the presence of a coronary artery stenosis. Circulation 1991;84:1796–1807.

77a. Smith AM, Gullberg GT, Christian PE, Datz FL: Kinetic modeling of teboroxime using dynamic SPECT imaging in a canine model. J Nucl Med 1994;35:484–495.

77b. Chiao P-C, Ficaro EP, Dayanikili F, Rogers WL, Schwaiger M: Compartmental analysis of technetium-99m–teboroxime kinetics employing fast dynamic SPECT at rest and stress. J Nucl Med 1994;35:1265–1273.

78. Rumsey WL, Rosenspire KC, Nunn AD: Myocardial extraction of teboroxime: Effects of teboroxime interaction with blood. J Nucl Med 1992;33:94–101.

79. Kelly JD, Forster AM, Higley B, Archer CM, Booker FS, Canning LR, Chiu KW, Edwards B, Gill HK, McPartlin M, et al.: Technetium-99m-tetrofosmin as a new radiopharmaceutical for myocardial perfusion imaging. J Nucl Med 1993;34:222–227.

79a. Dahlberg S, Gilmore M, Leppo J: Effect of coronary flow on the "uptake" of tetrofosmin in the isolated rabbit heart (Abstract). J Nucl Med 1992;33:846.

79b. Sinusas AJ, Shi QX, Saltzberg MT, Vitals P, Jain D, Wackers FJ Th, Zaret BL: Technetium-99m–tetrofosmin to assess myocardial blood flow: Experimental validation in an intact canine model of ischemia. J Nucl Med 1994;35:664–671.

79c. Nakajima K, Taki J, Shuke N, Bunko H, Takata S, Hisada K: Myocardial perfusion imaging and dynamic analysis with technetium-99m tetrofosmin. J Nucl Med 1993;34:1478–1484.

80. Gerson MC, Millard RW, Roszell NJ, et al.: Myocardial kinetics of Tc-99m Q12 in dogs (Abstract). Circulation 1992;86(suppl I):I-708.

80a. Gerson MC, Millard RW, Roszell et al: Kinetic properties of 99mTc-Q12 in canine myocardium. Circulation 1994;89:1291–1300.

81. Beller G: Nuclear cardiology: current indications and clinical usefulness. Curr Probl Cardiol 1985;10:1–76.

82. Parkey RW, Bonte FJ, Meyer SL, Atkins JM, Curry GL, Stokely EM, Willerson JT: A new method for radionuclide imaging of acute myocardial infarction in humans. Circulation 1974;50:540–546.

83. Aburano T, Taniguchi M, Hisada K, Miyazaki Y, Shiozaki J, Inoue H, Fujioka M: Aneurysmal dilatation of portal vein demonstrated on radionuclide hepatic scintiangiogram. Clin Nucl Med 1991;16:862–864.

84. Buja LM, Parkey RW, Dees JH, Stokely EM, Harris RA Jr, Bonte FJ, Willerson JT: Morphologic correlates of technetium-99m stannous pyrophosphate imaging of acute myocardial infarcts in dogs. Circulation 1975;52:596–607.

85. Buja LM, Parkey RW, Stokely EM, Bonte FJ, Willerson JT: Pathophysiology of technetium-99m stannous pyrophosphate and thallium-201 scintigraphy of acute anterior myocardial infarcts in dogs. J Clin Invest 1976;57:1508–1522.

86. Jansen DE, Corbett JR, Buja LM, Hansen C, Ugolini V, Parkey RW, Willerson JT: Quantification of myocardial injury produced by temporary coronary artery occlusion and reflow with technetium-99m pyrophosphate. Circulation 1987;75:611–617.

87. Achrafi H: Hypertrophic cardiomyopathy and myocardial bridging. Int J Cardiol 1992;37:111–112.

88. Khaw BA, Yasuda T, Gold HK, Leinbach RC, Johns JA, Kanke M, Barlai-Kovach M, Strauss HW, Haber E: Acute myocardial infarct imaging with indium-111–labeled monoclonal antimyosin Fab. J Nucl Med 1987;28:1671–1678.

88a. Maddahi J: Clinical applications of antimyosin monoclonal antibody imaging. Am J Cardiac Imag 1994;8:249–260.

88b. Khaw B-A, Narula J: Antibody imaging in the evaluation of cardiovascular diseases. J Nucl Cardiol 1994;1:457–476.

89. Beller GA, Khaw BA, Haber E, Smith TW: Localization of radiolabeled cardiac myosin-specific antibody in myocardial infarcts. Comparison with technetium-99m stannous pyrophosphate. Circulation 1977;55:74–78.

90. Adams ME, Antczak-Bouckoms A, Frazier HS, Lau J, Chalmers TC, Mosteller F: Assessing the effectiveness of ambulatory cardiac monitoring for specific clinical indications. Introduction. Int J Technol Assess Health Care 1993;9:97–101.

91. Ballinger JR, Gerson B, Gulenchyn KY: Technetium-99m diethyldithiocarbamate (DDC): Comparison with thallium-201 DDC as an agent for brain imaging. Int J Rad Appl Instrum [A]. 1987;38:665–668.

92. Adams BK, Fataar A, Boniaszczuk J, Kahn D: Equilibrium radionuclide angiocardiography in the detection of unsuspected mycotic aneurysms in cardiac transplantation. Transplantation 1992;53:681–683.

93. Takeda K, LaFrance ND, Weisman HF, Wagner HN Jr, Becker LC: Comparison of indium-111 antimyosin antibody and technetium-99m pyrophosphate localization in reperfused and nonreperfused myocardial infarction. J Am Coll Cardiol 1991;17:519–526.

94. Khaw BA, Strauss HW, Pohost GM, Fallon JT, Katus HA, Haber E: Relation between immediate and delayed thallium-201 distribution to localization of iodine-125 antimyosin antibody in acute experimental myocardial infarction. Am J Cardiol 1983;51:1428–1432.

94a. Morguet AJ, Munz DL, Klein HH, Pich S, Conrady A, Nebendahl K, Kreuzer H, Emrich D: Myocardial distribution of indium-111-antimyosin Fab and technetium-99m-sestamibi in experimental nontransmural infarction. J Nucl Med 1992;33:223–228.

95. Johnson LL, Cannon PJ: Antimyosin imaging in cardiac transplant rejection. Circulation 1991;84:I273–I279.

95a. Addonizio LJ, Michler RE, Marboe C, Esser PE, Johnson LL, Seldin DW, Gersony WM, Alderson PO, Rose EA, Cannon PJ: Imaging of cardiac allograft rejection in dogs using indium-111 monoclonal antimyosin Fab. J Am Coll Cardiol 1987;9:555–564.

96. Isobe M, Haber E, Khaw BA: Early detection of rejection and assessment of cyclosporine therapy by ^{111}In antimyosin imaging in mouse heart allografts. Circulation 1991;84:1246–1255.

97. Kishimoto C, Hung GL, Ishibashi M, Khaw BA, Kolodny GM, Abelmann WH, Yasuda T: Natural evolution of cardiac function, cardiac pathology and antimyosin scan in a murine myocarditis model. J Am Coll Cardiol 1991;17:821–827.

98. Yamada T, Matsumori A, Watanabe Y, Tamaki N, Yonekura Y, Endo K, Konishi J, Kawai C: Pharmacokinetics of indium-111–labeled antimyosin monoclonal antibody in murine experimental viral myocarditis. J Am Coll Cardiol 1990;16:1280–1286.

99. Hiroe M, Ohta Y, Fujita N, Nagata M, Toyozaki T, Kusakabe K, Sekiguchi M, Marumo F: Myocardial uptake of ^{111}In monoclonal antimyosin Fab in detecting doxorubicin cardiotoxicity in rats. Morphological and hemodynamic findings. Circulation 1992;86:1965–1972.

100. Carrío I, Lopez-Pousa A, Estorch M, Duncken D, Berná L, Torres G, de Andrés L: Detection of doxorubicin cardiotoxicity in patients with sarcomas by indium-111-antimyosin monoclonal antibody studies. J Nucl Med 1993;34:1503–1507.

101. Gould KL, Yoshida K, Hess MJ, Haynie M, Mullani N, Smalling RW: Myocardial metabolism of fluorodeoxyglucose compared to cell membrane integrity for the potassium analogue rubidium-82 for assessing infarct size in man by PET. J Nucl Med 1991;32:1–9.

102. Yano Y, Cahoon JL, Budinger TF: A precision flow-controlled Rb-82 generator for bolus or constant-infusion studies of the heart and brain. J Nucl Med 1981;22:1006–1010.

103. Mullani NA, Goldstein RA, Gould L, Marani SK, Fisher DJ, O'Brien A Jr, Loberg MD: Myocardial perfusion with rubidium-82. I. Measurement of extraction fraction and flow with external detectors. J Nucl Med 1983;24:898–906.

104. Gould KL, Yoshida K, Hess MJ, Haynie M, Mullani N, Smalling RW: Myocardial metabolism of fluorodeoxyglucose compared to cell membrane integrity for the potassium analogue rubidium-82 for assessing infarct size in man by PET. J Nucl Med 1991;32:1–9.

105. Niemeyer MG, Kuijper AF, Gerhards LJ, D'Haene EG, van der Wall EE: Nitrogen-13 ammonia perfusion imaging: Relation to metabolic imaging. Am Heart J 1993;125:848–854.

106. Hutchins GD, Schwaiger M, Rosenspire KC, Krivokapich J, Schelbert H, Kuhl DE: Noninvasive quantification of regional blood flow in the human heart using N-13 ammonia and dynamic positron emission tomographic imaging. J Am Coll Cardiol 1990;15:1032–1042.

107. Krivokapich J, Smith GT, Huang SC, Hoffman EJ, Ratib O, Phelps ME, Schelbert HR: 13N ammonia myocardial imaging at rest and with exercise in normal volunteers. Quantification of absolute myocardial perfusion with dynamic positron emission tomography. Circulation 1989;80:1328–1337.

108. Bellina CR, Parodi O, Camici P, Salvadori PA, Taddei L, Fusani L, Guzzardi R, Klassen GA, L'Abbate AL, Donato L: Simultaneous in vitro and in vivo validation of nitrogen-13-ammonia for the assessment of regional myocardial blood flow. J Nucl Med 1990;31:1335–1343.

109. Nienaber CA, Ratib O, Gambhir SS, Krivokapich J, Huang SC, Phelps ME, Schelbert HR: A quantitative index of regional blood flow in canine myocardium derived noninvasively with N-13 ammonia and dynamic positron emission tomography. J Am Coll Cardiol 1991;17:260–269.

110. Kuhle WG, Porenta G, Huang SC, Buxton D, Gambhir SS, Hansen H, Phelps ME, Schelbert HR: Quantification of regional myocardial blood flow using 13N-ammonia and reoriented dynamic positron emission tomographic imaging. Circulation 1992;86:1004–1017.

110a. Muzik O, Beanlands R, Wolfe E, Hutchins GD, Schwaiger M: Automated region definition for cardiac nitrogen-13-ammonia PET imaging. J Nucl Med 1993;34:336–344.

110b. Choi Y, Huang SC, Hawkins RA, Kuhle WG, Dahlbom M, Hoh CK, Czernin J, Phelps ME, Schelbert HR: A simplified method for quantification of myocardial blood flow using nitrogen-13-ammonia and dynamic PET. J Nucl Med 1993,34:488–497.

110c. Beanlands RSB, Muzik O, Hutchins GD, Wolfe ER Jr, Schwaiger M: Heterogeneity of regional nitrogen-13–labeled ammonia tracer distribution in the normal human heart: Comparison with rubidium 82 and copper 62–labeled PTSM. J Nucl Cardiol 1994;1:225–235.

111. Shah A, Schelbert HR, Schwaiger M, Henze E, Hansen H, Selin C, Huang SC: Measurement of regional myocardial blood flow with N-13 ammonia and positron-emission tomography in intact dogs. J Am Coll Cardiol 1985;5:92–100.

112. Bergmann SR, Fox KA, Rand AL, McElvany KD, Welch MJ, Markham J, Sobel BE: Quantification of regional myocardial blood flow in vivo with $H_2^{15}O$. Circulation 1984;70:724–733.

113. Bergmann SR, Herrero P, Markham J, Weinheimer CJ, Walsh MN: Noninvasive quantitation of myocardial blood flow in human subjects with oxygen-15–labeled water and positron emission tomography. J Am Coll Cardiol 1989;14:639–652.

114. Iida H, Kanno I, Takahashi A, Miura S, Murakami M, Takahashi K, Ono Y, Shishido F, Inugami A, Tomura N, et al.: Measurement of absolute myocardial blood flow with H2150 and dynamic positron-emission tomography. Strategy for quantification in relation to the partial-volume effect [published erratum appears in Circulation 1988, 78(4):1078]. Circulation 1988;78:104–115.

115. Araujo LI, Lammertsma AA, Rhodes CG, McFalls EO, Iida H, Rechavia E, Galassi A, de Silva R, Jones T, Maseri A: Noninvasive quantification of regional myocardial blood flow in coronary artery disease with oxygen-15–labeled carbon dioxide inhalation and positron emission tomography. Circulation 1991;83:875–885.

115a. Melon PG, Brihaye C, Degueldre C, et al: Myocardial kinetics of potassium-38 in humans and comparison with copper-62-PTSM. J Nucl Med 1994;35:1116–1122.

116. Walsh MN, Bergmann SR, Steele RL, Kenzora JL, Ter-Pogossian MM, Sobel BE, Geltman EM: Delineation of impaired regional myo-

cardial perfusion by positron emission tomography with $H_2^{15}O$. Circulation 1988;78:612–620.

117. Yamamoto Y, de Silva R, Rhodes CG, Araujo LI, Iida H, Rechavia E, Nihoyannopoulos P, Hackett D, Galassi AR, Taylor CJ, et al.: A new strategy for the assessment of viable myocardium and regional myocardial blood flow using ^{15}O-water and dynamic positron emission tomography. Circulation 1992;86:167–178.

118. Bergmann SR, Fox KA, Geltman EM, Sobel BE: Positron emission tomography of the heart. Prog Cardiovasc Dis 1985;28:165–194.

118a. Shelton ME, Senneff MJ, Ludbrook PA, Sobel BE, Bergmann SR: Concordance of nutritive myocardial perfusion reserve and flow velocity reserve in conductance vessels in patients with chest pain with angiographically normal coronary arteries. J Nucl Med 1993;34:717–722.

118b. Bol A, Melin JA, Vanoverschelde JL, Baudhuin T, Vogelaers D, De Pauw M, Michel C, Luxen A, Labar D, Cogneau M, et al.: Direct comparison of [^{13}N] ammonia and [^{15}O] water estimates of perfusion with quantification of regional myocardial blood flow by microspheres. Circulation 1993;87:512–525.

118c. Merlet P, Mazoyer B, Hittinger L, et al.: Assessment of coronary reserve in man: Comparison between positron emission tomography with oxygen-15–labeled water and intracoronary Doppler technique. J Nucl Med 1993;34:1899–1904.

119. Schelbert HR, Henze E, Keen R, Schon HR, Hansen H, Selin C, Huang SC, Barrio JR, Phelps ME: C-11 palmitate for the noninvasive evaluation of regional myocardial fatty acid metabolism with positron-computed tomography. IV. In vivo evaluation of acute demand-induced ischemia in dogs. Am Heart J 1983;106:736–750.

120. Schon HR, Schelbert HR, Robinson G, Najafi A, Huang SC, Hansen H, Barrio J, Kuhl DE, Phelps ME: C-11–labeled palmitic acid for the noninvasive evaluation of regional myocardial fatty acid metabolism with positron-computed tomography. I. Kinetics of C-11 palmitic acid in normal myocardium. Am Heart J 1982;103:532–547.

121. Schon HR, Schelbert HR, Najafi A, Hansen H, Huang H, Barrio J, Phelps ME: C-11–labeled palmitic acid for the noninvasive evaluation of regional myocardial fatty acid metabolism with positron-computed tomography. II. Kinetics of C-11 palmitic acid in acutely ischemic myocardium. Am Heart J 1982;103:548–561.

122. Klein MS, Goldstein RA, Welch MJ, Sobel BE: External assessment of myocardial metabolism with [^{11}C]palmitate in rabbit hearts. Am J Physiol 1979;237:H51–H58.

123. Schelbert HR: Current status and prospects of new radionuclides and radiopharmaceuticals for cardiovascular nuclear medicine. Semin Nucl Med 1987;17:145–181.

124. Lerch RA, Bergmann SR, Ambos HD, Welch MJ, Ter-Pogossian MM, Sobel BE: Effect of flow-independent reduction of metabolism on regional myocardial clearance of ^{11}C-palmitate. Circulation 1982;65:731–738.

125. Phelps ME, Hoffman EJ, Selin C, Huang SC, Robinson G, MacDonald N, Schelbert H, Kuhl DE: Investigation of [^{18}F]2-fluoro-2-deoxyglucose for the measure of myocardial glucose metabolism. J Nucl Med 1978;19:1311–1319.

126. Ratib O, Phelps ME, Huang SC, Henze E, Selin CE, Schelbert HR: Positron tomography with deoxyglucose for estimating local myocardial glucose metabolism. J Nucl Med 1982;23:577–586.

127. Krivokapich J, Huang SC, Phelps ME, Barrio JR, Watanabe CR, Selin CE, Shine KI: Estimation of rabbit myocardial metabolic rate for glucose using fluorodeoxyglucose. Am J Physiol 1982;243:H884–H895.

128. Brunken R, Tillisch J, Schwaiger M, Child JS, Marshall R, Mandelkern M, Phelps ME, Schelbert HR: Regional perfusion, glucose metabolism, and wall motion in patients with chronic electrocardiographic Q wave infarctions: Evidence for persistence of viable tissue in some infarct regions by positron emission tomography. Circulation 1986;73:951–963.

128a. Nienaber CA, Gambhir SS, Mody FV, Ratib O, Huang SC, Phelps ME, Schelbert HR: Regional myocardial blood flow and glucose utilization in symptomatic patients with hypertrophic cardiomyopathy. Circulation 1993;87:1580–1590.

129. Tillisch J, Brunken R, Marshall R, Schwaiger M, Mandelkern M, Phelps M, Schelbert H: Reversibility of cardiac wall-motion abnormalities predicted by positron tomography. N Engl J Med 1986;314:884–888.

130. Brunken R, Mody F, Hawkins R, Neinaber C, Phelps M, Shelbert H: Positron emission tomography detects metabolic viability in myocar-

131. dium with persistent 24-hour single-photon emissions tomography Tl-201 defects. Circulation 1992;86:1357–1369.

131. Schwaiger M, Schelbert HR, Ellison D, Hansen H, Yeatman L, Vinten-Johansen J, Selin C, Barrio J, Phelps ME: Sustained regional abnormalities in cardiac metabolism after transient ischemia in the chronic dog model. J Am Coll Cardiol 1985;6:336–347.

132. Brunken RC, Mody FV, Hawkins RA, Nienaber C, Phelps ME, Schelbert HR: Positron emission tomography detects metabolic viability in myocardium with persistent 24-hour single-photon emission computed tomography ^{201}Tl defects. Circulation 1992;86:1357–1369.

133. Tamaki N, Yonekura Y, Yamashita K, Saji H, Magata Y, Senda M, Konishi Y, Hirata K, Ban T, Konishi J: Positron emission tomography using fluorine-18 deoxyglucose in evaluation of coronary artery bypass grafting. Am J Cardiol 1989;64:860–865.

134. Baer FM, Voth E, Deutsch HJ, Schneider CA, Schicha H, Sechtem U: Assessment of viable myocardium by dobutamine transesophageal echocardiography and comparison with fluorine-18 fluorodeoxyglucose positron emission tomography. J Am Coll Cardiol 1994;24:343–353.

135. Brown M, Marshall DR, Sobel BE, Bergmann SR: Delineation of myocardial oxygen utilization with carbon-11–labeled acetate. Circulation 1987;76:687–696.

136. Buxton DB, Nienaber CA, Luxen A, Ratib O, Hansen H, Phelps ME, Schelbert HR: Noninvasive quantitation of regional myocardial oxygen consumption in vivo with [1-11C] acetate and dynamic positron emission tomography. Circulation 1989;79:134–142.

137. Walsh MN, Geltman EM, Brown MA, Henes CG, Weinheimer CJ, Sobel BE, Bergmann SR: Noninvasive estimation of regional myocardial oxygen consumption by positron emission tomography with carbon-11 acetate in patients with myocardial infarction. J Nucl Med 1989;30:1798–1808.

138. Henes CG, Bergmann SR, Walsh MN, Sobel BE, Geltman EM: Assessment of myocardial oxidative metabolic reserve with positron emission tomography and carbon-11 acetate. J Nucl Med 1989;30:1489–1499.

138a. Armbrecht JJ, Buxton DB, Brunken RC, Phelps ME, Schelbert HR: Regional myocardial oxygen consumption determined noninvasively in humans with [1-^{11}C] acetate and dynamic positron tomography. Circulation 1989;80:863–872.

139. Armbrecht JJ, Buxton DB, Schelbert HR: Validation of [1-11C]acetate as a tracer for noninvasive assessment of oxidative metabolism with positron emission tomography in normal, ischemic, postischemic, and hyperemic canine myocardium. Circulation 1990;81:1594–1605.

140. Hicks RJ, Herman WH, Kalff V, Molina E, Wolfe ER, Hutchins G, Schwaiger M: Quantitative evaluation of regional substrate metabolism in the human heart by positron emission tomography. J Am Coll Cardiol 1991;18:101–111.

141. Gropler RJ, Siegel BA, Sampathkumaran K, Perez JE, Sobel BE, Bergmann SR, Geltman EM: Dependence of recovery of contractile function on maintenance of oxidative metabolism after myocardial infarction. J Am Coll Cardiol 1992;19:989–997.

142. Gropler RJ, Siegel BA, Geltman EM: Myocardial uptake of carbon-11-acetate as an indirect estimate of regional myocardial blood flow. J Nucl Med 1991;32:245–251.

143. Vanoverschelde JL, Melin JA, Bol A, Vanbutsele R, Cogneau M, Labar D, Robert A, Michel C, Wijns W: Regional oxidative metabolism in patients after recovery from reperfused anterior myocardial infarction. Relation to regional blood flow and glucose uptake. Circulation 1992;85:9–21.

144. Gropler RJ, Geltman EM, Sampathkumaran K, Perez JE, Moerlein SM, Sobel BE, Bergmann SR, Siegel BA: Functional recovery after coronary revascularization for chronic coronary artery disease is dependent on maintenance of oxidative metabolism. J Am Coll Cardiol 1992;20:569–577.

145. Kalff V, Hicks RJ, Hutchins G, Topol E, Schwaiger M: Use of carbon-11 acetate and dynamic positron emission tomography to assess regional myocardial oxygen consumption in patients with acute myocardial infarction receiving thrombolysis or coronary angioplasty. Am J Cardiol 1993;71:529–535.

146. Buxton DB, Mody FV, Krivokapich J, Phelps ME, Schelbert HR: Quantitative assessment of prolonged metabolic abnormalities in reperfused canine myocardium. Circulation 1992;85:1842–1856.

147. Raylman RR, Hutchins GD, Beanlands RSB, Schwaiger M: Modeling of carbon-11-acetate kinetics by simultaneously fitting data from

multiple ROIs coupled by common parameters. J Nucl Med 1994;35:1286–1291.

148. Schwaiger M, Guibourg H, Rosenspire K, McClanahan T, Gallagher K, Hutchins G, Wieland DM: Effect of regional myocardial ischemia on sympathetic nervous system as assessed by fluorine-18-metaraminol. J Nucl Med 1990;31:1352–1357.

149. Schwaiger M, Kalff V, Rosenspire K, Haka MS, Molina E, Hutchins GD, Deeb M, Wolfe E Jr, Wieland DM: Noninvasive evaluation of sympathetic nervous system in human heart by positron emission tomography. Circulation 1990;82:457–464.

150. Wolpers HG, Nguyen N, Rosenspire K, Haka M, Wieland DM, Schwaiger M: C-11 hydroxyephedrine as marker for neuronal catecholamine retention in reperfused canine myocardium. Coronary Artery Disease 1991;2:923–929.

150a. Allman KC, Wieland DM, Muzik O, Degrado TR, Wolfe ER Jr, Schwaiger M: Carbon-11 hydroxyephedrine with positron emission tomography for serial assessment of cardiac adrenergic neuronal function after acute myocardial infarction in humans. J Am Coll Cardiol 1993;22:368–375.

150b. Allman KC, Stevens MJ, Wieland DM, Hutchins GD, Wolfe ER Jr, Greene DA, Schwaiger M: Noninvasive assessment of cardiac diabetic neuropathy by carbon-11 hydroxyephedrine and positron emission tomography. J Am Coll Cardiol 1993;22:1425–1432.

150c. Melon PG, Nguyen N, DeGrado TR, Mangner TJ, Wieland DM, Schwaiger M: Imaging of cardiac neuronal function after cocaine exposure using carbon-11 hydroxyephedrine and positron emission tomography. J Am Coll Cardiol 1994;23:1693–1699.

151. Calkins H, Lehmann MH, Allman K, Wieland D, Schwaiger M: Scintigraphic pattern of regional cardiac sympathetic innervation in patients with familial long QT syndrome using positron emission tomography. Circulation 1993;87:1616–1621.

152. Merlet P, Delforge J, Syrota A, Angevin E, Maziere B, Crouzel C, Valette H, Loisance D, Castaigne A, Rande JL: Positron emission tomography with ^{11}C CGP-12177 to assess beta-adrenergic receptor concentration in idiopathic dilated cardiomyopathy. Circulation 1993;87:1169–1178.

153. Goldstein DS, Chang PC, Eisenhofer G, Miletich R, Finn R, Bacher J, Kirk KL, Bacharach S, Kopin IJ: Positron emission tomographic imaging of cardiac sympathetic innervation and function. Circulation 1990;81:1606–1621.

153a. Valette H, Loc'h C, Marden K, et al.: Bromine-76-metabromobenzylguanidine: A PET radiotracer for mapping sympathetic nerves of the heart. J Nucl Med 1993;34:1739–1744.

154. Mudge GH, Jr., Mills RM Jr, Taegtmeyer H, Gorlin R, Lesch M: Alterations of myocardial amino acid metabolism in chronic ischemic heart disease. J Clin Invest 1976;58:1185–1192.

155. Gelbard AS, Benua RS, Reiman RE, McDonald JM, Vomero JJ, Laughlin JS: Imaging of the human heart after administration of L-(N-13)glutamate. J Nucl Med 1980;21:988–991.

156. Zimmermann R, Tillmanns H, Knapp WH, Helus F, Georgi P, Rauch B, Neumann FJ, Girgensohn S, Maier-Borst W, Kubler W: Regional myocardial nitrogen-13 glutamate uptake in patients with coronary artery disease: Inverse post-stress relation to thallium-201 uptake in ischemia. J Am Coll Cardiol 1988;11:549–556.

157. Shelton ME, Green MA, Mathias CJ, Welch MJ, Bergmann SR: Kinetics of copper-PTSM in isolated hearts: A novel tracer for measuring blood flow with positron emission tomography. J Nucl Med 1989;30:1843–1847.

158. Shelton ME, Green MA, Mathias CJ, Welch MJ, Bergmann SR: Assessment of regional myocardial and renal blood flow with copper-PTSM and positron emission tomography. Circulation 1990;82:990–997.

159. Beanlands RS, Muzik O, Mintun M, Mangner T, Lee K, Petry N, Hutchins GD, Schwaiger M: The kinetics of copper-62-PTSM in the normal human heart. J Nucl Med 1992;33:684–690.

160. Herrero P, Markham J, Weinheimer CJ, Anderson CJ, Welch MJ, Green MA, Bergmann SR: Quantification of regional myocardial perfusion with generator-produced ^{62}Cu-PTSM and positron emission tomography. Circulation 1993;87:173–183.

161. Martin GV, Caldwell JH, Rasey JS, Grunbaum Z, Cerqueira M, Krohn KA: Enhanced binding of the hypoxic cell marker [^{3}H]fluoromisonidazole in ischemic myocardium. J Nucl Med 1989;30:194–201.

162. Shelton ME, Dence CS, Hwang DR, Welch MJ, Bergmann SR: Myocardial kinetics of fluorine-18 misonidazole: A marker of hypoxic myocardium. J Nucl Med 1989;30:351–358.

163. Shelton ME, Dence CS, Hwang DR, Herrero P, Welch MJ, Bergmann SR: In vivo delineation of myocardial hypoxia during coronary occlusion using fluorine-18 fluoromisonidazole and positron emission tomography: A potential approach for identification of jeopardized myocardium. J Am Coll Cardiol 1990;16:477–485.

164. Martin GV, Caldwell JH, Graham MM, Grierson JR, Kroll K, Cowan MJ, Lewellen TK, Rasey JS, Casciari JJ, Krohn KA: Noninvasive detection of hypoxic myocardium using fluorine-18-fluoromisonidazole and positron emission tomography. J Nucl Med 1992;33:2202–2208.

165. Cerqueira M, Martin G, Embree L, Caldwell J, Krohn K, Rasey J: Enhanced binding of fluoromisonidazole in isolated adult rat myocytes during hypoxia (Abstract). J Nucl Med 1988;29:807–807.

166. Rasey JS, Krohn KA, Grunbaum Z, Conroy PJ, Bauer K, Sutherland RM: Further characterization of 4-bromomisonidazole as a potential detector of hypoxic cells. Radiation Res 1985;102:76–85.

166a. Martin GV, Biskupiak JE, Caldwell JH, Rasey JS, Krohn KA: Characterization of iodovinylmisonidazole as a marker for myocardial hypoxia. J Nucl Med 1993;34:918–924.

166b. Kusuoka H, Hashimoto K, Fukuchi K, Nishimura T: Kinetics of a putative hypoxic tissue marker, technetium-99m-nitroimidazole (BMS 181321), in normoxic, hypoxic, ischemic and stunned myocardium. J Nucl Med 1994;35:1371–1376.

167. Ezekowitz MD, Burrow RD, Heath PW, Streitz T, Smith EO, Parker DE: Diagnostic accuracy of indium-111 platelet scintigraphy in identifying left ventricular thrombi. Am J Cardiol 1983;51:1712–1716.

168. Fox KA, Bergmann SR, Mathias CJ, Powers WJ, Siegel BA, Welch MJ, Sobel BE: Scintigraphic detection of coronary artery thrombi in patients with acute myocardial infarction. J Am Coll Cardiol 1984;4:975–986.

169. Fuster V, Dewanjee MK, Kaye MP, Josa M, Metke MP, Chesebro JH: Noninvasive radioisotopic technique for detection of platelet deposition in coronary artery bypass grafts in dogs and its reduction with platelet inhibitors. Circulation 1979;60:1508–1512.

170. Stratton JR, Ritchie JL: ^{111}In platelet imaging of left ventricular thrombi. Predictive value for systemic emboli. Circulation 1990;81:1182–1189.

171. Sisson JC, Wieland DM, Sherman P, Mangner TJ, Tobes MC, Jacques S Jr.: Metaiodobenzylguanidine as an index of the adrenergic nervous system integrity and function. J Nucl Med 1987;28:1620–1624.

172. Sisson JC, Shapiro B, Meyers L, Mallette S, Mangner TJ, Wieland DM, Glowniak JV, Sherman P, Beierwaltes WH: Metaiodobenzylguanidine to map scintigraphically the adrenergic nervous system in man. J Nucl Med 1987;28:1625–1636.

173. Minardo JD, Tuli MM, Mock BH, Weiner RE, Pride HP, Wellman HN, Zipes DP: Scintigraphic and electrophysiological evidence of canine myocardial sympathetic denervation and reinnervation produced by myocardial infarction or phenol application. Circulation 1988;78:1008–1019.

174. Henderson EB, Kahn JK, Corbett JR, Jansen DE, Pippin JJ, Kulkarni P, Ugolini V, Akers MS, Hansen C, Buja LM, et al.: Abnormal I-123 metaiodobenzylguanidine myocardial washout and distribution may reflect myocardial adrenergic derangement in patients with congestive cardiomyopathy. Circulation 1988;78:1192–1199.

175. Schofer J, Spielmann R, Schuchert A, Weber K, Schluter M: Iodine-123 meta-iodobenzylguanidine scintigraphy: A noninvasive method to demonstrate myocardial adrenergic nervous system disintegrity in patients with idiopathic dilated cardiomyopathy. J Am Coll Cardiol 1988;12:1252–1258.

176. Dae MW, O'Connell JW, Botvinick EH, Ahearn T, Yee E, Huberty JP, Mori H, Chin MC, Hattner RS, Herre JM, et al.: Scintigraphic assessment of regional cardiac adrenergic innervation. Circulation 1989;79:634–644.

177. Stanton MS, Tuli MM, Radtke NL, Heger JJ, Miles WM, Mock BH, Burt RW, Wellman HN, Zipes DP: Regional sympathetic denervation after myocardial infarction in humans detected noninvasively using I-123-metaiodobenzylguanidine. J Am Coll Cardiol 1989;14:1519–1526.

178. Dae MW, Herre JM, O'Connell JW, Botvinick EH, Newman D, Munoz L: Scintigraphic assessment of sympathetic innervation after transmural versus nontransmural myocardial infarction. J Am Coll Cardiol 1991;17:1416–1423.

179. Merlet P, Valette H, Dubois-Rande JL, Moyse D, Duboc D, Dove P, Bourguignon MH, Benvenuti C, Duval AM, Agostini D, et al.: Prognostic value of cardiac metaiodobenzylguanidine imaging in patients with heart failure. J Nucl Med 1992;33:471–477.

180. Wakasugi S, Wada A, Hasegawa Y, Nakano S, Shibata N: Detection of abnormal cardiac adrenergic neuron activity in adriamycin-induced cardiomyopathy with iodine-125-metaiodobenzylguanidine. J Nucl Med 1992;33:208–214.

181. Mitrani RD, Klein LS, Miles WM, Hackett FK, Burt RW, Wellman HN, Zipes DP: Regional cardiac sympathetic denervation in patients with ventricular tachycardia in the absence of coronary artery disease. J Am Coll Cardiol 1993;22:1344–1353.

182. Wichter TW, Hindricks G, Lerch H, Bartenstein P, Borggrefe M, Schober O, Breithardt G: Regional myocardial sympathetic dysinnervation in arrhythmogenic right ventricular cardiomyopathy. An analysis using ^{123}I-*meta*-iodobenzylguanidine scintigraphy. Circulation 1994;89:667–683.

183. Fagret D, Wolf JE, Vanzetto G, Borrel E: Myocardial uptake of metaiodobenzylguanidine in patients with left ventricular hypertrophy secondary to valvular aortic stenosis. J Nucl Med 1993;34:57–60.

183a. Simmons WW, Freeman MR, Grima EA, Hsia TW, Armstrong PW: Abnormalities of cardiac sympathetic function in pacing-induced heart failure as assessed by [^{123}I] metaiodobenzylguanidine scintigraphy. Circulation 1994;89:2843–2851.

183b. Dae MW: Imaging of myocardial sympathetic innervation with metaiodobenzylguanidine. J Nucl Cardiol 1994;1:S23–S30.

184. Jansen D, Pippin J, Hansen C, Henderson E, Kulkarni P, Ugolni V, Corbett SR: Use of radioactive iodine-labeled fatty acids for myocardial imaging. Am J Cardiac Imaging 1987;1:132–144.

185. Rellas JS, Corbett JR, Kulkarni P, Morgan C, Devous MD, Buja LM, Bush L, Parkey RW, Willerson JT, Lewis SE: Iodine-123 phenylpentadecanoic acid: Detection of acute myocardial infarction and injury in dogs using an iodinated fatty acid and single-photon emission tomography. Am J Cardiol 1983;52:1326–1332.

186. Hansen CL, Corbett JR, Pippin JJ, Jansen DE, Kulkarni PV, Ugolini V, Henderson E, Akers M, Buja LM, Parkey RW, et al.: Iodine-123 phenylpentadecanoic acid and single photon emission computed tomography in identifying left ventricular regional metabolic abnormalities in patients with coronary heart disease: Comparison with thallium-201 myocardial tomography. J Am Coll Cardiol 1988;12:78–87.

187. Murray G, Schad N, Ladd W, Allie D, vander Zwagg R, Avet P, Rockett J: Metabolic cardiac imaging in severe coronary disease: Assessment of viability with iodine-123-iodophenylpentadecanoic acid and multicrystal gamma camera, and correlation with biopsy. J Nucl Med 1992;33:1269–1277.

187a. Corbett J: Clinical experience with iodine-123-iodophenylpentadecanoic acid. J Nucl Med 1994;35(suppl):325–375.

187b. Reske SN: Experimental and clinical experiences with iodine 123-labeled iodophenylpentadecanoic acid in cardiology. J Nucl Cardiol 1994;1:S58–S64.

188. Hansen CL, Heo J, Iskandrian AS: Prediction of improvement of left ventricular function after coronary revascularization from alterations in myocardial metabolic activity detected with I-123 phenylpentadecanoic and dynamic SPECT imaging (Abstract). J Am Coll Cardiol 1994;February:344A.

189. Chouraqui P, Maddahi J, Henkin R, Karesh SM, Galie E, Berman DS: Comparison of myocardial imaging with iodine-123-iodophenyl-9-methyl pentadecanoic acid and thallium-201-chloride for assessment of patients with exercise-induced myocardial ischemia. J Nucl Med 1991;32:447–452.

189a. Matsunari I, Saga T, Taki J, et al: Kinetics of iodine-123-BMIPP in patients with prior myocardial infarction: Assessment with dynamic rest and stress images compared with stress thallium-201 SPECT. J Nucl Med 1994;35:1279–1285.

190. Olexa S, Budzinski A: Evidence for four different polymerization sites involved in human fibrin formation. Proc Natl Acad Sci USA 1980;77:1374–1383.

191. Knight LC, Maurer AH, Robbins PS, Malmud LS, Budzynski AZ: Fragment E1 labeled with I-123 in the detection of venous thrombosis. Radiology 1985;156:509–514.

192. Knight LC, Abrams MJ, Schwartz DA, Hauser MM, Kollman M, Gaul FE, Rauh DA, Maurer AH: Preparation and preliminary evaluation of technetium-99m–labeled fragment E1 for thrombus imaging. J Nucl Med 1992;33:710–715.

193. Miller DD, Rivera FJ, Garcia OJ, Palmaz JC, Berger HJ, Weisman HF: Imaging of vascular injury with ^{99m}Tc-labeled monoclonal antiplatelet antibody S12. Preliminary experience in human percutaneous transluminal angioplasty. Circulation 1992;85:1354–1363.

194. Knight LC: Scintigraphic methods for detecting vascular thrombus. J Nucl Med 1993;34:554–561.

195. Morguet AJ, Munz DL, Ivančević V, Werner GS, Sandrock D, Bökemeier M, Kreuzer H: Immunoscintigraphy using technetium-99m-labeled anti-NCA-95 antigranulocyte antibodies as an adjunct to echocardiography in subacute infective endocarditis. J Am Coll Cardiol 1994;23:1171–1178.

Chapter 3

Detection of Coronary Artery Disease

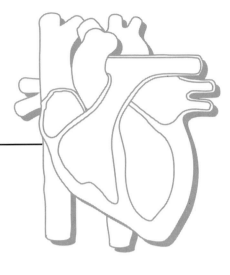

One of the major clinical applications of noninvasive cardiologic techniques is the detection of coronary artery disease (CAD) in patients who present with undiagnosed chest pain or in minimally symptomatic or asymptomatic patients who have multiple risk factors for premature development of CAD. The techniques for CAD detection all employ either exercise or pharmacologic stress to produce flow heterogeneity or functional or ECG alterations consequent to myocardial ischemia, or both. These alterations are detected by electrocardiographic (ECG) monitoring, with or without the concurrent assessment of regional myocardial perfusion or global and regional function. At present, regional myocardial perfusion in conjunction with exercise or pharmacologic stress is undertaken with either planar or single-photon emission computed tomography (SPECT) imaging techniques utilizing thallium-201 (Tl-201), technetium-99m (Tc-99m)–labeled sestamibi, Tc-99m teboroxime, Tc-99m tetrofosmin, or a positron-emitting flow tracer such as nitrogen-13 ammonia (N-13 ammonia) or rubidium-82 (Rb-82). Global and regional function during stress is evaluated with either first-pass or equilibrium radionuclide angiography or stress echocardiography employing Tc-99m–labeled red blood cells. The radionuclide techniques for detection of CAD are discussed in Chapter 1, and the radiopharmaceuticals used are described in Chapter 2.

The rationale for all of the stress-related noninvasive techniques for detection of CAD is that with an increase in oxygen demand or an increase in coronary blood flow, myocardial regions supplied by obstructed coronary vessels demonstrate regional hypoperfusion or regional dysfunction or generate ECG manifestations of ischemia. This occurs because of an imbalance between oxygen supply and demand and impaired flow reserve (Fig. 3–1).

CORONARY ANGIOGRAPHY AS THE "GOLD STANDARD"

Coronary angiography is presently considered the "gold standard" for establishing the diagnosis of CAD in patients with chest pain and for documenting its extent by delineating focal coronary obstructions that are considered significant (e.g., $\geq 50\%$ stenosis or $\geq 70\%$ stenosis). However, the angiographic evaluation of the epicardial segments of the three major coronary arteries cannot provide data relevant to the presence or degree of ischemia that may occur under such stress conditions as exercise, dipyridamole-induced vasodilation, or dobutamine-induced regional wall motion abnormalities. Some studies have shown considerable interobserver variability in the interpretation of coronary arteriograms: observers disagree about the number of major vessels involved with 70% stenosis approximately 30% of the time.[1] When compared with autopsy measurements of the degree of narrowing, stenotic lesions between 50% and 70% are usually underestimated by angiographers using visual or caliper grading. This most likely relates to the observation that the atherosclerotic process tends to be diffuse, and the measurement of percentage of narrowing may not indicate the true severity of the coronary obstruction. The new computer-assisted quantitative techniques using edge detection or video densitrometry of coronary stenoses with digital subtraction angiography may enhance the ac-

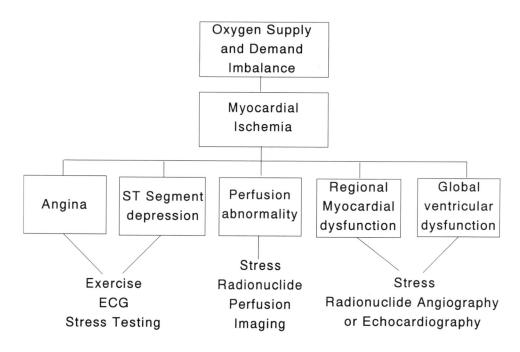

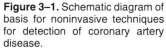

Figure 3–1. Schematic diagram of basis for noninvasive techniques for detection of coronary artery disease.

curacy of grading the severity of these lesions.[2] However, even if the extent of coronary artery stenoses could be measured more precisely by quantitative angiography, the functional or physiologic severity of CAD still would not be accurately determined, since "myocardium at risk" does not correlate well with the severity of stenosis, nor can coronary reserve capacity be predicted simply from a measurement of luminal narrowing.

The functional importance of visualized collaterals must also be taken into account. Angiographic demonstration of collaterals does not necessarily imply protection against exercise-induced ischemia, or even against myocardial infarction (MI) if the proximal stenosis should suddenly become totally occluded. The extent of myocardium in a risk region distal to a given stenotic vessel cannot easily be ascertained by coronary arteriographic assessment alone. Risk areas distal to given sites of coronary stenoses along any of the three epicardial coronary vessels may vary considerably from patient to patient. Obviously, some patients with single-vessel disease, particularly that involving the proximal portion of the left anterior descending (LAD) coronary artery, may be at high risk for an adverse outcome, because a large area of the anterior wall and septum is rendered ischemic, particularly at low levels of exercise. Certain patients with multivessel disease may have negative noninvasive stress test results or minimal abnormalities because of lack of substantial stress-induced hypoperfusion in risk regions in the distribution of the diseased vessels.

For the reasons cited above, the rationale for the diagnostic and prognostic applications of noninvasive stress testing is that physiologic and functional information, rather than just structural or anatomic information, are the ultimate "gold standard" for detection of prognostically important CAD. Myocardial perfusion scintigraphy, radionuclide an-

giography, or exercise echocardiography performed in conjunction with the exercise ECG provides clinically relevant data about the presence and extent of ischemia, which prognostically may be as important or moreso, than mere classification by the number of diseased vessels observed by angiography. The prognostic applications of stress radionuclide imaging are discussed in Chapter 4.

SENSITIVITY, SPECIFICITY, PREDICTIVE VALUES, AND BAYES' THEOREM

The accuracy of any test to diagnose CAD is measured by the *sensitivity* and *specificity* of the test.[3–6] Based on Bayes' theorem, the accuracy of any test that is not 100% sensitive and 100% specific depends on the pretest probability of disease in the patient population being studied. Bayes' theorem expresses the posttest likelihood of disease as a function of sensitivity and specificity of the test and the prevalence of the disease in question in the population being studied (e.g., a population of patients with nonanginal-type chest pain). Diamond states that Bayes' theorem is the "formal rule by which one integrates the interpretation of any combination of observations in light of past experience."[4] According to Bayes' theorem, if a test's sensitivity and specificity are known, the posttest probability of disease can be calculated for any pretest disease prevalence. This is important, since the critical aspect of making an accurate diagnosis of CAD is that the positive and negative predictive value of the test result must be known. The practicing clinician can use the principles of Bayes' theorem to help interpret tests aimed at detecting CAD. The clinician desires to know, if the test result is positive, what is the probability that the patient has CAD and, conversely,

Table 3–1. **Definitions of Measures of Test Accuracy for Any Diagnostic Procedure.**

Sensitivity:
$$\frac{\text{True positives}}{\text{True positives + False negatives}} = \frac{\text{True positives}}{\text{Total patients with disease}}$$

Specificity:
$$\frac{\text{True negatives}}{\text{True negatives + False positives}} = \frac{\text{True negatives}}{\text{Total patients without disease}}$$

False-positive rate:
$$\frac{\text{False positives}}{\text{True negatives + False positives}} = \frac{\text{False positives}}{\text{Total patients without disease}}$$

False-negative rate:
$$\frac{\text{False negatives}}{\text{True positives + False negatives}} = \frac{\text{False negatives}}{\text{Total patients with disease}}$$

Positive predictive value:
$$\frac{\text{True positives}}{\text{True positives + False ~~negatives~~} \; positives \; \rightarrow err}$$

Negative predictive value:
$$\frac{\text{True negatives}}{\text{True negatives + False negatives}}$$

if the result is negative, what is the probability that a particular patient does not have CAD?

Definition of Sensitivity, Specificity, and False-Negative and False-Positive Rates

The definitions of sensitivity, specificity, false-positive rate, and false-negative rate are summarized in Table 3–1. The sensitivity of a test, also referred to as a *true-positive rate,* measures a test's ability to correctly indicate the presence of the disease. It measures what fraction of patients with disease is detected by the test and is calculated as the number of true positives divided by the total number of patients with CAD, usually as determined by coronary an-

giography. The specificity of a test, commonly designated as the *true-negative rate,* indicates the test's ability correctly to identify the absence of disease. It reflects the frequency of a negative test result in a disease-free population and is calculated as the number of true negatives divided by the number of true negatives plus false positives. This denominator identifies the total number of patients tested who do not have CAD. The false-positive rate is calculated as *1 minus the specificity* and is expressed numerically as the number of false-positives divided by the sum of the true-negatives and the false-positives. The false-negative rate is equal to *1 minus the sensitivity.* This rate is determined numerically by dividing the number of false negatives by the number of true positives plus false negatives.

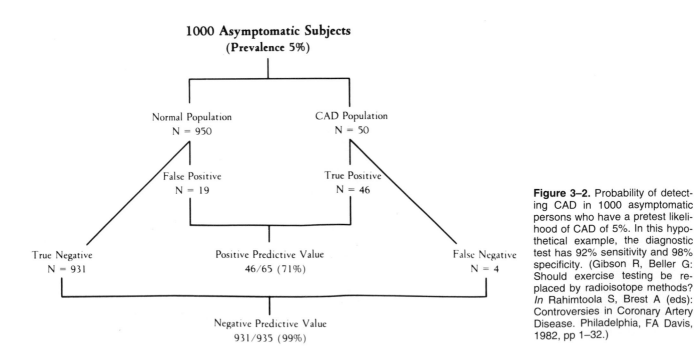

Figure 3–2. Probability of detecting CAD in 1000 asymptomatic persons who have a pretest likelihood of CAD of 5%. In this hypothetical example, the diagnostic test has 92% sensitivity and 98% specificity. (Gibson R, Beller G: Should exercise testing be replaced by radioisotope methods? *In* Rahimtoola S, Brest A (eds): Controversies in Coronary Artery Disease. Philadelphia, FA Davis, 1982, pp 1–32.)

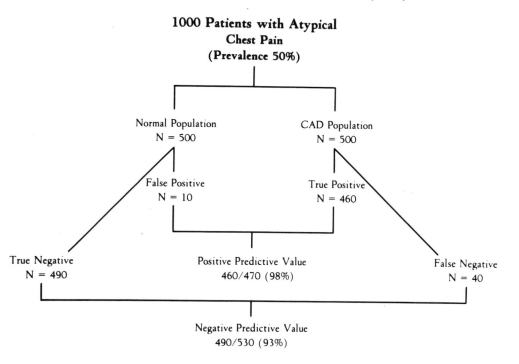

**1000 Patients with Atypical
Chest Pain
(Prevalence 50%)**

Normal Population
N = 500

CAD Population
N = 500

False Positive
N = 10

True Positive
N = 460

True Negative
N = 490

Positive Predictive Value
460/470 (98%)

False Negative
N = 40

Negative Predictive Value
490/530 (93%)

Figure 3–3. Probability of coronary artery disease in 1000 individuals with atypical chest pain who hypothetically have a 50% pretest likelihood of disease and the diagnostic test has 92% sensitivity and 98% specificity. (Gibson R, Beller G: Should exercise testing be replaced by radioisotope methods? *In* Rahimtoola S, Brest A (eds): Controversies in Coronary Artery Disease. Philadelphia, FA Davis, 1982, pp 1–32.)

Predictive Values of a Test Result

Although sensitivity and specificity values define the essential accuracy of a test, the interpretation of any individual patient's test results depends on the pretest likelihood of disease in that tested individual or in the overall population being tested. *Prevalence* is the percentage of patients with the disease in a particular population. The influence of disease prevalence in test interpretation is illustrated from the publication by Gibson and Beller.[7] Assume a test has 92% sensitivity (8% false-negative rate) and 98% specific-

ity (2% false-positive rate). Figure 3–2 considers the results when this test is applied to 1000 asymptomatic subjects whose pretest probability of having CAD is 5%, and Figure 3–3 considers the results of the test in 1000 patients with atypical chest pain and a presumed 50% prevalence of CAD. Finally, Figure 3–4 illustrates the interpretation of test results in 1000 patients with typical angina pectoris and presumed disease prevalence of 90%.

In the first example of 1000 asymptomatic subjects with a 5% probability of disease (see Fig. 3–2), there would be 950 normal subjects and 50 patients with CAD. Since the

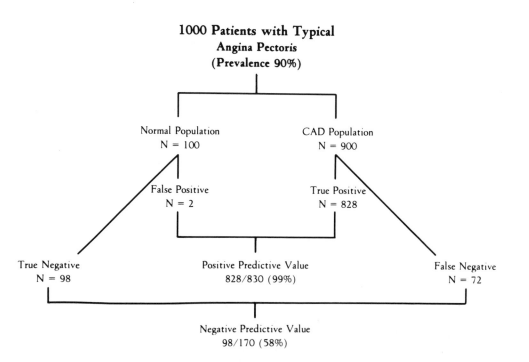

**1000 Patients with Typical
Angina Pectoris
(Prevalence 90%)**

Normal Population
N = 100

CAD Population
N = 900

False Positive
N = 2

True Positive
N = 828

True Negative
N = 98

Positive Predictive Value
828/830 (99%)

False Negative
N = 72

Negative Predictive Value
98/170 (58%)

Figure 3–4. Probability of CAD in 1000 patients with typical anginal chest pain who hypothetically have a pretest likelihood of CAD of 90% with a diagnostic test having a 92% sensitivity and 98% specificity. (Gibson R, Beller G: Should exercise testing be replaced by radioisotope methods? *In* Rahimtoola S, Brest A (eds): Controversies in Coronary Artery Disease. Philadelphia, FA Davis, 1982, pp 1–32.)

test has a 2% false-positive rate and an 8% false-negative rate, 19 of 950 normal subjects and 46 of 50 CAD patients would have a positive test result, yielding a positive predictive value of 71%. Misleading information would thus be provided to 29% of normal asymptomatic subjects in this population. A negative test result excludes the disease in 99% of subjects, which is of marginal additional benefit since the pretest likelihood of disease absence was already 95%.

In the second example (see Fig. 3–3) of 1000 persons with atypical chest pain and a 50% pretest likelihood of disease, the calculation of predictive values reveals definite test benefit. In this population of patients, CAD is identified correctly in 98%, a significant increase over the pretest probability of 50%. A negative test result reduces the probability of disease to 7%. In the third example (see Fig. 3–4) of 1000 patients with a 90% pretest probability of disease, a positive test result increases the posttest likelihood of CAD to 99%, whereas a negative result reduces the likelihood of disease to only an intermediate level. The negative predictive value is suboptimal at 58% because of the high pretest probability of disease in the population.

Diamond summarizes the important features of all diagnostic tests based on the principles of Bayesian analysis as reflected by the three patient examples described above.[8] First, a positive or abnormal test response does not establish presence of disease but only increases its probability. Second, a negative or normal test result does not rule out disease but only lessens the probability. Only if a diagnostic test were ideal, with 100% sensitivity and 100% specificity, could the test result be accepted without any question. Since no test is perfect, test results can be analyzed only by using probability analysis concepts. For any test an abnormal result is more likely to be "false positive" in patients with a low pretest likelihood of disease than in patients whose pretest likelihood of disease was high. Similarly, negative test results are more likely to be false negative in patients with a high pretest likelihood than in those with a low pretest likelihood of disease. When pretest likelihood of disease is greater than 90% or less than 10%, the test has limited diagnostic value but certainly may have prognostic value. All diagnostic tests are of greatest value when there is an intermediate probability of disease, in the range of 50%, and when uncertainty is greatest. In a high-prevalence-of-disease population (>90%), a positive test outcome merely confirms the presence of disease, though it can also provide information on the extent and severity of disease. In the instance of a negative test result in a high-prevalence population, disease is not excluded, and such a result indicates a better prognosis or a false-negative result. In a low-prevalence-of-disease population, a negative test result merely confirms the absence of disease suspected by clinical criteria, but a positive test result in this population does not establish the presence of disease with a high degree of confidence. This is because such a response may

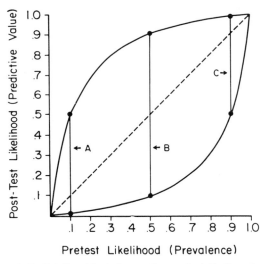

Figure 3–5. Relationship between the pretest likelihood and the posttest likelihood of disease for a hypothetical test with 90% sensitivity and 90% specificity. Line A represents a population with a 10% prevalence of disease, showing the poor predictive value of a positive test result. Line C represents a population with a 90% pretest likelihood of disease and shows that a negative test result also has a poor predictive value. The diagnostic value of this test is best for the population represented by line B, which has an intermediate pretest likelihood of disease of 50%. (Gibson RS, Watson DD: Progr Cardiol 1983;12:67–112.)

represent a false-positive result. These concepts are summarized in Figure 3–5, which depicts the posttest likelihood of CAD according to negative and positive test results in patients with different pretest likelihoods of CAD.[8] The hypothetical test has sensitivity of 90% and specificity of 90%. The line of identity in this figure represents sensitivity and specificity values of 50%. For all points along this line of identity, the posttest probability is equal to the pretest probability; therefore, a test with these characteristics should have no diagnostic value. The true diagnostic value of the test is reflected by the degree to which the upper and lower curves, representing abnormal and normal test outcomes respectively, deviate from the line of identity. At the extremes of pretest probability of disease (<5% and >90%), the abnormal and normal curves are less well separated than in the intermediate range of pretest probability (40% to 60%). Figure 3–5 shows that the predictive value of a positive test result is poor in the population with a 10% prevalence of disease (line A), whereas the predictive value of a negative test result is poor in the population with a 90% pretest prevalence of disease (line C). A family of curves can be depicted in this type of relationship, as shown in Figure 3–6, if different criteria for positive test results are used. In this example from a review by Epstein,[9] different criteria for abnormal ST-segment depression response are illustrated. As the criteria for an abnormal test result become more stringent (e.g., ST depression ≥2.5 mm, top curve), the predictive value of a positive result in a low-prevalence population improves.

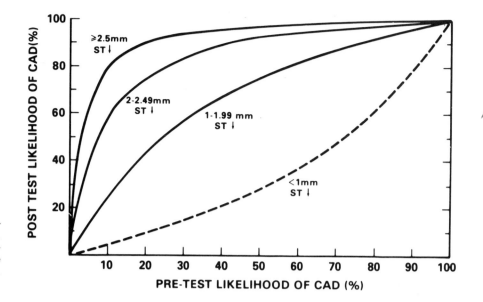

Figure 3–6. Family of ST-segment depression (ST ↓) curves and likelihood of CAD. (Reprinted with permission from the American College of Cardiology (Journal of the American College of Cardiology, 1980, Vol. 46, pp. 491–499).)

Estimating Probability of Coronary Artery Disease Based on Age, Sex, and Symptoms

The pretest likelihood of CAD can be well estimated from consideration of the patient's age, sex, and symptom classification. Knowledge of risk factors and findings on a resting ECG are also useful for estimating pretest probability. Diamond and Forrester[4] reviewed records of thousands of patients reported in the literature and developed tables showing that an asymptomatic male aged 50 to 59 years would have a posttest likelihood of CAD of only 18.5% with 1.0 to 1.5 mm of ST depression on the exercise ECG. A woman aged 40 to 49 with typical angina would have a posttest likelihood of CAD of 72.3% with 1.0 to 1.5 mm of ST depression, whereas a male in the same age range with typical angina and a comparable ECG stress test result would have a posttest likelihood of 93.6%.

There are substantial data that relate the prevalence of significant angiographic CAD to the type of chest pain manifested. Gibson and Beller[7] described the prevalence of significant angiographic CAD relative to the type of chest pain derived from five series in the literature comprising 3317 patients. Patients were classified as either being asymptomatic or having nonanginal chest pain, atypical angina, or typical angina. In patients classified as having typical angina, the pain must be substernal, provoked by exercise, and relieved by rest or relieved within 10 minutes by sublingual nitroglycerin. If only two of these three features are present, the chest pain is classified as atypical angina. If only one of the three is present, the pain is classified as nonanginal. There was an 11% prevalence of CAD in patients with nonanginal chest pain, compared to 54% prevalence of CAD and 88% prevalence of CAD in patients with atypical and typical angina pectoris, respectively.

Bayes' Theorem and Multiple Test Results

Diamond et al.[5] have indicated that, if individual test results are independent of one another, Bayes' theorem can be applied to more than one test. When several tests are performed (e.g., exercise ECG stress testing and Tl-201 scintigraphy), the probability of disease following the first test becomes the pretest probability of disease for the second test. This is commonly referred to as *sequential Bayesian analysis.* This approach would be significant when multiple tests are used in a low-prevalence population since a single positive test result in such a population is of limited diagnostic value. If two independent tests were concordantly positive, a higher posttest likelihood of disease in such a low-prevalence population would be calculated. Concordantly negative results for two independent tests in intermediate or high–pretest likelihood populations tend to produce a lower posttest probability than the results of a single test.

Discordant test results have to be carefully analyzed in conjunction with other factors that are known relevant to the tests (e.g., presence of left ventricular [LV] hypertrophy, which can cause false-positive ST-segment depression). Nevertheless, discordant test results would still yield an intermediate probability of disease. The exercise ECG is generally the first test employed, and a radionuclide stress test usually the second. If, for example, a patient is able to exercise only to a heart rate of 105 bpm, which would be less than 85% of the maximum predicted heart rate, and has a normal ST-segment response but a discrete anteroseptal redistribution defect, the posttest likelihood of CAD would still be in the range of 80% to 85%, despite a negative exercise ECG test result. On the other hand, if such a patient exercises to a heart rate of 180 bpm, has a normal Tl-201 perfusion scan but 1.0 mm of transient ST depres-

EFFECTS OF POPULATION PREVALENCE ON NON-INVASIVE PREDICTION OF CAD

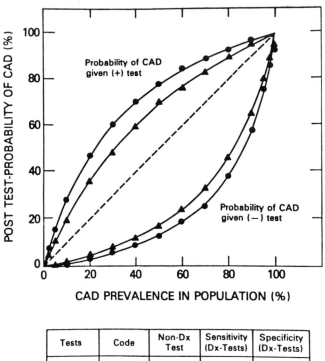

Tests	Code	Non-Dx Test	Sensitivity (Dx-Tests)	Specificity (Dx-Tests)
E_xECG	▲——▲	35	84%	62%
201_{Tl}	●——●	9	88%	74%

Figure 3–7. Graphic display of Bayes' theorem employing exercise electrocardiography and thallium 201 as the diagnostic tests. Note the increased or decreased posttest probability of CAD when test results are positive and negative, respectively. (Reprinted by permission from the American College of Cardiology (Journal of the American College of Cardiology, 1989, Vol. 13, pp. 1653–1655).)

sion that normalizes within 1 minute into the recovery period, the posttest probability of CAD would still be reduced to <15%, despite the positive ST-segment response. Figure 3–7 shows the posttest probability of CAD using the sequential Bayesian analysis approach from Patterson and Horowitz.[10] In this example, sensitivity values for the exercise ECG and Tl-201 scintigraphy are 84% and 88%, respectively. Specificity values for the two tests are 62% and 74%, respectively.

EXERCISE ELECTROCARDIOGRAPHIC STRESS TESTING

Physiologic Responses to Exercise

Dynamic exercise is preferred for testing because it puts a volume stress, rather than a pressure stress, on the heart and it can be graduated.[11] When exercise is begun, oxygen uptake by the lungs rapidly increases, but it reaches a steady state after 1 minute at each exercise intensity. That

is, during a steady-state condition, heart rate, cardiac output, blood pressure, and pulmonary ventilation are maintained at relatively constant levels. Maximal oxygen uptake (Vo_2max) is the greatest amount of oxygen that can be utilized while performing dynamic exercise. In stress-testing parlance, oxygen uptake is expressed in multiples of sitting, resting requirements. The metabolic equivalent (MET) is a unit of sitting, resting oxygen uptake at 3.5 ml oxygen (O_2) per kilogram of body weight per minute. A workload of 4 MET is equivalent to level walking at 4 mph. The maximal oxygen uptake (Vo_2) is equal to product of the maximum cardiac output and the maximum arterial venous oxygen difference. Since cardiac output is equal to the product of stroke volume and heart rate, Vo_2 is directly proportional to heart rate.

Myocardial oxygen uptake is determined by myocardial wall tension reflected by (1) LV systolic pressure multiplied by the end-diastolic volume and divided by LV wall thickness, (2) contractility, and (3) heart rate. The myocardial oxygen demand can be estimated during clinical exercise testing by the double product or rate-pressure product, which is the product of heart rate and systolic blood pressure. There is a direct relationship between myocardial oxygen uptake and myocardial blood flow during exercise. A patient with a coronary stenosis may not increase coronary blood flow sufficiently to fulfill the metabolic demands of the myocardium during exercise, in which case myocardial ischemia results.

As cardiac output increases with exercise, arterial blood pressure increases, owing to the increased cardiac output. There is an increase in heart rate with exercise attributed to diminished vagal tone, followed by an increase in sympathetic neural outflow to the heart and blood vessels. Heart rate during exercise is influenced by age, in that maximum heart rate decreases with age. Maximum heart rate is calculated by subtracting a subject's age from 220.

Safety of Exercise Stress Testing

Exercise stress testing is an extremely safe procedure. Risk of complications is greatest in postinfarction patients and in those being evaluated for complex ventricular arrhythmias. Table 3–2 lists absolute and relative contraindications to exercise testing.[11] All exercise testing should be undertaken under the supervision of a physician appropriately trained to conduct such tests. The American College of Physicians, American College of Cardiology, and American Heart Association Task Force has published the training recommendations for physicians conducting exercise stress tests.[12] Although the number of procedures necessary to ensure competence has not been definitively established by objective criteria, the opinion of the Task Force committee and its consultants was that a trainee should participate in at least 50 exercise procedures under supervision during training.

Table 3–2. Absolute and Relative Contraindications to Exercise Testing

Absolute	Relative*
Acute myocardial infarction or recent change on resting ECG	Less serious noncardiac disorder
Active unstable angina	Significant arterial or pulmonary hypertension
Serious cardiac arrhythmias	Tachyarrhythmias or bradyarrhythmias
Acute pericarditis	Moderate valvular or myocardial heart disease
Endocarditis	Drug effect or electrolyte abnormalities
Severe aortic stenosis	Left main coronary obstruction or its equivalent
Severe left ventricular dysfunction	Hypertrophic cardiomyopathy
Acute pulmonary embolus or pulmonary infarction	Psychiatric disease
Acute or serious noncardiac disorder	
Severe physical handicap or disability	

*Under certain circumstances, and with appropriate precautions, relative contraindications can be superseded.

(From Fletcher GF, et al.: Exercise standards. A statement for health professionals from the American Heart Association. Circulation 1990;82:2286–2322.)

Indications for Exercise Stress Testing and Technique of Testing

General indications for exercise testing have been comprehensively described.[12] Table 3–3 lists the class I (conditions for which there is general agreement that exercise testing is justified) indications for exercise testing, as determined by a task force of the American College of Cardiology and American Heart Association.[13]

All protocols for diagnostic exercise testing involve a warm-up low-load phase, followed by progressive uninterrupted exercise of finite duration at each level, and a recovery period. The most popular incremental exercise protocol used is the Bruce protocol.[14] The advantages of the Bruce protocol include a seventh or final stage that cannot be completed by most subjects and its use in many published studies. With the Bruce protocol, the fourth stage can be either run or walked. The optimal protocol should last 6 to 12 minutes.

The indications for terminating exercise testing have been well defined. Although ischemic chest pain induced by the exercise test is strongly predictive of CAD, ≥1.0 mm of horizontal or down-sloping ST-segment depression is considered a positive test endpoint for ischemia. This standard criterion involves a duration of horizontal or down-sloping ST depression of ≥80 msec. Figure 3–8 shows the rest and exercise ECGs of a patient with horizontal ST depression reflective of a positive response for ischemia. Rapid up-sloping ST depression is a normal ECG response to exercise. Slow up-sloping ST depression, where the ST segment is still depressed by ≥1.5 mm at 80 msec,

is considered a nondiagnostic test response (Fig. 3–9). In the presence of baseline ECG abnormalities, exercise-induced ST-segment depression is less specific for ischemia. Increasing or initial appearance of ST-segment elevation in leads where Q waves are present indicates exercise-induced LV dysfunction. ST-segment elevation observed in the situation of a normal ECG at rest without pathologic Q waves suggests severe stress-induced coronary vasospasm. Resting T-wave inversions may "pseudonormalize" during exercise. This finding is not highly predictive of underlying CAD. In normal subjects, there is an increase in R-wave amplitude during submaximal exercise but a fall in the height of the R wave at maximal stress.

Some abnormal ST-segment responses occur only during the postexercise recovery period. Monitoring is continued for a minimum of 5 minutes after exercise or until ST abnormalities resolve. Typical ischemic chest pain provoked during exercise testing is strongly predictive of CAD; however, atypical chest pain or nonanginal chest pain that can also be reproduced during testing has a low predictive value for CAD unless it is associated with other manifestations of ischemia (i.e., ST depression of myocardial perfusion abnormalities).

Detection of Coronary Artery Disease by Electrocardiographic Stress Testing

Gianrossi et al.[15] applied metaanalysis techniques to 147 consecutively published reports comparing exercise-induced ST-segment depression with coronary angiography. These published studies were of 24,074 patients who underwent both tests. Wide variability in sensitivity and specificity was observed (mean sensitivity, 68%; range, 23% to 100%, SD, 16%; mean specificity, 77%; range, 17% to 100%, SD, 17%; Fig. 3–10). There are a number of explanations for this wide range in published sensitivity and specificity results. In some studies, equivocal or nondiagnostic tests were considered normal results. Up-sloping ST depression was considered an abnormal finding in many

Table 3–3. Class I Indications for Exercise Testing

To assist in the diagnosis of CAD in male patients with symptoms that are atypical for myocardial ischemia
To assess functional capacity and to aid in assessing the prognosis of patients with known CAD
To evaluate the prognosis and functional capacity of patients with CAD soon after an uncomplicated myocardial infarction (before discharge or soon after discharge)
To evaluate patients after coronary artery revascularization by surgery or coronary angioplasty
To evaluate patients with symptoms consistent with recurrent, exercise-induced cardiac arrhythmias
To evaluate functional capacity of selected patients with congenital heart disease
To evaluate patients with rate-responsive pacemakers

(Adapted from Schlant RC, et al: Clinical competence in exercise testing. J Am Coll Cardiol 1990;16:1061–1065.)

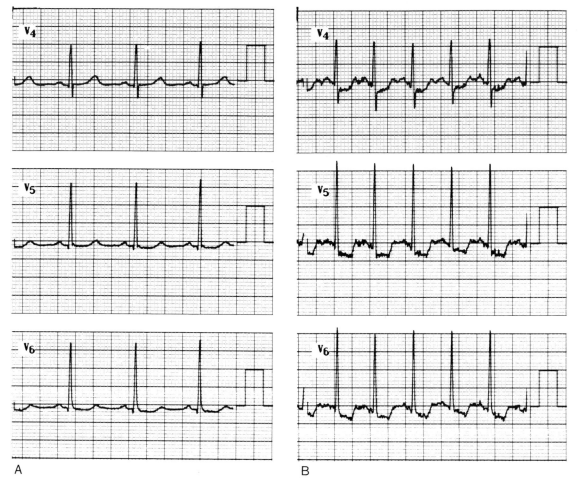

Figure 3–8. A. Baseline V_4, V_5, and V_6 leads in upright position prior to exercise stress. **B.** ECG tracings at peak exercise in same patient showing horizontal to downsloping ischemic ST depression in leads V_5 and V_6.

studies. Classifying up-sloping ST depression as abnormal can significantly lower specificity. Similarly, studies that exclude patients with a history of MI yield less specificity. As expected, increased specificity was observed in studies when patients with left bundle branch block (LBBB) were excluded.

The extent of CAD certainly may affect sensitivity of the exercise ECG. Sensitivity for CAD detection is in the range of 50% for patients with single-vessel disease and exceeds 85% for those with three-vessel CAD. Detrano et al.[16] sought to determine the accuracy of exercise-induced ST depression for predicting multivessel CAD, by metaanalysis to the world's literature. From 60 reports comprising 12,030 patients, 5174 of whom had multivessel CAD by angiography, sensitivity was 81% ± 12% and specificity 66% ± 16% for prediction of multivessel CAD. Right bundle branch block (RBBB) diminished sensitivity for detection of multivessel disease. A decreased sensitivity for predicting three-vessel or left main disease was associated with inclusion of patients who were receiving digitalis. The best independent variable for enhancing specificity for

either multivessel or "critical" CAD was heart rate adjustment of ST depression.

Causes of false-positive exercise ST-segment responses include ST-T–wave abnormalities on the resting ECG due to digitalis administration, LV hypertrophy, Wolff-Parkinson-White syndrome, electrolyte abnormalities, BBB, and hyperventilation syndrome. Other disorders, such as cardiomyopathy, hypertension, and pericardial disease, may be associated with false-positive ST-segment responses to exercise stress.

The administration of beta-blocking drugs may influence exercise stress test results, as they can prevent the patient from attaining the desired heart rate–blood pressure product at which ischemic ST-segment depression would appear. This would increase the prevalence of false-negative ST-segment responses. Similarly, other antianginal drugs (e.g., nitrates) may prevent the appearance of the abnormal ST-segment changes. The recommendation has been made that antianginal drugs should be withheld for at least 12 hours if the purpose of the exercise tests is to establish a diagnosis of ischemic heart disease.[13]

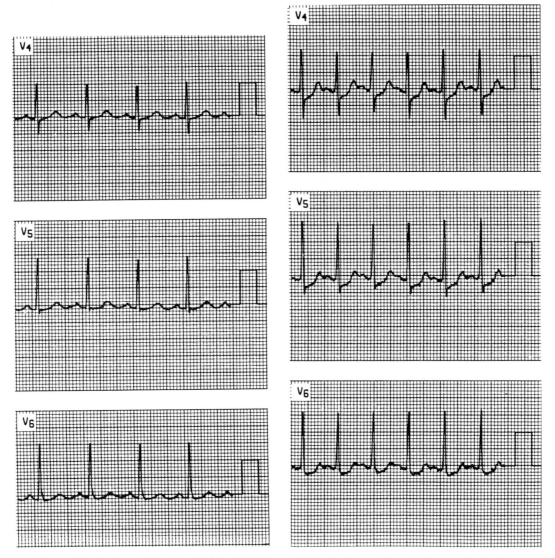

Figure 3–9. *Left panel:* Baseline ECG leads V$_4$, V$_5$, and V$_6$ in standing position prior to exercise testing. *Right panel:* The same ECG leads at a speed of 1.7 miles per hour and a grade of 10.0%. The tracings show slow upsloping ST depression in these leads. The patient had no accompanying chest pain and achieved a workload of 7.0 METS.

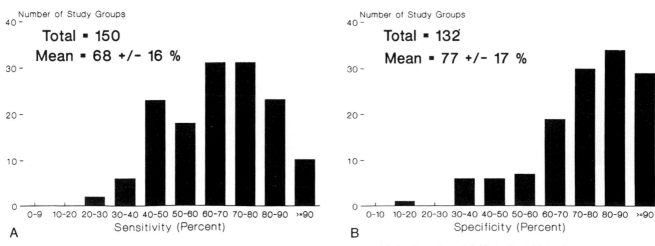

Figure 3–10. A. Distribution of sensitivities of the exercise ECG for detection of CAD in the 150 study groups identified in the literature (values are mean ± SD). Sensitivity of the exercise ECG was 68 ± 16% in this literature survey with a wide range of values reported. **B.** Distribution of specificities for CAD detection by exercise ECG stress testing in the 132 studies derived from the literature. The mean value for specificity for CAD detection was 77 ± 17% in this literature survey with a wide range of values reported. (Gianrossi R, et al.: Circulation 1989;80:87–98.)

Correlation of the maximal rate of progression of ST-segment depression relative to increases in heart rate (maximal ST/heart rate [HR] slope) has been reported to be a more precise indicator of stress-induced ischemia than ST-segment depression alone. Okin et al.[17] compared exercise ECG with exercise radionuclide cineangiography and coronary angiography in 35 patients with stable angina to assess the clinical value of the maximal ST/HR slope. They found that an ST/HR slope of 6.0 or more identified three-vessel disease with a sensitivity of 89% and a specificity of 88%. The exercise ST/HR slope was shown to be linearly related to the exercise change in LV ejection fraction (EF). Bobbio et al.[18] found only a small increase in accuracy by dividing exercise-induced ST depression by heart rate. In that study, sensitivities of ST depression and ST/HR index in detecting three-vessel or left main disease were 75% and 78%, respectively, in 401 patients analyzed. Figure 3–11 shows receiver operating characteristic (ROC) curves for the conventional measurement of ST depression and the heart rate–adjusted ST depression in this study.

Computer exercise ECG has also been evaluated to assist interpretation and enhance sensitivity and specificity of exercise stress testing. Hollenberg et al.[19] utilized a computer-derived treadmill exercise score that quantifies the ECG response to exercise. These authors found that the treadmill exercise score improved the diagnostic specificity of exercise ECG in the screening of a population with a low prevalence of CAD.

In summary, there is marked variability in the literature concerning sensitivity and specificity values for the detection of CAD by exercise ECG. Because of suboptimal sensitivity and specificity, efforts were made in the 1970s to develop alternative or supplementary noninvasive techniques aimed at enhancing the ability to accurately detect CAD with exercise testing. These techniques involved simultaneous assessment of either regional myocardial perfusion or cardiac function during exercise.

EXERCISE THALLIUM-201 SCINTIGRAPHY

The technical aspects of myocardial perfusion imaging are discussed in detail in Chapter 1, and the essentials of myocardial Tl-201 kinetics required for a comprehensive understanding of the use of this agent for stress imaging are summarized in Chapter 2. Myocardial perfusion imaging with radioactive tracers can be performed in patients who are asymptomatic, who have symptoms suggestive of CAD, or who have known CAD.[19a–19d] In the latter group, a physiologic assessment of the extent and severity of ischemia is desirable. Perfusion imaging can be undertaken utilizing planar imaging technology or with SPECT techniques. Quantitation of Tl-201 uptake and redistribution is required for optimal sensitivity and specificity for CAD detection.

Detection of Occult Coronary Artery Disease in the Asymptomatic Patient

Certain totally asymptomatic subjects with multiple CAD risk factors may manifest painless ischemia and, therefore, are at increased risk for subsequent cardiac events without premonitory warning signs (see Chap. 5). The exercise ECG alone generally is not clinically useful when applied to a patient population with a low (<10%) pretest likelihood of CAD.[20] Allen et al.[21] reported a 5-year follow-up study of 888 asymptomatic men and women without known CAD who had undergone maximal treadmill ECG testing. For the 105 patients who initially had an abnormal exercise test result and were followed up, there was only a 1.1% prevalence of CAD per year. Only two of 221 men 40 years of age or younger developed manifestations of heart disease, and neither patient had exercise-induced ST-segment abnormalities. That study concluded that the treadmill test did not accurately predict CAD in asymptomatic men 40 years of age or younger. Froelicher et al.[22] performed cardiac catheterization on 138 asymptomatic men with an abnormal treadmill test. Fewer than a third of them had at least one lesion of at least 50% narrowing. Borer et al.[23] found a 37% incidence of angiographic CAD in 30 asymptomatic persons with hyperlipidemia and an abnormal exercise test. Uhl et al.[24] found a 26% predictive value for the exercise ECG for detecting significant angiographic CAD in 255 apparently healthy men undergoing exercise stress testing.

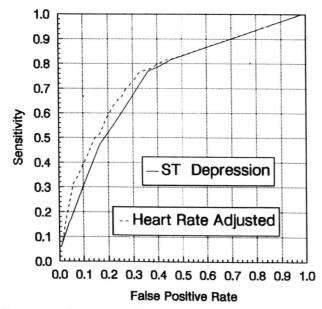

Figure 3–11. Receiver-operating characteristic curves for the conventional measurement of ST-segment depression *(solid line)* and the heart rate–adjusted ST-segment depression *(dotted line).* The endpoint is angiographic triple-vessel and left main CAD. The area under the curve for the heart rate–adjusted ST-segment depression was somewhat larger than that for ST depression alone. (Reprinted with permission from the American College of Cardiology (Journal of the American College of Cardiology, 1992, Vol. 19, pp. 11–18).)

The poor predictive value of the exercise ECG response for detection of CAD in totally asymptomatic subjects is not surprising. As discussed previously, the predictive accuracy of any test for CAD detection, such as the exercise ECG, is based not only on sensitivity and specificity values but also on the prevalence of the disease in the population under study (Bayes' theorem). In an asymptomatic male patient with less than a 10% pretest likelihood of CAD, 1.0 mm of ST-segment depression at peak exercise increases the likelihood of CAD after testing to only 35% because the false-positive rate is quite high for the mildly positive exercise ST response in this type of patient.

In the totally asymptomatic patient, Tl-201 stress imaging appears to identify more patients with asymptomatic ischemia than the exercise ECG test alone—probably because perfusion imaging is more sensitive than exercise ECG for detection of CAD.

An interesting study involved 130 asymptomatic Air Force pilots who had been referred for catheterization because of coronary risk factors or positive stress ECGs.[25] Of the 22 who had significant CAD—that is, more than 50% coronary stenosis—all had an abnormal Tl-201 scan. Twelve were deemed by angiography to have nonsignificant disease with lesions between 25% and 50%. Of these, eight had an abnormal Tl-201 scan. These data suggest that exercise Tl-201 imaging may be an appropriate second test to identify or confirm the presence of silent ischemia in a patient who demonstrates painless ST-segment depression on a screening exercise ECG. Another indication for stress perfusion imaging would be an asymptomatic patient with multiple risk factors and a strong family history of CAD but a normal exercise ECG at a suboptimal heart rate response. The addition of Tl-201 imaging to exercise stress testing in a low-prevalence population makes sense from the standpoint of conditional probability analysis.[5] In patients with a low pretest likelihood of CAD, multiple tests are required to enhance the predictive value of noninvasive stress testing for detection of silent ischemia.[10] Concordant positive findings indicative of asymptomatic ischemia would result in a significantly increased posttest likelihood of CAD.

Uhl et al.[26] examined the value of the addition of exercise Tl-201 imaging to the exercise ECG in 191 flight crewmen who exhibited an abnormal ST-segment response to exercise. The predictive value of the exercise ECG alone was 21%, versus 74% for Tl-201 scintigraphy. The specificity of Tl-201 imaging in that study was 90%. These investigators pointed out that if both an abnormal exercise ECG and an abnormal Tl-201 scintigram had been required before angiography was performed 136 subjects with ST depression and no underlying CAD would have been spared angiography. In another study of asymptomatic siblings of patients with premature CAD, both planar and tomographic Tl-201 scintigraphy identified more patients with silent ischemia than the exercise ECG stress test alone (Table 3–4).[27] Schwartz et al.[27a] determined the utility of Tl-201 ex-

Table 3–4. **Screening Asymptomatic Siblings of Patients with Coronary Artery Disease**

	Abnormal (definite or probable)	Borderline (%)	Total (%)
Tomographic thallium (N = 65)	23	5	28
Planar thallium (N = 79)	6	14	20
Exercise ECG (N = 83)	11	1	12
Treadmill chest pain (N = 83)	——	——	4

(From Becker LC, et al.: Screening of asymptomatic siblings of patients with premature coronary artery disease. Circulation 1987;75 [Suppl II]: II-14–II-17.)

ercise scintigraphy in 845 asymptomatic male military air crew who underwent coronary arteriography because abnormal noninvasive test results suggested possible ischemia. The prevalence of CAD in this population was 16.9%. Overall sensitivity and specificity of planar Tl-201 scintigraphy was 45% ± 4% and 78% ± 1%, respectively, in this cohort with a low prevalence of CAD. For patients younger than 45 years with a total cholesterol–high density lipoprotein (HDL) ratio less than 4.5 the probability that an abnormal scan was a false-positive result was 90%. A limitation of this study was that some patients were referred for coronary arteriography because of an abnormal Tl-201 scan.

Some basic guidelines, derived from clinical experience, may improve the efficiency and accuracy of diagnosing silent myocardial ischemia in totally asymptomatic subjects. For totally asymptomatic patients who require exercise stress testing for any of a variety of reasons, such as a strong family history, multiple risk factors, an unexplained resting ECG abnormality, or consideration for a large life insurance policy, the exercise ECG stress test is still cost effective as the first screening test (see Chap. 5). If the exercise ECG shows no ST-segment depression at a workload of 85% or more of maximal predicted heart rate or exceeds 10 MET, then risk-factor modification, without repeat testing with radionuclide imaging, would be appropriate because such a patient would have a low probability of having functionally important CAD. A positive ST-segment shift of 1 mm or more that occurs at less than 5 MET and is associated with either diminished exercise tolerance or an abnormal blood pressure response is probably a true-positive stress test response. This test result suggests a high probability of silent ischemia, and referral directly to cardiac catheterization would be appropriate. Absence of ST-segment depression at a low workload might imply a false-negative response as a result of inadequate exercise stress to induce ST depression and, therefore, repeat testing with radionuclide imaging is the appropriate next diagnostic step. Finally, ST-segment depression that appears at very high workload without associated chest pain and resolves rapidly during recovery might suggest a false-positive response. For such patients, repeat exercise Tl-201 or Tc-99m sestamibi scintigraphy is warranted. A normal scan at a high exercise heart rate or workload in the presence of 1.0 mm of ST-segment depression would indicate a low probability of significant underlying CAD.

Detection of Coronary Artery Disease in Patients with Chest Pain: Planar Scintigraphy

The earliest studies evaluating the additional benefit of Tl-201 imaging to exercise ECG stress testing used planar imaging techniques, most often employing anterior and several oblique projections.[28–51]

When only visual analysis of planar Tl-201 scintigrams is performed, sensitivity and specificity for CAD detection are approximately 80% to 85% and 80% to 90%, respectively. Kotler and Diamond, in their review of the literature, found an average sensitivity of 84% and a specificity of 87% when data from 33 published studies were pooled.[52] Gerson reviewed 30 studies published from 1976 to 1981 and found, on average, 83.6% sensitivity and 88.4% specificity for Tl-201 scintigraphy.[53] Only one of these 30 studies utilized quantitative scan analysis of serial Tl-201 images. In the review by Kotler and Diamond,[52] qualitative Tl-201 scintigraphy employing visual scan interpretation showed 78% sensitivity for detection of single-vessel disease, 89% sensitivity for two-vessel disease, and 92% sensitivity for three-vessel disease. In most studies, the sensitivity of Tl-201 scintigraphy for CAD detection was found to be greater than the sensitivity of exercise ECG. Gibson and Watson[54] reviewed data from 22 studies in the literature comprising 2048 patients. The average sensitivity and specificity for exercise ECG were 73% and 82%, respectively, compared with 83% and 90% for Tl-201 imaging. Only one of these studies utilized quantitative scan analysis. Port et al.[55] showed that planar Tl-201 scintigraphy was more sensitive than exercise ECG for detection of CAD. In a group of 46 patients with ≥70% luminal diameter obstruction of only one major coronary artery and no history of MI, exercise ECGs were abnormal in 52%. This contrasted with a 91% prevalence of abnormal planar Tl-201 images in the same patients. Results were similar for the right (RCA) and LAD coronary arteries, but sensitivity was lower for isolated circumflex (LCx) artery disease. This finding is different from that reported by Kaul et al.,[56] who showed comparable sensitivity for detecting single-vessel LCx, RCA, and LAD disease.

Quantitative Planar Thallium-201 Imaging

The sensitivity and specificity for Tl-201 scintigraphy are reported to be in the range of 90% or greater when serial postexercise images are analyzed quantitatively using computer-assisted techniques[57–60] (see Chap. 1). Quantitative planar techniques typically use either a circumferential profile analysis of Tl-201 distribution and washout or a horizontal profile, or "slice," approach, in which regional count profiles are delineated in various myocardial regions. Quantitation is undertaken both on spatial and temporal levels. Certain patients demonstrate abnormal net clearance of Tl-201 by quantitative criteria on postexercise images, even though no initial postexercise defect might be measured. However, an isolated regional washout abnormality without any defects elsewhere on a scintigram is often a false-positive finding and the result of an artifact. Crucial to the success of image analysis in many of these quantitative planar imaging techniques is the use of an interpolative background subtraction algorithm (see Chap. 1). Use of quantitative Tl-201 scan analysis diminishes the inter- and intraobserver variability well described for visual scan interpretation.

Table 3–5 shows the sensitivity and specificity of CAD detection by quantitative Tl-201 scintigraphy from papers published from 1981 to 1986 on data from 682 patients. The average sensitivity and specificity values for CAD detection were 91% and 89%, respectively. One of the major advantages of quantitative scan analysis is the enhancement of the individual stenosis detection rate in patients with CAD. Overall sensitivity for CAD detection is improved only 5% to 10% as compared with visual analysis, yet the detection rate for individual stenoses and multivessel disease identification may be enhanced to a far greater degree. In the study by Berger et al.,[57] quantitative planar Tl-201 scintigraphy yielded 91% sensitivity, 90% specificity, and 97% predictive accuracy for CAD detection. In this study, the sensitivity of ≥1.0 mm of ST depression for CAD detection was 62%. Specificity for both tests was comparable, at 90%. For patients without prior MI, the sensitivity of the exercise ECG was 66% and for Tl-201 imaging 88%. Comparison of qualitative and quantitative imaging analyses in a subset of these patients (Table 3–6) showed that both specificity and predictive power for multivessel disease were greater when the quantitation was used (90% vs. 73% and 78% vs. 39%, respectively). Interestingly, in that study sensitivity and specificity were not significantly different when the 95 patients with diagnostic (≥85% maximum predicted HR) and 45 patients with suboptimal (≤85% maximum HR) exercise tests were compared. Fig-

Table 3–5. **Sensitivity and Specificity of Quantitative Thallium-201 Scintigraphy for Detection of Coronary Artery Disease**

Investigator (year)	Patients (No.)	Sensitivity (%)	Specificity (%)
Berger[57] (1981)	140	91	90
Maddahi[58] (1981)	67	93	91
Wackers[59] (1985)	150	89	95
Kaul[60] (1986)	325	90	80
Total	682	91	89

(From Beller GA: Current status of nuclear cardiology techniques. Curr Probl Cardiol 1991;16 [7]:451–535.)

Table 3–6. **Comparison of Qualitative and Quantitative Thallium-201 Scintigraphy for Detection and Recognition of Multivessel Coronary Artery Disease (MVD)**

	Sensitivity (%) (No.)	Specificity (%) (No.)	MVD Recognition (%) (No.)
Qualitative	85% (60/70)	73% (22/30)	39% (20/51)
Quantitative	94% (66/70)	90% (27/30)	78% (40/51)
P value	<0.08	<0.08	<0.002

(Reprinted by permission of the Society of Nuclear Medicine from: Berger BC, et al.: Quantitative thallium-201 exercise scintigraphy for detection of coronary artery disease. J Nucl Med 1981;22:585–593.)

ures 3–12 and 3–13 show postexercise and delayed planar Tl-201 scintigrams with quantitative scan analysis in a patient with CAD.

Maddahi et al.[58] used the multiple-view maximum-count circumferential profile technique for planar image quantitation and found that the quantitative technique significantly increased sensitivity for CAD detection over the visual method in the LAD (56% to 80%), LCx (34% to 63%), and RCA (65% to 94%) without loss of specificity. For patients with one-vessel CAD, qualitative and quantitative scan analysis detected 86% of lesions, whereas for three-vessel CAD quantitative analysis detected 83% of lesions, compared with 53% for visual analysis. Quantitative planar imaging was shown to be significantly superior to exercise ECG in the detection of single-vessel CAD. Kaul et al.[56] observed 88% sensitivity for quantitative planar scintigraphy for detection of single-vessel CAD, as compared with 64% sensitivity for exercise-induced ST-segment depres-

sion. This is comparable to the observations of Berger and coworkers.[57]

Wackers et al.[59] also compared the sensitivity of visual and quantitative Tl-201 analysis for detection of CAD in patients with significant coronary stenoses on angiography. Table 3–7 summarizes the results of this analysis. Overall sensitivity for CAD detection was 65% with visual analysis and 89% with quantitative scan analysis. For single-vessel disease detection, visual and quantitative analysis yielded 55% and 84% sensitivity values, respectively. The predictive accuracy was 69% for predicting single-vessel disease, 34% for two-vessel disease, and 26% for three-vessel disease. The overall prediction rate for multivessel disease was 63%. This means that 37% of patients with "angiographic" multivessel CAD had perfusion defects in the supply region of only one diseased coronary vessel. Of 20 patients with three-vessel CAD, only six (30%) had defects in all three stenotic coronary supply regions. Of the 32 patients with angiographic two-vessel disease, nine (28%) had defects in the distribution of both stenotic arteries. Thus, even with quantitative scan analysis, less than a third of patients with either two-vessel or three-vessel disease demonstrate stress-induced perfusion defects in the distribution of all diseased vessels. Nevertheless, 85% or more have a positive scan, with an abnormality in the region of at least one major defect.

Quantitative scan analysis greatly enhances the ability to confirm the presence or absence of redistribution. This is accomplished by measuring the magnitude of the initial defect and the change in this magnitude in the delayed

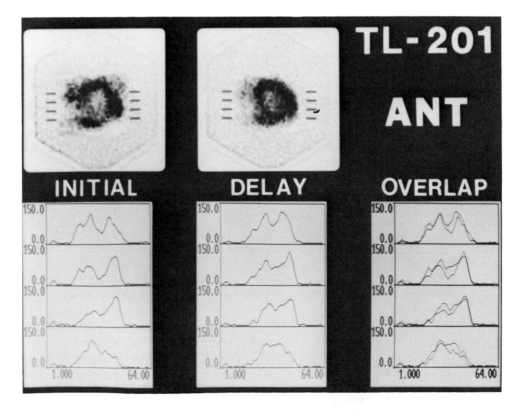

Figure 3–12. *Top panel:* Anterior *(ANT)* planar Tl-201 images postexercise *(INITIAL)* and 2.5-hour delayed *(DELAY)* images with corresponding horizontal count profiles shown below each image. The *OVERLAP* column depicts a superimposition of initial and delayed count profiles from the first two columns. Note the inferior defect with delayed redistribution characterized by increasing regional inferior wall counts over time. There is also an anterolateral defect showing delayed redistribution. Transient left ventricular cavity dilation from initial to delayed images is noted.

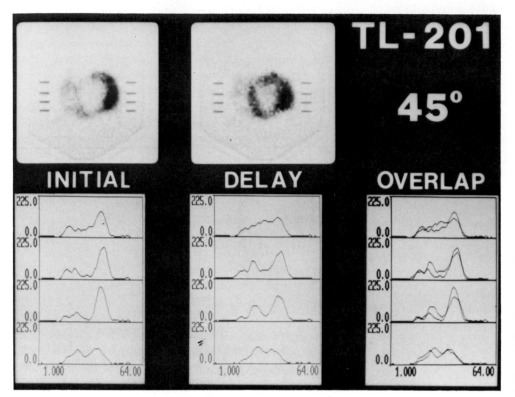

Figure 3–13. A 45-degree anterior oblique image from the same patient whose anterior projection images are shown in Figure 3–12, demonstrating severe septal and inferoapical defects on postexercise *(INITIAL)* images, which demonstrate partial redistribution on the delayed *(DELAY)* images. Increasing septal counts are apparent on the quantitative profiles.

images. Gray-scale images, which are a decidedly nonlinear representation of count density, do not provide a reliable estimate of either redistribution or the time dependence of Tl-201 uptake and washout. The interpretation of Tl-201 uptake and washout in a temporal sequence of images should be based on the underlying principles of Tl-201 kinetics (see Chap. 2).

Factors That Affect Sensitivity and Specificity

Certain factors can affect sensitivity and specificity of planar Tl-201 scintigraphy for CAD detection in patients with chest pain (Table 3–8). Some of them relate to technical considerations and others to physiologic issues.

The location of coronary artery stenoses appears to affect

Table 3–7. Sensitivity of Visual and Quantitative Tl-201 Analysis for Detection of Coronary Artery Disease

Angiographic CAD (N)	Visual Analysis (No.) (%)	Quantitative Analysis (No.) (%)
Any vessel (131)	85/131 (65)	117/131 (89)
One-vessel (77)	42/77 (55)	65/77 (84)
Two-vessel (34)	27/34 (79)	32/34 (94)
Three-vessel (20)	16/20 (80)	20/20 (100)
Multivessel (54)	43/54 (80)	52/54 (96)

(From Wackers FJT, et al.: Quantitative planar thallium-201 stress scintigraphy: A critical evaluation of method. Semin Nucl Med 1985;15:46–66.)

the sensitivity of Tl-201 scintigraphy for appropriately assessing extent of CAD. Circumflex coronary stenoses are more difficult to detect than LAD or RCA obstructions, even with quantitative imaging techniques.[57, 58] Stenoses of the diagonal branches of the LAD or LCx marginal narrowings are also more difficult to detect than the more proximal stenoses in the three major coronary vessels. The reason for the lower sensitivity for detecting LCx marginal or diagonal branch vessel stenoses is not readily obvious. LCx-perfused myocardial regions are located farther posterior and farther from the gamma camera positioned over the chest wall. Small defects in this region may be beyond the resolving capacity of the image method used. Another explanation might be that the amount of myocardium rendered underperfused in the risk area of a circumflex marginal artery narrowing may not be substantial and, therefore, is not well delineated on planar images because of superimposition of myocardial segments perfused by other coronary arteries. In contrast, the myocardial risk area for proximal LAD and proximal dominant LCx disease is proportionately greater, thus the detection rate by planar Tl-201 scintigraphy is higher.

In one study comparing scintigraphic and coronary angiographic findings in patients with isolated disease of the proximal LAD artery, with cutoff values of 0.30 for the pressure gradient and 80% for the reduction in cross-sectional area, the results of exercise Tl-201 scintigraphy were correctly predicted from the angiographic data in 83%.[61] When the pressure gradient was <0.30 and the area of

Table 3–8. **Variables That Affect Sensitivity of Tl-201 Scintigraphy for Detection of Coronary Artery Disease**

Sensitivity Enhancers
 Prior myocardial infarction
 Achieving high exercise heart rate
 Advanced age
 Left main and/or multivessel CAD
 High-grade coronary stenoses
 Proximal location of stenoses
 Associated ST-segment depression
 Regional wall motion abnormality
Sensitivity Diminishers
 Circumflex coronary stenoses
 Branch (e.g., diagonal) or distal stenoses
 Single-vessel CAD
 Nonjeopardized coronary collaterals
 Lesser degrees of coronary narrowing
 Low exercise workload without symptoms
 Antiangina drug therapy during testing
 Visual analysis of scintigrams

From Beller GA: Myocardial perfusion imaging with thallium-201. *In* ML Marcus, HR Schelbert, DJ Skorton, GL Wolf (eds): Cardiac Imaging: A companion to Braunwald's *Heart Disease.* Philadelphia, WB Saunders, 1991, pp 1047–1073.)

stenosis <80%, Tl-201 uptake was normal in 22 of 24 patients. Thus, in the presence of proximal LAD stenosis, abnormal Tl-201 uptake in anterior or septal zones suggests that the coronary narrowing is functionally significant.

Myocardial perfusion abnormalities are more likely to be seen in the distribution of vessels with severe stenoses (>75%) than in vessels with moderate stenoses (50% to 75%).[7, 58] The influence of angiographically demonstrated collateral vessels on sensitivity of Tl-201 imaging remains controversial.[62, 63] Rigo et al. reported that perfusion abnormalities are more frequently noted in the distribution of occluded arteries not fed by collateral vessels than in occluded arteries filled in a retrograde fashion by collaterals.[62]

Tl-201 uptake was normal with greater frequency in the distribution of an occluded artery fed by "nonjeopardized" collaterals compared with the uptake observed in the situation of collaterals that originate from feeding vessels with stenoses. Berger et al.[63] reported that collaterals were not protective in maintaining a normal perfusion response as measured by quantitative Tl-201 scintigraphic criteria during exercise but were associated with enhanced Tl-201 uptake at rest. In another study,[64] collateral flow did not prevent ischemia on exercise Tl-201 imaging in patients with Q-wave infarction.

Diminished sensitivity of Tl-201 scintigraphy could occur if a suboptimal level of exercise is achieved during testing. A minimal level of stress is required to increase coronary blood flow and induce maldistribution of flow; however, it appears that the level of exercise achieved during stress testing influences the exercise ECG response more than the Tl-201 scintigram. Esquivel et al.[65] found that, throughout the range of exercise workloads or peak heart rates achieved, the frequency of Tl-201 scan abnormalities was more prevalent than exercise ST-segment depression. A comparison of the prevalence of ST depression and Tl-201 scan abnormalities related to the intensity of exercise stress is shown in Figure 3–14. Flow heterogeneity is most likely induced early during the course of exercise stress, before either the myocardial metabolic abnormalities that mediate the ST-segment response or anginal chest pain is produced. Figure 3–15 depicts a proposed relationship between exercise intensity and the timing of the appearance of various abnormalities produced by exercise stress in the presence of significant coronary artery stenosis. Note that ST-segment depression and angina are rather late manifestations of ischemia, whereas a perfusion defect that can be detected on a Tl-201 scintigram appears earlier in the course of graded exercise stress.

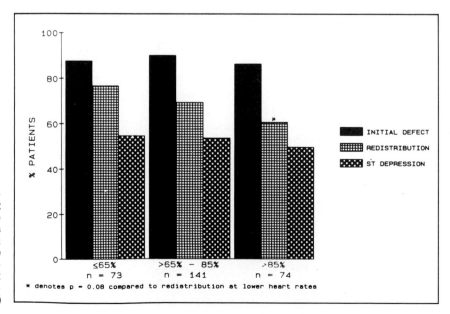

Figure 3–14. Overall prevalence of initial defects, redistribution, and ischemic ST-segment depression on exercise ECG based upon the maximal predicted heart rate in patients undergoing exercise testing for evaluation of a chest pain syndrome. Note that the prevalence of ST-segment depression is reduced compared to Tl-201 scintigraphic abnormalities at each level of exercise heart rate response. (Esquivel L, et al.: Am J Cardiol 1989;63:160–165.)

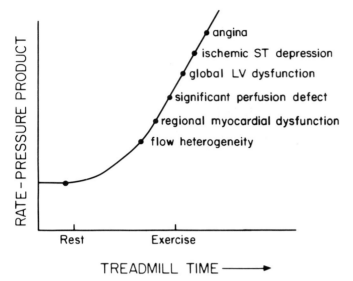

Figure 3–15. Relationship between exercise intensity (treadmill time) and appearance of various functional abnormalities of either myocardial blood flow or contraction. Note that ST-segment depression and exercise angina are rather late manifestations of ischemia, whereas appearance of a perfusion defect that can be detected on a Tl-201 scintigram occurs earlier in the course of graded exercise stress.

Certain drugs have the potential to affect the diagnostic accuracy of Tl-201 scintigraphy, yet, in clinical practice, influence of drugs on scintigraphic results does not seem to be a major obstacle. Pretreatment with isosorbide dinitrate improved Tl-201 uptake on exercise scintigraphy and, thus, diminished sensitivity.[66] In our experience, neither beta-blocker drugs[57] nor calcium antagonists seem to significantly affect sensitivity or specificity of planar Tl-201 scintigraphy for CAD detection. These antiangina drugs do, however, reduce the prevalence of exercise-induced angina and ST-segment depression. For maximum accuracy, it may be prudent to discontinue antiangina-type drugs before exercise testing of patients with an undiagnosed chest pain syndrome.

Age can be an important determinant of perfusion defect size in patients with similar coronary anatomy. A study by DePace et al.[67] found that more myocardium was rendered underperfused in the distribution of a 70% LAD stenosis in older patients than in younger ones.

The major factor promoting enhanced sensitivity in studies of the detection rate of CAD is a history of MI. Sensitivity for CAD detection is lower when patients with a history of MI or Q waves on a resting ECG are not included.[57] This is because a myocardial scar is relatively thin and avascular. Patients with chest pain and prior Q-wave infarction most often exhibit persistent Tl-201 defects on serial images (see Chap. 6).

Causes of Potential False-Positive Scans

There are a host of factors that, if not taken into account or recognized, can diminish specificity of either qualitative or quantitative planar Tl-201 imaging. Tl-201 scintigraphic interpretation can be difficult if one is not knowledgeable about image artifacts or variants of normal. Such knowledge is required to decrease false-positive interpretations of an overlying breast shadow, an altered position of either the inflow or outflow tract of the left ventricle, a greater than normal degree of apical thinning in certain individuals, an overlying diaphragm resulting in diminished relative activity of the inferior wall, or an enlarged right ventricular (RV) blood pool overlying the inferior wall on the anterior image. The major cause of false-positive Tl-201 interpretations in women is breast tissue attenuation. Figure 3–16 shows an example of a false-positive planar Tl-201 scintigraphic study due to breast attenuation in an obese woman. The Tc-99m sestamibi planar image shows markedly less attenuation of the anterior wall, and the SPECT sestamibi image (Fig. 3–16) shows minimal anterior wall attenuation.

In certain patients, the upper septum and upper posterolateral wall may be thin, which could be misinterpreted as perfusion defects or even a left main coronary pattern. In very obese persons, Tl-201 scintigrams of the heart may be of such poor quality because of significant attenuation of Tl-201 activity due to overlying adipose tissue. Applying quantitative analysis for assessing regional Tl-201 uptake, Watson et al.[68] reported that inferior wall segment Tl-201 activity on the anterior projection image can be reduced by as much as 35% and still be within normal limits. This is because the RV blood pool is situated between the gamma camera and the inferior wall of the left ventricle, resulting in attenuation.

Recognition of image artifacts and variants of normal reduces unnecessary referrals for coronary angiography for patients with false-positive Tl-201 scan results. In a study by Desmarais et al.,[69] only 4 of 93 patients with abnormal Tl-201 scans judged to be artifactual were ultimately referred to coronary angiography (Fig. 3–17). All four had normal coronary angiograms. Two underwent angiography because of clinical findings consistent with Prinzmetal's angina, and one was referred for cardiac catheterization because of aortic stenosis. The remaining patients with abnormal scans deemed secondary to image artifact had an excellent prognosis. In contrast, 96% of patients in this study who were referred for coronary angiography because their scans were judged to be truly abnormal and nonartifactual had documented CAD. Of interest, four of the six patients with abnormal scans and angiographically normal coronary arteries in this subgroup had ventriculographic evidence of prior MI. Thus, this study shows that it is important to render interpretations of Tl-201 scans that are unequivocal and do not hedge about what type of abnormality was identified. When attenuation artifacts are identified, the scan report should not be equivocal. The scan should be interpreted as showing no evidence of defects attributed to CAD. This reduces the false-positive rate, enhances the positive predictive accuracy of the test, and

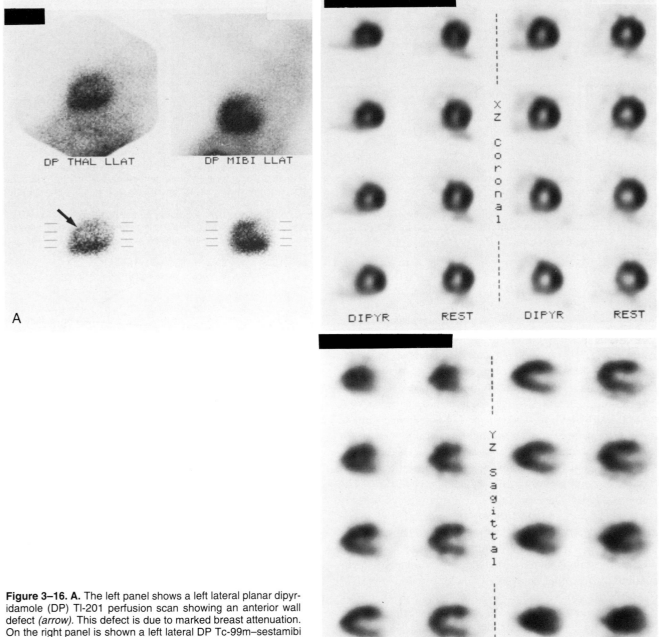

Figure 3–16. A. The left panel shows a left lateral planar dipyridamole (DP) Tl-201 perfusion scan showing an anterior wall defect *(arrow).* This defect is due to marked breast attenuation. On the right panel is shown a left lateral DP Tc-99m–sestamibi (MIBI) perfusion scan in the same patient showing significantly less attenuation in this region. **B.** SPECT Tc-99m–sestamibi images in the same patient show only slight evidence of an attenuation artifact in the anterior wall.

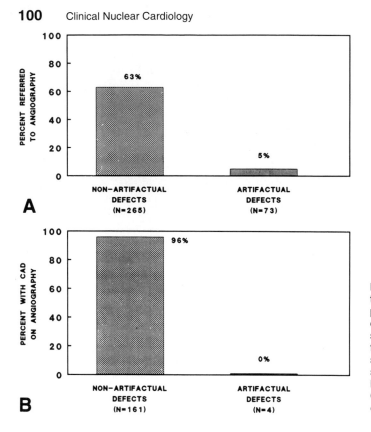

Figure 3–17. A. Percent of patients with nonartifactual and artifactual defects referred for coronary angiography. Note that very few patients with Tl-201 scintigrams interpreted as abnormal because of scan artifacts were referred by their physicians for further invasive evaluation. **B.** Percent of patients with nonartifactual and artifactual defects referred for coronary angiography who demonstrated significant angiographic coronary artery disease (≥50% stenosis). None of the patients with defects judged to be artifactual had significant CAD. (Reprinted with permission from the American College of Cardiology (Journal of the American College of Cardiology, 1993, Vol. 21, pp. 1058–1063).)

prevents unnecessary referrals for coronary angiography. Wackers et al.[69a] assessed the factors affecting interobserver agreement in interpretation of planar Tl-201 stress images in a multicenter trial. A total of 556 scans were interpreted in 24 clinical centers and at a Radionuclide Core Laboratory at Yale University School of Medicine. The clinical centers interpreted more stress studies as abnormal than the care laboratory, and agreement was poor (κ:0.27). Poor reproductivity was also found in the participating centers (κ:0.45) as compared with the core laboratory (κ:0.77). The poor agreement and reproducibility in the clinical centers was thought to be due to lack of standardization of image display and lack of criteria for image interpretation. Agreement improved between the centers and core laboratory with uniformity of image display and with quantitative circumferential profile analysis used for quantitation (see Chap. 1).

Virtually none of the studies of the determination of sensitivity and specificity of Tl-201 imaging techniques for CAD detection have utilized quantitative coronary angiographic criteria as a gold standard and/or employed direct measurements of coronary flow reserve in the cardiac catheterization laboratory. Certain patients deemed to have a false-positive Tl-201 scan may actually have angiographic stenoses that have been underestimated by coronary angiography or a previous infarction in which the infarct-related artery has almost totally "recanalized." Brown et al.[70] evaluated the incidence and causes of abnormal Tl-201 exercise

scintigrams in the absence of "significant" CAD. The group analyzed consisted of 100 consecutive patients undergoing exercise Tl-201 scintigraphy and coronary angiography who were found to have maximal coronary artery diameter stenosis of <50%. Fifty-nine percent of patients with stenoses of 21% to 40% had positive Tl-201 scan results. Tl-201 defects in this group of patients were more common when patients exercised to 85% of maximal heart rate than when slower exercise heart rates were achieved. Similarly, patients with an underlying 21% to 40% maximal stenosis who were taking propranolol were more likely to have a positive Tl-201 test response than patients who did not take propranolol. Kaul et al.[71] found a 35% prevalence of abnormal Tl-201 scans in patients with less than 50% coronary stenoses. According to Becker et al.,[72] dependency on measuring absolute Tl-201 clearance alone from myocardial segments for detection of a significant stenosis may lead to a false-positive scan interpretation. Clearance from normal zones was related to exercise heart rate and exercise duration. These authors observed faster washout from normally perfused regions in normal volunteers as compared with washout from "normal" regions in CAD patients. Differential Tl-201 washout, where one region exhibits significantly more rapid washout than another region in the same patient, may be a useful parameter for detecting ischemia.[57, 60, 73–78]

Finally, a number of noncoronary diseases of the heart or coronary circulation may yield an abnormal myocardial perfusion scan (e.g., scleroderma). These diseases that can cause a false-positive Tl-201 image for CAD are discussed in Chapter 11.

Thallium-201 Scintigraphy for Detection of Coronary Artery Disease: SPECT Techniques

A significant advance in the noninvasive detection of CAD by perfusion imaging techniques is the improved utilization of the SPECT technique. The instrumentation required and technical aspects of SPECT imaging are discussed in Chapter 1. The sensitivity for CAD detection and individual coronary stenosis identification may be superior with SPECT than with planar imaging techniques.[79] Interestingly, at the time of this writing, no prospective studies of a large number of patients comparing quantitative SPECT with quantitative planar imaging have been reported. As discussed in Chapter 1, the SPECT technique permits a more three-dimensional delineation of in vivo radiopharmaceutical distribution than planar imaging. SPECT images are interpreted free of background activity, and lesion contrast is higher. Localization of defects is more precise and more readily appreciated. The extent and size of defects are better defined by tomographic reconstructed views. Because reorientation is undertaken on all hearts, the scintigraphic views are more standardized with respect to cardiac orientation. With the higher image contrast for SPECT and the capability of separating overlying myocardial structures, individual coronary vascular territories (e.g., LAD, RCA, LCx) can be better differentiated. Figures 3–18 and 3–19 are examples of SPECT Tl-201 scintigrams in patients who presented with chest pain. Table 3–9 summarizes the pooled data on sensitivity and specificity of SPECT Tl-201 imaging for CAD detection from studies published in the literature.[80–85] As shown, the average sensitivity in the 1447 patients in this pooled analysis was 92%, and specificity, 68%. This low specificity may, in part, be related to an increasing referral bias in recent years, by which patients with predominantly abnormal scans tend to be referred for coronary angiography more often than patients with normal scans.[86] This would yield a higher

proportion of patients with false-positive Tl-201 scintigrams who undergo catheterization. Patients with normal coronary arteries and normal Tl-201 perfusion scans (true negatives) are not being referred for cardiac catheterization. A better assessment of the "specificity" of SPECT Tl-201 imaging is to use what is referred to as the "normalcy" rate. This value is derived from the Tl-201 scintigraphic results in patients presenting with a <5% pretest likelihood of CAD, most of whom have not been referred for coronary angiography. In the pooled analysis cited above, the normalcy rate for SPECT Tl-201 imaging was 84%.

SPECT Thallium-201 Quantitation

Quantitation of SPECT Tl-201 images can improve image interpretation and enhance the detection rate of individual coronary stenoses. The various methods for quantifying SPECT images are described in Chapter 1. Maddahi et al. evaluated 183 men who underwent Tl-201 SPECT imaging.[85] Quantitation of Tl-201 activity was undertaken on short-axis and apical portions of vertical long-axis images. A Butterworth filter with a frequency cutoff of 0.2 cycles-pixel was used in the back-projection algorithm for these studies. Normal limits were obtained from a group of 20 normal men. The overall detection rate of CAD was 96%, the normalcy rate, 86%. The sensitivity and specificity of Tl-201 SPECT imaging in this study for identification of individual stenotic vessels in 47 catheterized patients without history of infarction are shown in Figure 3–20. The sensitivity for detection of all vessels was 73%, and the specificity, 81%. Thus, utilizing a quantitative method for analysis of SPECT images yielded very high sensitivity while maintaining an adequate normalcy rate.

A multicenter trial comprised of 242 patients who underwent coronary angiography and 76 patients with a low pretest likelihood of CAD yielded a sensitivity of 94% and a normalcy rate of 82% for CAD detection.[84] The specificity of SPECT Tl-201 scintigraphy in patients with angiographically normal coronary arteries in this study was only 44%. Again, this reflects the referral bias—sending to cardiac catheterization predominantly patients who have abnormal scans. Display of the SPECT data in the form of a polar

Table 3–9. **Detection of Coronary Artery Disease with Exercise SPECT–Thallium-201 Scintigraphy**

Investigator	Patients (No.)	Sensitivity (%)	Specificity (%)	Normalcy Rate (%)
Maddahi[85]	183	96	56	86
Van Train[84]	318	94	44	82
Tamaki[80]	104	98	91	—
DePasquale[81]	210	95	71	—
Mahmarian[83]	360	87	87	—
Iskandrian[82]	272	82	62	—
Total	1447	92	68	84

(From Beller GA: Current status of nuclear cardiology techniques. Curr Probl Cardiol 1991;16[7]:451–535.)

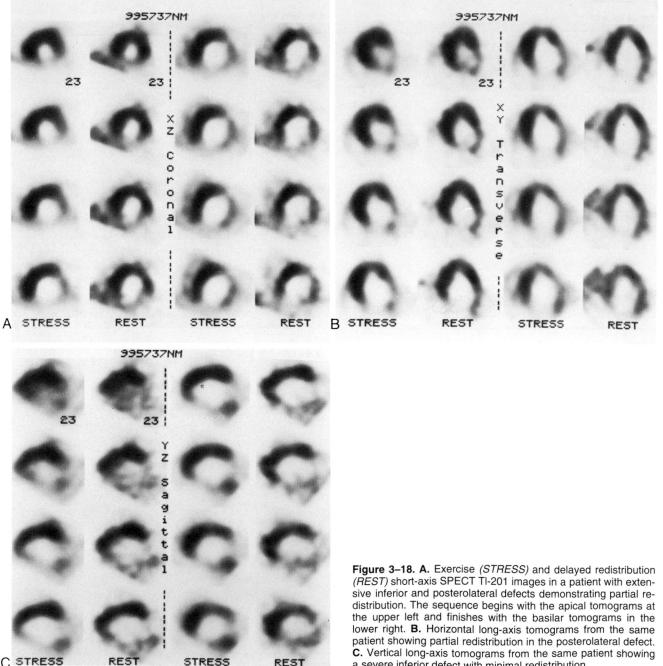

Figure 3–18. A. Exercise *(STRESS)* and delayed redistribution *(REST)* short-axis SPECT Tl-201 images in a patient with extensive inferior and posterolateral defects demonstrating partial redistribution. The sequence begins with the apical tomograms at the upper left and finishes with the basilar tomograms in the lower right. **B.** Horizontal long-axis tomograms from the same patient showing partial redistribution in the posterolateral defect. **C.** Vertical long-axis tomograms from the same patient showing a severe inferior defect with minimal redistribution.

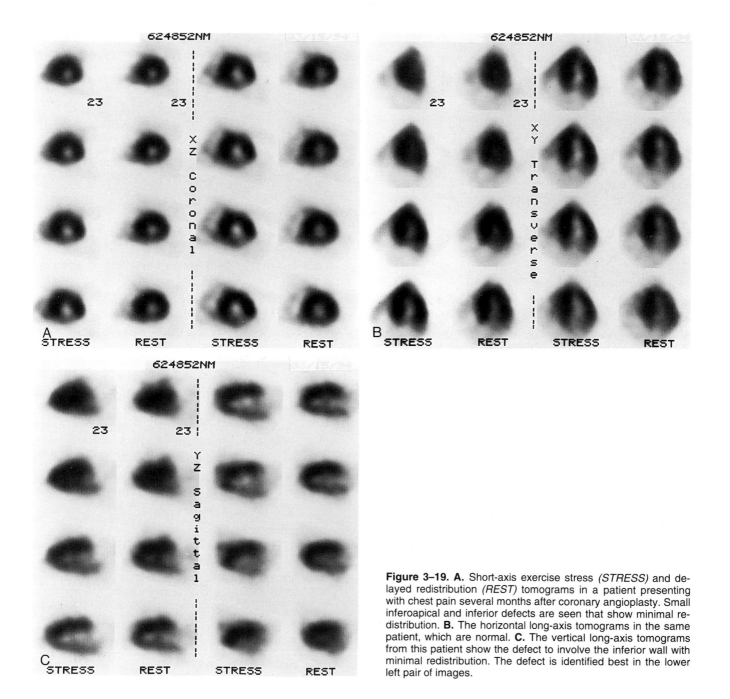

Figure 3–19. A. Short-axis exercise stress *(STRESS)* and delayed redistribution *(REST)* tomograms in a patient presenting with chest pain several months after coronary angioplasty. Small inferoapical and inferior defects are seen that show minimal redistribution. **B.** The horizontal long-axis tomograms in the same patient, which are normal. **C.** The vertical long-axis tomograms from this patient show the defect to involve the inferior wall with minimal redistribution. The defect is identified best in the lower left pair of images.

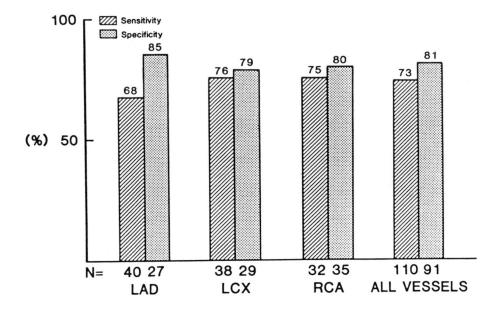

Figure 3–20. Sensitivity and specificity of SPECT Tl-201 imaging in identification of individual stenotic vessels in 47 catheterized patients who have no history of myocardial infarction. (Key: LAD, left anterior descending; LCX, left circumflex; RCA, right coronary artery.) (Reprinted with permission from the American College of Cardiology (Journal of the American College of Cardiology, 1989, Vol. 14, pp. 1689–1699).)

map, or bull's-eye plot, seems to aid in the detection of CAD and identifying Tl-201 redistribution (see Chap. 1).

As with planar Tl-201 scintigraphy, the detection rate for single-vessel disease by SPECT Tl-201 imaging is less than the detection rate for two- or three-vessel disease. Mahmarian and Verani,[87] in a review of the literature, found a sensitivity rate of 83% for detection of single-vessel disease by SPECT, as compared with 93% and 95% for detection of two-vessel and three-vessel disease, respectively. The normalcy rate in the six studies pooled for this analysis was 89%.

The sensitivity for CAD detection with SPECT Tl-201 imaging is somewhat less in patients without a history of MI (85%) than in patients who have such a history (99%).[83] Similarly, stenoses that are >70% narrowed are more likely to be detected by SPECT imaging than stenotic narrowing

of 50% to 70% (Table 3–10). Interestingly, in the study by Mahmarian et al.[83] all patients with >70% stenosis in at least one vessel and multivessel disease had an abnormal SPECT Tl-201 study, regardless of whether or not they had a history of infarction. Quantitative SPECT correctly predicted the presence of multivessel involvement in 65% of patients with two or more >50% stenotic arteries by identifying scan abnormalities in multiple vascular regions within the polar map. The pooled analysis from the literature[87] revealed that the overall individual detection rate for vessels narrowed ≥50% was 79%, with 84% specificity. In patients without a history of infarction the overall detection rate of individual stenoses was 76%.

SPECT perfusion defect size increases with increasing severity of stenosis. Patients with moderate stenosis (51% to 69% narrowing) tend to have smaller perfusion defects

Table 3–10. Sensitivity of Tl-201 Single-Photon Emission Computed Tomography for Detecting Patients with Coronary Artery Disease

Sensitivity	Visual SPECT (Sensitivity) (No.)	Quantitative SPECT (Sensitivity) (No.)
>50% Stenosis		
Total	87% (193/221)	87% (192/221)
No myocardial infarction	78% (67/86)	79% (68/86)
Myocardial infarction	99% (73/74)*	99% (73/74)*
≥70% Stenosis		
Total	95% (162/171)†	93% (159/171)†
No myocardial infarction	90% (56/62)†	87% (54/62)
Myocardial infarction	100% (64/64)*	100% (64/64)*

*P <0.01 myocardial infarction vs. no myocardial infarction; P <0.05 ≥70% stenosis vs. >50% stenosis.
(Reprinted with permission from the American College of Cardiology (Journal of the American College of Cardiology, 1990, Vol. 15, pp. 318–329).)

than those with more severe stenosis, regardless of which coronary artery is involved.[88] A proximal stenosis in the LAD artery produces a perfusion defect approximately twice as large as that produced by a proximal RCA or LCx artery stenosis. There is, however, marked variability in the size of perfusion defects within the classification of the three major coronary vessels, despite comparable severity of stenosis. The risk area on the SPECT scintigram for a mid-LAD lesion overlaps with the defect size in the proximal portion of that vessel (Fig. 3–21).[88] This observation again highlights the fact that the physiologic information from myocardial perfusion imaging gives a truer picture with respect to area of myocardium jeopardized than the site and location of a coronary stenosis on angiography. Presumably, prognosis is also more closely related to defect size than to delineation of the location, severity, and extent of a coronary anatomic lesion. That is, the extent of jeopardized myocardium is imprecisely determined from coronary angiography alone. Perfusion imaging data complements the anatomic information with respect to determining the extent of myocardium at jeopardy in the supply regions of stenotic coronary vessels. Long-acting nitrates have been reported to cause a reduction in SPECT Tl-201 perfusion defect size in patients with stable angina pectoris.[88a]

Intraobserver and interobserver variability are quite good for estimating SPECT Tl-201 defect size.[83] Paired perfusion defect sizes were 28.4% ± 19.1% versus 28.6% ± 18.5% when measured by the same observer and 28.3% ± 18.0% versus 27.8% ± 17.9% (P = not significant [NS]) when measured by two observers. Prigent et al.[89] also evaluated the reproducibility of SPECT Tl-201 imaging to quantitate extent of hypoperfused myocardium on exercise studies. Duplicate studies performed on different occasions with comparable levels of exercise stress were compared. Reproducibility was very high: mean absolute deviation was 2.9%

for patients without prior infarction. Similar findings were reported by Alazraki et al.[83a] with SPECT Tl-201 imaging repeated within 3 to 9 days in 20 stable patients. Tl-201 results were identical in 15 of 16 patients whose ECG/exercise tests were reproducible. Interobserver agreement was 95%.

Iskandrian et al.[82] investigated the effect of the level of exercise on SPECT Tl-201 scintigraphic results. The detection rate of one-, two-, and three-vessel CAD was higher in patients who achieved ≥85% of maximum predicted heart rate (74%, 88%, and 98%, respectively) than for those who achieved only submaximal exercise heart rates (52%, 84%, and 79%, respectively). Redistribution defects were also detected more frequently in patients who achieved adequate exercise heart rates.

Fintel and coworkers[90] identified certain factors that contributed to the improved imaging results with SPECT as compared with planar Tl-201 scintigraphy. SPECT was more accurate than planar imaging for overall detection or exclusion of CAD and for involvement of the LAD and LCx coronary arteries. Figure 3–22 shows the paired SPECT and planar ROC curves for the diagnosis of disease in the LAD, LCx, and RCA vascular territories and the effect of stenosis severity. In that study, tomography offered relatively greater advantages in male patients and in patients with milder forms of CAD who had no history of MI, only single-vessel disease or no stenoses in the range of ≥50% to 69%. For some reason, tomography did not appear to improve diagnostic accuracy in women or detection of disease of the RCA.

Factors That Affect the Specificity of SPECT

Despite the fact that SPECT offers higher defect contrast and better separation of overlying myocardial segments,

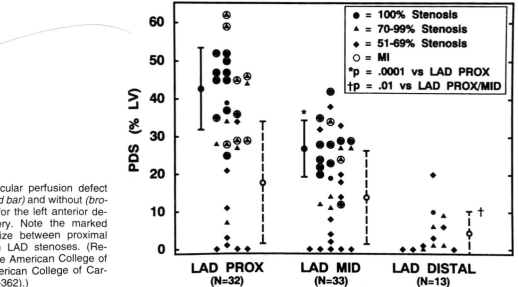

Figure 3–21. Mean left ventricular perfusion defect size (PDS) in patients with *(solid bar)* and without *(broken bar)* myocardial infarction for the left anterior descending (LAD) coronary artery. Note the marked overlap in perfusion defect size between proximal (PROX) and midportion (MID) LAD stenoses. (Reprinted with permission from the American College of Cardiology (Journal of the American College of Cardiology, 1991, Vol. 17, pp. 355–362).)

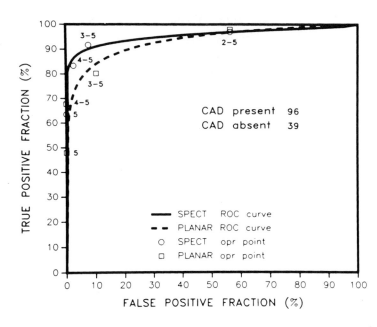

Figure 3–22. Paired ROC curves for the diagnosis of CAD. The solid line indicates the SPECT ROC curve, and the dotted line depicts the planar ROC curve. Individual operating points (circle, SPECT; square, planar) were obtained employing varying decision thresholds for a positive and a negative test. The SPECT ROC curve is shifted upward and to the left, implying improved diagnostic performance at each diagnostic threshold compared to planar imaging. (Reprinted by permission of the American College of Cardiology (Journal of the American College of Cardiology, 1989, Vol. 13, pp. 600–612).)

some pitfalls of this technique can lower its specificity. The patient is more likely to move during SPECT imaging than during planar imaging, since the patient remains in an awkward position for a rather long time. Patient motion is a source of artifactual defects on tomographic reconstruction.[91–91b] In one study, 17% of patients undergoing SPECT imaging moved enough to produce perfusion defect artifacts.[91] Germano et al.[91a] developed a method for detecting and correcting translational patient motion in dynamic and static myocardial SPECT studies using a low-activity Tc-99m point source designed especially for multidetector cameras. Cooper et al.[91b] found that visual inspection, cross-correlation, and two-dimensional fit most accurately detected axial patient motion, whereas cross-correlation most accurately detected lateral motion. Cross-correlation best localized the camera angle at which the motion occurred. Two-dimensional fit measured the distance of axial patient motion to ±1.1 mm and the distance of lateral motion to ±8.7 mm. There is a phenomenon encountered called *upward creep* of the heart.[92] In normal persons, an "upward creep" shift of ≥2 pixels is associated with a higher incidence of reversible inferior or septal perfusion defects in the absence of CAD. As expected, upward creep is more often observed in patients who exercise longer and achieve faster exercise heart rates, raising the possibility that this phenomenon is due to persistent hyperpnea following exhaustive stress. False-positive defects are most commonly observed in the inferoapical region toward the basilar segments of the left ventricle, owing to self-attenuation. Inferobasilar thinning can result from absorption by the heart of photons arising from deep within the LV myocardium. Attenuation artifacts in women due to breast attenuation are most often localized to the anterior wall and septum, whereas a high diaphragm can produce attenuation in inferior segments. Hypertension with left ventricular hypertro-

phy does not appear to cause perfusion defects in the absence of CAD.[92a] In this study, no patient had a defect, defined as a lateral/septal count ratio >2.0 standard deviations below the limits of normal. Watson and Smith give a superb review of the causes of artifacts of SPECT imaging.[93] DePuey also provides excellent reviews of this subject.[94, 94a]

To reduce false-positive interpretations, the multiple individual planar images obtained at each angle as the camera rotates around the patient should be reviewed for artifacts. Often, a motion artifact can be observed when reviewing each planar image that constitutes the input data to the computer, or a breast shadow that enters and then leaves the myocardium field of view can be perceived.[91b] Reconstruction artifacts caused by axis-of-rotation errors during the acquisition of tomographic information can also contribute to false-positive studies. Artifacts that can be observed on SPECT images are discussed in detail in Chapter 1.

Common artifacts encountered in cardiac Tl-201 SPECT are summarized in Table 3–11. The thinning seen in the posterobasal segments of the heart due to self-attenuation and breast attenuation causing anterior defects have been mentioned. If the long axis of the LV is selected incorrectly from either the middle short-axis or middle vertical long-axis slice, the geometry of the ventricle in reconstructed slices can be distorted. Polar maps reveal that this distortion results in apparently decreased Tl-201 activity in the basal myocardial regions at the periphery of the bull's-eye plot. The long axis should precisely bisect the ventricular cavity to avoid such basilar artifacts. The accurate determination of the gamma camera's center of rotation is important for SPECT image reconstruction. Errors in the center of rotation in the rightward or leftward direction create posteroapical or anteroapical artifacts, respectively. In horizontal long-axis images, these artifacts appear linear and extend through the thickness of the myocardium, and the anterior and posterior walls are misaligned. Ringlike artifacts on reconstructed tomographic slices can be observed with flood field nonuniformity. Concentric ring artifacts can also be identified on the bull's eye display with nonuniform flood fields. DePuey[94a] points out that with dual- and triple-headed SPECT cameras, misalignment of detector heads can lead to artifacts that could be misinterpreted as perfusion defects. DePuey further states that overlapping liver or intestinal activity on resting SPECT images can create "pseudo-redistribution," making a fixed defect appear reversible.

Distinguishing True-Positive from False-Positive Ischemic ST-Segment Responses with Thallium-201 Scintigraphy

Often, when an exercise ECG stress test is performed in a patient who has a low pretest likelihood of CAD, an unexpected ST-segment depression response consistent with ischemia is observed. These presumed false-positive ECG responses to exercise stress are more likely to be seen in patients with hypertension and LV hypertrophy, in patients receiving digitalis, or in patients who achieve a fast exercise heart rate or heavy workload. Botvinick et al.[34] studied 65 patients with exercise ECG and visual planar Tl-201 scintigraphy and correlated the results with coronary angiography findings. In that study, Tl-201 scintigraphy helped clarify the equivocal stress test result due to LBBB, LV hypertrophy, drugs that affect repolarization, hyperventilation, and other conditions and was more accurate than the stress ECG (89% vs. 53%), even in the presence of a depressed ST segment at rest. Iskandrian et al.[42] found that

Table 3–11. **Common Artifacts in SPECT Tl-201 Imaging**

Soft-tissue attenuation artifacts
Breast tissue
High diaphragm
Lateral chest wall fat
Overlying right ventricular blood pool
Inferobasilar self attenuation
Increased visceral tracer uptake
Upward creep
Patient motion
Cardiac rotation (normal variant)
Exaggerated apical thinning (normal variant)
Reconstruction error such as incorrect selection of long-axis of the left ventricle
Errors in center of rotation producing apical artifacts
Ringlike artifacts with flood field nonuniformity

54% of exercise ECGs were judged to be inconclusive in a group of patients undergoing exercise scintigraphy and subsequent coronary angiography. The causes of the inconclusive ECGs were submaximal exercise and ST-segment abnormalities at rest. In that study, 95% of patients with abnormal exercise images had CAD, and 82% of patients with normal images had normal coronary arteries.

Guiney et al.[95] studied 35 patients with a low pretest likelihood of CAD who were referred for coronary angiography because their exercise test was interpreted as positive for ischemic ST-segment depression (Fig. 3–23). These 35 patients underwent repeat exercise testing in conjunction with Tl-201 perfusion imaging just before angiography. Of these, 24 (69%) had normal exercise Tl-201 scintigrams and 11 (31%) demonstrated exercise-induced myocardial perfusion defects. Of the 24 with ST-segment depression and a normal Tl-201 study, 23 had no significant angiographic CAD (see Fig. 3–23). In contrast, of the 11 patients with ST depression and abnormal scintigrams, 8 were found

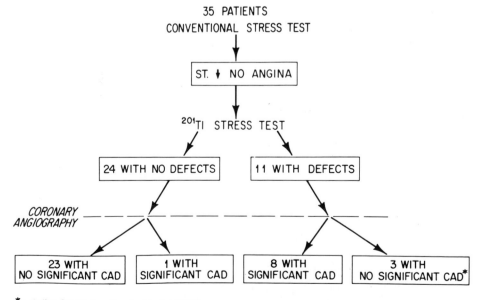

Figure 3–23. Correlation between Tl-201 exercise stress imaging results and coronary angiographic findings in 35 patients with ischemic ST-segment changes but no angina on exercise testing. The 24 patients with ST depression, no angina, and no inducible defects had an extremely low prevalence of CAD by angiography. (Guiney TE, et al.: Chest 1981; 80:4–10.)

to have ≥50% stenosis and 2 had stenosis between 30% and 50%. This study demonstrated that myocardial imaging utilizing Tl-201 was of considerable value in differentiating between true-positive and false-positive ST-segment responses to exercise stress.

Tl-201 scintigraphy may also be valuable in identifying which patients who exhibit T-wave normalization during exercise have underlying CAD.[96] The issues related to Tl-201 imaging in patients with LBBB and no history of CAD are discussed in Chapter 11.

Summary

From the Tl-201 data reviewed in this chapter, either planar or SPECT imaging enhances the chance of detecting CAD among patients who present with chest pain over that with exercise ECG alone. Specificity of Tl-201 scintigraphy is also superior to that of the exercise ECG, particularly in patients with resting ST-T abnormalities due to LV hypertrophy or digitalis use. Data from myocardial perfusion imaging provide unique physiologic information about the amount of myocardium at risk in the supply zones of stenotic coronary vessels. The more severe and extensive the CAD, the greater is the total area of hypoperfusion on exercise scintigrams. The risk area assessment by the radionuclide method may be superior to mere determination of number of diseased coronary vessels on angiography for identifying patients with multivessel CAD who are at the highest risk for an adverse outcome (see Chap. 4). As discussed in greater detail in the next chapter, prognosis for patients with chest pain is related to the extent of reversible hypoperfusion on Tl-201 scintigraphy. Quantitation of defect magnitude for identifying defects that are significant, as compared with defects that can be within range of normal, is mandatory for maximizing sensitivity, specificity, and the rate of detecting individual coronary stenoses. SPECT imaging has potential advantages over planar imaging, including higher lesion contrast, less background activity, and quantitation of the extent and size of lesions. Views are more standardized, and LCx disease is more readily identified. Nevertheless, SPECT imaging is difficult, and attenuation artifacts can be more difficult to recognize in reconstructed tomographic images than in planar images. In the future, attenuation correction techniques will be applied to SPECT imaging, which should improve specificity.

EXERCISE TECHNETIUM-99m–SESTAMIBI IMAGING

Several new Tc-99m–labeled myocardial perfusion agents have been introduced into clinical practice. The one that has gained most widespread attention is Tc-99m sestamibi (Cardiolite).[97–102a] The kinetics of this radiopharmaceutical are described in detail in Chapter 2. Briefly, myocar-

dial uptake of Tc-99m sestamibi is proportional to regional blood flow, and nonviable cells cannot concentrate the tracer.[103] Image quality with Tc-99m sestamibi is superior to that obtained with Tl-201, because of the more favorable physical characteristics of Tc-99m for imaging with a gamma camera. Approximately 10 to 20 times larger doses can be administered than are feasible with Tl-201, yielding a higher count density in both planar and SPECT images. Tc-99m produces less scatter and attenuation than Tl-201. Gating is permitted because of the high count rate, which also improves resolution. Similarly, first-pass acquisition to assess ventricular function is feasible.

Exercise Imaging Protocols

Since Tc-99m sestamibi does not redistribute over time after intravenous injection, separate injections of the radionuclide have to be administered during stress and resting states. These separate injections are required to differentiate defects that represent stress-induced ischemia from those that represent myocardial scar. At this writing, a variety of protocols for exercise perfusion imaging with Tc-99m sestamibi have been advocated or are under investigation.[103a, 103b] Perhaps the most optimal protocol using this radionuclide is performance of, first, the exercise study and then the resting study 24 hours later. Each imaging procedure employs 20 to 30 mCi of Tc-99m sestamibi. It seems logical to perform the stress study first with the 2-day protocol, since if regional myocardial perfusion is unequivocally normal the resting study could be cancelled. This might particularly be the case when gated perfusion images are acquired, permitting simultaneous assessment of perfusion and regional systolic thickening. The combination of uniform Tc-99m–sestamibi uptake with normal regional thickening from end-diastole to systole would provide confidence that the study was, indeed, within normal limits. One advantage of the 2-day imaging procedure is that it avoids "cross-talk" between the exercise and resting images as might occur when they are performed several hours apart during a 1-day protocol. This is because residual Tc-99m activity from the first image persists when the views are acquired for the second image.

In clinical practice, a protocol involving separate rest and stress injections separated by 24 hours may not be very practical. To overcome this limitation of Tc-99m sestamibi, several abbreviated protocols have been proposed. One "same-day" protocol involves performing a rest-stress sequence.[104] In this protocol, the rest image, utilizing 8 to 10 mCi with imaging performed 60 minutes later, is performed first. A dose of 22 to 30 mCi is then injected during peak exercise, and images are acquired 30 to 45 minutes postinjection. The exercise injection should be administered about 4 hours after the resting injection, in order to perform quantitative scan analysis. This same-day rest-stress imaging procedure permits the entire study to be completed within 4.5 to 5 hours. Some advocated that the patient drink a glass of whole milk or eat a fatty meal 15 minutes before commencing image acquisition, to stimulate enhanced Tc-99m–sestamibi clearance from the gallbladder.

Like Tl-201, Tc-99m sestamibi is injected at symptom-limited endpoints, and exercise is encouraged for at least another minute. Some have advocated continuing exercise for another 1 to 2 minutes at a rate several stages lower than the stage that corresponds to peak exercise, to allow more complete initial uptake in the myocardium. The rationale for continuing exercise for another minute at this submaximal level is that there is slightly slower initial blood clearance for Tc-99m sestamibi than for Tl-201. Figure 3–24 shows stress and rest Tc-99m–sestamibi images in two patients with CAD. These images were obtained using the same-day protocol: the rest images first, followed by exercise images.

Taillefer et al. compared a same-day, split-dose planar Tc-99m–sestamibi imaging protocol with a 2-day imaging protocol among 15 patients with CAD.[104] Among the 225 planar segments (15 segments per patient) analyzed qualitatively, the detection of reversible and fixed defects was identical for the same-day and the 2-day Tc-99m–sestamibi protocol. Also in that study, the normal-ischemic segment ratios were practically identical for the same-day (1.33) and the 2-day (1.28) protocol.

Performing the exercise imaging study in the afternoon employing the same-day, split-dose protocol for Tc-99m sestamibi imaging may be somewhat inconvenient for some laboratories. Taillefer examined the feasibility of performing the stress study first, with a 9-mCi dose of Tc-99m sestamibi, then waiting 3 to 4 hours to perform a resting study with a 22-mCi dose. The prospectively compared protocols used rest-stress and stress-rest sequences in a group of 18 patients. He reported that the detection of ischemia was underestimated when the exercise study with the small dose of Tc-99m sestamibi was performed first. The explanation for this underestimation was the cross-talk from the stress dose, which prevented observers from identifying ''reversibility'' on the subsequent resting study. He showed that 7.4% of defects judged to be reversible using the rest-stress sequence were misinterpreted to be irreversible with the stress-rest sequence. Agreement between protocols was still not bad: 87% of segments analyzed showed agreement for detection of reversible and fixed defects. From this study and others, the rest-stress imaging sequence for Tc-99m sestamibi same-day imaging was judged to be preferable. Heo et al.[105] compared the rest-exercise and the exercise-rest same-day protocols using SPECT Tc-99m–sestamibi imaging, and found 93% concordance between the two protocols when 640 segments were classified as normal, ischemia, or scar (Fig. 3–25). The rest-stress protocol showed greater count differences between abnormal and normal zones in stress images, with better defect normalization on rest images.

Preliminary data from a multicenter trial yet unpublished suggest that the stress-rest sequence for same-day Tc-99m sestamibi–imaging may yield detection rates of defect reversibility comparable to those achieved with the rest-stress sequence.

Detection of Coronary Artery Disease: Planar Imaging

The technical aspects of planar imaging with Tc-99m sestamibi and the recommended acquisition parameters for planar imaging performed with this radionuclide are described in detail in Chapter 2. Gated planar imaging can be performed using available multiple-gated acquisition (MUGA) software and hardware. Adding this wall motion assessment to the evaluation of regional myocardial perfusion requires no supplementary imaging time, because the gated image set can be summed to obtain a static image for quantitative image analysis.[106]

Quantitation of Tl-201 uptake and washout are required to optimally assess the extent and severity of regional myocardial perfusion abnormalities and to distinguish ischemia from infarction. Undoubtedly, quantitation of Tc-99m sestamibi planar images also becomes important for optimal differentiation between ischemia and scar. Crucial to the success of quantitative planar perfusion imaging is a valid method of background subtraction. The magnitude of a Tl-201 or Tc-99m–sestamibi defect will be underestimated if insufficient background is subtracted. Conversely, defect magnitude will be overestimated if too much background is subtracted. Injection of Tc-99m sestamibi under stress and rest conditions produces differences in the distribution of the radionuclide in body organs. Splanchnic activity is significantly higher on resting Tc-99m–sestamibi images than on either stress Tc-99m–sestamibi or Tl-201 images.

Sinusas et al.[107] developed a new method of generating the background reference plane, which was a modification of a previously validated interpolative background subtraction algorithm. The new method provides more rapid fall-off of the background reference plane as it moves beneath the heart, away from a region of intense extracardiac activity, and provides a better approximation of the shape of the actual edge of the extracardiac organ. These investigators compared myocardial uptake of Tc-99m sestamibi and Tl-201, employing quantitative analysis in both patients with documented CAD and subjects with a low pretest likelihood of disease. There was a close correlation between Tc-99m–sestamibi and Tl-201 segmental activity in the patients with CAD, using the modified background subtraction algorithm. There was no significant difference in defect magnitude for either stress ($P = 0.91$) or rest ($P = 0.20$) images, and no evidence of oversubtraction. Utilizing the previous quantitative algorithm designed for Tl-201 scintigraphy, perfusion defects of greater relative magnitude were

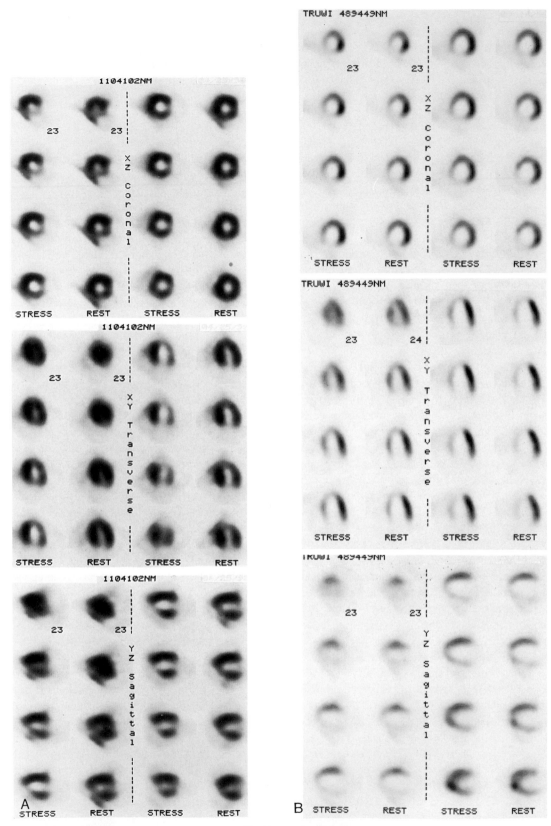

Figure 3–24. A. *Top panel,* Stress and rest Tc-99m–sestamibi short-axis tomograms from apex (upper left pair of images) to base (lower right pair of images) showing a reversible defect in the mid posterolateral wall. *Middle panel,* Stress and rest horizontal long-axis tomograms from the same patient showing an extensive totally reversible posterolateral defect extending from the midventricular slice (lower left pair of images) to the inferior region (lower right pair of images). *Lower panel,* Vertical long-axis tomograms from this patient demonstrating a reversible inferoapical defect. **B.** *Upper panel:* Stress and rest Tc-99m–sestamibi tomograms from apex (upper left pair of images) to base (lower right pair of images) showing apical, anterior, septal, and inferior defects, which appear nonreversible. *Middle panel:* Horizontal long-axis tomograms from the same patient showing apical and septal defects, which are nonreversible. *Lower panel:* Vertical long-axis tomograms showing extensive nonreversible anteroapical and inferior defects.

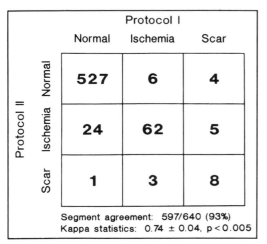

Figure 3–25. Comparison of the rest-exercise sequence (protocol 1) and the exercise-rest sequence (protocol 2) with same-day Tc-99m–sestamibi imaging in the same patients. Among the protocols, there was a concordance in 93% of the segments. Reprinted by permission of the Society of Nuclear Medicine from: Heo J, et al.: J Nucl Med 1992;33:186–191.)

Within figure:

Protocol I

	Normal	Ischemia	Scar
Protocol II — Normal	527	6	4
Protocol II — Ischemia	24	62	5
Protocol II — Scar	1	3	8

Segment agreement: 597/640 (93%)
Kappa statistics: 0.74 ± 0.04, p < 0.005

---

observed on resting images with Tc-99m sestamibi than with Tl-201 images. With the modified algorithm, in which proper account is taken for extracardiac background on resting Tc-99m–sestamibi images, defect magnitudes for Tc-99m sestamibi and Tl-201 were comparable. Thus, the modification of the standard interpolative background subtraction algorithm optimizes quantitative planar Tc-99m–sestamibi imaging. This modification allows for the difference in extracardiac activity of planar Tc-99m–sestamibi images and provides a simple quantitative method for assessing regional myocardial perfusion. When applying this algorithm, the myocardial uptake patterns for Tc-99m sestamibi and Tl-201 appeared to be comparable.

Koster et al.[108] utilized the modified background subtraction algorithm described above in 16 patients who were studied with both exercise-delayed Tl-201 and exercise-rest Tc-99m–sestamibi imaging. They compared their imaging results to those obtained using the standard background subtraction algorithm designed for Tl-201 imaging. Using the standard background subtraction, mean defect reversibility was significantly underestimated by Tc-99m sestamibi as compared with Tl-201 (2.8 ± 4.9 vs −1.8 ± 8.4).

Using the modified background subtraction algorithm of Sinusas et al.,[107] mean defect reversibility on Tl-201 and Tc-99m–sestamibi images was comparable (2.8 ± 4.9 vs 1.7 ± 5.2; $P = $ NS). A new normal database to be used with circumferential profile analysis was generated. In the normal population, there was a small but significant difference between Tl-201 and Tc-99m activities at the valve planes in the anterior and left anterior oblique (LAO) views. The authors stated that this was consistent with the observation that less scatter gives better resolution of valve plane ''defects'' with Tc-99m sestamibi. Apical thinning was also better defined with Tc-99m sestamibi.

Several groups have evaluated the sensitivity and specificity of planar Tc-99m–sestamibi imaging for detection of CAD, comparing values obtained with Tl-201 exercise scintigraphy in the same patients.[109-116] Table 3–12 summarizes the results of these studies.

The clinical efficacy of Tc-99m–sestamibi planar stress and rest imaging was evaluated in a multicenter phase II clinical trial involving 38 patients.[110] Of the patients with CAD, 35 (97%) had abnormal Tl-201 stress images and 32 (89%) had abnormal Tc-99m–sestamibi stress images. This difference was not statistically significant. The two patients with insignificant CAD had both normal Tl-201 and Tc-99m–sestamibi images. Of a total of 114 arteries analyzed, 65 had significant stenoses and 49 had no lesions or insignificant ones (<50% stenosis). Of 65 regions supplied by vessels with significant stenoses, 45 (69%) were abnormal by Tl-201 and 39 (60%) by Tc-99m–sestamibi stress imaging ($P = $ NS). Of 49 coronary supply regions supplied by normal vessels, 40 (82%) were normal by Tl-201 and 38 (78%) by Tc-99m–sestamibi imaging. No significant difference was observed between Tl-201 and Tc-99m sestamibi in the detection rate of disease in the LAD, RCA, or LCx artery (Fig. 3–26). Tc-99m–sestamibi and Tl-201 images were concordant in 86% of patients with respect to differentiating ischemia from scar. By segmental analysis, concordance with respect to ischemia and scar was seen in 81% of myocardial segments. In this phase II study, the investigators concluded that Tc-99m–sestamibi images were equal in quality to, and frequently better than (i.e., less granular and with sharper myocardial walls), their companion Tl-201 images. As expected, resting Tc-99m–sesta-

---

Table 3–12. Sensitivity and Specificity of Planar Tc-99m Sestamibi Versus Planar Tl-201 for Detection of Coronary Artery Disease

Investigator	Sensitivity (%) Tl-201	Sensitivity (%) Tc-99m Sestamibi	Specificity (%) Tl-201	Specificity (%) Tc-99m Sestamibi	Normalcy (%) Tl-201	Normalcy (%) Tc-99m Sestamibi
Wackers[110]	97	89	100	100	—	—
Kiat[109]	73	73	50	75	88	94
Najm[114]	70	88	—	—	100	100
Maisey[113]	98	96	—	—	—	—
Overall	88	90	67	83	93	97

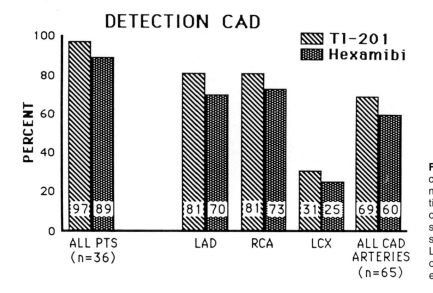

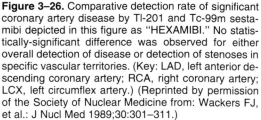

Figure 3–26. Comparative detection rate of significant coronary artery disease by Tl-201 and Tc-99m sestamibi depicted in this figure as "HEXAMIBI." No statistically-significant difference was observed for either overall detection of disease or detection of stenoses in specific vascular territories. (Key: LAD, left anterior descending coronary artery; RCA, right coronary artery; LCX, left circumflex artery.) (Reprinted by permission of the Society of Nuclear Medicine from: Wackers FJ, et al.: J Nucl Med 1989;30:301–311.)

mibi images showed significantly more liver uptake than Tl-201 delayed images. This increased uptake was judged not to interfere with image interpretation. The authors pointed out that at times the intense subdiaphragmatic activity had the potential to interfere with detection of inferior wall defects, particularly in images obtained within 1 hour after injection of the isotope.

Kiat et al.[109] reported an overall sensitivity rate of 73% for CAD detection by both Tl-201 and Tc-99m–sestamibi planar imaging. The normalcy rates were 94% for Tc-99m sestamibi and 88% for Tl-201 in these studies. There was no difference between Tc-99m sestamibi and Tl-201 for detection of individual vessel stenoses (60% vs. 54%). For the pattern of reversibility in myocardial segments with stress defects, agreement was 91% for the planar approach, not very different from what was observed in the phase II trial reviewed above.

Taillefer et al.[115] performed qualitative assessment of both Tl-201 and Tc-99m–sestamibi uptake in 297 myocardial segments in 33 patients with chest pain who underwent two exercise stress tests, one with Tl-201 and one with Tc-99m sestamibi. There was good correlation for the presence of normality, scar, or ischemia with the two radionuclides, both on a segment-by-segment (259 of 297, 87.2%) and patient-by-patient basis (29 of 33, 87.9%). These investigators found that the number of ischemic segments detected with Tl-201 and with Tc-99m–sestamibi imaging were nearly equal. In a subsequent study,[111] Taillefer et al. showed an overall agreement in 88.4% of segments in 65 patients undergoing Tc-99m–sestamibi and Tl-201 imaging at least 1 week apart. Tl-201 scintigraphy detected 74.2% of all significantly stenotic coronary arteries, and Tc-99m–sestamibi imaging detected 70.1% of stenotic arteries. This difference was not statistically significant. Thus, in this expanded population, the results again show a good correlation between Tl-201 and Tc-99m–sestamibi imaging for detection of significant CAD using the planar approach.

Maddahi et al.[116] reported the preliminary results of the phase III multicenter trial in which 24 centers participated in an open-label study designed to compare Tc-99m–sestamibi with Tl-201 imaging in patients undergoing coronary angiography. With planar imaging, there was 92% agreement between the two agents for classifying patients as normal or abnormal. A total of 4622 segments were analyzed, of which 4358 (94%) were concordantly designated as normal or abnormal by the two agents. Sensitivity, specificity, and normalcy rates for Tc-99m sestamibi were 85%, 95%, and 100%, respectively. For Tl-201, these values were 87%, 55%, and 100%, respectively. As expected, the sensitivity for detecting one-vessel disease was lower for Tc-99m sestamibi (73%) and Tl-201 (77%) than for detection of two-vessel or three-vessel disease. For three-vessel disease, sensitivities for Tc-99m sestamibi and Tl-201 were 92% and 95%, respectively. Tc-99m sestamibi and Tl-201 were also compared for their ability to differentiate between ischemia and scar. Seventy-eight percent of 734 segments corresponding to stress defects were concordant in differentiating ischemia from scar.

A European multicenter comparison of Tc-99m–sestamibi and Tl-201 imaging for detection of CAD was undertaken.[113] In 56 patients who comprised the study cohort, a high degree of concordance (81%) of myocardial segments classified as either normal, reversible, or persistent was observed. Overall detection of CAD in patients was 98% for Tl-201 and 96% for Tc-99m sestamibi. The individual stenosis detection rate was 68% for both tracers.

Watson et al.[112] determined how well interpreters experienced in Tl-201 imaging could read Tc-99m–sestamibi studies with the aid of quantitative image processing in terms of sensitivity and specificity for CAD detection, interinterpreter agreement, agreement with coronary angiographic findings, and comparison to computer interpretation of images totally devoid of observer input. Two interpreters performed entirely blinded readings of 44 planar Tc-99m–

Table 3–13. **Predictive Accuracy for Detection of Coronary Artery Disease by Two Observers Independently Interpreting Planar Tc-99m–Sestamibi Exercise and Rest Perfusion Studies**

	Predictive Accuracy	Observer 1	Observer 2
All patients	Positive	0.96	0.93
	Negative	0.79	0.93
Excluding prior MI	Positive	0.91	0.86
	Negative	0.83	0.93

(Reprinted by permission of the Society of Nuclear Medicine from: Watson DD, et al.: Blinded evaluation of planar technetium-99m-sestamibi myocardial perfusion studies. J Nucl Med 1992;33:668–675.)

sestamibi exercise and rest scintigrams from patients imaged at Hotel Dieu de Montreal. As shown in Table 3–13, observer 1 had 96% predictive accuracy for a positive test result and 79% predictive accuracy for a negative one. Observer 2 had corresponding predictive accuracies of 93% and 93%, respectively. The concordance between the interpreters for the 660 segments graded in the study was 90.2% (595 of 660). Figure 3–27 shows a conventional ROC curve from this study, demonstrating how sensitivity and specificity vary when different thresholds for detection of CAD are used. Plotted on this graph are the sensitivity and specificity for CAD detection derived from the interpreters of the study. Interestingly, the interpreters scored somewhat higher than the computer alone, presumably by exercising judgment in image analysis that was not programmed into the computer.

In summary, planar Tc-99m–sestamibi imaging is highly sensitive and specific for CAD detection and is comparable to values obtained from Tl-201 imaging in the same patients. As with Tl-201 imaging, quantitation of scintigrams is recommended to maximize predictive accuracy. Although Tc-99m sestamibi does not redistribute over time after injection, differentiation between ischemia and scar can be achieved with a high degree of accuracy by comparing stress and rest images. Like planar Tl-201 imaging, circumflex stenoses are detected less well than RCA or LAD lesions with Tc-99m sestamibi. The individual stenosis detection rate is also comparable for both radionuclides, though it is somewhat lower than that for SPECT imaging.

Detection of Coronary Artery Disease: SPECT

The higher photon energy, enhanced count rate, and decreased attenuation and scatter compared with Tl-201 make Tc-99m sestamibi most suitable for SPECT imaging. Table 3–14 summarizes the sensitivity, specificity, and normalcy results for detecting significant CAD by Tc-99m sestamibi.[109, 116–119] A pooled analysis of 81 patients from these studies collated by Maddahi et al.[116] yielded 90% sensitivity for Tc-99m sestamibi and 83% sensitivity for Tl-201 for detection of CAD. Specificity for SPECT Tc-99m sestamibi was 93%, as compared with 80% for SPECT Tl-201, whereas the normalcy rate was 100% for Tc-99m sestamibi and 77% for Tl-201. The number of patients in each of these studies was rather small. Kahn et al.,[118] who used quantitative SPECT imaging analysis with computer quantitation of regional tracer distribution, reported that the quality of reconstructed images with Tc-99m sestamibi judged visually was superior to that of Tl-201 in 88% of all

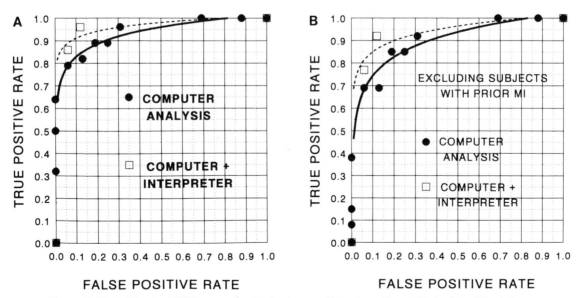

Figure 3–27. A. Standard ROC curve showing the true-positive rate on the vertical axis and the false-positive rate (1 − specificity) on the horizontal axis. The solid dots represent computer results at various detection thresholds. The open squares are the result of the interpretation by two experienced observers. **B.** ROC curve obtained after excluding all patients with history of myocardial infarction. (Reprinted by permission of the Society of Nuclear Medicine from: Watson DD, et al.: J Nucl Med 1992;33:668–675.)

Table 3–14. **Sensitivity and Specificity of SPECT Tc-99m Sestamibi Versus SPECT Tl-201 for Detection of Coronary Artery Disease**

Investigator	Sensitivity (%)		Specificity (%)		Normalcy (%)	
	Tl-201	Tc-99m Sestamibi	Tl-201	Tc-99m Sestamibi	Tl-201	Tc-99m Sestamibi
Kiat[109]	80	93	75	75	77	100
Iskandrian[117]	82	82	82	100	—	—
Kahn[118]	84	95	—	—	—	—
Overall	83	90	80	93	77	100

studies performed and was comparable to Tl-201 in the others. Tl-201 SPECT identified 60% and Tc-99m sestamibi identified 79% of all stenosed coronary arteries ($P <$ 0.05). Tc-99m sestamibi identified significantly more reversible defects than Tl-201. Seventy-nine percent of all individually stenosed arteries ($>50\%$ stenosis) were detected by Tc-99m sestamibi, as compared with a 60% individual stenosis detection rate for Tl-201 ($P < 0.05$). The enhanced detection rate of individual stenoses was greatest in arteries with 50% to 75% diminution in luminal diameter. Of these subcritical lesions, 65% were detected by Tc-99m sestamibi and 35% by Tl-201. Iskandrian et al.[117] found concordance between the SPECT Tc-99m–sestamibi and SPECT Tl-201 images in 93% of all segments. These authors considered the Tc-99m–sestamibi images to be of better quality than the Tl-201 images. Kiat et al.[109] found that more individually stenosed arteries were detected by SPECT (89%) than by planar Tc-99m–sestamibi imaging (60%) (Fig. 3–28). No difference was seen between SPECT and planar techniques with respect to vessel specificity when coronary vessels with $<50\%$ stenosis were analyzed. The individual vessel stenosis detection rate was slightly, but significantly, higher for Tc-99m sestamibi than for Tl-201 (87% vs. 77%) (see Fig. 3–28).

Quantitative Tc-99m–sestamibi SPECT imaging was performed in a population of 61 patients from two different institutions using different camera-computer systems in another study undertaken by Kiat et al.[119] The overall sensitivity for detection of CAD was 94%, with a normalcy rate of 88%. No difference was observed in sensitivity for normalcy rates between the two institutions participating in this trial (Cedars-Sinai Medical Center and the University of Texas Southwestern Medical Center). Individual vessel sensitivity was 85%; vessel specificity, 71%. This study revealed no difference in sensitivity and specificity for CAD detection between male and female patient subgroups. Thus, a quantitative method for image analysis developed at one institution can provide similar diagnostic accuracy for detection of CAD when applied to imaging data acquired in a different institution using a different camera-computer system. In a second multicenter trial composed of 161 patients from seven institutions, quantitative SPECT sestamibi with exercise stress yielded an overall sensitivity of 87%, specificity of 36%, and normalcy rate of 81%.[119a]

Sensitivity for CAD detection in patients without prior myocardial infarction (89%) was similar to the sensitivity value (90%) for patients with previous infarction. Sensitivities and specificities for individual-vessel stenosis detection rate were, respectively, 69% and 76% for LAD, 70% and 80% for LCX, and 77% and 85% for RCA. Figure 3–28B summarizes the results of this trial.

In the phase III multicenter SPECT trial comparing Tc-99m–sestamibi and Tl-201 imaging in 294 patients, the overall sensitivities of SPECT Tc-99m–sestamibi and SPECT Tl-201 imaging for CAD detection were 92% and 90%, respectively.[116] Because of referral bias with respect to which patients underwent coronary angiography, the specificities determined in patients with normal coronary arteriograms ($N = 45$) were 50% for Tc-99m sestamibi and 39% for Tl-201. In contrast, the normalcy rates in the 79 patients with $<5\%$ likelihood of CAD were 92% for Tc-99m sestamibi and 94% for Tl-201. Detection of one-vessel disease was 90% for both Tc-99m sestamibi and Tl-201, which was nearly 20% higher for detection of single-vessel disease using the planar approach in this phase III trial.[116] As expected, the sensitivity for detecting three-vessel disease was 98% for Tc-99m sestamibi and 96% for Tl-201. Thus, as observed with planar imaging, both Tl-201 and Tc-99m sestamibi have comparable sensitivity and specificity for CAD detection. However, the SPECT technique was more sensitive than planar imaging in detecting stress-induced hypoperfusion but had lower specificity. Of 7011 SPECT myocardial segments analyzed in this trial, there was precise agreement between Tc-99m sestamibi and Tl-201 for distinguishing normal, reversible, and persistent defect patterns in 89% of segments. Of 1285 segments that showed perfusion abnormalities following exercise stress by both agents, 84% were concordant for differentiating between ischemia and scar.

Narahara et al.[120] performed a comparison of Tl-201 and Tc-99m–sestamibi SPECT imaging for estimating the extent of myocardial ischemia and infarction in 24 patients with CAD. Tc-99–sestamibi defects were significantly smaller during exercise than the Tl-201 defects in the same patients. Interestingly, the resting Tc-99m–SPECT defect size was not different from the defect size evaluated on the redistribution Tl-201–SPECT images in the same patients. The authors speculated that the smaller Tc-99m defect sizes

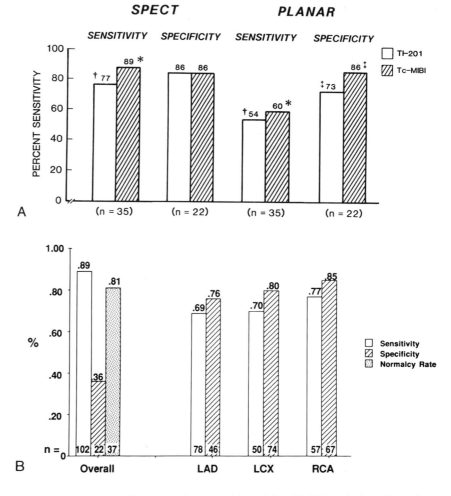

Figure 3–28. A. Sensitivity and specificity for identification of individual diseased coronary arteries. Comparisons are between SPECT and planar imaging and between Tl-201 *(open bars)* and Tc-99m sestamibi (Tc-MIBI, *crosshatched bars).* (Key: *, †, P < 0.005 vs. each other; ‡, p = NS vs. each other; *vs. †, p = NS for both planar and SPECT.) (Kiat H, et al.: Am Heart J 1989;117:1–11.) **B.** Overall sensitivity, specificity, normalcy rate, and sensitivity and specificity for detection of stenoses in the left anterior descending (LAD), left circumflex (LCX), and right coronary artery (RCA) in a multicenter trial composed of patients from seven centers. (Reprinted by permission of the Society of Nuclear Medicine from: Van Train KF, et al.: J Nucl Med 1994;35:609–618.)

were due to a lower myocardial extraction of the tracer during exercise and some slight redistribution, which might have occurred between the time of injection and the time of imaging, which in this trial was 2 hours later.

Maublant et al.[121] compared defect size on SPECT Tc-99m–sestamibi images with defect size on Tl-201 SPECT images performed 4 days apart and matched for the same workload in the same patient group. In patients with CAD, the mean defect size on the stress images was significantly larger with Tl-201 than with Tc-99m sestamibi. Redistribution Tl-201 images yielded a larger defect size than the resting Tc-99m–sestamibi images ($5.1\% \pm 4.4\%$ vs. $2.8\% \pm 3.2\%$; $P < 0.05$). Interestingly, no difference in resting defect size was seen in patients with MI who underwent only resting Tl-201 or resting Tc-99m–sestamibi imaging ($11.2\% \pm 10.4\%$ vs. $12.0\% \pm 11.5\%$). The authors proposed that the differences in defect size observed at exercise and redistribution in patients with CAD were likely due to differences in tissue tracer distribution rather than to artifacts of the imaging procedure. Smaller defect size with Tc-99m sestamibi may again be due to some redistribution that occurs between the time of injection and the time of imaging or to other factors such as lower extraction of the tracer relative to increased blood flow as compared with Tl-201.

Cuocolo et al.[122] reported that detection of reversible

defects was better achieved by Tl-201 scintigraphy using the reinjection technique compared with the detection of defect reversibility with stress-rest Tc-99m–sestamibi imaging performed in the same patients. All patients had LV dysfunction at rest. After Tl-201 reinjection, 27% of the perfusion defects were judged to be reversible, as compared with 15% of these segments demonstrating reversibility on the Tc-99m–sestamibi sequence of images (Fig. 3–29). This study conflicts with some of the earlier studies summarized in this chapter that showed that conventional serial Tl-201 imaging and rest-stress Tc-99m sestamibi imaging yielded comparable results for distinguishing between ischemia and scar.

Technetium-99m–Sestamibi Redistribution

Tc-99m sestamibi can show some slight degree of delayed redistribution, though far less than that observed with serial Tl-201 imaging. Franceschi et al.[123] reported that some redistribution of Tc-99m sestamibi will occur over time and that if imaging is delayed 4 hours or more after injection, defect magnitude may be less than when imaging is performed earlier. These authors found significant differences between the clearance rates from normal and ische-

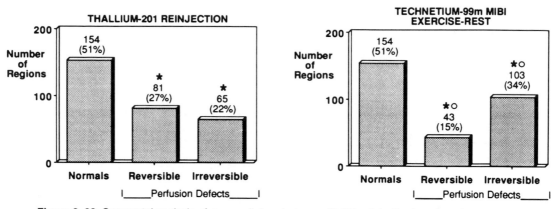

Figure 3–29. Segmental analysis of myocardial perfusion on Tl-201 reinjection imaging after exercise and Tc-99m–sestamibi imaging with exercise-rest separate studies. More reversible segments were detected on Tl-201 reinjection imaging compared to exercise-rest Tc-99m–sestamibi imaging in this patient population. (Key: *, $P < 0.001$ compared to reversibility on Tl-201 redistribution imaging (not shown); °, $P < 0.01$ when Tc-99m sestamibi is compared to Tl-201 reinjection with respect to reversibility.) (Reprinted by permission of the Society of Nuclear Medicine from: Cuocolo A, et al.: J Nucl Med 1992;33:505–511.)

mic myocardium in nine patients with angiographic or scintigraphic evidence of CAD. Tc-99m–sestamibi clearance from normal myocardium was 27% ± 8% by 6 hours after injection. Clearance from mild myocardial defects was 16% by 6 hours. The ischemic-normal ratio of activity increased from 0.7 to 0.84 from 4 to 6 hours after injection in patients with mild defects, indicating redistribution.

Similar findings were reported by Taillefer et al.,[124] who evaluated the myocardial clearance of Tc-99m sestamibi and ischemic:normal wall ratios 1 and 3 hours after injection in patients with significant CAD. The ischemic:normal wall ratios were 0.73 and 0.83 ($P < 0.05$) at 1 and 3 hours, respectively. This ratio was 0.98 on the resting Tc-99m

scintigrams. Myocardial washout was 26% from normal myocardium and 15% from ischemic segments. Figure 3–30 shows partial redistribution of Tc-99m sestamibi in the septum in a patient with a 95% stenosis of the LAD from this study. Only a few ischemic segments were missed when imaging was delayed 3 hours after Tc-99m–sestamibi injection.

The results of these studies suggest that one reason for a smaller Tc-99m–sestamibi defect size, as compared with Tl-201 in the same patient, may be some redistribution of Tc-99m sestamibi that occurs between the time of tracer injection and the time of imaging. These clinical observations are consistent with the experimental data of Sinusas

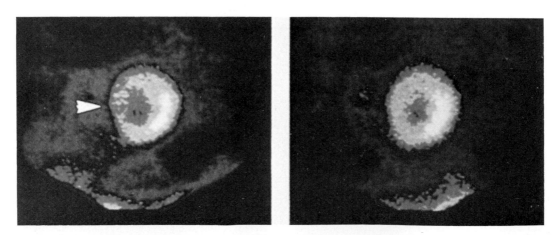

See Color Figure 3–30.

Figure 3–30. One-hour stress and 3-hour delayed 45-degree left anterior oblique Tc-99m–sestamibi images obtained in a patient with 95% left anterior descending coronary artery stenosis. The septal wall defect *(arrow)* observed 1 hour after Tc-99m–sestamibi injection at stress shows mild partial redistribution at 3 hours poststress (see Color Figure 3–30). (Reprinted by permission of the Society of Nuclear Medicine from: Taillefer R, et al.: J Nucl Med 1991;32:1961–1965.)

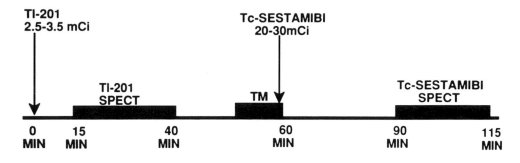

Figure 3–31. Injection and acquisition protocol for dual-isotope myocardial perfusion SPECT imaging employing rest Tl-201 and stress Tc-99m–sestamibi imaging sequence. (Reprinted with permission from the American College of Cardiology (Journal of the American College of Cardiology, 1993, Vol. 22, pp. 1455–1464).)

et al.,[125] which showed redistribution of Tc-99m sestamibi in a canine model of a severe coronary stenosis. The degree of redistribution was significantly less than that observed for Tl-201 in the same animals.

Dual-Isotope Rest Thallium-201–Stress Tc-99m–Sestamibi SPECT Imaging

Berman et al.[125a] evaluated the sensitivity and specificity of a novel dual-isotope procedure characterized by injection of 3.5 mCi of Tl-201 at rest with images acquired 10 minutes later, followed by immediate exercise sestamibi imaging utilizing 20 to 30 mCi of tracer injected at peak exercise. Sestamibi images were then acquired 30 minutes after isotope injection (Fig. 3–31). As shown in Figure 3–32, sensitivity and specificity for this technique for CAD detection (≥50% stenosis) were 91% and 75%, respectively. These values were 96% and 82% when ≥70% stenosis was used as a criterion for CAD detection. The normalcy rate for 107 patients with a low likelihood of CAD was 95%. Defect reversibility was comparable for the dual-isotope rest Tl-201–stress Tc-99m–sestamibi technique and the standard rest-stress sestamibi SPECT technique. Figure 3–33 is an example of a dual-isotope study in a patient with a reversible defect. The authors state that the major advantage

of this technique is more rapid completion of imaging studies than with conventional rest-exercise sestamibi studies, where typically 3 to 4 hours is the interval between rest and stress procedures. Heo et al.[125b] found that the entire dual-isotope imaging study could be completed in 2 hours. They found a 77% sensitivity, 65% specificity, and 97% normalcy rate using this imaging protocol. Sensitivity was 56%, 83%, and 90%, respectively, in patients with one-vessel, two-vessel, and three-vessel CAD. In 386 segments with no wall motion abnormality on ventriculography, 357 (92%) had a normal perfusion pattern or reversible defects. The authors commented that the lower sensitivity for CAD detection found in this study was because many patients with mild coronary stenoses were included. The indication for the stress imaging test was to determine the hemodynamic significance of borderline lesions observed on coronary angiography. Tl-201 imaging should be performed first in this dual-isotope protocol because of substantial Tc-99m crosstalk into Tl-201 windows.[125c] In this study, Tc-99m crosstalk contributed 26.7% to the dual Tl-201 images.

Electrocardiographic-Gated Technetium-99m–Sestamibi Imaging

Since the dose of Tc-99m sestamibi that is injected for imaging contains at least 10 times more radioactivity than a comparable imaging dose of Tl-201, ECG-gated perfusion images can be more easily acquired. Gating allows for simultaneous assessment of myocardial perfusion during stress and resting regional systolic function at rest. A comparison between the perfusion pattern during stress and systolic function at rest can be undertaken because initial Tc-99m–sestamibi images acquired are usually obtained at least 30 to 60 minutes after cessation of exercise. A perfusion abnormality seen on the exercise scintigram demonstrating preserved regional systolic thickening at rest would imply transient ischemia and preserved viability. In contrast, a significant perfusion defect associated with absence of regional thickening at rest might represent either irreversible cellular injury or hibernating or stunned myocardium. In a study by Verzijlbergen et al.,[126] interpretation of gated diastolic Tc-99m–sestamibi images was no different than interpretation of static images with respect to sensitivity and specificity of CAD detection. Overall sensitivity for detecting significant CAD was 86% using static image

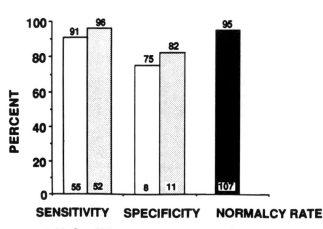

Figure 3–32. Sensitivity, specificity, and normalcy rate for dual-isotope SPECT imaging utilizing 50% stenosis *(open bars)* and at least 70% stenosis *(stippled bars)* as criteria for significant coronary artery disease. (Reprinted with permission from the American College of Cardiology (Journal of the American College of Cardiology, 1993, Vol. 22, pp. 1455–1464).)

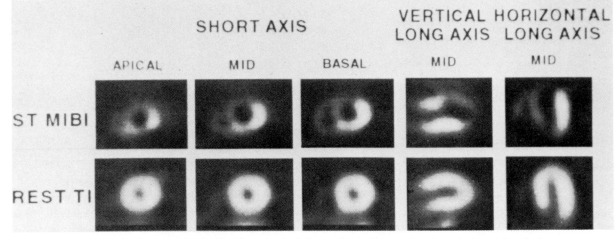

Figure 3–33. An example of a dual-isotope study in a patient with an extensive anteroseptal perfusion abnormality. The stress (ST) Tc-99m–sestamibi (MIBI) images are shown in the top row, and the rest Tl-201 (Tl) images in the same region are shown in the bottom row. (Reprinted with permission of the American College of Cardiology (Journal of the American College of Cardiology, 1993, Vol. 22, pp. 1455–1464).)

interpretation and 89% when diastolic images were interpreted. Specificity was 78% and 70%, respectively, using the two approaches to analysis. Najm et al.[126a] reported that measurement of radionuclide fractional shortening on the anterior Tc-99m–sestamibi images derived from analysis of diastolic and systolic images correlated closely ($r = 0.89$) with echocardiographic fractional shortening. Mannting and Morgan-Mannting[127] reported that the right ventricle appeared more distinct in diastolic frames of gated Tc-99m–sestamibi images than in nongated images. In that study, extent and degree of perfusion abnormalities in rest and stress studies correlated highly in nongated and diastolic images ($r = 0.98$).

In a preliminary report, Wackers et al.[128] compared regional wall motion on planar-gated Tc-99m–sestamibi images to regional wall motion as assessed by standard radionuclide-gated ventriculography. Visual evaluation of endocardial and epicardial motion on the ECG-gated Tc-99m–sestamibi images were compared directly with endocardial motion on the MUGA scans. These investigators found that endocardial motion significantly underestimated regional dysfunction as compared with the gated blood pool studies. Of 111 segments that were abnormal on the gated radionuclide ventriculograms, only 43% were abnormal by analysis of endocardial Tc-99m–sestamibi motion, compared with 85% by analysis of epicardial motion. They concluded that, if gated imaging is performed, then analysis of epicardial motion on video images is more accurate than endocardial motion on Tc-99m–sestamibi images. Marcassa et al.[129] described a new method of noninvasive quantitation of segmental myocardial wall thickening on Tc-99m–sestamibi planar images. Analysis of regional systolic thickening using a circumferential profile approach revealed maximum and minimal values of 35% and 27% located to the inferoapical and the proximal anterior wall, respectively.

The thickening analysis was obtained from the end-diastolic and end-systolic count distribution profiles.

Tischler et al.[128a] reported excellent interobserver and intraobserver agreement for global and segmental Tc-99m–sestamibi wall motion analysis. These investigators also shared excellent agreement with echocardiographic wall motion assessment.

DePuey et al.[128b] devised a method to calculate the left ventricular ejection fraction (LVEF) from gated SPECT Tc-99m–sestamibi tomograms. They used 8 frames/cycle gated 180-degree SPECT imaging using 6.4-mm thick midventricular vertical and horizontal long-axis slices from end-diastolic and end-systolic frames. Endocardial borders were manually drawn at a count level of 34% of the maximum. Using the Simpson's rule method, LVEF ranged from 0.21 to 0.73 and correlated linearly with values from gated blood pool radionuclide imaging (0.79 to 0.88).

Simultaneous Technetium-99m–Sestamibi First-Pass Radionuclide Ventriculography and Myocardial Perfusion Imaging

A significant advantage of the Tc-99m–labeled myocardial perfusion agents is the capability of evaluating myocardial perfusion and function simultaneously using a single intravenous injection of the radionuclide. A two-day study is preferred for this dual-imaging technique, since 25 mCi of Tc-99m sestamibi permits a high-quality first-pass acquisition. A minimum count rate of 125,000 counts per second is required for satisfactory first-pass studies, but most often 250,000 counts is exceeded with conventional tracer doses. Dynamic acquisition at 25 to 30 milliseconds per frame for at least 800 frames using a matrix of 32 by 32 or smaller are recommended. LVEF determined by quantitating Tc-99m activity in the LV blood pool with the first pass of Tc-

99m sestamibi through the central circulation correlates well with LVEF as determined by the first-pass technique (see Chap. 1) using a conventional multicrystal camera and Tc-99m–labeled red blood cells. Hassan[130] reported a significant correlation between LVEF measured by Tc-99m sestamibi first-pass radionuclide angiography and by contrast ventriculography ($r = 0.85$). Baillet et al.[131] compared resting first-pass radionuclide angiography using Tc-99m sestamibi with Tc-99m diethylenetriaminepentaacetic acid (DTPA) first-pass studies in 27 patients undergoing both procedures. A significant correlation was seen for LVEFs measured with both radiopharmaceuticals.

Boucher et al.[132] reported the results of a multicenter trial assessing first-pass RVEF and LVEF with Tc-99m sestamibi in 85 patients. As shown in Figure 3–34, there was an excellent correlation (0.96) between the standard Tc-99m first-pass LVEF determination and the Tc-99m–sestamibi LVEF. Larock et al.[133] also found an excellent correlation between first-pass LVEF obtained with Tc-99m sestamibi and equilibrium LVEF obtained with Tc-99m red blood cells ($r = 0.96$); however, these investigators did not find

as good a correlation for RVEF ($r = 0.75$). Iskandrian et al.[117] reported that 8 of 10 patients with CAD had both abnormal Tc-99m–sestamibi myocardial perfusion images and abnormal EF responses to exercise when both perfusion and function were evaluated with a single injection of the radionuclide. One patient had abnormal perfusion images but a normal EF response to exercise, whereas the other patient had an abnormal EF response to exercise but normal Tc-99m–sestamibi perfusion images. Thus, all 10 CAD patients had either abnormal perfusion images or an abnormal EF response to exercise.

Regional myocardial wall motion can also be evaluated during first-pass Tc-99m–sestamibi radionuclide ventriculography. Villanueva-Meyer et al.[134] compared regional wall motion at stress and rest after first-pass Tc-99m sestamibi ventriculography with myocardial perfusion assessed with SPECT imaging in the same patients after a single administered injection of the radionuclide. Complete agreement between LV wall motion and myocardial perfusion imaging was observed in 68% of myocardial segments. Segmental wall motion analysis showed the best correlation with inferior wall myocardial perfusion, and the most frequent disagreement was found at the apex.

Borges-Neto et al.[135] showed good concordance between myocardial perfusion and ventricular function with Tc-99m sestamibi first-pass ventriculography/perfusion imaging. There was a significant correlation between tomographic Tc-99m–sestamibi perfusion defect size and EF ($P < 0.001$, $r = 0.75$ at rest; $P < 0.0001$, $r = 0.76$ during exercise; Fig. 3–35). Multivariate analysis demonstrated that Tc-99m–sestamibi SPECT provided more diagnostic information than exercise ECG testing alone or radionuclide angiography alone for detecting one or more 60% stenoses.

Williams et al.[135a] found that Tc-99m–sestamibi first-pass radionuclide angiography was superior to Tc-99m teboroxime first-pass angiography secondary to greater pulmonary uptake with the latter tracer. Greater background during the levo phase of tracer transit was seen with Tc-99m teboroxime, and the final ejection fraction was lower. Also, there was poorer image quality, which compromised assessment of regional wall motion. The gold standard for first-pass imaging was Tc-99m DTPA. As mentioned in the previous section, De Puey et al.[128b] measured the LVEF from gated sestamibi SPECT imaging using manually drawn endocardial borders on midventricular and horizontal long-axis slices on end-diastolic and end-systolic frames. The measurements of LVEF correlated well with standard gated blood pool imaging.

The ability to measure exercise EF and regional myocardial perfusion simultaneously with Tc-99m sestamibi may significantly enhance the prognostic value of this imaging agent. Many studies have shown that the exercise LVEF is an important prognostic variable in identifying high-risk patients with CAD (see Chap. 4). Measuring the first-pass EF may serve as a surrogate for lung Tl-201 uptake in the

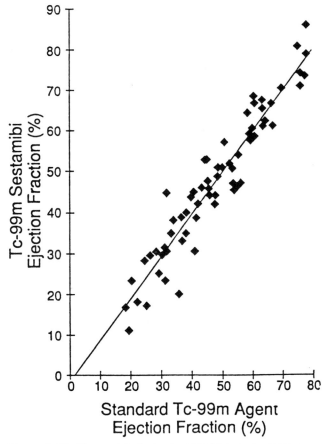

Figure 3–34. Linear plot of standard Tc-99m–sestamibi first-pass left ventricular ejection fraction (LVEF; *horizontal axis*) and Tc-99m–sestamibi LVEF *(vertical axis).* The correlation coefficient was 0.96. (Reprinted with permission from the American College of Cardiology (Journal of the American College of Cardiology, 1992, Vol. 69, pp. 22–27).)

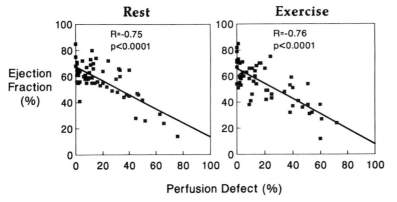

Figure 3–35. Correlation between percentage of myocardium with a Tc-99m–sestamibi perfusion defect and left ventricular ejection fraction calculated after first-pass Tc-99m–sestamibi ventriculography. There was a significant correlation between tomographic Tc-99m–sestamibi perfusion defect size and ejection fraction at rest and during exercise. (Borges-Neto S, et al.: Semin Nucl Med 1991; 21:223–229.)

assessment of prognosis using Tc-99m–sestamibi imaging. The lung-heart Tc-99m–sestamibi ratio has not yet been shown to be of prognostic value, and the lack of measurement of this variable is a potential limitation of Tc-99m–sestamibi perfusion imaging. One encouraging report[135b] suggests that reliable first-pass radionuclide angiography can be achieved using a large field-of-view tomographic single-crystal gamma camera employing an ultra–high-sensitivity collimator. First-pass LVEF values correlated linearly with multicrystal camera values (V = 0.94; slope = 1.05; intercept = 1.3; SE = 5.3%).

Right Ventricular Perfusion Imaging with Technetium-99m Sestamibi

Visualization of the right ventricle with Tc-99m–sestamibi perfusion imaging is superior to that with Tl-201 imaging.[136] Using RV polar maps, 7 of 11 patients (64%) with RCA disease had fixed or reversible RV defects. None of the 25 volunteers or patients without an RCA stenosis had RV defects on SPECT images. Thus, RV perfusion can adequately be assessed with SPECT Tc-99m–sestamibi imaging.

Mental Stress and Myocardial Technetium-99m–Sestamibi Imaging

Giubbini et al.[137] found that 20 of 24 patients with a recent MI had reversible perfusion defects after mental arithmetic (Fig. 3–36). All had exercise-induced defects. Of the 360 pooled segments, 99 corresponded to exercise-induced defects, and 48 of these showed the same defects during mental stress.

Summary

Tc-99m–sestamibi imaging is replacing Tl-201 scintigraphy in many institutions as the perfusion imaging technique of choice for detection of CAD. It offers several

distinct advantages over Tl-201. Because it is labeled with Tc-99m, it can be available day and night without requiring periodic delivery from a cyclotron distribution center. The 140-keV energy is ideal for gamma camera imaging and should result in improved resolution, owing to less scatter and attenuation. Because of its smaller radiation dose, a significantly greater amount of radioactivity can be administered than with Tl-201, resulting in increased count density, making feasible gated imaging and first-pass ventriculography. The minimal redistribution of Tc-99m sestamibi permits greater flexibility and increased convenience, since one can uncouple the time of injection with the time of imaging. This would allow injection of Tc-99m sestamibi during an exercise stress test in one location in an office or hospital setting and performance of imaging at a distant site. Since, ideally, a 30- to 60-minute period is required for clearance of early hepatic and pulmonary uptake, sufficient time is available to transport the patient without loss of significant defect resolution. Nevertheless, several studies cited in this chapter suggest that waiting as along as 3 to 4 hours after Tc-99m–sestamibi injection could result in some diminution in defect resolution. Some investigators in the field have found that imaging can commence as early as 15 minutes after Tc-99m–sestamibi injection during exercise without much interference from pulmonary or hepatic activity.

Patients who could benefit most from imaging with Tc-99m sestamibi rather than Tl-201 are obese females. Soft-tissue attenuation artifacts common in women because of overlying breast tissue may be minimized with the Tc-99m–labeled agent.

Some limitations of Tc-99m–sestamibi imaging deserve mention. First, there is some question as to whether viability detection in hibernating myocardium is as good as that achieved with Tl-201 imaging (see Chap. 9). Preliminary data on this issue show that the amount of Tc-99m–sestamibi uptake alone has excellent predictive value for viability determination. Lack of lung uptake data with Tc-99m–sestamibi imaging results in loss of an excellent prognostic variable; however, a large reversible defect on SPECT images may be all that is required for identifying CAD patients at high risk. Determination of LVEF using first-pass

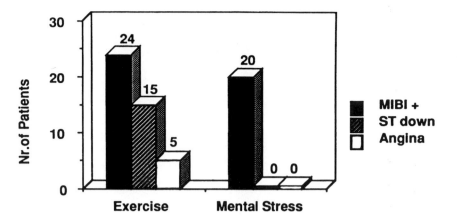

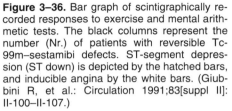

Figure 3–36. Bar graph of scintigraphically recorded responses to exercise and mental arithmetic tests. The black columns represent the number (Nr.) of patients with reversible Tc-99m–sestamibi defects. ST-segment depression (ST down) is depicted by the hatched bars, and inducible angina by the white bars. (Giubbini R, et al.: Circulation 1991;83[suppl II]: II-100–II-107.)

ventriculographic approaches may also assist in the risk stratification process using this radionuclide.

EXERCISE TECHNETIUM-99m–TEBOROXIME IMAGING

Exercise Imaging Protocol

The kinetics and basic properties of Tc-99m teboroxime are summarized in Chapter 2. Tc-99m teboroxime is a BATO compound that is a neutral lipophilic agent with high initial myocardial extraction, rapid myocardial clearance, and enterohepatic excretion. With respect to its molecular size, Tc-99m teboroxime is larger than Tl-201 but smaller than Tc-99m sestamibi. Tc-99m teboroxime rapidly diffuses across cell membranes; it is not yet known whether it is transported intracellularly or remains bound to the phospholipid layers of the membrane. The myocardial washout of Tc-99m teboroxime is biexponential, the first rapid component having a half-time of 5 to 10 minutes. This rapid component, which is the major clearance component, correlates with regional myocardial blood flow. As with Tc-99m sestamibi, separate stress and rest injections are required to differentiate ischemia from scar. Tc-99m teboroxime may be clinically useful for imaging protocols where acquisition of images begins very soon after injection.[137a]

Planar Imaging with Tc-99m Teboroxime

Because of its rapid myocardial clearance, all imaging protocols using Tc-99m teboroxime must be performed rapidly. Ideally, no more than 1 to 2 minutes should elapse between Tc-99m–teboroxime injection and the commencement of imaging. This can be accomplished either by having the patient perform bicycle exercise while positioned in front of the gamma camera or by having the camera prepared to begin acquisition before treadmill exercise commences and transporting the patient rapidly from the treadmill to the camera. The exercise imaging protocol described by Hendel et al.[138] involved treadmill exercise after which patients were positioned seated upright in front of the gamma camera in order to minimize the interference by hepatic uptake of the tracer. Data collection using this approach was initiated within 1 minute of the discontinuation of exercise. For planar imaging, a rapid dynamic acquisition protocol was used with a frame rate of 20 seconds per frame with data acquired in a 64 by 64 matrix, initially in the anterior view. Each view was continuously monitored, and 40 to 80 seconds (2 to 4 frames) of data were accumulated in the anterior position after blood pool clearance. With this protocol, subjects were then sequentially rotated in the chair to the 45-degree left anterior oblique position, and later the left lateral, and data were acquired for 40 to 80 seconds per view. Imaging was repeated in the same fashion at rest after a second injection of Tc-99m teboroxime. Tc-99m–teboroxime scans are summated during image processing and analysis; 2 or 3 frames are used for each view (40 to 60 seconds). Images that show significant amounts of blood pool activity or motion artifact due to repositioning can be excluded. Figure 3–37 shows stress and rest planar Tc-99m–teboroxime images in a patient with CAD.

Seldin et al.[139] employed upright bicycle exercise in a standard-field-of-view camera positioned in front of the patient's chest for Tc-99m–teboroxime imaging. Dynamic imaging at 10 seconds per frame on a 128 by 128 matrix for 5 minutes in the anterior projection, 6 minutes in the shallow, and 9 minutes in the steep left anterior oblique projections for total imaging time of 20 minutes was accomplished. With this approach, the dynamic images are summed to produce three planar views for interpretation. A second rest injection with this protocol was performed 2 hours after exercise stress.

A third approach to Tc-99m–teboroxime imaging has been described by Johnson.[140] With this method, a high count-rate multicrystal scintillation camera with a small field of view is used for rapid imaging. This camera was originally designed for first-pass radionuclide ventriculography. Johnson equipped the instrument with a 1-inch collimator for Tc-99m–sestamibi imaging. Patients are exer-

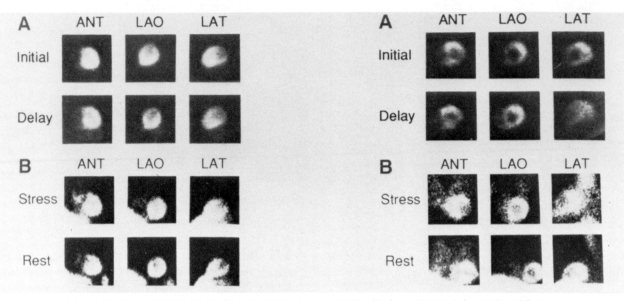

Figure 3–37. A. Normal planar Tl-201 images in the anterior (Ant), 40-degree left anterior oblique (LAO) and left lateral (LAT) images showing uniform Tl-201 uptake on both initial and delayed images. **B.** Planar teboroxime images from the same patient in the same projections. Note that there is greater hepatic uptake of activity on the teboroxime images compared with the Tl-201 images. (Reprinted with permission from the American College of Cardiology (Journal of the American College of Cardiology, 1990, Vol. 16, pp. 855–861).)

cised with their chest against the detector face with an americium-241 (Am-241) point source marker over the sternum for motion correction. Dynamic dual isotope (Tc-99m–Am-241) acquisition is performed following injection of 15 mCi of Tc-99m teboroxime at peak exercise. Two minutes later, while the patient is still standing on a motionless treadmill, three or four 30- to 60-second static images are required in the anterior, shallow and steep left anterior oblique projections. In the first 30-second image, before hepatic uptake occurs, there are typically 400,000 to 700,000 counts in the field of view, predominantly in the myocardium. Patients are reinjected in the resting state 1 hour later while standing in front of the camera, and the same dynamic-static acquisition protocol is repeated.

Johnson comments that the best approach to performing planar imaging with a standard gamma camera utilizes moving the patient rapidly from the treadmill to the camera for imaging beginning 2 minutes after injection. Dynamic imaging is performed at 20 seconds per frame using a general all-purpose collimator and terminated after 2 to 4 frames, depending on the count rate. The steep left anterior oblique view is obtained first, before accumulation of significant liver activity. The major drawback of Tc-99m–teboroxime imaging, which must be avoided, is starting the imaging sequence too late, when myocardial Tc-99m–teboroxime clearance has been substantial and liver activity is high.

SPECT Imaging with Technetium-99m Teboroxime

SPECT imaging of Tc-99m teboroxime must be performed rapidly with a total short acquisition time of no more than 7 to 9 minutes. Leppo et al.[141] advise that, to get the greatest number of counts using the SPECT approach, either the camera dead time must be short or the camera must have the option for continuous step-and-shoot acquisition. Either a general all-purpose collimator or a high-resolution collimator can be employed for SPECT Tc-99m–teboroxime imaging. The acquisition protocol suggested by these authors is continuous acquisition or step-and-shoot with total live time plus stepping time <7 minutes, beginning in the left posterior oblique and finishing in the right anterior oblique projection. Because of the need for a short acquisition time following Tc-99m teboroxime injection, a three-headed camera is preferable.

Detection of Coronary Artery Disease: Planar and SPECT

In one of the first large studies reported,[141] the diagnostic accuracy of Tc-99m–teboroxime imaging was shown to be high in 177 patients, some of whom had coronary arteriography, or stress Tl-201 scintigraphy, or both. In that study, sensitivity was 84% and specificity 91% for detection of CAD. These data were derived from a phase III trial, and the results of Tc-99m–teboroxime scans were compared against ''overall clinical impression based on results of angiography and other imaging studies.'' In the 123 patients who had coronary angiography and Tc-99m–teboroxime imaging, sensitivity and specificity were 83% and 91%, respectively, for CAD detection. Dahlberg et al.,[142] using planar Tc-99m teboroxime imaging with a rapid-acquisition protocol, reported 86% agreement between Tc-99m–teboroxime and Tl-201 scans for determining presence or absence of CAD, 80% agreement in individual vessel stenosis detection rate, and 78% segmental agreement for normal versus abnormal perfusion. Tc-99m teboroxime showed more ischemic segments (66%) than did Tl-201 (54%, $P <$ 0.05). Iskandrian et al.[143] found 89% agreement in identifying normal or abnormal perfusion zones when comparing Tc-99m–teboroxime and Tl-201 results. In only one of 22 patients studied were Tc-99m–teboroxime and Tl-201 results discordant. Fleming et al.[144] compared Tc-99m–teboroxime SPECT imaging with quantitative coronary angiography and Tl-201 imaging. In this SPECT study involving 30 patients with suspected CAD, there was no difference between Tc-99m teboroxime and Tl-201 for detection of presence or absence of disease using quantitative coronary angiography as the gold standard. All patients with multivessel disease were detected by both imaging techniques. One-vessel disease was detected with Tc-99m teboroxime in 9 of 10 patients, and with Tl-201 in 8 of 10 patients (difference not significant). Similar findings were reported by Hendel et al.,[138] in which diagnostic agreement (abnormal vs. normal) was achieved for 28 of 30 patients undergoing planar Tc-99m–teboroxime imaging and Tl-201 scintigraphy. Seldin et al.[139] found that hepatic uptake of Tc-99m teboroxime obscured the inferoapical region in some views in 14 of 20 patients but apparently did not interfere with detection of coronary lesions. In that study, Tc-99m teboroxime detected 16 of 20 cases and Tl-201 17 of 20 in patients who had CAD by angiographic criteria.

Serafini et al.,[145] using a single-detector SPECT camera with a continuous-acquisition imaging protocol in 17 patients with suspected or known CAD, found 94% concordance in patient classification between Tc-99m–teboroxime and Tl-201 exercise studies performed within a 2-week period. Comparison of scintigraphic findings between Tl-201 and Tc-99m teboroxime on a segment-by-segment basis showed concordance in 90% (107 of 119) of segments. Table 3–15 summarizes this analysis. Interestingly, of 14 segments judged to be ischemic on Tl-201 imaging, only seven were designated as reversible in Tc-99m teboroxime images.

A direct comparison of planar Tc-99m–teboroxime and Tc-99m–sestamibi imaging was made by Taillefer et al.[146] in 17 patients who also underwent Tl-201 imaging. Patients

achieved similar levels of exercise on all three tests. Segmental comparison showed agreement in 85% of segments between Tl-201 and Tc-99m teboroxime, in 92% between Tl-201 and Tc-99m sestamibi, and in 84% between Tc-99m sestamibi and Tc-99m teboroxime. Ischemic-normal wall ratios were 0.75, 0.73, and 0.78 for Tl-201, Tc-99m sestamibi, and Tc-99m teboroxime, respectively. Thus, a good correlation among the three imaging agents for detection of significant CAD was observed in a "high–pretest likelihood" population. A comparison was made between Tl-201 and Tc-99m teboroxime with respect to segmental analysis of identifying normal, reversible, and fixed defects. Thirteen segments showed redistribution on Tl-201 images but were normal on Tc-99m–teboroxime scans, indicating superior results for ischemia detection using Tl-201. Only one segment showed reversibility on Tc-99m–teboroxime images and was normal on Tl-201 scan interpretation. In Figure 3–38 are Tl-201, Tc-99m–sestamibi, and Tc-99m–teboroxime images from a representative patient in this study. Note the marked hepatic tracer uptake on the resting Tc-99m–teboroxime images.

Weinstein et al.[146a] reported rapid redistribution of Tc-99m teboroxime on 5-minute postinjection images, which was attributed to differential washout of the tracer from normal and ischemic zones. Defect intensity improved from 0.79 with stress to 0.88 on early delayed images ($P < 0.005$) in ischemic scintigrams. Sublingual isosorbide dinitrate administration before injecting Tc-99m teboroxime at rest improved the detection of reversibility in exercise-induced perfusion defects.[146b]

Simultaneous Assessment of Perfusion and Function

As with Tc-99m sestamibi, first-pass LV radionuclide angiography can be undertaken with Tc-99m teboroxime before acquisition of perfusion imaging data. Johnson et al.[147] used a small field of view, portable multicrystal camera to perform stress-rest combined first-pass LV function and perfusion studies in 26 patients with abnormal Tl-201 scans and in eight healthy volunteers. The agreement was 92% for detection of CAD and 83% for identifying abnormal vascular territories, when compared with Tl-201 images. Fourteen patients had an exercise LVEF <50%. All had a history of infarction, infarction and ischemia, or ischemia alone in the territory of the LAD.

Summary

Tc-99m teboroxime has certain features that make it attractive for the assessment of regional myocardial perfusion under conditions of stress. The Tc-99m label permits high count rates with the possibility of dynamic imaging to quantitate regional differences in washout that may reflect

Table 3–15. **Segmental Analysis of Tl-201 and Tc-99m Teboroxime SPECT in 17 Patients**

	Tl-201	Tc-99m Teboroxime
Normal	77	77
Ischemic	14	11
Infarcted	8	28
Ischemia plus infarction	14	0
Equivocal	6	3
Total	119	119

(Reprinted by permission of the Society of Nuclear Medicine from: Serafini AN, et al.: J Nucl Med 1992;33:1304–1311.)

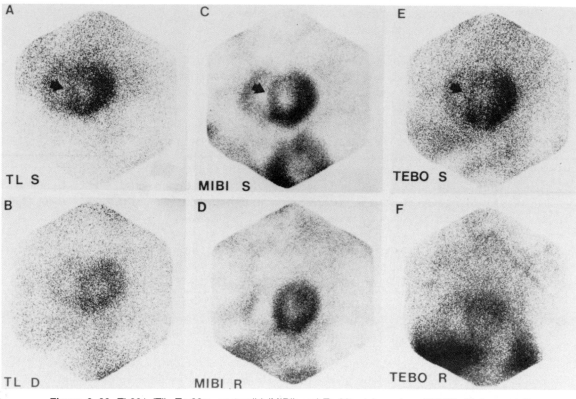

Figure 3–38. Tl-201 (Tl), Tc-99m–sestamibi (MIBI) and Tc-99m teboroxime (TEBO) 45-degree left anterior oblique (LAO) images obtained in a patient who had a 95% stenosis of the left anterior descending coronary artery. A reversible anteroseptal defect *(arrow)* is seen on all images. (Key: S, stress; R, rest; D, delayed.) (Reprinted by permission of the Society of Nuclear Medicine from: Taillefer R, et al.: J Nucl Med 1992;33:1091–1098.)

the magnitude of stress-induced ischemia. The rapid clearance of the radionuclide could permit serial imaging, which could shorten an entire stress-rest study to less than an hour. Certainly, first-pass LVEF and RVEF can be measured with Tc-99m teboroxime similarly to the method described earlier in this chapter for Tc-99m sestamibi. There are certain limitations to Tc-99m–teboroxime imaging that deserve mention despite its good initial myocardial extraction. There can be logistic difficulties in moving a patient rapidly from a treadmill to a camera to commence image acquisition within 2 minutes after tracer injection. Imaging must be complete within 6 minutes. Some studies are difficult to interpret because of high splanchnic activity due to intense liver uptake early after tracer administration. Scattered activity into the inferior wall from anatomic overlap and hepatic uptake on planar scans can interfere with adequate assessment of inferior zone perfusion. Performing planar imaging solely with the patient in the upright, erect position could improve the diagnostic quality of the images by lowering the liver.

Pharmacologic stress imaging may be more suitable for this radionuclide, since a patient can be placed under the imaging camera at the time of drug infusion (see Chap. 8). SPECT techniques may be more difficult to employ with Tc-99m teboroxime because of the need to complete the Tc-99m–teboroxime perfusion scan within 6 to 8 minutes.

Perhaps the approach with a continuous-rotation acquisition using a three-headed camera will prove most acceptable in this regard.

Exercise Tc-99m–Tetrofosmin Imaging

Tc-99m tetrofosmin is a compound of the diphosphine group that is rapidly cleared from the blood pool after intravenous injection and taken up by the myocardium in proportion to blood flow.[147a–147c] The biology and pharmacokinetics of this tracer are described in Chapter 2. Preliminary reports suggest that its ability to detect CAD with exercise imaging is comparable to that achieved with Tl-201.[147c–147e] With rest imaging, cardiac activity exceeds activity in the gallbladder, liver, and gastrointestinal tract by 30 to 60 minutes after injection.[147a] Figure 3–39 shows stress and redistribution Tl-201 and Tc-99m–tetrofosmin planar images from a patient with atypical chest pain in this study.[147a] Sridhara et al.[147e] reported no evidence of Tc-99m–tetrofosmin redistribution over 240 minutes after intravenous injection during exercise stress. No increased lung uptake was seen with this radionuclide as compared with Tl-201 in the same patients in that study. Stress and reinjection Tc-99m–tetrofosmin images from one of the patients in this study with an ischemic response is shown

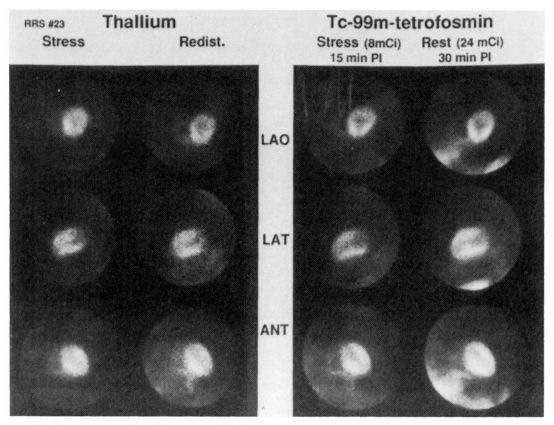

Figure 3–39. Left anterior oblique (LAO), left lateral (LAT) and anterior (ANT) planar thallium *(left panel)* and Tc-99m tetrofosmin *(right panel)* images at stress and at rest in a patient with atypical chest pain. Both sets of images show normal regional myocardial perfusion. (Reprinted by permission of the Society of Nuclear Medicine from: Jain D, et al.: J Nucl Med 1993;34:1254–1259.)

in Figure 3–40. The sensitivity for CAD detection in another multicenter trial was 86% for both same-day stress-rest and separate-day rest protocols with Tc-99m tetrofosmin.[147f] Of a total of 396 segments studied, 107 abnormal segments were detected on the exercise scintigrams. Of these 76 and 81 were also abnormal on the same-day and separate-day resting scintigrams, respectively. Assessment of regional wall motion by first-pass radionuclide angiography combined with assessment of perfusion with Tc-99m tetrofosmin can increase sensitivity for CAD detection.[147g]

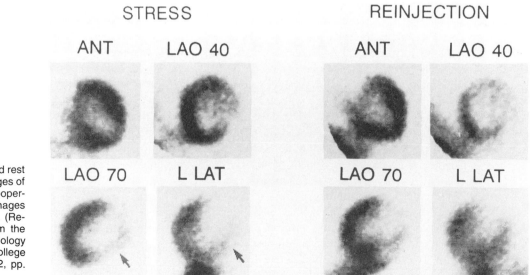

Figure 3–40. Stress *(left)* and rest reinjection *(right)* planar images of Tc-99m tetrofosmin. The hypoperfused area on the stress images are indicated by the arrows. (Reprinted with permission from the American College of Cardiology (Journal of the American College of Cardiology, 1993, Vol. 72, pp. 1015–1019).)

All indications to date are that Tc-99m–tetrofosmin imaging yields the same diagnostic accuracy for CAD detection as Tc-99m sestamibi and Tl-201.[147i]

EXERCISE TECHNETIUM-99m-Q3 IMAGING

Tc-99m-Q3 is a cationic diphosphine complex that has also been tested for use as a radionuclide perfusion agent.[147h] With this agent 5 to 7 mCi is injected at rest, with imaging performed 15 minutes later. Exercise imaging is undertaken 10 minutes after acquisition of the resting study with a 23-mCi dose. The heart-to-lung ratio of uptake was 1.88 during exercise, slightly less than the Tl-201 ratio of 2.33. Overall accuracy for CAD detection was 78% for Tl-201 versus 89% for Tc-99m-Q3 using tomographic imaging. Accuracy for detection of individual coronary stenoses was 75% for Tl-201 imaging and 83% for Tc-99m-Q3 imaging (P = not significant). Interobserver agreement concerning the presence or absence of a defect in an individual myocardial segment was 88% (141 of 160). The major feature of the Tc-99m agent is the rapid hepatic clearance.

EXERCISE RADIONUCLIDE ANGIOGRAPHY

Technique and Criteria for an Abnormal Test Response

Techniques for assessing global and regional function using either first-pass or equilibrium radionuclide angiography are discussed in Chapter 1. The Tc-99m red cell–labeling technique required for gated cardiac blood pool imaging is reviewed in Chapter 2. The exercise radionuclide angiographic protocol employing the equilibrium technique first involves obtaining gated blood pool images at rest and calculating the resting EF (see Chap. 1). A recording of regional motion dynamics is also made. Patients in a supine position then begin to pedal a bicycle ergometer, with the camera placed to obtain a 45- to 50-degree left anterior oblique image. Exercise workloads are increased by 25-W increments at 3-minute intervals, culminating in exercise levels that produce symptom-limited endpoints. Heart rates achieved at peak supine exercise are considerably slower than those achieved with upright exercise. Imaging is begun after 1 minute of exercise at each workload and continued to the end of the session. Measurements of EF are made using the count-based method described in Chapter 1, and a comparison of global and regional ventricular function during rest and exercise is performed. Ventricular function studies during exercise can also be obtained by first-pass radionuclide angiography. When using Tc-99m, the resting study is often performed with Tc-99m pentetate, whereas the peak exercise study is undertaken with Tc-99m sodium pertechnetate following clearance from the blood pool through the kidneys of the first technetium-labeled agent. The resting study is per-

formed initially with the patient positioned in front of the detector, usually in an upright position. The exercise protocol is similar to that described for the gated method. At peak exercise, the bolus injection is made while the chest wall is stabilized but while the patient is still exercising maximally.

On the basis of studies performed in subjects who showed no evidence of underlying cardiopulmonary disease, the normal ventricular response to exercise has been defined as an absolute increment of at least 5% in the RVEF and LVEF without the development of new regional wall motion abnormalities.[148–150] Figure 3–41 shows the EF at rest and at peak exercise in normal patients and patients with CAD from the study of Borer et al.[150] The physiologic response to exercise is associated with a small increase in the LV end-diastolic volume. An increase of more than 5% in the end-systolic volume during exercise is considered an abnormal response. The definition of a normal response—requiring a 5% or greater increase in LVEF during exercise—has been somewhat disputed.[151] This is because a change in LVEF from rest to exercise is influenced by variables other than the intrinsic systolic performance of the left ventricle under stress conditions. Variables that influence this response include resting EF, gender, the change in end-diastolic volume index from rest to exercise, the resting pulse pressure, the presence of ECG changes induced with exercise, and the extent of CAD.[151]

Other investigators have defined the normal response of the LVEF to exercise by the absolute level of EF achieved.[152, 153] In apparently normal subjects who were 60 years of age, the LVEF was shown not to increase normally with exercise and actually to decrease in some patients.[154] This phenomenon may represent an intrinsic property of the aging process. Gibbons et al.[155] found that, for patients whose resting LVEF was at least 75%, the normal response should be defined as no diminution in LVEF with exercise. These patients with hyperdynamic LV performance at rest, cannot be expected to exhibit a further decrease in end-systolic volume with exercise. Inadequate stress secondary to physical limitations may be associated with a normal response in spite of underlying CAD.[150] Normal patients without underlying cardiac disease receiving beta-blocking agents may also fail to demonstrate the appropriate increase in LVEF with exercise.[156]

Gender can certainly affect the response of the LVEF to exercise. Jones et al.[152] found that approximately 30% of women who have chest pain but normal coronary arteries demonstrate either a decrease in or failure to increase the radionuclide LVEF during exercise. Higginbotham et al.[157] found a basic difference between men and women with respect to the mechanism by which they achieve a normal response of stroke volume to exercise. In women, decreases in LVEF during exercise were matched by increases in end-diastolic counts, and the relative increases in stroke counts and cardiac output by the count-based method were the same for men and women. Hanley et al.[158] found that the gender difference reported for the LVEF response to exer-

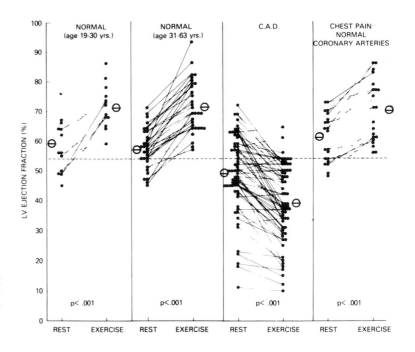

Figure 3–41. Left ventricular (LV) ejection fraction at rest and during exercise in normal subjects, patients with coronary artery disease (CAD) and patients with chest pain in angiographic normal coronary arteries. (Borer J, et al.: Circulation 1979;60:572–580.)

cise may be related more to the fact that women tend to have smaller hearts than men, even when adjustment is made for body size and weight. A smaller heart can certainly influence analysis of radionuclide angiographic results, particularly if an increase of 5% or more is the criterion for a normal response. As shown in Figure 3–42, for both men and women, the peak exercise ejection fraction was found to be a better variable than the change in ejection fraction from rest to exercise from CAD detection.[151]

Sensitivity and Specificity for Detection of Coronary Artery Disease

Gibbons[151] reviewed the data in the literature that compared exercise radionuclide angiography with ECG stress testing for detection of CAD. A total of 424 patients de-

rived from four studies were the source of his pooled analysis.[150, 152, 159, 160] Sensitivity and specificity for radionuclide angiography were 86% and 79%, respectively. The values for exercise ECG stress testing in the same patient cohort were 58% and 91%, respectively. In a study by Weishammer et al.,[161] the conventional criterion that normal subjects have an increase in LVEF of ≥5% with exercise provided only 78% sensitivity and 57% specificity. In the report by Jones et al.,[152] when EF-oriented criteria alone were used with criteria based on absolute volumes, radionuclide angiography was 90% sensitive and 58% specific. These data are not surprising, since the EF is a nonspecific indicator of LV function and any myocardial disorder could affect systolic performance both at rest and during exercise.

No studies reported in the literature used a large number of patients and adequately compared the accuracy of exercise radionuclide angiography with exercise Tl-201 scintig-

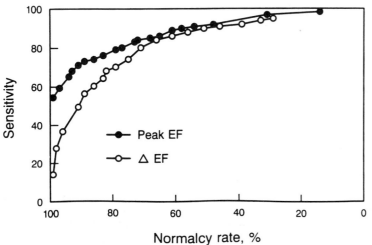

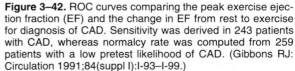

Figure 3–42. ROC curves comparing the peak exercise ejection fraction (EF) and the change in EF from rest to exercise for diagnosis of CAD. Sensitivity was derived in 243 patients with CAD, whereas normalcy rate was computed from 259 patients with a low pretest likelihood of CAD. (Gibbons RJ: Circulation 1991;84(suppl I):I-93–I-99.)

raphy for detection of CAD. Most comparison studies were reported in the era before quantitative myocardial perfusion imaging and before the emergence of SPECT Tl-201 scintigraphy as the preferred approach for stress imaging. Nevertheless, data referable to the comparison of the two techniques suggested comparable sensitivity but lower specificity for radionuclide angiography.[162–165]

As with Tl-201 scintigraphic studies, the sensitivity of exercise radionuclide angiography for CAD detection improves with higher levels of stress achieved and when underlying CAD is more severe. In patients who failed to achieve a rate-pressure product $>250 \times 10^3$, the sensitivity of the exercise radionuclide angiogram was shown to be only 62%, as compared with 94% when patients exceeded this workload.[166] Pretreatment with nitrates may prevent the abnormal functional response to stress in patients with CAD.[167] If propranolol improves the oxygen supply-demand ratio, myocardial ischemia may be prevented during exercise and a normal or flat EF response will be observed.[168] Beta-adrenergic blockade effectively improved the reduction in exercise regional EF usually seen in CAD patients with silent myocardial ischemia.[169] The coexistence of hypertension may influence the specificity of exercise radionuclide angiography. Wasserman et al.[170] found that exercise radionuclide angiography was inadequate as a screening test for CAD in hypertensive patients with chest pain. In this study, no difference in EF at rest was observed in hypertensive patients with CAD and hypertensive patients without CAD. Neither subgroup had a significant mean change in EF from rest to exercise. Interestingly, a wall motion abnormality developed during exercise in five of the 17 hypertensive patients with CAD (29%) and in four of the 20 without CAD (20%; P = NS). In contrast, nonhypertensive patients who had CAD had a mean *decrease* in LVEF of 3.6% as compared with an *increase* of 6% in nonhypertensive patients who did not have CAD ($P < 0.001$).

The LVEF response to exercise can be abnormal in patients with chest pain and angiographically normal coronary arteries.[171] In such patients, who may have syndrome X (angina with normal coronary arteries), coronary flow reserve can be significantly impaired. Legrand et al.[171] showed that coronary flow reserve in the arterial distributions supplying regions with abnormal function on radionuclide angiography was significantly lower than in the arterial distributions associated with normal systolic functional responses.

Kimchi et al. made the observation that segmental wall motion that is abnormal at rest can sometimes improve with exercise.[172] Myocardial segments that show enhanced systolic function with exercise most often show preserved Tl-201 uptake. Also, such segments are rarely associated with pathologic Q waves. Johnson et al.[173] found that proximal RCA lesions were associated with a drop in LVEF during exercise but no change in RVEF. In contrast, CAD that did not involve the proximal RCA resulted in a drop in LVEF

but a rise in RVEF. The RVEF is most difficult to quantify on equilibrium-gated radionuclide angiography and is more accurately determined on first-pass studies.

Summary

Most nuclear cardiology laboratories do not prefer exercise radionuclide angiography as the first technique for use in detection of CAD in patients with undiagnosed chest pain. The major reason that perfusion imaging is more popular relates to the fact that it is performed using treadmill rather than bicycle exercise, has a better diagnostic accuracy than exercise radionuclide angiography, and has a higher specificity in women and patients of advanced age. Anti-ischemic medications have a greater influence on exercise radionuclide angiographic responses than on perfusion. Failure to increase LVEF with exercise by 5% or more is a sensitive but not very specific criterion, whereas the appearance of regional dysfunction consequent to exercise stress is quite specific for CAD but not very sensitive and rather subjective.[173a]

EXERCISE STRESS ECHOCARDIOGRAPHY

An alternative to radionuclide-based methods for CAD detection is assessment of regional myocardial systolic function by echocardiography during or immediately after exercise stress. Echocardiographic imaging can be performed continuously during bicycle ergometer stress or immediately after treadmill exercise when body motion ceases and hyperventilation diminishes. The basis for this approach is this: When there is a mismatch between myocardial oxygen demand and blood flow, ischemic wall motion abnormalities appear in the presence of physiologically significant coronary artery stenosis. A major technologic development that has yielded improved sensitivity and specificity for CAD detection with exercise echocardiography is digital recording and storage of echocardiographic images. Using computer-assisted approaches, echocardiograms can be stored, and continuous loop cinerecordings of individual cardiac cycles can be displayed in either split- or quad-screen formats. This permits resting and exercise images to be juxtaposed on one screen for comparative visual analysis. The images are synchronized to the R wave of the ECG, allowing for synchronization of the continuous cineloop.

Sensitivity and Specificity for Detection of Coronary Artery Disease

Not all patients are suitable for echocardiographic image acquisition during stress. In most institutions where the technique has been perfected, studies appropriate for interpretation are obtained for approximately 90% of subjects.[174] The overall sensitivity of exercise echocardiography for CAD detection is in the range of 75% to 85%, which is a somewhat lower sensitivity rate than that for exercise myocardial perfusion imaging.[175-185] Specificity in these studies was reported to be in the 90% range. Quinones et al.[186] reported the results of exercise echocardiography and Tl-201–SPECT imaging performed simultaneously in 292 patients being evaluated for CAD. There was 88% agreement between the two tests. The two tests demonstrated 82% agreement in detecting the same type of finding within the regions analyzed. SPECT, however, detected more reversible abnormalities than did echocardiography. Regions that on echocardiography showed an abnormality that persisted throughout rest and exercise often showed partial Tl-201 redistribution on SPECT. In contrast, approximately a third of regions with persistent Tl-201 defects on SPECT showed normal resting function or reversible abnormalities by two-dimensional echocardiography. The sensitivity for detecting a stenosis of at least 50% was similar for the two tests (Fig. 3–43). Sensitivity for echocardiography was 58% and for SPECT Tl-201 was 61%, respectively, for single-vessel disease, and 94% for both tests for detecting patients with three-vessel disease. Specificity of the two noninvasive techniques was also comparable: 88% for echocardiography and 81% for SPECT.

Marwick et al.[183] identified certain factors that affected sensitivity and specificity of the exercise echocardiogram. False-negative results correlated with the performance of submaximal exercise, single-vessel disease, and mild stenosis (50% to 70% reduction of luminal diameter). As expected, exercise echocardiography was significantly more sensitive for detection of CAD than the exercise ECG (87% vs. 63%; $P = 0.01$). Also, in that study the technique produced more accurate results when patients exceeded 85% of their age-predicted maximal heart rate and when they had more severe disease in multiple coronary vessels.

Sheikh et al.[187] correlated quantitative angiographic findings with echocardiographic demonstration of ischemia in a group of 34 patients with isolated, single-vessel CAD and normal wall motion at rest. All 11 patients with at least 75% stenosis as judged by visual assessment had an ischemic response, whereas 10 of 11 patients (91%) with no more than 25% visually estimated stenosis had a normal echocardiographic response to exercise. Among 12 patients whose visually estimated stenosis was 50%, 6 (50%) had an ischemic echocardiographic response and the remaining 6 demonstrated a normal response to exercise. Also, the smaller the minimal luminal diameter by quantitative angiography, and the smaller the minimal cross-sectional area of the stenosis, the greater was the likelihood of an ischemic echocardiographic response to exercise stress. Hecht et al.[187a] found that, in 222 patients, digital supine bicycle stress echocardiography yielded 93% sensitivity, 86% specificity, and 92% accuracy for detection of CAD. In this study, images were obtained at peak exercise intensity. Interestingly, sensitivity was comparable regardless of whether subjects (1) had a history of infarction or (2) achieved at least 85% of maximum predicted heart rate. LCx stenoses were less readily detected (78%) than were LAD (95%) or RCA (81%) lesions ($P < 0.01$). Sensitivity was 81% for patients with 50% to 70% stenosis, as compared with 91% for 90% to 100% lesions. Mertes et al.,[187b] who also employed digital bicycle exercise echocardiography to evaluate patients after nonsurgical coronary revascularization, reported 83% sensitivity and 85% specificity for detection of significant CAD. When an additional analysis, using an increase in end-systolic volume index or a decrease in EF during stress as an additional variable for ischemia was conducted, sensitivity increased to 90%. Marangelli et al.[187c] reported a high sensitivity (89%) and specificity (91%) for digital exercise echocardiography in 104 consecutive patients with no previous myocardial infarction or resting LV wall motion abnormalities. However, in that study, feasibility of exercise echocardiography was only 84%, and 8 patients were withdrawn from the study because of inadequate exercise or imaging. This may have led to a selection bias that enhanced sensitivity of the test.

From review of published studies, it appears that the specificity of exercise echocardiography for CAD detection is similar to that for exercise myocardial perfusion imaging.

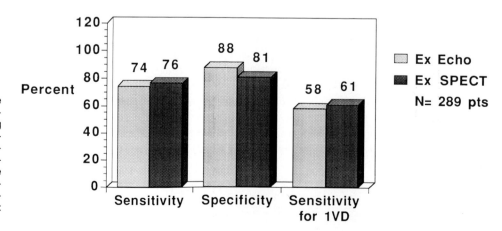

Figure 3–43. Comparison of exercise echocardiography (Ex Echo) and exercise thallium 201 SPECT imaging (Ex SPECT) for sensitivity and specificity for detecting CAD in 289 patients undergoing both tests. Sensitivity for detection of one-vessel disease (1VD) is lower for both tests compared with the overall values. (Quinones MA, et al.: Circulation 1992;85: 1026–1031.)

However, the sensitivity for CAD detection is approximately 10% lower with echocardiography than with radionuclide perfusion imaging. One explanation for the lower sensitivity may relate to the acquisition of stress echocardiographic images immediately after exercise, rather than during exercise. Some patients with single-vessel disease or lesser degrees of stenosis (50% to 70%) may experience rapid reversal of ischemia in the immediate recovery period. The detection rate of CAD by exercise echocardiography may depend more on the level of exercise stress achieved than does exercise perfusion imaging. Another potential limitation of exercise echocardiography is the lack of an operator-independent quantitative analytical method for identifying new regional wall motion abnormalities. The interpretation of echocardiographic studies is a very subjective exercise. Another possible limitation of exercise echocardiography is the detection of residual ischemia in an area of infarction that on the resting echocardiographic study displays severe asynergy. Tl-201 imaging permits the detection of partial redistribution in zones of infarction, suggesting preserved viability and some remaining myocardium at jeopardy. With exercise echocardiography, this infarct zone may already be akinetic or dyskinetic at rest owing to myocardial stunning or hibernation. Nevertheless, exercise echocardiography has certain advantages over SPECT myocardial perfusion imaging. One relates to the lower cost of exercise echocardiography and the less complex equipment required. Exercise echocardiographic stress testing can be performed in the office setting and does not require extensive space and support staff.

EXERCISE POSITRON EMISSION TOMOGRAPHIC IMAGING

Positron emission tomography (PET) has been used principally in conjunction with pharmacologic stress for detection of CAD (see Chap. 8). PET instrumentation and the radiopharmaceuticals employed are reviewed in Chapters 1 and 2, respectively. Tamaki et al.[188] evaluated the use of exercise PET imaging with N-13 ammonia for CAD detection: they reported 88% sensitivity and 90% specificity. Because N-13 ammonia has a half-life of 10 minutes, stress and rest imaging studies can be completed within 1½ hours. In recent years, exercise stress has not often been employed in conjunction with PET imaging with short-lived tracers. Most clinical imaging studies for detection of CAD are undertaken with intravenous dipyridamole or adenosine in conjunction with N-13 ammonia or Rb-82—the preferred radiopharmaceuticals (see Chap. 8). Oxygen-15 water, a diffusible and metabolically inert flow tracer, has also been used for quantification of regional blood flow, at rest and after pharmacologic stress.

REFERENCES

1. DeRouen T, Murray J, Owen W: Variability in the analysis of coronary arteriograms. Circulation 1977;55:324–328.
2. Mancini GB, Simon SB, McGillem MJ, LeFree MT, Friedman HZ, Vogel RA: Automated quantitative coronary arteriography: Morphologic and physiologic validation in vivo of a rapid digital angiographic method. Circulation 1987;75:452–460.
3. Rifkin RD, Hood WB Jr: Bayesian analysis of electrocardiographic exercise stress testing. N Engl J Med 1977;297:681–686.
4. Diamond GA, Forrester JS: Analysis of probability as an aid in the clinical diagnosis of coronary-artery disease. N Engl J Med 1979;300:1350–1358.
5. Diamond GA, Forrester JS, Hirsch M, Staniloff HM, Vas R, Berman DS, Swan HJ: Application of conditional probability analysis to the clinical diagnosis of coronary artery disease. J Clin Invest 1980;65:1210–1221.
6. Weintraub WS, Madeira SW Jr, Bodenheimer MM, Seelaus PA, Katz RI, Feldman MS, Agarwal JB, Banka VS, Helfant RH: Critical analysis of the application of Bayes' theorem to sequential testing in the noninvasive diagnosis of coronary artery disease. Am J Cardiol 1984;54:43–49.
7. Gibson R, Beller G: Should exercise ECG testing be replaced by radioisotope methods? In Rahimtoola S, Brest A (eds): Controversies in Coronary Artery Disease. Philadelphia, FA Davis, 1982, pp 1–32.
8. Diamond G: Clinical diagnosis of coronary artery disease using Bayes' theorem. Myocardium 1989;1:9–11.
8a. Gibson RS, Watson DD: Clinical applications of myocardial perfusion scentography with thallium-201. In Yu PN, Goodwin JF (eds): Progress in Cardiology, Vol 12. Philadelphia, Lea & Febiger, 1983, pp 67–112.
9. Epstein SE: Implications of probability analysis on the strategy used for noninvasive detection of coronary artery disease. Role of single or combined use of exercise electrocardiographic testing, radionuclide cineangiography and myocardial perfusion imaging. Am J Cardiol 1980;46:491–499.
10. Patterson RE, Horowitz SF: Importance of epidemiology and biostatistics in deciding clinical strategies for using diagnostic tests: a simplified approach using examples from coronary artery disease. J Am Coll Cardiol 1989;13:1653–1665.
11. Fletcher GF, Froelicher VF, Hartley LH, Haskell WL, Pollock ML: Exercise standards. A statement for health professionals from the American Heart Association. Circulation 1990;82:2286–2322.
12. Schlant RC, Friesinger GC, Leonard JJ: Clinical competence in exercise testing. A statement for physicians from the ACP/ACC/AHA Task Force on Clinical Privileges in Cardiology. J Am Coll Cardiol 1990;16:1061–1065.
13. Firsch C, DeSanctis R, Dodge H, Reeves T, Weinberg S: Guidelines for exercise testing: A report of the American College of Cardiology/American Heart Association Task Force on Assessment of Cardiovascular Procedures (subcommittee on exercise testing). J Am Coll Cardiol 1986;8:725–738.
14. Bruce R: Exercise testing of patients with coronary heart disease: Principles and normal standards for evaluation. Ann Clin Res 1971;3:323–332.
15. Gianrossi R, Detrano R, Mulvihill D, Lehmann K, Dubach P, Colombo A, McArthur D, Froelicher V: Exercise-induced ST depression in the diagnosis of coronary artery disease. A meta-analysis. Circulation 1989;80:87–98.
16. Detrano R, Gianrossi R, Mulvihill D, Lehmann K, Dubach P, Colombo A, Froelicher V: Exercise-induced ST segment depression in the diagnosis of multivessel coronary disease: A meta analysis. J Am Coll Cardiol 1989;14:1501–1508.
17. Okin P, Klingfield P, Amerson O, Goldberg H, Borer J: Improved accuracy of the exercise electrocardiograph: Identification of three-vessel coronary disease in stable angina pectoris by analysis of peak rate-related changes in ST segments. Am J Cardiol 1985;55:271–276.
18. Bobbio M, Detrano R, Schmid JJ, Janosi A, Righetti A, Pfisterer M, Steinbrunn W, Guppy KH, Abi-Mansour P, Deckers JW, et al.: Exercise-induced ST depression and ST/heart rate index to predict triple-vessel or left main coronary disease: A multicenter analysis. J Am Coll Cardiol 1992;19:11–18.
19. Hollenberg M, Zoltick JM, Go M, Yaney SF, Daniels W, Davis RC Jr, Bedynek JL: Comparison of a quantitative treadmill exercise score with standard electrocardiographic criteria in screening asymptomatic young men for coronary artery disease. N Engl J Med 1985;313:600–606.
19a. Beller GA: Myocardial perfusion imaging with thallium-201. J Nucl Med 1994;35:674–680.

19b. Wackers FJ Th: Exercise myocardial perfusion imaging. J Nucl Med 1994;35:726–729.

19c. Beller GA: Current status of nuclear cardiology techniques. Curr Prob Cardiol 1991;16[7]:447–535.

19d. Botvinick EH: A consideration of current clinical options for stress imaging in the diagnosis and evaluation of coronary artery disease. J Nucl Cardiol 1994;1:S147–S170.

20. Sox HC Jr, Griner P: An invitation to join a controversy. Ann Intern Med 1992;116:422–423.

21. Allen WH, Aronow WS, Goodman P, Stinson P: Five-year follow-up of maximal treadmill stress test in asymptomatic men and women. Circulation 1980;62:522–527.

22. Froelicher VF Jr, Thompson AJ, Wolthuis R, Fuchs R, Balusek R, Longo MR Jr, Triebwasser JH, Lancaster MC: Angiographic findings in asymptomatic aircrewmen with electrocardiographic abnormalities. Am J Cardiol 1977;39:32–38.

23. Borer J, Brensike J, Redwood D, Itscoitz S, Pessamani E, Stone N, Richardson J, Levi R, Epstein S: Limitations of electrocardiographic response to exercise in predicting coronary artery disease. N Engl J Med 1975;293:367–371.

24. Uhl GS, Froelicher V: Screening for asymptomatic coronary artery disease. J Am Coll Cardiol 1983;1:946–955.

25. Uhl GS, Kay TN, Hickman JR Jr, Montgomery MA, McGranahan GM: Detection of coronary artery disease in asymptomatic aircrew members with thallium-201 scintigraphy. Aviation Space Environ Med 1980;51:1250–1255.

26. Uhl GS, Kay TN, Hickman JR Jr: Computer-enhanced thallium scintigrams in asymptomatic men with abnormal exercise tests. Am J Cardiol 1981;48:1037–1043.

27. Becker LC, Becker DM, Pearson TA, Fintel DJ, Links J, Frank TL: Screening of asymptomatic siblings of patients with premature coronary artery disease. Circulation 1987;75:II14–II17.

27a. Schwartz RS, Jackson WG, Celio PV, Richardson LA, Hickman JR Jr: Accuracy of exercise ^{201}Tl myocardial scintigraphy in asymptomatic young men. Circulation 1993;87:165–172.

28. Hamilton GW, Trobaugh GB, Ritchie JL, Williams DL, Weaver WD, Gould KL: Myocardial imaging with intravenously injected thallium-201 in patients with suspected coronary artery disease: Analysis of technique and correlation with electrocardiographic, coronary anatomic and ventriculographic findings. Am J Cardiol 1977;39:347–354.

29. Bailey IK, Griffith LS, Rouleau J, Strauss W, Pitt B: Thallium-201 myocardial perfusion imaging at rest and during exercise. Comparative sensitivity to electrocardiography in coronary artery disease. Circulation 1977;55:79–87.

30. Ritchie JL, Trobaugh GB, Hamilton GW, Gould KL, Narahara KA, Murray JA, Williams DL: Myocardial imaging with thallium-201 at rest and during exercise. Comparison with coronary arteriography and resting and stress electrocardiography. Circulation 1977;56:66–71.

31. Ritchie JL, Zaret BL, Strauss HW, Pitt B, Berman DS, Schelbert HR, Ashburn WL, Berger HJ, Hamilton GW: Myocardial imaging with thallium-201: A multicenter study in patients with angina pectoris or acute myocardial infarction. Am J Cardiol 1978;42:345–350.

32. Blood DK, McCarthy DM, Sciacca RR, Cannon PJ: Comparison of single-dose and double-dose thallium-201 myocardial perfusion scintigraphy for the detection of coronary artery disease and prior myocardial infarction. Circulation 1978;58:777–788.

33. McCarthy DM, Blood DK, Sciacca RR, Cannon PJ: Single dose myocardial perfusion imaging with thallium-201: Application in patients with nondiagnostic electrocardiographic stress tests. Am J Cardiol 1979;43:899–906.

34. Botvinick EH, Taradash MR, Shames DM, Parmley WW: Thallium-201 myocardial perfusion scintigraphy for the clinical clarification of normal, abnormal and equivocal electrocardiographic stress tests. Am J Cardiol 1978;41:43–51.

35. Murray RG, McKillop JH, Bessent RG, Turner JG, Lorimer AR, Hutton I, Greig WR, Lawrie TD: Evaluation of thallium-201 exercise scintigraphy in coronary heart disease. Br Heart J 1979;41:568–574.

36. Carillo A, Marks D, Pickard S, Khaja F, Goldstein S: Correlation of exercise Tl-201 myocardial scan with coronary arteriograms and the maximal exercise test. Chest 1978;73:321.

37. Sonnemaker RE, Floyd JL, Nusynowitz ML, Bode RF, Spicer MJ, Waliszewski JA: Single injection thallium-201 stress and redistribution myocardial perfusion imaging: comparison with stress electro-cardiography and coronary arteriography. Radiology 1979;131:199–203.

38. Verani MS, Marcus ML, Razzak MA, Ehrhardt JC: Sensitivity and specificity of thallium-201 perfusion scintigrams under exercise in the diagnosis of coronary artery disease. J Nucl Med 1978;19:773–782.

39. Verani MS, Jhingran S, Attar M, Rizk A, Quinones MA, Miller RR: Poststress redistribution of thallium-201 in patients with coronary artery disease, with and without prior myocardial infarction. Am J Cardiol 1979;43:1114–1122.

40. Corne RA, Gotsman MS, Weiss A, Enlander D, Samuels LD, Salomon JA, Warshaw B, Atlan H: Thallium-201 scintigraphy in diagnosis of coronary stenosis. Comparison with electrocardiography and coronary arteriography. Br Heart J 1979;41:575–583.

41. Caralis DG, Bailey I, Kennedy HL, Pitt B: Thallium-201 myocardial imaging in evaluation of asymptomatic individuals with ischaemic ST segment depression on exercise electrocardiogram. Br Heart J 1979;42:562–567.

42. Iskandrian AS, Wasserman LA, Anderson GS, Hakki H, Segal BL, Kane S: Merits of stress thallium-201 myocardial perfusion imaging in patients with inconclusive exercise electrocardiograms: correlation with coronary arteriograms. Am J Cardiol 1980;46:553–558.

43. Rigo P, Bailey IK, Griffith LS, Pitt B, Wagner HN Jr, Becker LC: Stress thallium-201 myocardial scintigraphy for the detection of individual coronary arterial lesions in patients with and without previous myocardial infarction. Am J Cardiol 1981;48:209–216.

44. Melin JA, Piret LJ, Vanbutsele RJ, Rousseau MF, Cosyns J, Brasseur LA, Beckers C, Detry JM: Diagnostic value of exercise electrocardiography and thallium myocardial scintigraphy in patients without previous myocardial infarction: A Bayesian approach. Circulation 1981;63:1019–1024.

45. Jengo JA, Freeman R, Brizendine M, Mena I: Detection of coronary artery disease: Comparison of exercise stress radionuclide angiocardiography and thallium stress perfusion scanning. Am J Cardiol 1980;45:535–541.

46. Elkayam U, Weinstein M, Berman D, Maddahi J, Staniloff H, Freeman M, Waxman A, Swan HJ, Forrester J: Stress thallium-201 myocardial scintigraphy and exercise technetium ventriculography in the detection and location of chronic coronary artery disease: Comparison of sensitivity and specificity of these noninvasive tests alone and in combination. Am Heart J 1981;101:657–666.

47. Rigo P, Bailey IK, Griffith LS, Pitt B, Burow RD, Wagner HN Jr, Becker LC: Value and limitations of segmental analysis of stress thallium myocardial imaging for localization of coronary artery disease. Circulation 1980;61:973–981.

48. Hung J, Chaitman BR, Lam J, Lesperance J, Dupras G, Fines P, Bourassa MG: Noninvasive diagnostic test choices for the evaluation of coronary artery disease in women: A multivariate comparison of cardiac fluoroscopy, exercise electrocardiography and exercise thallium myocardial perfusion scintigraphy. J Am Coll Cardiol 1984;4:8–16.

49. Caldwell JH, Hamilton GW, Sorensen SG, Ritchie JL, Williams DL, Kennedy JW: The detection of coronary artery disease with radionuclide techniques: A comparison of rest-exercise thallium imaging and ejection fraction response. Circulation 1980;61:610–619.

50. Bodenheimer MM, Banka VS, Fooshee CM, Helfant RH: Comparative sensitivity of the exercise electrocardiogram, thallium imaging and stress radionuclide angiography to detect the presence and severity of coronary heart disease. Circulation 1979;60:1270–1278.

51. McKillop JH, Murray RG, Turner JG, Bessent RG, Lorimer AR, Greig WR: Can the extent of coronary artery disease be predicted from thallium-201 myocardial images? J Nucl Med 1979;20:714–719.

52. Kotler TS, Diamond GA: Exercise thallium-201 scintigraphy in the diagnosis and prognosis of coronary artery disease. Ann Intern Med 1990;113:684–702.

53. Gerson M: Test accuracy, test selection and test result interpretation in chronic coronary artery disease. *In* Gerson M (ed): Cardiac Nuclear Medicine. Newark, McGraw Hill, 1987, pp 309–348.

54. Gibson R, Watson D: Clinical applications of myocardial perfusion scintigraphy with thallium-201. Progr Cardiol 1983;12:67–112.

55. Port SC, Oshima M, Ray G, McNamee P, Schmidt DH: Assessment of single vessel coronary artery disease: Results of exercise electrocardiography, thallium-201 myocardial perfusion imaging and radionuclide angiography. J Am Coll Cardiol 1985;6:75–83.

56. Kaul S, Kiess M, Liu P, Guiney TE, Pohost GM, Okada RD, Boucher CA: Comparison of exercise electrocardiography and quantitative thallium imaging for one-vessel coronary artery disease. Am J Cardiol 1985;56:257–261.

57. Berger BC, Watson DD, Taylor GJ, Craddock GB, Martin RP, Teates CD, Beller GA: Quantitative thallium-201 exercise scintigraphy for detection of coronary artery disease. J Nucl Med 1981;22:585–593.

58. Maddahi J, Garcia EV, Berman DS, Waxman A, Swan HJ, Forrester J: Improved noninvasive assessment of coronary artery disease by quantitative analysis of regional stress myocardial distribution and washout of thallium-201. Circulation 1981;64:924–935.

59. Wackers FJ, Fetterman RC, Mattera JA, Clements JP: Quantitative planar thallium-201 stress scintigraphy: A critical evaluation of the method. Semin Nucl Med 1985;15:46–66.

60. Kaul S, Boucher CA, Newell JB, Chesler DA, Greenberg JM, Okada RD, Strauss HW, Dinsmore RE, Pohost GM: Determination of the quantitative thallium imaging variables that optimize detection of coronary artery disease. J Am Coll Cardiol 1986;7:527–537.

61. Wijns W, Serruys PW, Reiber JH, van den Brand M, Simoons ML, Kooijman CJ, Balakumaran K, Hugenholtz PG: Quantitative angiography of the left anterior descending coronary artery: Correlations with pressure gradient and results of exercise thallium scintigraphy. Circulation 1985;71:273–279.

62. Rigo P, Becker LC, Griffith LS, Alderson PO, Bailey IK, Pitt B, Burow RD, Wagner HN Jr: Influence of coronary collateral vessels on the results of thallium-201 myocardial stress imaging. Am J Cardiol 1979;44:452–458.

63. Berger BC, Watson DD, Taylor GJ, Burwell LR, Martin RP, Beller GA: Effect of coronary collateral circulation on regional myocardial perfusion assessed with quantitative thallium-201 scintigraphy. Am J Cardiol 1980;46:365–370.

64. Freedman SB, Dunn RF, Bernstein L, Morris J, Kelly DT: Influence of coronary collateral blood flow on the development of exertional ischemia and Q wave infarction in patients with severe single-vessel disease. Circulation 1985;71:681–686.

65. Esquivel L, Pollock SG, Beller GA, Gibson RS, Watson DD, Kaul S: Effect of the degree of effort on the sensitivity of the exercise thallium-201 stress test in symptomatic coronary artery disease. Am J Cardiol 1989;63:160–165.

66. Tono I, Satoh S, Kanaya T, Komatani A, Takahashi K, Tsuiki K, Asui S: Alterations in myocardial perfusion during exercise after isosorbide dinitrate infusion in patients with coronary disease: Assessment by thallium-201 scintigraphy. Am Heart J 1986;111:525–533.

67. DePace NL, Iskandrian AS, Nadell R, Colby J, Hakki AH: Variation in the size of jeopardized myocardium in patients with isolated left anterior descending coronary artery disease. Circulation 1983;67:988–994.

68. Watson DD, Campbell NP, Read EK, Gibson RS, Teates CD, Beller GA: Spatial and temporal quantitation of plane thallium myocardial images. J Nucl Med 1981;22:577–584.

69. Desmarais R, Kaul S, Watson D, Beller G: Do false positive thallium-201 scans lead to unnecessary catheterization? Outcome of patients with perfusion defects on quantitative planar thallium-201 scintigraphy. J Am Coll Cardiol 1993;21:1058–1063.

69a. Wackers FJ, Bodenheimer M, Fleiss JL, Brown M: Factors affecting uniformity in interpretation of planar thallium-201 imaging in a multicenter trial. The Multicenter Study on Silent Myocardial Ischemia (MSSMI) Thallium-201 Investigators. J Am Coll Cardiol 1993;21:1064–1074.

70. Brown KA, Osbakken M, Boucher CA, Strauss HW, Pohost GM, Okada RD: Positive exercise thallium-201 test responses in patients with less than 50% maximal coronary stenosis: Angiographic and clinical predictors. Am J Cardiol 1985;55:54–57.

71. Kaul S, Newell JB, Chesler DA, Pohost GM, Okada RD, Boucher CA: Quantitative thallium imaging findings in patients with normal coronary angiographic findings and in clinically normal subjects. Am J Cardiol 1986;57:509–512.

72. Becker LC, Rogers WJ Jr, Links JM, Corn C: Limitations of regional myocardial thallium clearance for identification of disease in individual coronary arteries. J Am Coll Cardiol 1989;14:1491–1500.

73. Sklar J, Kirch D, Johnson T, Hasegawa B, Peck S, Steele P: Slow late myocardial clearance of thallium: A characteristic phenomenon in coronary artery disease. Circulation 1982;65:1504–1510.

74. Kaul S, Chesler DA, Newell JB, Pohost GM, Okada RD, Boucher CA: Regional variability in the myocardial clearance of thallium-201 and its importance in determining the presence or absence of coronary artery disease. J Am Coll Cardiol 1986;8:95–100.

75. Botvinick EH, O'Connell WJ, Dae MW, Hattner RS, Schechtmann NM: Analysis of thallium-201 "washout" from parametric color coded images. J Nucl Med 1988;29:302–310.

76. Bateman TM, Maddahi J, Gray RJ, Murphy FL, Garcia EV, Conklin CM, Raymond MJ, Stewart ME, Swan HJ, Berman DS: Diffuse slow washout of myocardial thallium-201: A new scintigraphic indicator of extensive coronary artery disease. J Am Coll Cardiol 1984;4:55–64.

77. Maddahi J, Abdulla A, Garcia EV, Swan HJ, Berman DS: Noninvasive identification of left main and triple vessel coronary artery disease: Improved accuracy using quantitative analysis of regional myocardial stress distribution and washout of thallium-201. J Am Coll Cardiol 1986;7:53–60.

78. Abdulla A, Maddahi J, Garcia E, Rozanski A, Swan HJ, Berman DS: Slow regional clearance of myocardial thallium-201 in the absence of perfusion defect: Contribution to detection of individual coronary artery stenoses and mechanism for occurrence. Circulation 1985;71:72–79.

79. Verani MS: Thallium-201 single-photon emission computed tomography (SPECT) in the assessment of coronary artery disease. Am J Cardiol 1992;70:3E–9E.

80. Tamaki N, Yonekura Y, Mukai T, Kodama S, Kadota K, Kambara H, Kawai C, Torizuka K: Stress thallium-201 transaxial emission computed tomography: Quantitative versus qualitative analysis for evaluation of coronary artery disease. J Am Coll Cardiol 1984;4:1213–1221.

81. DePasquale EE, Nody AC, DePuey EG, Garcia EV, Pilcher G, Bredlau C, Roubin G, Gober A, Gruentzig A, D'Amato P, et al.: Quantitative rotational thallium-201 tomography for identifying and localizing coronary artery disease. Circulation 1988;77:316–327.

82. Iskandrian AS, Heo J, Kong B, Lyons E: Effect of exercise level on the ability of thallium-201 tomographic imaging in detecting coronary artery disease: Analysis of 461 patients. J Am Coll Cardiol 1989;14:1477–1486.

83. Mahmarian JJ, Boyce TM, Goldberg RK, Cocanougher MK, Roberts R, Verani MS: Quantitative exercise thallium-201 single photon emission computed tomography for the enhanced diagnosis of ischemic heart disease. J Am Coll Cardiol 1990;15:318–329.

83a. Alazraki NP, Krawczynska EG, DePuey EG, Ziffer JA, Vansant JP, Pettigrew RI, Taylor A, King SB III, Garcia EV: Reproducibility of thallium-201 exercise SPECT studies. J Nucl Med 1994;35:1237–1244.

84. Van Train KF, Maddahi J, Berman DS, Kiat H, Areeda J, Prigent F, Friedman J: Quantitative analysis of tomographic stress thallium-201 myocardial scintigrams: A multicenter trial. J Nucl Med 1990;31:1168–1179.

85. Maddahi J, Van Train K, Prigent F, Garcia EV, Friedman J, Ostrzega E, Berman D: Quantitative single photon emission computed thallium-201 tomography for detection and localization of coronary artery disease: Optimization and prospective validation of a new technique. J Am Coll Cardiol 1989;14:1689–1699.

86. Rozanski A: Referral bias and the efficacy of radionuclide stress tests: Problems and solutions. J Nucl Med 1992;33:2074–2079.

87. Mahmarian JJ, Verani MS: Exercise thallium-201 perfusion scintigraphy in the assessment of coronary artery disease. Am J Cardiol 1991;67:2D–11D.

88. Mahmarian JJ, Pratt CM, Boyce TM, Verani MS: The variable extent of jeopardized myocardium in patients with single vessel coronary artery disease: Quantification by thallium-201 single photon emission computed tomography. J Am Coll Cardiol 1991;17:355–362.

88a. Mahmarian JJ, Fenimore NL, Marks GF, Francis MJ, Morales-Ballejo H, Verani MS, Pratt CM: Transdermal nitroglycerin patch therapy reduces the extent of exercise-induced myocardial ischemia: Results of a double-blind, placebo controlled trial using quantitative thallium-201 tomography. J Am Coll Cardiol 1994;24:25–32.

89. Prigent FM, Berman DS, Elashoff J, Rozanski A, Maddahi J, Friedman J, Dwyer JH: Reproducibility of stress redistribution thallium-201 SPECT quantitative indexes of hypoperfused myocardium secondary to coronary artery disease. Am J Cardiol 1992;70:1255–1263.

90. Fintel DJ, Links JM, Brinker JA, Frank TL, Parker M, Becker LC:

Improved diagnostic performance of exercise thallium-201 single photon emission computed tomography over planar imaging in the diagnosis of coronary artery disease: A receiver operating characteristic analysis. J Am Coll Cardiol 1989;13:600–612.

91. Friedman J, Berman DS, Van Train K, Garcia EV, Bietendorf J, Prigent F, Rozanski A, Waxman A, Maddahi J: Patient motion in thallium-201 myocardial SPECT imaging. An easily identified frequent source of artifactual defect. Clin Nucl Med 1988;13:321–324.

91a. Germano G, Chua T, Kavanaugh P, Kiat H, Berman D: Detection and correction of patient motion in dynamic and static myocardial SPECT using a multi-media detector camera. J Nucl Medicine 1993;34:1349–1355.

91b. Cooper JA: Detection of patient motion during tomographic myocardial perfusion imaging. J Nucl Med 1993;34:1341–1348.

92. Friedman J, Van Train K, Maddahi J, Rozanski A, Prigent F, Bietendorf J, Waxman A, Berman DS: "Upward creep" of the heart: A frequent source of false-positive reversible defects during thallium-201 stress-redistribution SPECT. J Nucl Med 1989;30:1718–1722.

92a. Cecil MP, Pilcher WC, Eisner RL, Chu TH, Merlino JD, Patterson RE: Absence of defects in SPECT thallium-201 myocardial images in patients with systemic hypertension and left ventricular hypertrophy. Am J Cardiol 1994;74:43–46.

93. Watson DD, Smith WH: SPECT: Current and future developments. J Nucl Biol Med 1992;36:108–112.

94. DePuey EG, Garcia EV: Optimal specificity of thallium-201 SPECT through recognition of imaging artifacts. J Nucl Med 1989;30:441–449.

94a. DePuey EG: How to detect and avoid myocardial perfusion SPECT artifacts. J Nucl Med 1994;35:699–702.

95. Guiney TE, Pohost GM, McKusick KA, Beller GA: Differentiation of false- from true-positive ECG responses to exercise stress by thallium 201 perfusion imaging. Chest 1981;80:4–10.

96. Lee W, Zhu, Morris L, Bhatia S, Botvinick E, Dae M, O'Connell J, Chatterjee K, Goldschlager N: The value of perfusion scintigraphy to assess exercise-induced T-wave normalization. Am J Cardiac Imaging 1988;2:148.

97. Berman DS, Kiat H, Van Train K, Garcia E, Friedman J, Maddahi J: Technetium 99m sestamibi in the assessment of chronic coronary artery disease. Semin Nucl Med 1991;21:190–212.

98. Sinusas AJ, Beller GA, Watson DD: Cardiac imaging with technetium 99m-labeled isonitriles. J Thoracic Imaging 1990;5:20–30.

99. Leppo JA, DePuey EG, Johnson LL: A review of cardiac imaging with sestamibi and teboroxime. J Nucl Med 1991;32:2012–2022.

100. Gibbons RJ: Technetium-99m sestamibi in the assessment of acute myocardial infarction. Semin Nucl Med 1991;21:213–222.

101. Blackburn T, Beller G: Scintigraphic assessment of myocardial perfusion using thallium-201 and Tc-99m imaging. Coronary Artery Dis 1992;3:274.

102. Berman D: Stress testing and the new technetium-99m cardiac imaging agents. Am J Cardiac Imaging 1991;5:32–36.

102a. Udelson JE: Choosing a thallium-201 or technetium-99m sestamibi imaging protocol. J Nucl Cardiol 1994;1:S99–S108.

103. Beller GA, Watson DD: Physiological basis of myocardial perfusion imaging with the technetium-99m agents. Semin Nucl Med 1991;21:173–181.

103a. Wackers FJ Th: The maze of myocardial perfusion imaging protocols in 1994. J Nucl Cardiol 1994;1:180–188.

103b. Taillefer R, Lambert R, Bisson G, Benjamin C, Phaneuf D-C: Myocardial technetium 99m–labeled sestamibi single-photon emission computed tomographic imaging in the detection of coronary artery disease: Comparison between early (15 minutes) and delayed (60 minutes) imaging. J Nucl Cardiol 1994;1:441–448.

104. Taillefer R, Gagnon A, Laflamme L, Gregoire J, Leveille J, Phaneuf DC: Same day injections of Tc-99m methoxy isobutyl isonitrile (hexamibi) for myocardial tomographic imaging: Comparison between rest-stress and stress-rest injection sequences. Eur J Nucl Med 1989;15:113–117.

105. Heo J, Kegel J, Iskandrian AS, Cave V, Iskandrian BB: Comparison of same-day protocols using technetium-99m-sestamibi myocardial imaging. J Nucl Med 1992;33:186–191.

106. Smith WH, Watson DD: Technical aspects of myocardial planar imaging with technetium- 99m sestamibi. Am J Cardiol 1990;66:16E–22E.

107. Sinusas AJ, Beller GA, Smith WH, Vinson EL, Brookeman V, Watson DD: Quantitative planar imaging with technetium-99m methoxy-isobutyl isonitrile: Comparison of uptake patterns with thallium-201. J Nucl Med 1989;30:1456–1463.

108. Koster K, Wackers FJ, Mattera JA, Fetterman RC: Quantitative analysis of planar technetium-99m-sestamibi myocardial perfusion images using modified background subtraction. J Nucl Med 1990;31:1400–1408.

109. Kiat H, Maddahi J, Roy LT, Van Train K, Friedman J, Resser K, Berman DS: Comparison of technetium 99m methoxy isobutyl isonitrile and thallium 201 for evaluation of coronary artery disease by planar and tomographic methods. Am Heart J 1989;117:1–11.

110. Wackers FJ, Berman DS, Maddahi J, Watson DD, Beller GA, Strauss HW, Boucher CA, Picard M, Holman BL, Fridrich R, et al.: Technetium-99m hexakis 2-methoxyisobutyl isonitrile: Human biodistribution, dosimetry, safety, and preliminary comparison to thallium-201 for myocardial perfusion imaging. J Nucl Med 1989;30:301–311.

111. Taillefer R, Lambert R, Dupras G, Gregoire J, Leveille J, Essiambre R, Phaneuf DC: Clinical comparison between thallium-201 and Tc-99m-methoxy isobutyl isonitrile (hexamibi) myocardial perfusion imaging for detection of coronary artery disease. Eur J Nucl Med 1989;15:280–286.

112. Watson DD, Smith WH, Beller GA, Vinson EL, Taillefer R: Blinded evaluation of planar technetium-99m-sestamibi myocardial perfusion studies. J Nucl Med 1992;33:668–675.

113. Maisey MN, Lowry A, Bischof-Delaloye A, Fridrich R, Inglese E, Khalil MN, van der Schoot JB: European multi-centre comparison of thallium 201 and technetium 99m methoxyisobutylisonitrile in ischaemic heart disease. Eur J Nucl Med 1990;16:869–872.

114. Najm C, Maisey MN, Clarke SM, Fogelman I, Curry PV, Sowton E: Exercise myocardial perfusion scintigraphy with technetium-99m methoxy isobutylisonitrile: A comparative study with thallium-201. Int J Cardiol 1990;26:93–102.

115. Taillefer R, Dupras G, Sporn V, Rigo P, Leveille J, Boucher P, Perez-Balino N, Camin LL, McKusick KA: Myocardial perfusion imaging with a new radiotracer, technetium- 99m-hexamibi (methoxy isobutyl isonitrile): Comparison with thallium-201 imaging. Clin Nucl Med 1989;14:89–96.

116. Maddahi J, Kiat H, Friedman G, Berman D, Van Trian K, Garcia E: Tc-99m sestamibi myocardial perfusion imaging for evaluation of coronary artery disease. *In* Zaret B, Beller G (eds): Nuclear Cardiology. St. Louis, CV Mosby, 1992.

117. Iskandrian AS, Heo J, Kong B, Lyons E, Marsch S: Use of technetium-99m isonitrile (RP-30A) in assessing left ventricular perfusion and function at rest and during exercise in coronary artery disease, and comparison with coronary arteriography and exercise thallium-201 SPECT imaging. Am J Cardiol 1989;64:270–275.

118. Kahn JK, McGhie I, Akers MS, Sills MN, Faber TL, Kulkarni PV, Willerson JT, Corbett JR: Quantitative rotational tomography with ^{201}Tl and ^{99m}Tc 2- methoxy-isobutyl-isonitrile. A direct comparison in normal individuals and patients with coronary artery disease. Circulation 1989;79:1282–1293.

119. Kiat H, Van Train KF, Maddahi J, Corbett JR, Nichols K, McGhie AI, Akers MS, Friedman JD, Roy L, Berman DS: Development and prospective application of quantitative 2-day stress-rest Tc-99m methoxy isobutyl isonitrile SPECT for the diagnosis of coronary artery disease. Am Heart J 1990;120:1255–1266.

119a. Van Train KF, Maddahi J, Areeda J, Cooke CD, Kiat H, Silagan G, Folks R, Friedman J, Matzer L, Germano G, Bateman T, Ziffer J, DePuey EG, Fink-Bennett D, Cloninger K, Berman DS: Multicenter trial validation for quantitative analysis of same-day rest-stress technetium-99m-sestamibi myocardial tomograms. J Nucl Med 1994;35:609–618.

120. Narahara KA, Villanueva-Meyer J, Thompson CJ, Brizendine M, Mena I: Comparison of thallium-201 and technetium-99m hexakis 2-methoxyisobutyl isonitrile single-photon emission computed tomography for estimating the extent of myocardial ischemia and infarction in coronary artery disease. Am J Cardiol 1990;66:1438–1444.

121. Maublant JC, Marcaggi X, Lusson JR, Boire JY, Cauvin JC, Jacob P, Veyre A, Cassagnes J: Comparison between thallium-201 and technetium-99m methoxyisobutyl isonitrile defect size in single-photon emission computed tomography at rest, exercise and redistribution in coronary artery disease. Am J Cardiol 1992;69:183–187.

122. Cuocolo A, Pace L, Ricciardelli B, Chiariello M, Trimarco B, Salvatore M: Identification of viable myocardium in patients with

chronic coronary artery disease: Comparison of thallium-201 scintigraphy with reinjection and technetium-99m-methoxyisobutyl isonitrile. J Nucl Med 1992;33:505–511.

123. Franceschi M, Guimond J, Zimmerman RE, Picard MV, English RJ, Carvalho PA, Tumeh SS, Holman BL: Myocardial clearance of Tc-99m hexakis-2-methoxy-2-methylpropyl isonitrile (MIBI) in patients with coronary artery disease. Clin Nucl Med 1990;15:307–312.

124. Taillefer R, Primeau M, Costi P, Lambert R, Leveille J, Latour: Technetium-99m-sestamibi myocardial perfusion imaging in detection of coronary artery disease: Comparison between initial (1-hour) and delayed (3-hour) postexercise images. J Nucl Med 1991;32:1961–1965.

125. Sinusas A, Bergin JD, Edwards NC, Watson DD, Ruiz M, Makuch RW, Smith WH, Beller GA: Redistribution of ^{99m}Tc-sestamibi and ^{201}Tl in the presence of a severe coronary artery stenosis. Circulation 1994;89:2332–2341.

125a. Berman DS, Kiat H, Friedman JD, Wang FP, Van Train K, Matzer L, Maddahi J, Germano G: Separate acquisition rest thallium-201/technetium-99m sestamibi dual-isotope myocardial perfusion single-photon emission computed tomography. A clinical validation study. J Am Coll Cardiol 1993;22:1455–1464.

125b. Heo J, Wolmer I, Kegel J, Iskandrian AS: Sequential dual-isotope SPECT imaging with thallium-201 and technetium-99m-sestamibi. J Nucl Med 1994;35:549–553.

125c. Kiat H, Germano G, Friedman J, Van Train K, Silagan G, Wang FP, Maddahi J, Berman D: Comparative feasibility of separate or simultaneous rest thallium-201/stress technetium-99m-sestamibi dual-isotope myocardial perfusion SPECT. J Nucl Med 1994;35:542–548.

126. Verzijlbergen JF, Suttorp MJ, Ascoop CA, Zwinderman AH, Niemeyer MG, van der Wall EE, Pauwels EK: Combined assessment of technetium-99m SESTAMIBI planar myocardial perfusion images at rest and during exercise with rest/exercise left ventricular wall motion studies evaluated from gated myocardial perfusion studies. Am Heart J 1992;123:59–68.

126a. Najm YC, Timmis AD, Maisey MN, Ellam SV, Mistry R, Curry PV, Sowton E: The evaluation of ventricular function using gated myocardial imaging with Tc-99m MIBI. Eur Heart J 1989;10:142–148.

127. Mannting F, Morgan-Mannting MG: Gated SPECT with technetium-99m-sestamibi for assessment of myocardial perfusion abnormalities. J Nucl Med 1993;34:601–608.

128. Wackers F, Mattera J, Bowman L, Zaret B: Gated Tc-99-isonitrile myocardial perfusion imaging: Disparity between endo-, epicardial wall motion. Circulation 1987;76(S4):203–207.

128a. Tischler MD, Niggel JB, Battle RW, Fairbank JT, Brown KA: Validation of global and segmented left ventricular contractile function using gated planar technetium-99m sestamibi myocardial perfusion imaging. J Am Coll Cardiol 1994;23:141–145.

128b. DePuey EG, Nichols K, Dobrinsky C: Left ventricular ejection fraction assessed from gated technetium-99m sestamibi SPECT. J Nucl Med 1993;34:1871–1876.

129. Marcassa C, Marzullo P, Parodi O, Sambuceti G, L'Abbate A: A new method for noninvasive quantitation of segmental myocardial wall thickening using technetium-99m 2-methoxy-isobutyl-isonitrile scintigraphy—results in normal subjects. J Nucl Med 1990;31:173–177.

130. Hassan IM, Mohammed MM, Constantinides C, Sadek S, Nair M, Belani N, Yousef AM, Abdel-Dayem HM: Segmental analysis of SPECT 99mTc-methoxy isobutyl isonitrile and 201Tl myocardial imaging in ischaemic heart disease. Eur J Nucl Med 1990;16:705–711.

131. Baillet GY, Mena IG, Kuperus JH, Robertson JM, French WJ: Simultaneous technetium-99m MIBI angiography and myocardial perfusion imaging. J Nucl Med 1989;30:38–44.

132. Boucher CA, Wackers FJ, Zaret BL, Mena IG: Technetium-99m sestamibi myocardial imaging at rest for assessment of myocardial infarction and first-pass ejection fraction. Multicenter Cardiolite Study Group. Am J Cardiol 1992;69:22–27.

133. Larock MP, Cantineau R, Legrand V, Kulbertus H, Rigo P: 99mTc-MIBI (RP-30) to define the extent of myocardial ischemia and evaluate ventricular function. Eur J Nucl Med 1990;16:223–230.

134. Villanueva-Meyer J, Mena I, Narahara KA: Simultaneous assessment of left ventricular wall motion and myocardial perfusion with

technetium-99m-methoxy isobutyl isonitrile at stress and rest in patients with angina: Comparison with thallium-201 SPECT. J Nucl Med 1990;31:457–463.

135. Borges-Neto S, Coleman RE, Potts JM, Jones RH: Combined exercise radionuclide angiocardiography and single photon emission computed tomography perfusion studies for assessment of coronary artery disease. Semin Nucl Med 1991;21:223–229.

135a. Williams KA, Taillon LA, Draho JM, Foisy MF: First-pass radionuclide angiographic studies of left ventricular function with technetium-99m-teboroxime, technetium-99m-sestamibi and technetium-99m-DTPA. J Nucl Med 1993;34:394–399.

135b. Nichols K, DePuey EG, Gooneratne N, Salensky H, Friedman M, Cochoff S: First-pass ventricular ejection fraction using a single-crystal nuclear camera. J Nucl Med 1994;35:1292–1300.

136. DePuey EG, Jones ME, Garcia EV: Evaluation of right ventricular regional perfusion with technetium-99m-sestamibi SPECT. J Nucl Med 1991;32:1199–1205.

137. Giubbini R, Galli M, Campini R, Bosimini E, Bencivelli W, Tavazzi L: Effects of mental stress on myocardial perfusion in patients with ischemic heart disease. Circulation 1991;83:II100–107.

137a. Johnson LL: Myocardial perfusion imaging with technetium-99m-teboroxime. J Nucl Med 1994;35:689–692.

138. Hendel RC, McSherry B, Karimeddini M, Leppo JA: Diagnostic value of a new myocardial perfusion agent, teboroxime (SQ 30,217), utilizing a rapid planar imaging protocol: Preliminary results. J Am Coll Cardiol 1990;16:855–861.

139. Seldin DW, Johnson LL, Blood DK, Muschel MJ, Smith KF, Wall RM, Cannon PJ: Myocardial perfusion imaging with technetium-99m SQ30217: Comparison with thallium-201 and coronary anatomy. J Nucl Med 1989;30:312–319.

140. Johnson LL: Clinical experience with technetium 99m teboroxime. Semin Nucl Med 1991;21:182–189.

141. Leppo JA, DePuey EG, Johnson LL: A review of cardiac imaging with sestamibi and teboroxime. J Nucl Med 1991;32:2012–2022.

142. Dahlberg ST, Weinstein H, Hendel RC, McSherry B, Leppo JA: Planar myocardial perfusion imaging with technetium-99m-teboroxime: Comparison by vascular territory with thallium-201 and coronary angiography. J Nucl Med 1992;33:1783–1788.

143. Iskandrian AS, Heo J, Nguyen T, Mercuro J: Myocardial imaging with Tc-99m teboroxime: Technique and initial results. Am Heart J 1991;121:889–894.

144. Fleming RM, Kirkeeide RL, Taegtmeyer H, Adyanthaya A, Cassidy DB, Goldstein RA: Comparison of technetium-99m teboroxime tomography with automated quantitative coronary arteriography and thallium-201 tomographic imaging. J Am Coll Cardiol 1991;17:1297–1302.

145. Serafini AN, Topchik S, Jimenez H, Friden A, Ganz WI, Sfakianakis GN: Clinical comparison of technetium-99m teboroxime and thallium-201 utilizing a continuous SPECT imaging protocol. J Nucl Med 1992;33:1304–1311.

146. Taillefer R, Lambert R, Essiambre R, Phaneuf DC, Leveille J: Comparison between thallium-201, technetium-99m-sestamibi and technetium-99m-teboroxime planar myocardial perfusion imaging in detection of coronary artery disease. J Nucl Med 1992;33:1091–1098.

146a. Weinstein H, Dahlberg ST, McSherry BA, Hendel RC, Cappo JA: Rapid redistribution of teboroxime. Am J Cardiol 1993;71:848–852.

146b. Bisi G, Sciagra R, Santoro GM, Zerauschek F, Fazzini PF: Sublingual isosorbide dinitrate to improve technetium-99m-teboroxime perfusion defect reversibility. J Nucl Med 1994;35:1274–1278.

147. Johnson LL, Rodney RA, Vaccarino RA, Egbe P, Wasserman L, Esser PD, Posniakoff TA, Seldin DW: Left ventricular perfusion and performance from a single radiopharmaceutical and one camera. J Nucl Med 1992;33:1411–1416.

147a. Jain D, Wackers F, Mattera J, Mcmahon M, Sinusas A, Zaret B: Biokinetics of technetium-99m-tetrofosmin: Myocardial perfusion imaging agent: Implications for a one-day imaging protocol. J Nucl Med 1993;34:1254–1259.

147b. Kelly JD, Forster AM, Higley B, Archer CM, Booker FS, Canning LR, Chiu KW, Edwards B, Gill HK, McPartlin M, et al.: Technetium-99m-tetrofosmin as a new radiopharmaceutical for myocardial perfusion imaging. J Nucl Med 1993;34:222–227.

147c. The Tetrofosmin Study Group: Comparative myocardial perfusion imaging with Tc-99m tetrofosmin and thallium-201: Results of phase III international trial (Abstract). Circulation 1992;86(I):506–506.

147d. Nakajima K, Taki J, Shuke N, Bunko H, Takata S, Hisada K: Myocardial perfusion imaging and dynamic analysis with the technetium-99m tetrofosmin. J Nucl Med 1993;34:1478–1484.

147e. Sridhara BS, Braat S, Rigo P, Itti R, Cload P, Lahiri A: Comparison of myocardial perfusion imaging with technetium-99m tetrofosmin versus thallium-201 in coronary artery disease. Am J Cardiol 1993;72:1015–1019.

147f. Sridhara B, Sochor H, Rigo P, Braat S, Itti R, Martinez-Duncker D, Cload P, Lahiri A: Myocardial single-photon emission computed tomographic imaging with technetium-99m-tetrofosmin: Stress-rest imaging with same-day and separate-day rest imaging. J Nucl Cardiol 1994;1:138–143.

147g. Takahashi N, Tamaki N, Tadamura E, et al: Combined assessment of regional perfusion and wall motion in patients with coronary artery disease with technetium-99m-tetrofosmin. J Nucl Cardiol 1994;1:29–38.

147h. Gerson MC, Lukes J, Deutsch E, Biniakiewicz D, Washburn LC, Elgazzar AH, Elder RC, Walsh RA: Comparison of technetium-99m-Q3 and thallium-201 for detection of coronary artery disease in humans. J Nucl Med 1994;35:580–586.

147i. Braat SH, Leclercq B, Itti R, Lahiri A, Sridhara B, Rigo P: Myocardial imaging with technetium-99m-tetrofosmin: Comparison of one-day and two-day protocols. J Nucl Med 1994;35:1581–1585.

148. Borer JS, Bacharach SL, Green MV, Hochreiter C, Wallis J, Holmes J: Assessment of ventricular function by radionuclide angiography: Applications and results. Cardiology 1984;71:136–161.

149. Borer JS, Bacharach SL, Green MV, Kent KM, Epstein SE, Johnston GS: Real-time radionuclide cineangiography in the noninvasive evaluation of global and regional left ventricular function at rest and during exercise in patients with coronary-artery disease. N Engl J Med 1977;296:839–844.

150. Borer J, Kant K, Bacharach S, Green M, Rosing D, Sedes S, Epstein S, Johnson G: Sensitivity, specificity and predictive accuracy of radionuclide cineangiography during exercise in patients with coronary artery disease. Comparison with exercise electrocardiography. Circulation 1979;60:572–580.

151. Gibbons RJ: Rest and exercise radionuclide angiography for diagnosis in chronic ischemic heart disease. Circulation 1991;84:I93–I99.

152. Jones RH, McEwan P, Newman GE, Port S, Rerych SK, Scholz PM, Upton MT, Peter CA, Austin EH, Leong KH, Gibbons RJ, Cobb FR, Coleman RE, Sabiston DC Jr: Accuracy of diagnosis of coronary artery disease by radionuclide management of left ventricular function during rest and exercise. Circulation 1981;64:586–601.

153. Campos CT, Chu HW, D'Agostino HJ Jr, Jones RH: Comparison of rest and exercise radionuclide angiocardiography and exercise treadmill testing for diagnosis of anatomically extensive coronary artery disease. Circulation 1983;67:1204–1210.

154. Port S, Cobb FR, Coleman RE, Jones RH: Effect of age on the response of the left ventricular ejection fraction to exercise. N Engl J Med 1980;303:1133–1137.

155. Gibbons RJ, Lee KL, Cobb F, Jones RH: Ejection fraction response to exercise in patients with chest pain and normal coronary arteriograms. Circulation 1981;64:952–957.

156. Marshall RC, Wisenberg G, Schelbert HR, Henze E: Effect of oral propranolol on rest, exercise and postexercise left ventricular performance in normal subjects and patients with coronary artery disease. Circulation 1981;63:572–583.

157. Higginbotham MB, Morris KG, Coleman RE, Cobb FR: Sex-related differences in the normal cardiac response to upright exercise. Circulation 1984;70:357–366.

158. Hanley PC, Zinsmeister AR, Clements IP, Bove AA, Brown ML, Gibbons RJ: Gender-related differences in cardiac response to supine exercise assessed by radionuclide angiography. J Am Coll Cardiol 1989;13:624–629.

159. Berger HJ, Reduto LA, Johnstone DE, Borkowski H, Sands JM, Cohen LS, Langou RA, Gottschalk A, Zaret BL, Pytlik L: Global and regional left ventricular response to bicycle exercise in coronary artery disease. Assessment by quantitative radionuclide angiocardiography. Am J Med 1979;66:13–21.

160. Jengo JA, Oren V, Conant R, Brizendine M, Nelson T, Uszler JM, Mena I: Effects of maximal exercise stress on left ventricular function in patients with coronary artery disease using first pass radionuclide angiocardiography: A rapid, noninvasive technique for determining ejection fraction and segmental wall motion. Circulation 1979;59:60–65.

161. Wieshammer S, Delagardelle C, Sigel HA, Henze E, Kress P, Bitter F, Lippert R, Seibold H, Adam WE, Stauch M: Limitations of radionuclide ventriculography in the non-invasive diagnosis of coronary artery disease. A correlation with right heart haemodynamic values during exercise. Br Heart J 1985;53:603–610.

162. Johnstone DE, Sands MJ, Berger HJ, Reduto LA, Lachman AS, Wackers FJ, Cohen LS, Gottschalk A, Zaret BL: Comparison of exercise radionuclide angiocardiography and thallium-201 myocardial perfusion imaging in coronary artery disease. Am J Cardiol 1980;45:1113–1119.

163. Jengo JA, Freeman R, Brizendine M, Mena I: Detection of coronary artery disease: Comparison of exercise stress radionuclide angiocardiography and thallium stress perfusion scanning. Am J Cardiol 1980;45:535–541.

164. Bodenheimer MM, Banka VS, Fooshee CM, Helfant RH: Comparative sensitivity of the exercise electrocardiogram, thallium imaging and stress radionuclide angiography to detect the presence and severity of coronary heart disease. Circulation 1979;60:1270–1278.

165. Caldwell JH, Hamilton GW, Sorenson SG, Ritchie JL, Williams DL, Kennedy JW: The detection of coronary artery disease with radionuclide techniques: A comparison of rest-exercise thallium imaging and ejection fraction response. Circulation 1980;61:610–619.

166. Brady TJ, Thrall JH, Lo K, Pitt B: The importance of adequate exercise in the detection of coronary heart disease by radionuclide ventriculography. J Nucl Med 1980;21:1125–1130.

167. Borer JS, Bacharach SL, Green MV, Kent KM, Johnston GS, Epstein SE: Effect of nitroglycerin on exercise-induced abnormalities of left ventricular regional function and ejection fraction in coronary artery disease. Assessment by radionuclide cineangiography in symptomatic and asymptomatic patients. Circulation 1978;57:314–320.

168. Cohn PF, Brown EJ Jr, Swinford R, Atkins HL: Effect of beta blockade on silent regional left ventricular wall motion abnormalities. Am J Cardiol 1986;57:521–526.

169. Gibbons R, Lee K, Pryor D, Harrell F, Coleman R, Cobb F, Rosati R, Jones R: The use of radionuclide angiography in the diagnosis of coronary artery disease—a logistic regression analysis. Circulation 1983;68:740–746.

170. Wasserman AG, Katz RJ, Varghese PJ, Leiboff RH, Bren GG, Schlesselman S, Varma VM, Reba RC, Ross AM: Exercise radionuclide ventriculographic responses in hypertensive patients with chest pain. N Engl J Med 1984;311:1276–1280.

171. Legrand V, Hodgson JM, Bates ER, Aueron FM, Mancini GB, Smith JS, Gross MD, Vogel RA: Abnormal coronary flow reserve and abnormal radionuclide exercise test results in patients with normal coronary angiograms. J Am Coll Cardiol 1985;6:1245–1253.

172. Kimchi A, Rozanski A, Fletcher C, Maddahi J, Swan HJ, Berman DS: Reversal of rest myocardial asynergy during exercise: A radionuclide scintigraphic study. J Am Coll Cardiol 1985;6:1004–1010.

173. Johnson LL, McCarthy DM, Sciacca RR, Cannon PJ: Right ventricular ejection fraction during exercise in patients with coronary artery disease. Circulation 1979;60:1284–1291.

173a. Port SC: Radionuclide angiography. Am J Cardiac Imaging 1994;8:240–248.

174. Quinones M: Exercise two-dimensional echocardiography. Echocardiography 1984;1:151–163.

175. Maurer G, Nanda NC: Two dimensional echocardiographic evaluation of exercise-induced left and right ventricular asynergy: Correlation with thallium scanning. Am J Cardiol 1981;48:720–727.

176. Limacher MC, Quinones MA, Poliner LR, Nelson JG, Winters WL Jr, Waggoner AD: Detection of coronary artery disease with exercise two-dimensional echocardiography. Description of a clinically applicable method and comparison with radionuclide ventriculography. Circulation 1983;67:1211–1218.

177. Armstrong W, O'Donnell J, Dillon J, Mchenry P, Morris S, Feigenbaum H: Complementary value of two-dimensional exercise echocardiography to routine treadmill testing. Ann Intern Med 1986;105:829–835.

178. Ryan T, Vasey CG, Presti CF, O'Donnell JA, Feigenbaum H, Armstrong WF: Exercise echocardiography: Detection of coronary artery disease in patients with normal left ventricular wall motion at rest. J Am Coll Cardiol 1988;11:993–999.

179. Sawada SG, Ryan T, Fineberg NS, Armstrong WF, Judson WE, McHenry PL, Feigenbaum H: Exercise echocardiographic detection of coronary artery disease in women. J Am Coll Cardiol 1989;14:1440–1447.

180. Heng MK, Simard M, Lake R, Udhoji VH: Exercise two-dimensional echocardiography for diagnosis of coronary artery disease. Am J Cardiol 1984;54:502–507.

181. Robertson WS, Feigenbaum H, Armstrong WF, Dillon JC, O'Donnell J, McHenry PW: Exercise echocardiography: A clinically practical addition in the evaluation of coronary artery disease. J Am Coll Cardiol 1983;2:1085–1091.

182. Armstrong WF, O'Donnell J, Dillon JC, McHenry PL, Morris SN, Feigenbaum H: Complementary value of two-dimensional exercise echocardiography to routine treadmill exercise testing. Ann Intern Med 1986;105:829–835.

183. Marwick TH, Nemec JJ, Pashkow FJ, Stewart WJ, Salcedo EE: Accuracy and limitations of exercise echocardiography in a routine clinical setting. J Am Coll Cardiol 1992;19:74–81.

184. Crouse LJ, Harbrecht JJ, Vacek JL, Rosamond TL, Kramer PH: Exercise echocardiography as a screen test for coronary artery disease and correlation with coronary arteriography. Am J Cardiol 1991;67:1213–1218.

185. Salustri A, Pozzoli MM, Reijs AE, Fioretti PM, Roelandt JR: Comparison of exercise echocardiography with myocardial perfusion scintigraphy for the diagnosis of coronary artery disease. Herz 1991;16:388–394.

186. Quinones MA, Verani MS, Haichin RM, Mahmarian JJ, Suarez J, Zoghbi WA: Exercise echocardiography versus 201T1 single-photon emission computed tomography in evaluation of coronary artery disease. Analysis of 292 patients. Circulation 1992;85:1026–1031.

187. Sheikh KH, Bengtson JR, Helmy S, Juarez C, Burgess R, Bashore TM, Kisslo J: Relation of quantitative coronary lesion measurements to the development of exercise-induced ischemia assessed by exercise echocardiography. J Am Coll Cardiol 1990;15:1043–1051.

187a. Hecht HS, DeBord L, Shaw R, Dunlap R, Ryan C, Stertzer SH, Myler RK: Digital supine bicycle stress echocardiography: A new technique for evaluating coronary artery disease. J Am Coll Cardiol 1993;21:950–956.

187b. Mertes H, Erbel R, Nixdorff U, Mohr-Kahaly S, Kruger S, Meyer J: Exercise echocardiography for the evaluation of patients after nonsurgical coronary artery revascularization. J Am Coll Cardiol 1993;21:1087–1093.

187c. Marangelli V, Iliceto S, Piccinni G, DeMartino G, Sorgente L, Rizzon P: Detection of coronary artery disease by digital stress echocardiography: Comparison of exercise, transesophageal atrial pacing and dipyridamole echocardiography. J Am Coll Cardiol 1994;24:117–124.

188. Tamaki N, Yonekura Y, Senda M, Kureshi SA, Saji H, Kodama S, Konishi, Ban T, Kambara H, Kawai C, et al.: Myocardial positron computed tomography with 13N-ammonia at rest and during exercise. Eur J Nucl Med 1985;11:246–251.

Chapter 4

Radionuclide Assessment of Prognosis

One of the principal applications of noninvasive cardiologic techniques is to identify patients at high risk for future cardiac events. The rationale for the use of noninvasive methods that evaluate either myocardial perfusion or function for risk stratification is that physiologic or functional alterations may be more sensitive than knowledge of coronary anatomy alone in separating high- and low-risk subgroups of coronary artery disease (CAD) patients. Cerqueira and Ritchie[1] stated in an editorial, "Optimal management of patients with symptomatic CAD, either suspected in those with chest pain or confirmed in those who have had a myocardial infarction, requires accurate, safe, and inexpensive assessment of risk for subsequent adverse events or need for intervention." Before entering into a discussion of the role of radionuclide imaging for risk assessment, some background information regarding high-risk clinical, angiographic, and exercise stress test variables indicative of a poor prognosis is warranted. "Prognosis" is defined as "a prediction of the probable course and outcome of a disease." Accurate prognostication is an inherent element of clinical decision making. The selection of both diagnostic tests and subsequent therapeutic options in an individual patient is based on cumulative information that relates to prognosis. Table 4–1 lists the major determinants of prognosis in CAD. In broad terms, they are (1) the degree of left ventricular (LV) dysfunction, which is manifested by diminution in LV ejection fraction (LVEF) and the extent of regional wall motion abnormalities; (2) the extent of jeopardized myocardium and the number of significantly stenotic coronary arteries, which are manifested by indices reflecting extent and severity of ischemia and the extent of anatomic CAD, respectively; and (3) arrhythmogenicity, which is evidenced by complex ventricular ectopy, an abnormal signal-averaged electrocardiogram (ECG), and abnormal heart rate variability. The impact of the first two major determinants of prognosis is greater when associated with certain clinical and resting ECG variables. They include history of myocardial infarction (MI), advanced age, clinical signs of congestive heart failure, history of progressive angina, diabetes, resting ECG ST-T–wave abnormalities, hypertension with LV hypertrophy, peripheral vascular disease, and untreated hyperlipidemia. Figure 4–1 illustrates the interaction of these prognostic variables.

Much of our modern knowledge of the natural history of CAD and the identification of important prognostic variables comes from large institutional or multicenter databases

Table 4–1. **Major Determinants of Prognosis in Coronary Artery Disease**

Degree of LV dysfunction
  Depressed LVEF
  Multiple regional wall motion abnormalities
  Clinical congestive heart failure
Extent of myocardium at jeopardy
  Multivessel CAD
  Extensive zone of inducible ischemia
  Severe hypoperfusion or regional asynergy
Arrhythmogenicity
  Complex ventricular ectopy
  Abnormal signal-averaged ECG
  Abnormal heart rate variability

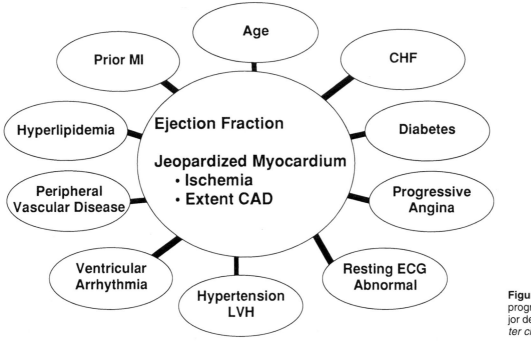

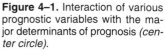

Figure 4–1. Interaction of various prognostic variables with the major determinants of prognosis *(center circle).*

established in the early 1970s.[2–5] From some of these large clinical trials and databases, we have learned that CAD patients with multivessel disease have a worse prognosis than patients with single-vessel disease, particularly when it is associated with LV dysfunction and inducible ischemia. Figure 4–2 lists the variables that were most predictive of survival in the 550 medically treated patients from the Seattle Heart Watch database.[2] As shown, LVEF was the best predictor of survival, followed by age, number of vessels with more than 70% stenosis, and ventricular arrhythmias on the rest ECG. Data from Duke University[3] also demonstrated that the worse the left ventricular function and the greater the extent of CAD, the lower was the survival rate (Fig. 4–3). In a survival analysis from the 7-year Duke follow-up study, more than 50% of patients with three-vessel CAD who were treated medically were still alive after 7 years' follow-up. The challenge of noninvasive

cardiology is to identify those high-risk three-vessel–disease patients destined for premature death if treated only with medical therapy and to intervene early with revascularization. Patients with three-vessel disease who succumb while receiving medical therapy surely have more myocardium at jeopardy than those who survive despite angiographic evidence of disease of similar extent observed at cardiac catheterization.

Two hypotheses can be proposed that form the basis of the physiologic approach to risk assessment in CAD. The first is that patients with multivessel CAD and a normal or depressed EF enjoy a survival benefit from coronary bypass surgery because viable but jeopardized myocardium is revascularized. This reduces the probability of fatal ischemic arrhythmias and development of irreversible myocardial damage. The greater the depression of LVEF, the greater the advantage of surgery versus medical therapy.[6] The second hypothesis is that patients with multivessel CAD and significant myocardium at jeopardy can be identified noninvasively by assessment of LV function at rest and extent and severity of inducible ischemia during stress. Patients with multivessel disease and normal LV function are at increased risk of future events and are benefited by coronary bypass surgery if inducible ischemia is elicited. The greater the extent and severity of the ischemia that is provoked, the greater is the risk of subsequent cardiac events. A lower incidence of events on medical therapy, and thus less benefit from revascularization, would be expected if there were minimal inducible ischemia or none, even though angiography might demonstrate multivessel CAD. Earlier studies addressing this issue employed exercise electrocardiography as the sole means of detecting ischemia in populations of patients with CAD. Rahimtoola[7] has pro-

Cox Regression for Survival

n = 550 Medically Treated Patients

Variables	χ^2
Ejection fraction	48.54
Age	17.16
# vessels with ≥70% stenoses	7.36
Ventricular arrhythmias	4.46

Figure 4–2. Variables most predictive of survival in 550 medically treated patients from the Seattle Heart Watch database. (Adapted from Hammermeister KE, et al.: Circulation 1979;59:421–430.)

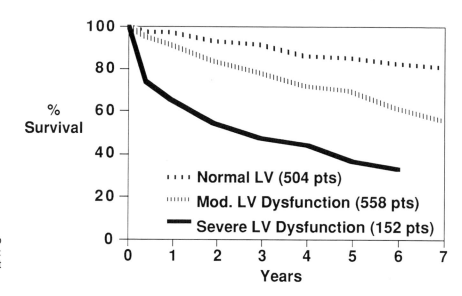

Figure 4–3. Percent survival during follow-up related to extent of LV dysfunction. (Key: Mod., moderate.) (Adapted from Harris PJ, et al.: Circulation 1979;60:1259–1269.)

posed that, for any given amount of apparent CAD and status of LV function, patient subgroups range from those at low risk to those at high risk. The major determinant of their status within the range is the presence or absence of ischemia. Not only is the qualitative presence or absence of ischemia important, but so is the extent of myocardium that is at risk.

The interaction between extent of CAD, status of LV function, and presence or absence of ischemia for determining prognosis is illustrated by analysis of the Coronary Artery Surgery Study (CASS) nonrandomized patient data bank.[8] A cohort of 1249 nonrandomized patients with three-vessel CAD from the CASS registry who underwent exercise testing as well as cardiac catheterization was studied. Among patients with normal LV function, those with at least 1 mm of ischemic ST depression or low exercise capacity had better 7-year survival when treated by surgical rather than medical therapy. Survival was not different between the medical and surgical groups of three-vessel–disease patients without ischemic ST depression with good exercise capacity. For patients with poor LV function and three-vessel disease, coronary bypass surgery was not associated with improved survival in those who were able to achieve an exercise level of stage III or greater with absence of ischemic ST depression. Thus, physiologic assessment of exercise capacity and ischemic potential were able to separate high- and low-risk subsets, whereas mere delineation of coronary anatomic disease and degree of LV dysfunction could not.

The European Coronary Surgery Study examined the relationship between survival and the magnitude of exertional ST-segment depression.[9] As shown in Figure 4–4, there was no significant difference between surgical and medical therapy in patients who showed no more than 1 mm of ST-segment depression on exercise testing. In contrast, surgery conferred significant survival benefit for patients who exhibited more than 1.5 mm of ST-segment

depression. Thus, without demonstrable objective evidence of significant ischemia, revascularization did not enhance survival.

EXERCISE ELECTROCARDIOGRAPHIC STRESS TESTING FOR RISK STRATIFICATION

As discussed briefly in the previous section, exercise ECG stress testing without radionuclide imaging has been shown to be useful for identifying high-risk patients with CAD who have severe, functionally important underlying CAD.[10] Table 4–2 lists the high-risk exercise test variables associated with an increased cardiac event rate and more severe underlying anatomic CAD. Patients with at least 2.0 mm of ST-segment depression, particularly when it is manifested at a low exercise heart rate or workload, have a higher incidence of left main and three-vessel disease than patients with lesser degrees of ST-segment depression.[11] Patients who are unable to exercise to stage III of the Bruce protocol have a higher annual mortality rate on follow-up than patients who can exceed this exercise level.[12] Similarly, patients who are unable to achieve greater than 4 metabolic equivalents (METs) are at higher risk for subsequent cardiac events than those who can exceed this workload. Normally, the systolic blood pressure increases with

Table 4–2. **High-Risk Exercise ECG Stress Test Variables**

ST depression >2.0 mm
ST depression at low exercise heart rate or light workload
ST depression lasting >5 minutes into recovery
Little change in heart rate from rest to exercise
Abnormal exercise blood pressure response
Achieved <4 METs workload
Exercise-induced ventricular ectopy

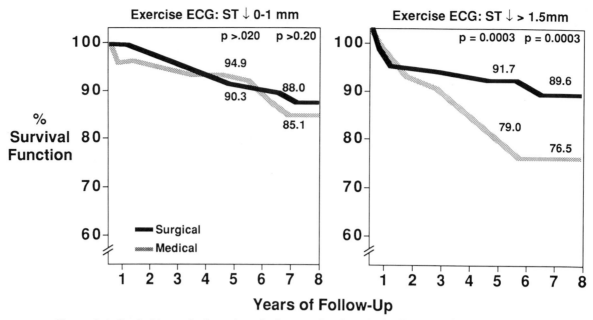

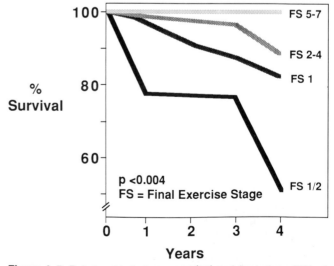

Figure 4–4. Survival in medically and surgically treated patients in the European Coronary Surgery study. **Left.** Survival with the exercise ECG demonstrating ST depression (↓) of no more than 1 mm. **Right.** Medical and surgical survival for patients demonstrating more than 1.5 mm of ST depression. (European Coronary Study Group: Lancet 1982;2:1173–1180 © by The Lancet Ltd. 1982.)

exercise because of the increased cardiac output with maintenance of stroke volume under normal physiologic conditions. Exercise-induced mechanical dysfunction resulting in impaired systolic contraction due to ischemia results in failure to increase the systolic blood pressure by at least 10 mm Hg or may actually cause exercise hypotension. A fall in systolic blood pressure of 10 mm Hg or more during exercise has been shown to be predictive of left main or three-vessel CAD.[13] Finally, the demonstration of complex ventricular ectopy at peak exercise is associated with increased risk of subsequent cardiac events.[14]

Exercise capacity is, perhaps, a more important prognostic variable than ST-segment changes for separating high- and low-risk subgroups of patients with the same anatomic classification. As shown in Figure 4–5, Wiener and coworkers[14a] reported that, in a group of 572 patients with three-vessel disease and relatively preserved LV function in the CASS registry, the probability of survival at 4 years ranged from 53% for patients who were able to achieve only stage ½ of exercise to 100% for patients who could exercise into the final stages 5 to 7. In that study, the final exercise stage was the most important exercise test predictor of outcome and ranked third after congestive heart failure and history of MI as predictors of survival. The ST-segment response ranked considerably lower.

Peak exercise heart rate, alone, is related to survival. McNeer et al.,[15] in their catheterized subgroup of patients with documented CAD, showed that patients who achieved a heart rate of 120 bpm or less on exercise testing had a significantly worse survival rate than patients whose heart rate reached 120 to 159 or exceeded 160 bpm (Fig. 4–6).

Based on their earlier observations, the Duke group developed a treadmill score derived from the duration of exercise, the maximal ST-segment deviation, and the treadmill angina index.[16] The treadmill score provided additive prognostic information to the readily obtainable clinical data (Fig. 4–7). The treadmill score was actually a stronger prognostic factor by itself than all of the available clinical variables, including history of MI, congestive heart failure, and age. Sixty-two percent of outpatients in this study had

Figure 4–5. Relationship between survival and final stage (FS) of exercise in patients with angiographic three-vessel disease and relatively preserved left ventricular function. (Reprinted with permission from the American College of Cardiology (Journal of the American College of Cardiology, 1984, Vol. 3, pp. 772–779).)

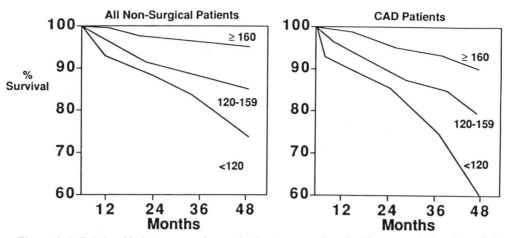

Figure 4–6. Relationship between peak exercise heart rate and survival in nonsurgical patients *(left panel)* and patients with documented coronary artery disease (CAD) *(right panel)*. Note that with peak exercise heart rate values less than 120/min, survival with medical therapy is significantly reduced. (McNeer JF, et al.: Circulation 1978;57:64–70.)

a low-risk treadmill score. For that group 4-year survival was 99%.

Morrow et al.[17] derived a prognostic score that also included a history of congestive heart failure and/or taking digoxin, in addition to the exercise test variables of ST depression, exercise capacity in METs, and the exercise blood pressure response. A simple score based on these four factors stratified approximately 2500 male patients from low risk (less than 1% annual cardiac death rate) to high risk (annual mortality rate 7%).

Thus, exercise ECG stress testing alone provides useful prognostic information on patients with suspected or documented CAD. Marked ST-segment depression of more than 2.0 mm at a low exercise workload or heart rate identifies high-risk patients with functionally significant left main or multivessel CAD.

MYOCARDIAL PERFUSION IMAGING FOR RISK STRATIFICATION

Rationale for Myocardial Perfusion Imaging for Prognostication

Myocardial perfusion imaging is increasingly being utilized in conjunction with treadmill exercise ECG stress testing to identify patients with suspected or known CAD who are at increased risk for future cardiac events.[18–19a] In addition to enhancing the diagnostic accuracy of conventional exercise ECG stress testing, myocardial perfusion imaging provides information about the extent and severity of stress-induced ischemia, variables that are significant for short- and long-term prognosis. The demonstration of ischemia by either planar or single-photon emission computed tomogra-

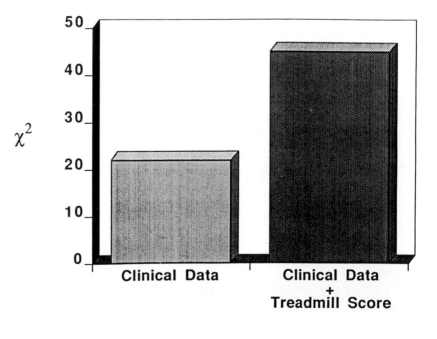

Figure 4–7. Additional prognostic value of treadmill score to readily obtainable clinical data. The Duke treadmill score is derived from the variables of duration of exercise, the maximal ST-segment deviation and the treadmill angina index. (Reprinted by permission of *The New England Journal of Medicine* from Mark DB, et al.: Prognostic value of a treadmill exercise score in outpatients with suspected coronary artery disease. N Engl J Med 325:849–853, Copyright 1991, Massachusetts Medical Society.)

phy (SPECT) perfusion imaging techniques are likely more important in the risk stratification process than the mere demonstration of the extent of coronary narrowings detected on angiography during cardiac catheterization. For example, patients with two-vessel disease and proximal left anterior descending (LAD) coronary stenosis who exhibit an ischemic response on testing survive longer if treated with revascularization than with medical therapy.[9] This is true whether LV dysfunction is present or not. Patients with two-vessel disease that includes a proximal LAD coronary stenosis are surely at greater risk for an adverse outcome than those whose two-vessel disease involves the right and left circumflex (LCx) coronary arteries. The exercise ECG alone cannot provide precise localization of ischemia, whereas exercise perfusion imaging can delineate the location of hypoperfused myocardial regions appropriate to the three major coronary vessels.

There are some potential advantages to myocardial perfusion imaging over exercise ECG stress testing alone for identifying high-risk CAD patients by noninvasive stress testing (Table 4–3). First, sensitivity for detection of ischemia by scintigraphic criteria may be increased by as much as 30% to 35% as compared with exercise ST depression in patients with underlying CAD (see Chap. 3).[18, 19a] This enhanced sensitivity is more evident in patients who fail to achieve at least 85% of maximum predicted heart rate for age during stress.[20] Suboptimal exercise heart rates may occur because of limiting noncardiac conditions, beta-blockade therapy, exercise-induced LV dysfunction producing dyspnea as an endpoint, poor motivation, or deconditioning.

Second, myocardial perfusion imaging is superior to exercise ECG stress testing alone for localization of myocardial regions that are rendered ischemic during stress. As mentioned above, this is an important feature of myocardial perfusion scintigraphy, since defects observed in the anterior wall and septum are almost always due to a coronary stenosis in the supply zone of the LAD coronary artery. Because prognosis in patients with two- or three-vessel disease is, in part, related to the existence of a proximal LAD coronary lesion, it would be important to identify such physiologically significant proximal stenoses by noninvasive means.

Third, multivessel ischemia can be well identified by

Table 4–3. Advantages of Exercise Myocardial Perfusion Imaging Over Exercise Electrocardiographic Testing for Prognosis

Greater sensitivity for detecting inducible ischemia
Better localization of site of ischemia
Better identification of multivessel ischemia
Better identification of ischemia in the supply zone of the left anterior descending coronary artery
Fewer nondiagnostic studies
Supplementary variables, such as increased lung Tl-201 uptake, can be utilized for risk assessment.

perfusion imaging techniques, as compared with ECG stress test findings alone. If defects are observed simultaneously in the inferior wall and in the anteroseptal regions, hypoperfusion most likely developed in the risk areas of the right and LAD coronary vessels. The prognosis is worse for a multivessel perfusion scan defect pattern is than for perfusion defects localized to a perfusion zone of only one of the three major coronary vessels.[21–26a] As will be discussed subsequently, the greater the number of segments that show perfusion abnormalities, the worse the prognosis with medical therapy. If those segments span more than one coronary supply region, the prognosis may be even worse.

Another important role of myocardial perfusion imaging for risk stratification is the ability to detect ischemia within a zone of MI or scar (see Chap. 6). Peri-infarction ischemia is demonstrated more easily with perfusion imaging than with exercise ECG. Resting ST-T–wave abnormalities in association with Q waves on the baseline resting ECG may preclude accurate interpretation of exercise ST-segment responses. Patients with resting ST-T abnormalities have more extensive hypoperfusion on exercise Tl-201 scintigraphy than patients without these resting ECG abnormalities.[27] Figure 4–8 summarizes these findings by Taylor et al.[27] Only 28% of patients with resting ST-T abnormalities had a normal scan, as compared with 60% of patients without resting ST-T abnormalities who had a normal scan. The prevalence of redistribution defects was higher in those with resting ECG abnormalities. Such patients could not adequately be risk stratified by ECG testing alone.

Thallium-201 Scintigraphic Variables Associated with High Risk

Thallium-201 (Tl-201) scintigraphy has been the predominant myocardial perfusion imaging technique applied for risk stratification. Table 4–4 lists the high-risk Tl-201 scintigraphic variables that have been shown to identify patients at increased risk for subsequent cardiac events. On the initial postexercise images, high-risk scan findings include multiple Tl-201 defects and/or washout abnormalities in one or more coronary supply regions, increased lung Tl-201 uptake that can be quantitated by measuring the lung-heart ratio,[25] and exercise-induced cardiac dilatation, with the LV cavity size appearing larger on the initial image than on the subsequent delayed image.[28, 28a] Presence of redistribution compared to solely persistent defects is also indicative of a higher risk of an adverse outcome.

Increased Lung Thallium-201 Uptake

Increased lung Tl-201 uptake on the initial postexercise image is a reflection of stress-induced LV dysfunction with consequent pulmonary interstitial edema.[29, 30] The LV dysfunction results from myocardial ischemia causing both di-

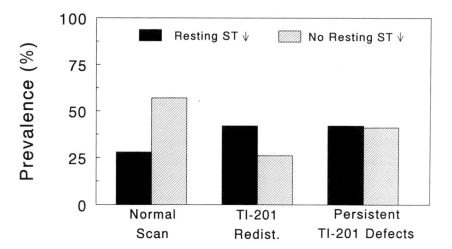

Figure 4–8. Comparison of patients with and without resting ST-segment depression with respect to exercise Tl-201 scintigraphic results. (Data from Taylor AJ, Beller GA: Am J Cardiol 1994;74:211–215.)

astolic and systolic dysfunction. This results in a sudden elevation of the LV filling pressure, which is transmitted to the pulmonary capillaries resulting in transient transudation of plasma into the lung parenchyma. When exercise ceases and ischemia resolves with a subsequent drop in the LV end-diastolic pressure, there is a movement of this interstitial fluid back to the pulmonary blood compartment. Figure 4–9 shows stress and delayed Tl-201 images in a patient with increased lung Tl-201 uptake.

Boucher et al.[29] determined the clinical significance of increased lung Tl-201 activity after exercise stress in 227 patients who also underwent cardiac catheterization. Increased lung activity was related to (1) a greater number of myocardial segmental Tl-201 defects and (2) increased severity and extent of CAD. A marked increase in lung Tl-201 activity was associated with a greater prevalence of prior myocardial infarction and a lower angiographic EF at rest. Supine stress Tl-201 imaging was performed during cardiac catheterization in a subgroup of 12 patients in that study. Five patients with increased lung Tl-201 activity had a mean pulmonary capillary wedge pressure that increased during exercise from 12 ± 1 to 24 ± 3 mm Hg without an associated increase in cardiac index. In contrast, the remaining seven patients who did not demonstrate increased lung Tl-201 uptake showed a rise in cardiac index during exercise but no associated alteration in the pulmonary capillary wedge pressure (rest, 10 ± 3 mm Hg; stress, 12 ± 2 mm Hg).

Ilmer et al.[31] assessed the relationships between the lung-heart Tl-201 ratio and the extent of ischemia on SPECT Tl-201 scintigrams and the extent of CAD on angiography. They showed that the lung-heart ratio was not significantly

different between patients with and without ischemia during exercise or between patients with single- and those with multivessel disease. In contrast, Kurata et al.[32] found that patients with increased lung-heart Tl-201 ratios had more

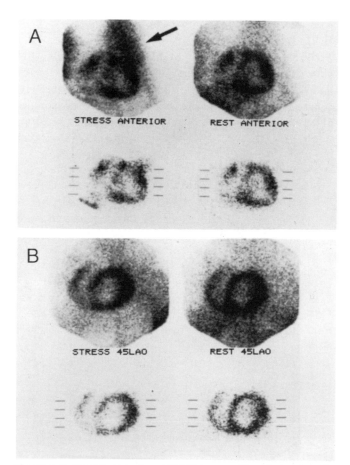

Figure 4–9. Poststress and rest Tl-201 images (**A,** anterior view; **B,** 45-degree left anterior oblique view) in a patient with increased lung Tl-201 uptake on the stress anterior projection image *(arrow)*. Increased lung Tl-201 uptake is reflective of exercise-induced pulmonary edema and indicative of high-risk coronary artery disease. The background-subtracted images are shown below the unprocessed images. Note the anterolateral, apical, and septal redistribution defects.

Table 4–4. **Tl-201 Scintigraphic Variables Associated with High-Risk Coronary Artery Disease**

Multiple defects and/or washout abnormalities
Multivessel disease scan pattern
Increased lung Tl-201 uptake
Transient ischemic LV cavity dilatation

multivessel disease, more severe LV dysfunction, and more Tl-201 defects than patients with normal ratios. Those patients with markedly increased lung-heart ratios had three-vessel disease more frequently than those with slight or moderate increases in ratios (67% vs. 14% and 35%, respectively; Fig. 4–10). These authors concluded that measurement of the lung/heart ratio provided useful information on the severity of CAD.

Homma et al.[33] sought to determine which of 23 clinical, exercise, Tl-201, and angiographic variables best discriminated between patients with an increased lung-heart ratio and those with a normal ratio. These authors found that the number of diseased vessels on coronary angiography was the best discriminator. Double product at peak exercise, number of segments with abnormal wall motion, patient gender, and duration of exercise were also significant discriminators. Table 4–5 summarizes the results of stepwise discriminant function analysis for identification of the variables that best correlated with an increased lung-heart ratio of Tl-201 in this study.

Kushner et al.[34] found that patients with multivessel disease had increased lung Tl-201 uptake, whereas patients with single-vessel disease did not differ significantly from controls. Patients with an abnormal lung-heart ratio in that study had significantly reduced resting EFs as compared with patients with CAD and normal lung Tl-201 uptake. Patients with four or five of a total of six abnormal segments on the initial Tl-201 exercise scans had a higher prevalence of abnormal lung Tl-201 uptake than CAD patients with one or no abnormal segments on the initial postexercise scans. Thus, the finding of elevated lung Tl-201 activity on exercise images correlated with increased severity of underlying CAD and degree of LV dysfunction.

Lahiri et al.[35] also reported a consistent increase in lung

Table 4–5. Stepwise Discriminant Function Analysis of the Correlates of an Increased Lung-Heart Tl-201 Ratio (>0.51)

Variable	F Value	P Value
Number of diseased vessels	47.99	<0.001
Peak double product	19.34	<0.001
Number of scan segments with normal wall motion	8.80	<0.01
Patient gender	7.19	<0.01
Exercise duration	5.77	<0.01

(Reprinted by permission of the Society of Nuclear Medicine from: Homma S, et al.: Correlates of lung/heart ratio of thallium-201 in coronary artery disease. J Nucl Med 1987; 28:1531–1535.)

Tl-201 uptake with the number of diseased coronary arteries. Patients with a history of MI had greater pulmonary Tl-201 activity than patients without infarction, and patients with ST-segment elevation on exercise had more pulmonary Tl-201 uptake than those with ST-segment depression or with no ST-segment shifts during stress. Increased lung Tl-201 can be observed on rest Tl-201 images after acute myocardial infarction.[36] This finding correlates with a greater number of perfusion defects, a lower LVEF, higher peak creatine kinase values, more extensive regional wall motion abnormalities, and an increased incidence of clinical in-hospital congestive heart failure. By stepwise discriminant function analysis, Jain et al.[36] found that congestive heart failure was the most important determinant and Tl-201 defect score the most important correlate of abnormal lung Tl-201 uptake. Thus, it is not surprising that increased lung Tl-201 activity is a potent predictor in CAD patients. It is a synthesis of multiple other variables well known to be associated with an adverse outcome and an increased incidence of future cardiac events. The most important determinants of lung Tl-201 uptake in this regard are multivessel CAD, depressed LV function, and extent of ischemia.

Detection of Left Main Coronary Artery Disease

Patients with a significant stenosis (at least 50%) of the left main coronary artery survive significantly longer when treated with surgery than with medical therapy.[37] Thus, one principal goal of noninvasive testing in patients with known or suspected CAD (e.g., chest pain) is to identify patients with a critical stenosis of the left main trunk. Several clinical studies have sought to determine whether or not patients with left main CAD could be identified by stress perfusion variables, which could supplement the ECG stress test findings. Figure 4–11 summarizes the Tl-201 scintigraphic patterns in 43 patients with left main CAD (at least 50% stenosis) reported by Nygaard et al.[38] First, 95% of patients with left main CAD had an abnormal scan (at least one perfusion abnormality). Sixty-seven percent of patients with left main disease had a multivessel CAD scan pattern, with defects demonstrated in multiple coronary supply zones.

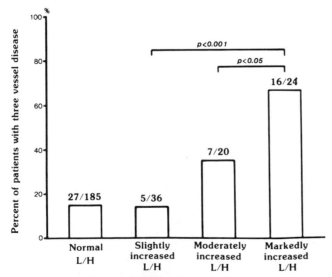

Figure 4–10. Percent of patients with three-vessel disease among normal, slightly increased, moderately increased, and markedly increased lung-heart (L/H) ratios in 265 patients with coronary artery disease. (Reprinted by permission of the Society of Nuclear Medicine from: Kurata C, et al.: J Nucl Med 1991;32:417–423.)

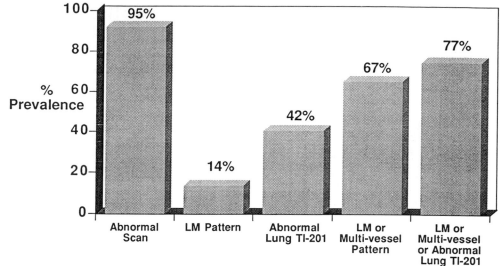

Figure 4–11. Prevalence of various scintigraphic variables in 43 patients with at least 50% stenosis of the left main coronary artery who underwent symptom-limited exercise Tl-201 stress testing. A left main (LM) scan pattern was defined as a uniform decrease in Tl-201 uptake in septal and posterolateral scan segments on the 45-degree left anterior oblique projection. A multivessel disease pattern is defined as perfusion defects in more than one coronary vascular supply region. (Reprinted from American Journal of Cardiology: 53:4; February 1, 1984; 462–469.)

Also, 42% of these patients had abnormal lung Tl-201 uptake. Seventy-seven percent of patients with left main CAD had either a multivessel scan pattern or abnormal lung Tl-201 uptake. In this study, only 14% of patients with left main CAD had what would be described as a "typical" left main Tl-201 scan pattern (see Fig. 4–11). That is, few patients with left main CAD had a homogeneous diminution in Tl-201 uptake in the middle and upper septum and the middle and upper posterolateral wall, the supply zones of the LAD and LCx vessels, respectively. One explanation for the low incidence of this typical left main scan pattern is that only 7% of the left main CAD patients in this study had an isolated stenosis confined to the left main trunk. Fourteen percent had associated single-vessel disease, 39.5% had two-vessel disease, and the remaining 39.5% had associated three-vessel disease. The high prevalence of

left main and multivessel CAD accounts for the more heterogeneous defect patterns that are more consistent with multivessel disease than with disease isolated to the left main coronary artery. Figure 4–12 shows the prevalence of a left main scan pattern, multivessel disease, pattern and increased lung Tl-201 uptake in patients with left main, three-vessel, two-vessel, and one-vessel CAD in this study.

In the Nygaard study,[38] a high-risk ECG stress test was defined as one that had at least two of the following characteristics: (1) at least 2.0 mm of ST depression; (2) horizontal or downward sloping (more than 1.0 mm) ST depression persisting 5 minutes or longer after exercise; (3) appearance of ST depression within 5 minutes of exercise; and (4) a decrease in systolic blood pressure of 10 mm Hg or more during exercise. The prevalence of a high-risk ECG stress test was 58% in patients with left main CAD, signif-

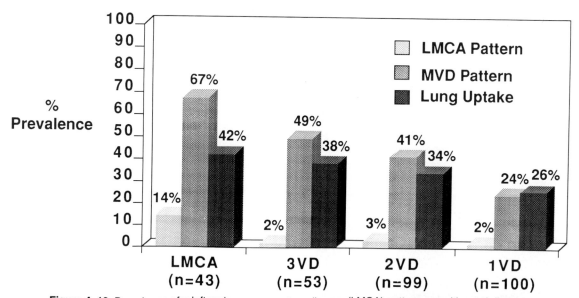

Figure 4–12. Prevalence of a left main coronary artery disease (LMCA) pattern, a multivessel disease (MVD) pattern and increased lung Tl-201 uptake in patients with angiographic LMCA, three-vessel disease (3VD), 2VD, and 1VD. (Reprinted from American Journal of Cardiology: 53:4; February 1, 1984; 462–469.)

icantly lower than the prevalence of a high-risk Tl-201 scintigram. The combination of the Tl-201 scintigraphic and exercise ECG stress variables was no better than scintigraphic variables alone (86% vs. 77%) in detecting high-risk CAD but did improve the overall detection rate as compared with exercise ECG testing alone (86% vs. 58%, P = 0.04). A high-risk scintigram (left main and/or multivessel disease pattern and/or increased lung Tl-201 uptake) was seen in 58% of patients with three-vessel disease, 60% of patients with two-vessel disease, and 41% of patients with one-vessel disease. This prevalence was significantly higher than the prevalence of a high-risk ECG stress test (defined as the presence of at least 2 variables) in the three angiographic subsets, which was 32%, 31%, and 16%, respectively, for three-vessel, two-vessel, and one-vessel disease.

Rehn et al.[39] also found that the prevalence of a "left main scan pattern" was infrequent (13%) in patients with left main CAD and was also seen in 33% of patients with combined LAD and LCx disease. They concluded that the perfusion defect pattern observed in patients with left main CAD was more determined by the location and severity of associated significant coronary stenoses downstream from the left main lesion.

Detection of Multivessel Coronary Artery Disease

In addition to detection of high-grade left main CAD, myocardial perfusion imaging can be used to distinguish patients with a high probability of angiographic multivessel CAD from patients with angiographic single-vessel disease. Figures 4–13 and 4–14 are examples of multivessel disease scan patterns. Defects can be observed in more than one coronary supply region in both of these examples. Multivariate analysis performed in a cohort of 383 consecutive patients who underwent exercise Tl-201 scintigraphy and coronary angiography reported by Pollock et al.[40] revealed that only age, ST depression and number of Tl-201 defects were independent predictors of multivessel disease. A joint effect of these three variables was demonstrated (Figure 4–15). The observed rate of angiographic multivessel disease increases as the number of initial Tl-201 defects increases, regardless of age or the presence of ST-segment depression. The lowest rate of multivessel disease (less than 5%) was seen in patients younger than 58 years with no initial Tl-201 defects and no ST depression. The highest rate of multivessel disease (more than 80%) was noted in patients older than 58 years who had more than one postexercise Tl-201 defect and associated stress-induced ischemic ST-segment depression. Christian et al.[41] determined the ability to predict left main or three-vessel disease employing SPECT Tl-201 imaging in 688 patients who underwent both exercise Tl-201 scintigraphy and coronary angiography. The magnitude of exercise-induced ST depression, the

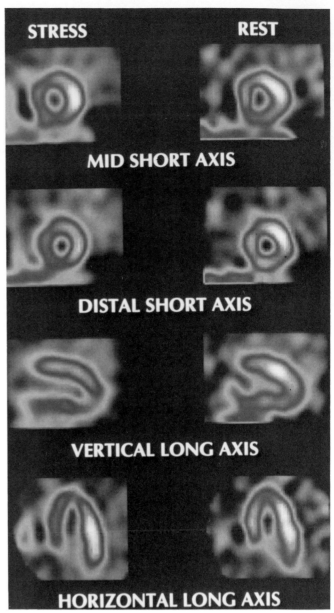

See Color Figure 4–13.

Figure 4–13. Example of a high-risk SPECT myocardial perfusion scan in a patient who underwent exercise sestamibi imaging for evaluation of chest pain. The exercise images are shown on the left and rest images on the right. Representative short-axis tomograms demonstrate reversible anteroseptal and inferior defects. The vertical long-axis tomogram reveals a partially reversible inferior defect and a persistent apical defect. Increased activity is also seen in the anterior wall when comparing rest and stress images. The horizontal long-axis image reveals a reversible septal defect and a persistent apical defect. These scintigraphic findings are consistent with LAD and right CAD. (See Color Figure 4–13.)

number of abnormal short-axis Tl-201 scan segments, the presence or absence of diabetes mellitus, and the change in systolic blood pressure with exercise were identified as the variables that were independently predictive of left main or three-vessel disease (Table 4–6). Thus, these studies, utilizing either planar or SPECT imaging techniques, are consistent in showing that the combination of multiple Tl-201

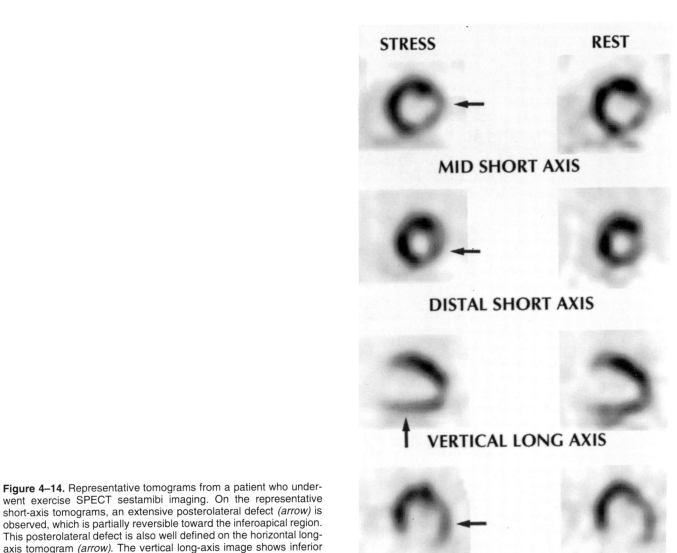

STRESS   REST

MID SHORT AXIS

DISTAL SHORT AXIS

VERTICAL LONG AXIS

HORIZONTAL LONG AXIS

Figure 4–14. Representative tomograms from a patient who underwent exercise SPECT sestamibi imaging. On the representative short-axis tomograms, an extensive posterolateral defect *(arrow)* is observed, which is partially reversible toward the inferoapical region. This posterolateral defect is also well defined on the horizontal long-axis tomogram *(arrow)*. The vertical long-axis image shows inferior *(arrow)* and apical defects with partial reversibility in the inferoapical region. These findings are consistent with a stenosis in a dominant left circumflex coronary artery or disease in both right and left circumflex vessels. The LV cavity also appears dilated.

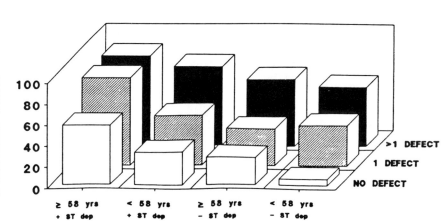

Figure 4–15. Combined effect of age over 58 years, ischemic ST-segment depression (+ST dep) and numbers of Tl-201 defects on the prevalence of angiographic multivessel CAD in 383 consecutive patients who underwent exercise Tl-201 scintigraphy in coronary angiography. Note that the highest prevalence of multivessel CAD is in patients aged 58 years and older who have ST depression and more than one Tl-201 defect (bar in upper left corner). (Pollock SG, et al.: Am J Med 1991;90:345–352.)

Table 4–6. Variables Independently Predictive of Three-Vessel or Left Main Coronary Artery Disease in 688 Patients Undergoing SPECT Tl-201 Imaging and Coronary Angiography

Variable	χ^2	P Value
Magnitude of ST depression	16.6	<0.0001
Number of abnormal Tl-201 segments	17.5	<0.0001
Diabetes	11.0	0.0009
Peak minus resting blood pressure	14.7	0.0001

(From Christian TF, et al.: Noninvasive identification of severe coronary artery disease using exercise thallium-201 imaging. Am J Cardiol 1992; 70:14–20.)

defects that span at the vascular supply zones of at least two of the major coronary arteries and ST depression is predictive of high-risk coronary anatomic disease.

Iskandrian et al.[41a] found only three variables that were independent predictors of left main or three-vessel CAD in 834 patients by stepwise descriminant analysis of clinical, exercise, and Tl-201 SPECT scintigraphic data. These included multivessel Tl-201 scan abnormality ($P < 0.001$), exercise heart rate ($P < 0.001$), and ST-segment depression ($P < 0.01$). The Tl-201 data were far more powerful for prognostication than the clinical or treadmill exercise data.

Transient Left Ventricular Cavity Dilatation

Transient dilatation of the LV cavity when the initial postexercise and delayed images are compared is another marker of high-risk CAD. Figure 4–16 shows an example of a patient with marked LV cavity dilatation on the postexercise image, which then improves on the image obtained several hours later. Weiss et al.[28] found that abnormal transient dilatation of the left ventricle was 60% sensitive and 95% specific for identifying patients with multivessel stenosis and was more specific than other known markers of high-risk CAD such as multiple perfusion defects, washout abnormalities, or both. Transient dilatation of the left ventricle was not observed in the group of patients with "noncritical" CAD (defined as no more than 50% to 89% stenosis). Figure 4–17 shows the relation between degree of transient LV dilatation measured by dividing the computer-derived LV area of the immediate postexercise anterior image by the area of the 4-hour redistribution image, and the extent and severity of CAD in this study. As shown, patients with three-vessel disease and at least 90% stenosis had significantly higher transient dilatation ratios than the group with one-vessel disease or the group with mild CAD. At present, inspection of serial scintigrams for detection of transient dilatation of the left ventricle involves viewing the anterior projection image. The enlarged LV cavity size on the poststress images may reflect diffuse subendocardial flow diminution rather than an acute increase in LV volume secondary to stress-induced LV dysfunction. Since both lung Tl-201 activity and LV cavity size are derived from the anterior planar image, this planar projection should be obtained before acquisition of SPECT perfusion images.

SPECT imaging appears to be more sensitive than planar imaging for detecting individual coronary stenosis (see Chap. 3), particularly LCx lesions or branch lesions (see Chap. 3). Defect size on SPECT images better reflects the extent of hypoperfusion than planar imaging because of absence of overlapping myocardial segments. Despite better defect contrast with SPECT imaging and improved resolution of small defects, the anterior view planar image should initially be acquired to evaluate pulmonary Tl-201 activity and LV cavity size. These scintigraphic variables supplement the evaluation of defect extent and severity for separation of high- and low-risk subsets of CAD patients. A quantitative index relating Tl-201 activity in the LV cavity to that in the myocardium (C-M ratio) on exercise scans was found to correlate linearly with the ejection fraction ($r = 0.65$).[28a] A C-M exercise ratio of no more than 0.40 identified 26 of 31 patients whose EF was not more than 50%.

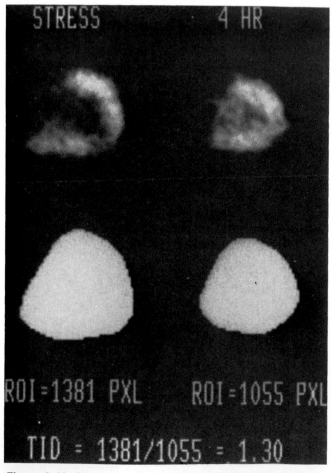

Figure 4–16. Example of transient ischemic left ventricular cavity dilatation from the exercise *(left image)* to the resting *(right image)* scintigram. Below the anterior view images are the computer display used for calculation of a transient dilatation ratio. The example is from a patient with three-vessel CAD. (Reprinted with permission from the American College of Cardiology (Journal of the American College of Cardiology, 1987, Vol. 9, pp. 752–759).)

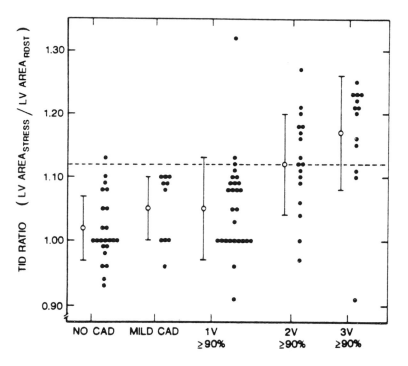

Figure 4–17. Relation between the transient dilatation ratio (TID) and the presence and extent and severity of CAD. Mean ±1 SD values are shown to the left of the individual values in each group. The horizontal line represents the upper limit of normal for the TID. (Key: LV, left ventricular; RDST, redistribution; 1V, 2V, 3V, one-, two-, and three-vessel disease; ≥90%, ≥90% coronary stenosis.) (Reprinted with permission from the American College of Cardiology (Journal of the American College of Cardiology, 1987, Vol. 9, pp. 752–759).)

Exercise Thallium-201 Scintigraphy and Prediction of Future Cardiac Events

Studies of Short-Term Follow-Up

Since multiple perfusion defects of the redistribution type, increased lung Tl-201 uptake, and transient LV cavity dilatation are markers of high risk for CAD, it would stand to reason that demonstration of one or more of these scintigraphic variables should be associated with an increased subsequent cardiac event rate in medically treated patients. Many studies in the literature have investigated the prognostic utility of exercise Tl-201 scintigraphy in patients with chest pain who are referred for noninvasive evaluation.[21–26a, 42–52d] A discussion of the prognostic value of exercise Tl-201 imaging in postinfarction patients is found in Chapter 6.

One of the first published studies evaluating the prognostic utility of exercise Tl-201 scintigraphy, by Brown et al.,[21] showed that the number of Tl-201 redistribution defects was the best predictor of future cardiac events as determined by logistic regression analysis in CAD patients without prior infarction (Table 4–7). Although the number of vessels with significant stenoses was a univariate predictor of cardiac events, it added no significant prognostic value to the extent of hypoperfused myocardium, as judged from the Tl-201 study. Also, data from the exercise ECG stress test did not provide additive prognostic information to the imaging data. In a similar study from Cedars-Sinai Medical Center in Los Angeles,[22] stepwise logistic regression analysis identified the number of myocardial regions with redistribution defects, the maximum magnitude of hypoperfusion, and the exercise heart rate as the only independent

predictors of future cardiac events in 1689 patients with CAD and no history of MI. Figure 4–18 shows the relation between cardiac event rate and number of reversible Tl-201 defects in this patient cohort. Note the dramatic rise in event rate with more than three reversible defects on scintigraphic analysis.

In another report from Cedars-Sinai, by Staniloff et al.,[48] as the magnitude of hypoperfusion increased, so did the event rate ($P = 0.0001$). The probability of an event also increased with the number of abnormal vascular scan territories. By combining results of the exercise test and Tl-201 scan, a risk ratio of 20.5:1 was observed using discriminate function analysis.

Iskandrian et al. also found that the number of myocardial scan segments with abnormal perfusion (redistribution or persistent type) was the single best predictor of future cardiac events.[23] Both extent and severity of hypoperfusion were correlated exponentially with event rate. In a subsequent study by Iskandrian et al.,[43] the presence of redistri-

Table 4–7. Predictors of Cardiac Death or Nonfatal Myocardial Infarction in 100 Patients with No History of Infarction

Predictor	χ^2	P Value
Number of redistribution defects	6.66	<0.01
Total number of defects	4.83	<0.05
Number of diseased vessels on angiography	3.57	<0.10
Left ventricular ejection fraction	0.86	NS
Number of persistent defects	0.03	NS
Abnormal exercise ECG	0.01	NS

Key: NS, not significant.
(Reprinted with permission from the American College of Cardiology (Journal of the American College of Cardiology, 1983, Vol. 1, pp. 994–1001).)

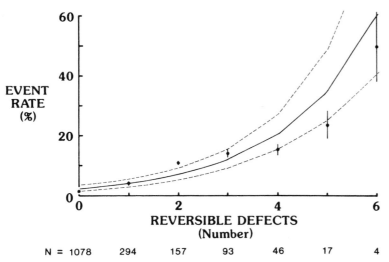

Figure 4–18. Relation between coronary event rate (cardiac death, nonfatal infarction, or coronary bypass surgery more than 60 days after testing) in patients with symptoms suggestive of CAD with no prior infarction versus the number of reversible defects. The reversibility of defects is exponentially related to the event rate ($r=0.97$, $P<0.001$). (Reprinted with permission from the American College of Cardiology (Journal of the American College of Cardiology, 1986, Vol. 7, pp. 464–471).)

bution Tl-201 defects, extent of perfusion abnormalities, and perfusion defects in a multivessel distribution each had significant univariate predictive power for cardiovascular death or nonfatal infarction. In this cohort of patients, whose mean age was 65 years, multivariate analysis identified abnormal Tl-201 images and a multivessel Tl-201 scan abnormality as independent predictors of events. The risk of a cardiac event was less than 1% for patients with normal images, 5% for patients with a one-vessel Tl-201 abnormality, and 13% for patients with multivessel Tl-201 abnormality (Mantel-Cox, $P < 0.0001$). One limitation of this particular study is that there were only eight deaths during follow-up, and more than half of the events were nonfatal infarctions ($N = 10$). Hilton et al.[44] assessed the prognostic value of exercise Tl-201 scintigraphy in patients at least 70 years of age who were followed for a mean of 36 ± 12 months after testing. Multivariate stepwise logistic regression analysis identified the combination of peak exercise at or below stage 1 and any Tl-201 perfusion defect as the most powerful predictor of subsequent cardiac events (relative risk, 5.3 at 1 year). Patients with a normal scan had a 2% cardiac event rate, as compared with 18% ($P = 0.004$) for those who had a fixed or redistribution defect. There were only six cardiac deaths in this study and one nonfatal infarction. Nevertheless, the findings of this study and the previous one by Iskandrian et al. show that exercise Tl-201 scintigraphy is useful for assessing prognosis in elderly patients with known or suspected CAD.

Bairey et al.[50] performed a retrospective analysis of the prognostic utility of exercise-induced Tl-201 redistribution. Tl-201 scintigraphy was performed in 190 patients who had a history of typical angina but a negative exercise ECG stress test. Findings were compared with a second group of 203 patients with typical angina who had a positive exercise ECG characterized by ischemic ST-segment depression. In patients with a negative exercise ECG but an abnormal Tl-201 scan, the subsequent cardiac event rate was increased threefold over that for patients with a negative exercise

ECG and a normal scan. Multivariate analysis revealed that an abnormal Tl-201 test result was the only significant correlate of future cardiac events. Petretta et al.[50b] confirmed the observation that among patients with nondiagnostic ECG stress tests, the cardiac event rate is higher in those with abnormal Tl-201 scintigraphic results. Both extent and severity of hypoperfusion or Tl-201 scintigraphy were significantly related to outcome. These studies point out that useful prognostic information is derived from Tl-201 scintigraphic data even when the exercise ECG stress test is within normal limits.

Long-Term Follow-Up Prognostic Studies

With respect to the University of Virginia experience, Kaul et al.[24] reported a follow-up study of 382 patients who underwent exercise ECG stress testing, exercise Tl-201 scintigraphy, and coronary arteriography. Eighty-three patients who had bypass surgery within 3 months of testing were excluded from further analysis. Of the remaining 299 patients, 210 had no events and 89 had events (41 deaths, 9 nonfatal infarctions, and 39 late coronary bypass procedures after 3 months) during follow-up. When all clinical, exercise, scintigraphic, and catheterization variables were analyzed by Cox regression analysis, the number of diseased vessels was the single most important predictor of subsequent events (Table 4–8). When the number of diseased vessels was excluded from analysis, the number of segments with Tl-201 redistribution became the single best predictor of future events. Other variables independently predicting future events in this cohort included the change in heart rate from rest to exercise, exercise-induced ST depression, and ventricular ectopy recorded during stress. Although the number of diseased vessels was the single most important determinant of future events ($\chi^2 = 38.1$), the combination of scintigraphic and exercise test variables when considered as a whole was equally powerful ($\chi^2 = 41.6$). Combination of both catheterization and exercise Tl-

Table 4–8. **Cox Regression Analysis of Clinical, Exercise, Tl-201, and Catheterization Variables**

Variables Selected	χ^2	P Value
All variables used		
Number stenoses ≥50%	38.1	<0.001
Number of diseased vessels excluded		
Number of Tl-201 redistribution segments	16.3	<0.0001
Change in heart rate	10.3	0.01
ST depression on exercise	9.1	0.003
Exercise arrhythmias	4.9	0.026

(From Kaul S, et al.: Prognostic utility of the exercise thallium-201 test in ambulatory patients with chest pain: A comparison with cardiac catheterization. Circulation 1988; 77:745–758.)

201 scintigraphic data was superior to either alone ($\chi^2 = 57$) for predicting future events.

The study by Kaul et al.[24] also revealed that patients with redistribution anywhere on their exercise scintigram had a significantly higher rate of cardiac events during follow-up than patients without redistribution (Fig. 4–19). Separation of high- and low-risk subgroups was better achieved when Tl-201 redistribution was used as a marker of ischemia than when ST-segment depression was used. Thus, these data show that information derived from coronary angiography and from noninvasive exercise Tl-201 scintigraphy are complementary in identifying patients at high risk for CAD. As expected, Tl-201 scan variables were more powerful predictors of events than were exercise ECG stress test variables considered alone. These findings confirm those of Brown et al.,[21] Ladenheim et al.,[22] and Iskandrian et al.,[23] in that the number of redistribution defects reflecting the extent of myocardium at risk is a powerful predictor of subsequent events, particularly when observed in association with ST-segment depression and an inadequate exercise heart rate during exercise.

The data from the study by Kaul et al.[24] were reanalyzed by Pollock et al.[51] to assess the incremental prognostic value of information obtained in succession (clinical, exercise ECG stress testing, Tl-201 scintigraphy, and coronary angiography) in patients suspected to have CAD. Both univariate and multivariate Cox regression analyses were performed to assess the individual and incremental prognostic value of the tests.[51] Patients who underwent coronary artery bypass surgery later than 3 months after testing were censored at the time of these events. That is, follow-up was stopped with the surgical procedure, which was considered an endpoint. The use of beta blockers was the only significant clinical predictor of cardiac events. Patients treated with beta blockers had nearly double the risk of those who did not take these medications, after adjustment was made for age, history of infarction, and type of chest pain. A suboptimal heart rate response during exercise stress was associated with a worse prognosis. A patient whose heart rate rose 20 bpm less than an otherwise similar patient had a nearly twofold risk of an event. The inability to exercise for a longer time was a significant predictor of events on univariate analysis but not on multivariate analysis. Neither ST-segment depression nor an abnormal systolic blood pressure response (fall or failure to rise during exercise) was a predictor of events.

In the earlier analysis, the number of segments that exhibited redistribution was the best Tl-201 predictor of hard cardiac events.[24] Pollock et al.[51] further showed in this patient population that a two-segment difference in the number of redistributing segments increased the risk of an event more than twofold. The number of diseased coronary arteries was also a significant predictor of events. A twofold increase in the event rate was noted for each additional diseased artery.

The incremental prognostic value of tests performed in a

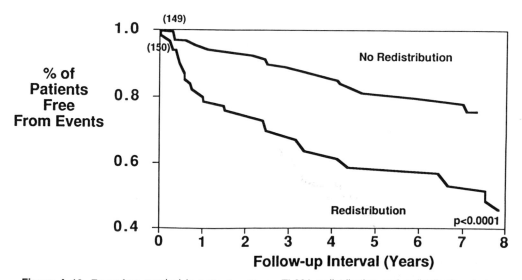

Figure 4–19. Event-free survival in patients with no Tl-201 redistribution and redistribution during follow-up while receiving medical therapy. (Kaul S, et al.: Circulation 1988;77:745–758.)

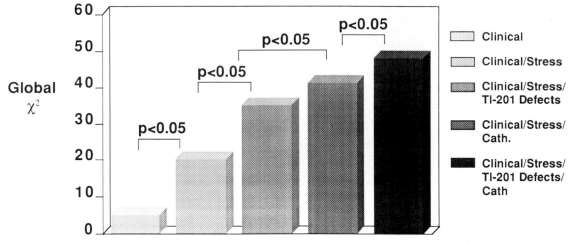

Figure 4–20. Incremental prognostic value of tests performed in a hierarchic order. Note significant incremental value when stress test variables (stress) are added to clinical information (clinical) and further increased prognostic information when the number of Tl-201 defects is added to clinical and ECG stress test information. Prognostic information provided by a combination of clinical, ECG stress test, and cardiac catheterization (Cath.) variables is slightly but significantly greater than the prognostic information provided from the combination of clinical, ECG stress test, and scintigraphic variables. (Pollock SG, et al.: Circulation 1992;85:237–248.)

hierarchical order in the study by Pollock et al.[51] is illustrated in Figure 4–20. When the additional value of sequentially performed tests was analyzed, the exercise stress test data added significant prognostic information to clinical data. The inclusion of the number of segments that showed redistribution on Tl-201 scintigraphy improved the prognostic information beyond that provided by clinical and exercise stress data alone. Coronary angiography added significant prognostic value to that obtained from the combination of clinical, exercise stress tests, and Tl-201 data; however, more than 80% of the prognostic information was already obtained from the clinical data, stress tests data, and number of Tl-201 redistribution segments. One limitation of this study was that lung Tl-201 uptake by quantitative derivation of the lung-heart ratio was not assessed as a prognostic variable.

Several follow-up studies in patients with CAD who underwent exercise Tl-201 scintigraphy have indicated that abnormal lung Tl-201 uptake is perhaps a better predictor than the number of redistribution defects.[25, 42] Gill et al. determined the value of pulmonary Tl-201 uptake as a prognostic variable as evaluated in 525 consecutive patients referred for exercise testing.[42] Cardiac events were monitored in these patients over a 5-year period after testing. Of the 105 cardiac events experienced in the 467 patients that were followed up, there were 25 deaths, 33 nonfatal infarctions, and 47 coronary bypass surgical procedures. Table 4–9 summarizes the significant univariate predictors of future cardiac events in this study. Cox regression analysis identified increased Tl-201 uptake as the best predictor of a cardiac event (relative risk ratio, 3.5). The next most powerful predictors were a history of typical angina, history of myocardial infarction, and ST-segment depression during

exercise. One limitation of this study was that coronary angiography was not performed in all patients, and the prognostic value of increased lung Tl-201 uptake relative to the number of stenotic arteries was not examined.

In a subsequent study from the Massachusetts General Hospital reported by Kaul et al.,[25] in which only patients who underwent Tl-201 scintigraphy and coronary angiography were evaluated, a lung-heart ratio of Tl-201 uptake of at least 0.52 was found to be the single best predictor of subsequent cardiac events (Table 4–10). A total of 293 patients followed from 4 to 9 years were included. Interestingly, 17 of the 20 patients who died during follow-up had an abnormal lung-heart Tl-201 ratio. Figure 4–21 shows the survival curves for patients with a normal or increased lung-heart ratio in this study. Note that the curves are significantly different: the chance of event-free survival was significantly worse for the group whose lung-heart Tl-201 ratio was abnormal. Although the number of diseased coronary vessels by angiography was a significant univariate

Table 4–9. Univariate Predictors of Cardiac Events in 467 Patients Undergoing Exercise Tl-201 Scintigraphy

Variables	χ^2	P Value
Increased lung Tl-201	73.5	0.0001
Number of initial defects	52.1	0.0001
Tl-201 redistribution	41.7	0.0001
Number of redistribution defects	41.5	0.0001
Typical angina	36.2	0.0001
Exercise duration	35.4	0.0001

(Reprinted by permission of *The New England Journal of Medicine* from Gill JB, et al.: Prognostic importance of thallium uptake by the lung during exercise in coronary artery disease. N Engl J Med 317:1486–1489, copyright 1987, Massachusetts Medical Society.)

Table 4–10. **Results of Cox Regression Analysis for Cardiac Events Versus No Events**

All Variables Used	χ^2	*P* Value
Lung-heart Tl-201 ratio	40.21	<0.0001
Number of diseased vessels	17.11	<0.0001
Patient gender	9.43	0.002
Change in heart rate from rest to exercise	4.19	0.04

(Reprinted with permission from the American College of Cardiology (Journal of the American College of Cardiology, 1988, Vol. 12, pp. 25–34).)

predictor of events, it did not add to the overall ability of the exercise perfusion scan to predict future events. In this study, patients with a history of infarction suffered an event more than twice as often as those without such a history, after adjusting for age. A suboptimal heart rate response during exercise stress was also associated with a worse prognosis. A patient whose heart rate rose 20 bpm less than an otherwise similar patient had a 30% excess risk of an event.

In this study from the Massachusetts General Hospital,[25] the lung-heart Tl-201 ratio superseded the other variables by multivariate analysis. A difference in this ratio of 0.15 translated into a greater than twofold increase in the risk for events. As expected, when this ratio was excluded from analysis, the number of segments that demonstrated Tl-201 redistribution emerged as the most powerful scintigraphic predictor of events. Tl-201 imaging improved the prognostic information beyond that provided by clinical and exercise stress test data alone. The information from coronary angiography did not provide additive prognostic information to the combined information obtained from the clinical, exercise stress test, and Tl-201 imaging data when the lung-heart Tl-201 ratio was included in the analysis (Fig. 4–22). Of interest, the combination of clinical, exercise stress test, and coronary angiographic variables was not more prog-

nostically powerful than the combination of clinical, exercise stress test, and lung-heart Tl-201 ratio variables. Thus, knowledge of extent of angiographic CAD did not add incremental prognostic information to that derived from the clinical, stress test, and lung-heart ratio data. When the lung-heart ratio was excluded from analysis and the number of segments with Tl-201 redistribution was used instead, coronary angiography did provide some additional prognostic information to that available from clinical, stress test, and Tl-201 data. In that respect, the findings of the Massachusetts General Hospital study[25] and the University of Virginia study[24] are comparable.

Travin et al[25a] reviewed the exercise Tl-201 test results of 268 patients from the Massachusetts General Hospital who had unequivocal Tl-201 redistribution on exercise scintigraphy. At a follow-up of 25 $\pm$ 19 months, occurrence of MI was most closely related to the extent and severity of ischemia by Tl-201 scintigraphy ($P = 0.0086$), whereas cardiac death was associated with abnormal lung Tl-201 uptake ($P = 0.0082$) and an inability to exercise to 9.6 METs ($P = 0.0144$). These data suggest that cardiac death is best predicted by variables that reflect poor LV function and that nonfatal infarction is best predicted by variables indicative of ischemia.

All the studies cited in this section clearly demonstrate the powerful prognostic value of stress perfusion imaging. The extent of ischemia reflected by the number of reversible defects and exercise-induced LV dysfunction evidenced by an increased lung-heart ratio of Tl-201 uptake identifies a subgroup of CAD patients who would certainly benefit from revascularization as compared to medical therapy. Figure 4–23 depicts an example of a high-risk exercise planar Tl-201 perfusion scan showing both increased lung Tl-201 uptake and multiple defects in more than one coronary supply region. A patient with these scintigraphic findings often manifests three-vessel or left main CAD and should be referred for coronary angiography.

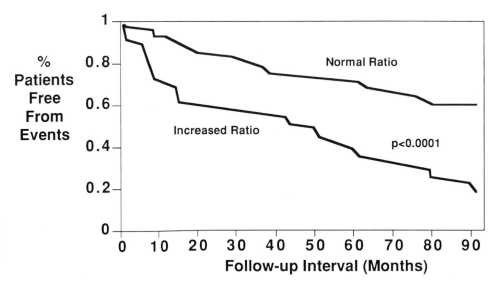

Figure 4–21. Event-free survival in patients with either a normal or an increased lung-heart ratio of Tl-201 activity. (Reprinted with permission from the American College of Cardiology (Journal of the American College of Cardiology, 1988, Vol. 12, pp. 25–34).)

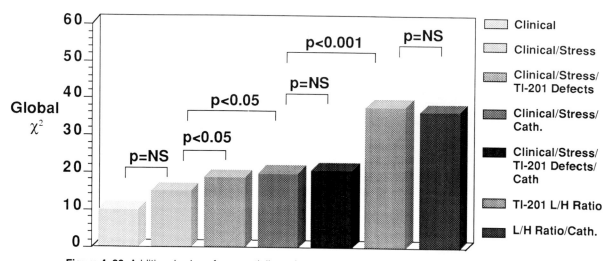

Figure 4–22. Additional value of sequentially performed tests. Exercise test (Stress) data in this cohort of patients did not add significant additional prognostic information to clinical data. When the lung-heart (L/H) TI-201 ratio was used in lieu of the number of segments with TI-201 redistribution (6th bar vs 3rd bar), the improvement in the prognostic information was greater than that afforded by the inclusion of the number of segments with redistribution in the University of Virginia cohort (see Fig. 4–20). Note that in this cohort from the Massachusetts General Hospital, information from coronary angiography (Cath.) did not add to the combined information from L/H ratio data (7th bar). (Pollock SG, et al.: Circulation 1992;85:237–248.)

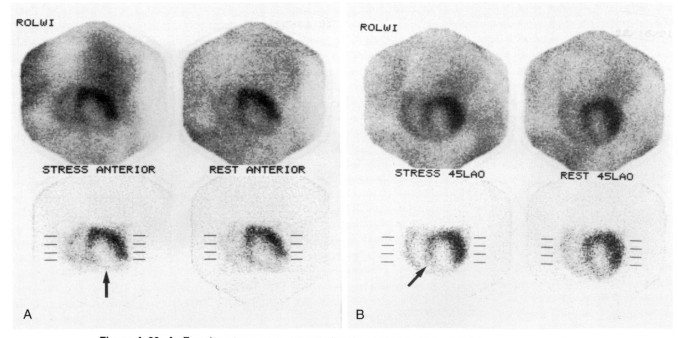

Figure 4–23. A. Exercise stress and rest anterior view images obtained 2.5 hours apart showing abnormal increase in lung TI-201 uptake as well as a severe inferior defect *(arrow)* with negligible delayed redistribution. The unprocessed images are shown on top and background-subtracted images on the bottom. **B.** Exercise stress and rest 45-degree left anterior oblique (LAO) images obtained in the same patient showing severe anteroseptal *(arrow)* and inferoapical defects with partial redistribution. This scintigraphic study is consistent with disease in the right and left anterior descending coronary arteries and exercise-induced left ventricular dysfunction characterized by lung pulmonary TI-201 uptake in pulmonary edema fluid.

Prognosis for Patients with Normal Thallium-201 Scintigrams

Several reports have indicated that patients who have chest pain but a normal myocardial exercise Tl-201 perfusion scan on symptom-limited exercise testing have an excellent prognosis during follow-up.[45, 47, 49–49d] In a study by Pamelia et al.,[49] the yearly mortality rate for 345 patients with chest pain and a normal quantitative planar myocardial Tl-201 perfusion scan was 0.5%. The nonfatal infarction rate was only 0.6% per year. Of interest in that study, 29% of the patients were unable to achieve 85% or more of maximal predicted heart rate adjusted for age, and 9% developed ischemic ST depression (at least 1.0 mm) during exercise. At the time of exercise testing, 45% of patients were taking nitrates and 38% were receiving beta-blocking drugs. Two of the five patients who died during follow-up had normal coronary arteries, as determined by angiography in one and at post mortem examination in the other. Thus, at most, three of the 345 patients with a normal Tl-201 perfusion scan who were followed died with underlying significant CAD. Another interesting finding in that study was that patients with chest pain and normal Tl-201 scintigrams who had a cardiac event were not predominantly males, nor did they have a higher prevalence of typical angina, exercise-induced ST depression, or inability to achieve 85% or more of maximal predicted heart rate normalized for age, than those who had no cardiac events. The conclusion of that study was that patients with chest pain and normal Tl-201 exercise scintigrams have a very low cardiac event rate during follow-up. The event rate is comparable to that reported for patients with chest pain and angiographically normal coronary arteries. Brown and Rowen[49a] studied 261 patients who had a normal exercise Tl-201 scan and were followed for 23 ± 6 months. Cardiac death or nonfatal infarction occurred in six patients, yielding a "hard" event rate of 1.2% per year, comparable to the findings of Pamelia et al.[49] Also, these investigators found no significant relationship between cardiac event rate and antiangina medication use, peak exercise heart rate, blood pressure, or exercise workload. Steinberg et al.[49b] found that a normal exercise Tl-201 scan retains its high negative predictive value for death at least 10 years after initial testing. Cardiac mortality was 1% at 10 years in 309 patients with a normal scan.

Wackers et al.[47] evaluated the outcome for 95 patients with unequivocally normal exercise Tl-201 scans by quantitative criteria. During a mean follow-up of 22 ± 3 months, no patient died and two had a nonfatal MI. One patient subsequently required coronary angioplasty. The Yale group extended these earlier observations in the investigation of the incidence of subsequent cardiac events in 236 consecutive patients who had a normal exercise Tl-201 scintigram but an abnormal exercise ECG.[52] Length of follow-up averaged 21 months and was available for 209 patients, of whom 80 (38%) had clinical evidence of CAD

demonstrated by angiography, enzyme-confirmed MI, or a history of typical angina. Cardiac events—defined as death, nonfatal infarction, unstable angina, subsequent bypass surgery, or angioplasty or hospitalization for any cardiac reason—occurred in 11% of the patients overall. Events occurred in 22.5% of patients with "clinical" CAD and 5.4% in those who did not previously have evidence of clinical CAD. Thus, patients with a normal exercise Tl-201 scintigram who have clinical evidence of CAD and an abnormal exercise ECG stress test probably should be evaluated further, since their risk of subsequent events is intermediate between those of patients with a normal Tl-201 scan and a normal exercise ECG and those of patients with an abnormal Tl-201 scintigraphic study and an abnormal exercise ECG. The latter group would represent the highest-risk subgroups of patients with known or suspected CAD.

Finally, Brown[52a] undertook a pooled analysis of studies published in the literature and found a 0.9% rate of cardiac death or nonfatal infarction in 3594 patients with normal Tl-201 scintigrams who were followed for an average of 29 months. Even patients with angiographic CAD and normal exercise Tl-201 studies have and excellent prognosis.[52c]

SPECT Thallium-201 Imaging and Prognosis

There are scant data in the literature on the prognostic value of SPECT Tl-201 imaging. Most of the studies cited in this chapter utilized planar Tl-201 scintigraphy for diagnostic and prognostic purposes. Nevertheless, there is no reason to think that SPECT imaging would not be even more sensitive than planar imaging for identifying high-risk patients with functionally important CAD. Compared with planar imaging, the SPECT technique is capable of identifying a greater number of stenotic vessels, with an enhanced detection rate of LCx stenoses (see Chap. 3). Similarly, the extent of hypoperfusion can be better evaluated using SPECT imaging than planar imaging because of the elimination of superimposition of various myocardial zones. Machecourt et al.[26a] followed 1926 patients who underwent stress SPECT Tl-201 imaging for 33 ± 10 (standard deviation) months. Exercise stress was performed in 1121 patients and 805 underwent dipyridamole infusion. The cardiac mortality rate was 0.42% per year in patients with a normal SPECT scan and 2.1% per year in those with an abnormal scan. There was a significant relation between the number of abnormal scan segments and cardiovascular mortality during follow-up ($P < 0.02$). The extent of the SPECT defect on the initial scan provided the best imaging variable for long-term prognosis. Iskandrian et al.[52b] examined the independent and incremental prognostic value of exercise SPECT Tl-201 imaging in patients with angiographic evidence of CAD. By Cox regression analysis of multiple variables in 316 medically treated patients (follow-up, 28 months), the extent of the perfusion abnormality was the single best predictor of prognosis ($\chi^2 = 4$). By univariate analysis, gender, exercise workload, extent of CAD,

Table 4–11. **Comparison of No Event and Event Groups with Respect to Univariate Analysis of Prognostic Variables**

Variables	No Event (N = 281)	Event (N = 35)	P Value
METs	7.4	6.3	0.05
LVEF (%)	61	53	0.07
Tl-201 variables			
Defect size (%)	16	25	0.0001
Number of abnormal segments	7.4	11	0.0005
Number of redistribution segments	4.9	7.8	0.006
Multivessel scan abnormality (%)	51	77	0.01
Left ventricular dilatation (%)	17	37	0.01

(Reprinted with permission from the American College of Cardiology (Journal of the American College of Cardiology, 1993, Vol. 22, pp. 665–670).)

and LVEF and Tl-201 variables were prognostically important (Table 4–11). The Tl-201 information provided incremental prognostic value to catheterization data ($\chi^2 = 33.7$; $P < 0.01$). The larger the perfusion abnormality, the worse was the prognosis. Figure 4–24 is a summary of these data showing the incremental prognostic value of SPECT Tl-201 imaging to clinical and exercise test variables. In another study by this group, exercise SPECT Tl-201 imaging was superior to the treadmill exercise score in risk assessment in medically treated patients with CAD.[52d]

Caution should be exercised in using the SPECT technique with respect to the specificity of correctly identifying patients with multivessel ischemia on stress imaging. Attenuation artifacts and variants of normal must also be well detected on SPECT scintigraphy to avoid "overreading"

the nuclear study in a particular patient.[53, 54] Relying solely on the quantitative polar maps (bull's-eye image) may result in an unacceptable false-positive rate—both for detecting CAD and for incorrectly designating patients at high risk. Image artifacts such as those due to attenuation or patient motion are incorporated in the polar map, and it is important to look at the raw images as well when rendering a final scan interpretation.

Summary

Taken together, the results of all of the prognostic studies cited above suggest that, even when cardiac catheterization findings are known, scintigraphic information obtained from stress myocardial perfusion imaging provides important supplementary physiologic information for identifying subgroups of patients with CAD who are at high risk. The extent of myocardial hypoperfusion reflected by the number of Tl-201 scan segments demonstrating initial defects with delayed redistribution, and the degree of exercise ischemic LV dysfunction reflected by abnormal lung Tl-201 uptake and LV cavity dilatation appeared to be important variables for predicting future cardiac events. Scintigraphic variables are more predictive of outcome than variables derived solely from exercise stress ECG. Similarly, scintigraphic variables have additional prognostic value to variables that can be identified from clinical evaluations such as history of myocardial infarction or beta-blocker use. Risk stratification using exercise perfusion imaging is as valuable in patients who are symptomatic as in those who are asymp-

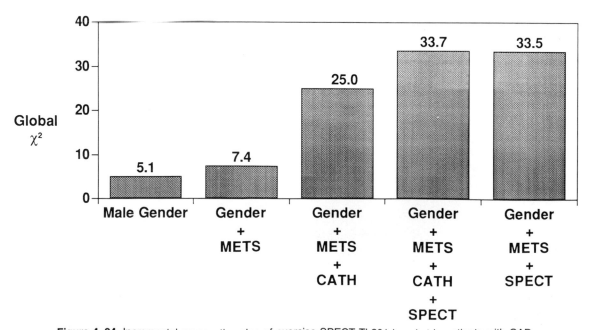

Figure 4–24. Incremental prognostic value of exercise SPECT Tl-201 imaging in patients with CAD. Note that the prognostic information provided by knowledge of patient gender, METs achieved at peak exercise, and SPECT Tl-201 variables was greater than the prognostic information provided by knowledge of gender, METs achieved, and catheterization variables. (Reprinted with permission from the American College of Cardiology (Journal of the American College of Cardiology, 1993, Vol. 22, pp. 665–670).)

tomatic while receiving medical therapy. Most patients who demonstrate high-risk Tl-201 scintigraphic variables have functionally important underlying multivessel CAD. Patients with multivessel disease and normal scans or only a single irreversible perfusion abnormality have a better prognosis than those with similar anatomic findings who demonstrate large areas of myocardium at risk, as evidenced by multiple defects, some showing redistribution, particularly when observed with increased lung Tl-201 uptake and limited exercise tolerance.

There are certainly limitations to the use of exercise Tl-201 scintigraphy for assessing prognosis and separating patients into high- and low-risk subsets. As with the diagnostic application of myocardial perfusion imaging, the prognostic value of this test is related to the quality of the nuclear cardiology laboratory performing the test and the skill and experience of the interpreters of images. Quantitation of both planar and SPECT Tl-201 scintigrams enhances the individual coronary stenosis detection rate (see Chap. 3). With quantitative planar imaging, regional washout abnormalities in association with perfusion defects elsewhere may be indicative of an ischemic response in another vascular territory. Identification of abnormal lung Tl-201 uptake is enhanced when the quantitative lung-heart ratio is employed. This is particularly true for the specificity of this finding, since certain patients with LV hypertrophy and no significant CAD may have visually increased lung Tl-201 uptake but a lung-heart ratio below 0.50. Specificity of detection of high-risk CAD may be a problem in situations where variants are normal and image artifacts are not well identified. For example, a patient with single-vessel LAD disease may have exercise-induced perfusion abnormalities localized to the anterior wall, apex, and septum. Such a patient may also have an inferior wall attenuation artifact because of a high-lying diaphragm. If this attenuation artifact is not correctly identified, the interpreter will report that the patient has an inferior wall perfusion defect and, thus, could have underlying multivessel CAD (LAD and right coronary artery narrowing). This may result in premature or unwarranted referral for coronary angiography.

Exercise Technetium-99m Sestamibi Scintigraphy and Prediction of Future Cardiac Events

SPECT exercise Tc-99m–sestamibi scintigraphy appears to provide useful prognostic information on patients with stable chest pain.[54a–54d] Of 521 patients followed for 13 ± 5 months after same-day "rest-stress" sestamibi perfusion studies, 11 had a nonfatal infarction and 11 experienced cardiac death.[54a] Multivariate analysis revealed that both exercise sestamibi perfusion abnormalities (RR = 11.9; 95% CI, 1.6 to 89.4) and reversible sestamibi defects (RR = 2.9; 95% CI, 1.2 to 7.0) had independent predictive value. During follow-up, cardiac events occurred in 0.5%

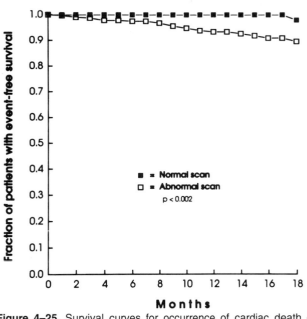

Figure 4–25. Survival curves for occurrence of cardiac death or nonfatal infarction in patients with normal and abnormal Tc-99m–sestamibi exercise SPECT studies. (Stratmann HG, et al.: Circulation 1994;89:615–622.)

of patients with abnormal scan and 7% of those with an abnormal scan. Event-free survival curves are shown in Figure 4–25. Patients with a normal stress Tc-99m sestamibi myocardial perfusion scan have an excellent prognosis, with a combined cardiac death and nonfatal infarction rate of 0.5% per year,[54b] which is similar to the event rate for patients with a normal stress Tl-201 perfusion scan. Figure 4–26 is an example of a patient with a high-risk exercise Tc-99m–sestamibi myocardial perfusion scan with inducible defects observed in the apex, septum, and inferior wall suggestive of multivessel CAD. A limitation of Tc-99m–sestamibi perfusion imaging for prognostication is the inability of using the amount of lung uptake of the tracer as a high-risk imaging variable. Saha et al.[54c] found that the lung-heart ratio of Tc-99m–sestamibi uptake on an anterior view image obtained with exercise stress had no relation to clinical, exercise stress test, hemodynamic, or perfusion variables. Also, the lung-heart ratio did not correlate with extent of resting echocardiographic wall motion abnormalities.

EXERCISE RADIONUCLIDE ANGIOGRAPHY FOR ASSESSING PROGNOSIS

Detection of High-Risk Coronary Artery Disease

The role and utility of exercise radionuclide angiography for detection of CAD is reviewed in Chapter 3. The functional severity of coronary artery stenoses and, thus, the

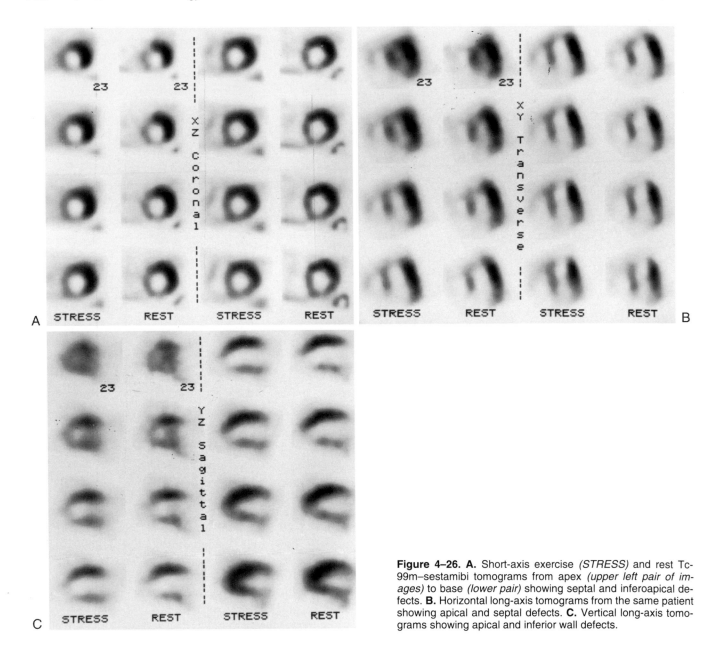

Figure 4–26. A. Short-axis exercise *(STRESS)* and rest Tc-99m–sestamibi tomograms from apex *(upper left pair of images)* to base *(lower pair)* showing septal and inferoapical defects. **B.** Horizontal long-axis tomograms from the same patient showing apical and septal defects. **C.** Vertical long-axis tomograms showing apical and inferior wall defects.

ability to identify high-risk subsets, can be determined with exercise radionuclide angiography in a manner similar to that described for exercise Tl-201 scintigraphy.[55–75] However, changes in function consequent to inducible ischemia, rather than perfusion, are assessed. Radionuclide angiography, like myocardial perfusion imaging, has the ability to distinguish between patients with single-vessel disease and those with multivessel disease. Results of some early studies indicated that the change in EF with exercise was related to the number of significant underlying coronary stenoses. DePace et al.[61] found that the change in EF from rest to exercise correlated weakly ($r = -0.42$) with a CAD score that was based on site and severity of coronary stenoses. The peak radionuclide EF during exercise correlated better with the coronary disease score ($r = 0.70$), particularly with an exercise heart rate of at least 130 bpm. In that

study, the peak EF correlated well with the extent of coronary disease if the patient exercised for at least 8 minutes or was younger than 50 years. Figure 4–27 shows exercise LVEF values in this study relative to extent of CAD. A follow-up study by DePace et al.[72] found that the peak exercise EF, the peak exercise heart rate, the presence of Q waves on the resting ECG, and age were all independently significant predictors of the extent of underlying CAD. Low- and high-risk subsets could be identified using a discriminate function based on these four variables. Only 9% of patients in the low-risk subgroup had three-vessel or left main disease, as compared with 43% in the high-risk subgroup who had three-vessel or left main disease.

Identification of patients with a high likelihood of left main or proximal three-vessel disease is enhanced when variables derived from the exercise ECG stress tests are

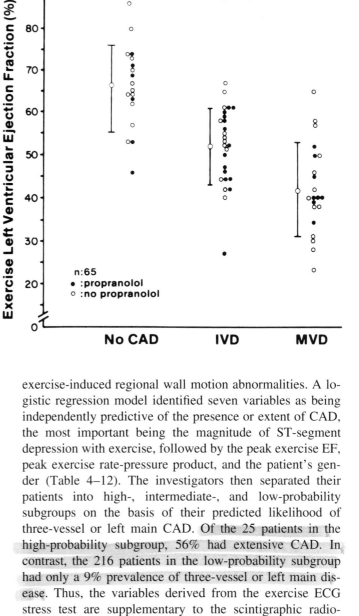

Figure 4–27. Exercise left ventricular ejection fraction in patients with no CAD, patients with one-vessel disease (1VD), and patients with multivessel disease (MVD). Note the considerable overlap in values among the groups with CAD. (Reprinted with permission from the American College of Cardiology (Journal of the American College of Cardiology, 1983, Vol. 1, pp. 1002–1010).)

combined with the radionuclide ventriculographic information. When stepwise linear discriminate analysis was undertaken by Weintraub et al.[70] to predict the extent of CAD in 185 patients undergoing exercise radionuclide angiography, the most important variables were the exercise EF, the magnitude of ST-segment depression, and the peak heart rate achieved during exercise. They were able to separate high- and low-risk subsets which had 64% and 11% risks of three-vessel or left main disease, respectively. Campos et al.[71] reported that the likelihood of extensive CAD increased significantly in patients who had both an abnormal EF response to exercise and ST-segment depression, as compared with those who had only an abnormal radionuclide ventriculographic response. Bonow et al.[73] found that the likelihood of left main or three-vessel disease increased from 60% to 75% in patients who exhibited both an abnormal EF response and ST-segment depression with exercise, as compared with 60% whose EF decreased with exercise alone.

The ability of exercise radionuclide angiography to predict the risk of having significant left main or three-vessel CAD was examined by the Mayo Clinic group in 681 patients who underwent both radionuclide ventriculography and coronary angiography.[56] Patients with left main or three-vessel CAD were found to be older and more likely male, to exhibit a significantly lower exercise heart rate–blood pressure product and a lower exercise workload, to have more chest pain with exercise, to demonstrate more ST-segment depression with exercise, and to manifest a lower exercise EF, a greater increase in the systolic blood pressure–end-systolic volume ratio with exercise, and more

exercise-induced regional wall motion abnormalities. A logistic regression model identified seven variables as being independently predictive of the presence or extent of CAD, the most important being the magnitude of ST-segment depression with exercise, followed by the peak exercise EF, peak exercise rate-pressure product, and the patient's gender (Table 4–12). The investigators then separated their patients into high-, intermediate-, and low-probability subgroups on the basis of their predicted likelihood of three-vessel or left main CAD. Of the 25 patients in the high-probability subgroup, 56% had extensive CAD. In contrast, the 216 patients in the low-probability subgroup had only a 9% prevalence of three-vessel or left main disease. Thus, the variables derived from the exercise ECG stress test are supplementary to the scintigraphic radio-

Table 4–12. **Logistic Regression Model to Identify Left Main or Three-Vessel Coronary Artery Disease**

Variables*	P Value
Magnitude of ST-segment depression	<0.0001
Exercise ejection fraction	<0.0001
Exercise heart rate–blood pressure product	<0.0001
Sex	0.0001
Exercise end-systolic volume index	0.001
Exercise pressure–volume ratio:rest pressure–volume ratio	0.01
METs of exercise	0.02

*Variables listed in order of importance
(Reprinted with permission from the American College of Cardiology (Journal of the American College of Cardiology, 1988, Vol. 11, pp. 28–34).)

nuclide ventriculographic data for increased noninvasive identification of patients with left main or three-vessel disease.

A more recent study from the Mayo group of investigators[74] showed that the magnitude of the additional value of exercise radionuclide angiography to the standard exercise ECG stress test for detection of high-risk anatomic CAD has been brought into question. They found that, in patients with no resting ECG abnormalities who were not taking digoxin, the exercise radionuclide stress test model generated from patient gender, peak exercise heart rate, and magnitude of ST-segment depression successfully segregated patients into low-, intermediate-, and high-likelihood subgroups (6%, 23%, and 60%, respectively) for detection of three-vessel or left main disease. The addition of variables from the exercise radionuclide angiogram did not significantly change the prevalence of left main or three-vessel disease in either the low- or high-risk subgroup.

Patients with a proximal LAD stenosis exhibit a greater drop in the exercise EF, as a group, as compared with patients with more distal disease in that vessel.[57] A fall in LVEF of 10% or more from rest to exercise is a strong indicator of the presence of underlying severe left main or proximal three-vessel disease. In contrast, the absence of a fall in EF indicates a low probability of such lesions. Miller et al.[74a] reported that severe exercise-induced ischemia failed to identify a high-risk subgroup among patients with normal left ventricular function and one- or two-vessel disease who are treated initially with medical therapy. *Severe ischemia* was defined as the triad of (1) peak exercise workload at least 600 kg-m/min, (2) exercise ECG with at least 1.0 mm ST segment depression, and (3) decrease in exercise LVEF. Figure 4–28 shows the event-free survival in patients with and without severe ischemia.

Like Tl-201 scintigraphy, exercise radionuclide angiography has been employed for determination of prognosis in

patients with known or suspected CAD.[74b, 74c] The prognostic value of the resting EF, determined by either first-pass or equilibrium radionuclide angiographic techniques, has been well established, as discussed earlier in this chapter. The magnitude of the depression in resting LVEF is one of the most important determinants of prognosis in patients with chronic CAD who have previously experienced an MI. The CASS study clearly indicated that the mortality rate increases progressively as the EF decreases.[4] More debate has been conducted on whether or not the exercise EF provides additional useful prognostic information, particularly when the resting EF is known to be abnormal. Since the exercise EF is a reflection of the extent of ischemia during stress, it should provide useful prognostic information.

Bonow et al.[58] reported 71% survival at 4 years for patients with three-vessel disease who had both ischemic ST-segment depression, an abnormal EF response during exercise, and an exercise tolerance of 120 W or less (Fig. 4–29). All deaths occurred in this subgroup, whereas no patient with three-vessel disease who demonstrated an unchanged or increased EF with exercise, a negative ST-segment response, or both, died while receiving medical therapy. Thus, both high- and low-risk subgroups of patients with three-vessel CAD were identified by the combination of ST depression and an abnormal exercise EF. From a prognostic standpoint, the three-vessel disease patients who demonstrate an abnormal functional response to exercise may be those for whom intervention with revascularization is most beneficial. This concept is similar to the one introduced earlier with respect to benefit of revascularization for three-vessel disease patients with multiple perfusion abnormalities. Detection of "all patients" with three-vessel disease by the noninvasive stress testing approach described may not be critical. Similarly, there are patients with one- and two-vessel disease who demonstrate as profound an

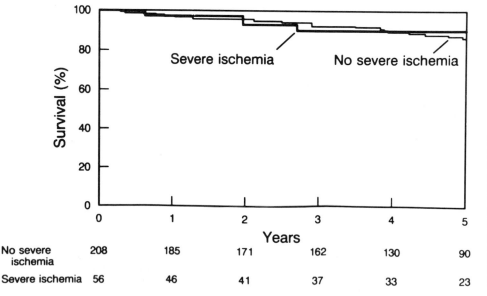

Figure 4–28. Event-free survival in patients with one- or two-vessel CAD with an LVEF of at least 50% who did and did not have severe ischemia on exercise radionuclide angiography. The numbers at bottom depict the number of patients available for analysis at each follow-up point. (Reprinted with permission from the American College of Cardiology (Journal of the American College of Cardiology, 1994, Vol. 23, pp. 219–224).)

	0	1	2	3	4	5
No severe ischemia	208	185	171	162	130	90
Severe ischemia	56	46	41	37	33	23

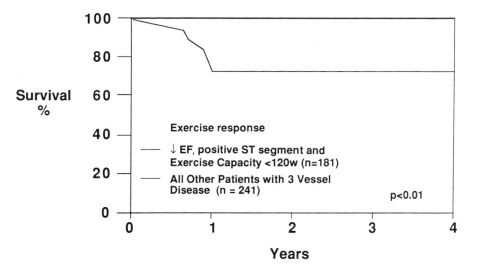

Figure 4–29. Survival rate based on exercise response during exercise radionuclide angiography. The high-risk group *(bottom curve)* includes those who exhibit a decreased (↓) ejection fraction (EF) during exercise, a positive ischemic ST-segment response, and an exercise capacity less than 120 W. The other patients with three-vessel disease not showing this abnormal response had a 100% survival during the follow-up period *(top line).* (Adapted from Bonow RO, et al.: N Engl J Med 1984;311:1339–1345. Copyright 1984, Massachusetts Medical Society. All rights reserved.)

abnormal functional response to exercise as some patients with three-vessel disease who exhibit an abnormal EF and/or ST-segment response. Although those patients have less extensive anatomic disease, they may be, from a prognostic standpoint, at just as high risk for future events as patients with three-vessel disease who exhibit a comparable abnormal EF response to exercise stress. A patient with a proximal LAD stenosis may have as marked a fall in EF during exercise as a patient with three-vessel disease and could be at the same risk for future cardiac events based on a large area of myocardium at risk.

The Duke University group has extensively investigated the prognostic utility of exercise radionuclide angiography for patients with chronic CAD or chest pain. In 1983, Jones et al.[75] from Duke reported that regardless of coronary anatomy, patients who demonstrated the greatest amount of exercise-induced LV dysfunction before surgery appeared to have had the most favorable outcome with myocardial revascularization. In that report, patients with chest pain who had a normal EF response to exercise fared no better, in terms of survival or pain relief, with surgery than with medical therapy. On the other hand, CAD patients who demonstrated an abnormal EF response to exercise before surgery had a better outcome with surgery. In a subsequent study from Duke, Pryor et al.[59] found that the exercise EF was the variable most closely associated with future cardiac events in 386 patients with symptomatic CAD followed for up to 4.5 years. They found that once the exercise EF was known, no other radionuclide variable, including the EF at rest or presence of wall motion abnormalities, contributed independent information about the likelihood of future events. In that study, the percentage of patients who were event free at 2 years diminished dramatically as the exercise EF fell below 50% (Fig. 4–30).

In a subsequent expanded report from the Duke group,[63] the prognostic utility of exercise radionuclide angiography relative to clinical and catheterization data was studied in 571 stable patients with symptomatic CAD who underwent

upright rest-exercise first-pass radionuclide angiography within 3 months of catheterization and were treated medically. This study had a median follow-up of 5.4 years, and during follow-up 90 patients died of cardiovascular causes. As shown in Table 4–13, using the Cox regression model the most important radionuclide angiographic predictor of mortality was the exercise EF ($\chi^2 = 81$). Neither rest EF nor the change in EF from rest to exercise contributed supplementary prognostic information. It should be pointed out that in this study a significant stenosis was defined as at least 75% and that only 20% of patients were women. Radionuclide angiographic variables were more predictive of subsequent mortality than clinical data derived from the history, physical examination, the resting ECG, and the chest x-ray. In fact, as depicted in Figure 4–31, the radionuclide angiographic variables were equivalent to the set of

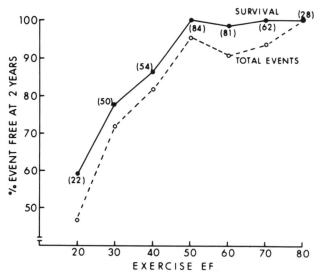

Figure 4–30. Two-year survival and survival free of total cardiac events as a function of the exercise EF. Numbers in parentheses delineate number of patients in each exercise EF group. (Reprinted from American Journal of Cardiology: 53:1; January 1, 1984; 18–22.).

Table 4–13. **Independent Prognostic Value of Exercise Radionuclide Angiography by Cox Regression Model**

Variables	Adjusted χ^2
Cardiovascular death	
Exercise ejection fraction	81
Change in heart rate	16
Rest end-diastolic volume index	7
Total cardiovascular events	
Exercise ejection fraction	45
Exercise heart rate	12
Rest end-diastolic volume index	9

(From Lee KL, et al.: Prognostic value of radionuclide angiography in medically treated patients with coronary artery disease. A comparison with clinical and catheterization variables. Circulation 1990;82:1705–1717.)

cardiac catheterization variables with respect to prognosis ($\chi^2 = 104$ for radionuclide angiography vs. $\chi^2 = 102$ for catheterization). The radionuclide angiographic variables contained 84% of the prognostic information provided by clinical and catheterization descriptors combined. Radionuclide angiography contributed significant additional prognostic information to the combination of clinical and catheterization data. Thus, functional and physiologic information provided by the radionuclide angiogram performed during exercise was shown to supplement the anatomic and structural abnormalities determined by coronary arteriography. Exercise radionuclide angiography was shown to be prognostically useful in defining risk, even when clinical and catheterization data were available. The radionuclide angiogram was also useful in further stratifying risk of patients with three-vessel disease and depressed LV function. Those with an exercise EF of 30% or less had significantly greater risk than those with an EF greater than 30%. Taliercio et al.,[64] using equilibrium-gated radionuclide angiography, also showed that patients with an EF of less than 30% during exercise had a significantly lower rate of event-free survival than patients with an EF of at least 30% (Fig. 4–32). In patients with an exercise EF of less than 30%, the cardiac event rate was nearly 50% over 4 years' follow-up. All had an angiographic EF of no more than 45%.

Figure 4–33 shows survival at 5 years after exercise radionuclide angiography predicted by the Cox model in an expanded population of 1663 patients in the Duke data bank.[66] In both catheterized and noncatheterized patients, the strength of the relation of radionuclide angiographic variables to mortality was equivalent to the strength of the relation of cardiac catheterization variables to mortality. This figure shows that late mortality increases significantly as the EF falls below 50% during exercise.

Iskandrian et al.[60] also found that the exercise LVEF was the best predictor of total major events, and that the resting EF was the best predictor of death or nonfatal infarction in patients with chest pain. Mazzotta et al.[62] reported that, among patients with one- or two-vessel CAD, survival at 6 years was 97% $\pm$ 3% for those with an exercise EF of at least 30%, as compared with survival of 62% $\pm$ 14% for those whose EF was less than 30%. All patients in that study were either asymptomatic or mildly symptomatic during medical therapy. Survival is reduced in patients with one-vessel or two-vessel disease if severe ischemia is demonstrated on exercise radionuclide angiography.[67] The definition of a severe ischemic response in this study by Miller et al. was a decrease in EF with exercise, at least 1.0 mm of ST-segment depression, and a peak exercise workload of not greater than 600 kg-m/min. Thirty-six percent of the patients with severely ischemic exercise radionuclide angiograms had events, compared to 13% without such a re-

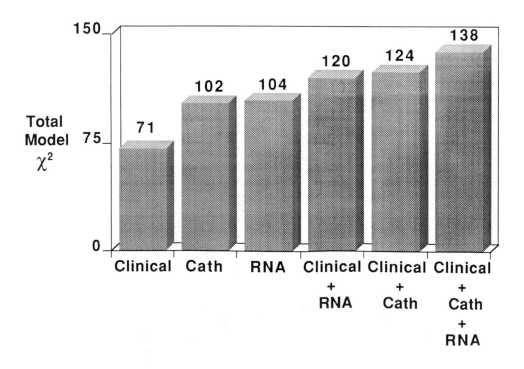

Figure 4–31. Relative prognostic importance of radionuclide angiographic (RNA), clinical, and catheterization (Cath) variables for cardiovascular death employing Cox-model multivariate analysis. RNA provided prognostic information considerably exceeding that of clinical variables and even slightly exceeding that of catheterization variables alone. RNA contained 84% of the information provided by the combination of clinical and catheterization descriptors. (Adapted from Lee KL, et al.: Circulation 1990;82:1705–1717.)

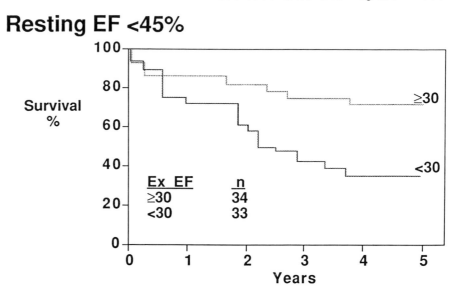

Resting EF <45%

Figure 4–32. Survival rate in patients with an exercise EF of ≥30% or <30% whose resting EF was ≤45%. (Taliercio CP, et al.: Mayo Clin Proc 1988;63:573–582.)

sponse. In this study, all patients had a resting EF of less than 50%.

Simari et al.[65] investigated the ability of supine exercise ECG and exercise radionuclide angiography to predict time to subsequent cardiac death, nonfatal infarction, or late revascularization. This study was undertaken in 256 patients with normal resting ECGs who were not taking digoxin. All had undergone coronary angiography and were treated medically. At a median 15 months' follow-up, separate logistic regression models developed previously to predict three-vessel or left main CAD were compared using Cox regression analysis. The exercise ECG model, consisting of the magnitude of ST depression, exercise heart rate, and patient gender, was a powerful predictor ($\chi^2 = 30.8$) of subsequent events. The exercise radionuclide angiographic model, which included the exercise response of the pressure-volume ratio in addition to exercise ECG variables, had similar prognostic power ($\chi^2 = 31.8$). None of the radionuclide angiography variables added significantly to

the prognostic power of the exercise ECG model. The conclusion of this study was that, in patients with a normal resting ECG, the supine exercise ECG model that predicts three-vessel or left main CAD also predicts future cardiac events. Furthermore, exercise radionuclide angiography did not provide any additional prognostic information in such patients. This finding seems to be at variance with the data previously summarized from the Duke studies.[65, 66] One possible explanation for this difference may be that of the 38 total number of cardiac events, only six were cardiac deaths. In addition, the study population was highly selective, since nearly a third of the original patient population was treated with early revascularization, perhaps because of the accepted notion that abnormal radionuclide responses identify a high-risk subset. Thus, the patients at highest risk crossed over immediately to revascularization, leaving a rather low-risk subgroup for follow-up. If such patients had not crossed over early to revascularization and a natural history study had been undertaken, it is likely that the

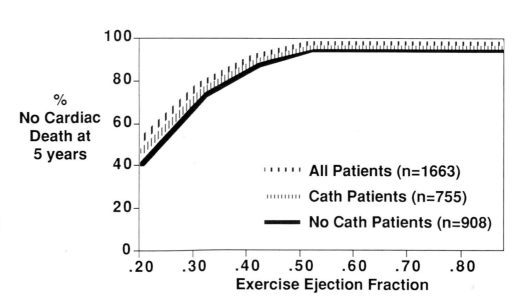

Figure 4–33. Survival at 5 years after exercise radionuclide angiography predicted by the Cox model. Late mortality increases significantly as the exercise ejection fraction falls below 50% during exercise. (Jones RH, et al.: Circulation 1991;84(suppl I):I-52–I-58.)

radionuclide angiographic information would have added additional supplementary variables to the risk stratification process that were not available from the ECG stress test model alone.

In a perhaps more homogeneous population, Johnson et al.[68] determined the prognostic value of radionuclide angiography in 908 patients with suspected CAD who underwent rest and exercise radionuclide angiography without subsequent cardiac catheterization. These patients, followed for a median of 4.6 years, suffered 52 cardiovascular deaths and 28 nonfatal infarctions during follow-up. Univariate analysis identified the exercise EF as the best predictor of cardiovascular death (total cardiac events, $\chi^2 = 84$; death from all causes, $\chi^2 = 66$). Three variables—exercise EF, exercise change in heart rate, and gender—contained independent prognostic information determined by multivariable analysis. The exercise EF was the strongest independent predictor ($P < 0.0001$) for every endpoint. The conclusion of this study was that the measurement of ventricular function during exercise provides important independent prognostic information for patients with suspected CAD. In a population-based cohort from Olmsted County, Minnesota, 71 of 536 residents who underwent supine exercise radionuclide angiography experienced death or nonfatal infarction at a median follow-up of 46 months.[68a] Four-year infarct-free survival was 98% for the 152 patients with a peak exercise heart rate of at least 122 beats/minute and an exercise EF of 58% or greater. In the 150 patients with a peak heart rate of less than 122 beats/minute and an exercise EF of less than 58%, 4-year infarct-free survival was 68%. In the aggregate, these clinical studies clearly demonstrate the prognostic utility of exercise radionuclide angiography in patients with suspected or known CAD. Failure to increase LVEF adequately, particularly when associated with suboptimal heart responses to exercise, identifies a high-risk subgroup with an increased future cardiac event rate.

Comparison with Prognostic Application of Thallium-201 Scintigraphy

At present, exercise Tl-201 scintigraphy is performed more frequently than exercise radionuclide angiography for detection of CAD and for assessment of prognosis. In patients who are unable to exercise, pharmacologic stress perfusion imaging is the preferred approach to detecting occult CAD and for risk stratification (see Chap. 8). In the United States, the mode of exercise testing is symptom-limited graded treadmill exercise stress, which provides information useful to the prognostication process and to assessing the efficacy of medical management. Supine or upright bicycle exercise, which must be performed with either first-pass or equilibrium radionuclide angiography, is less attractive to practitioners in the United States. Similarly, there is a perception that the radionuclide angiographic response is not as specific as an abnormal perfusion scan (see Chap. 3).

This is because non-CAD patients with other forms of heart disease (e.g., dilated cardiomyopathy, hypertensive heart disease) may manifest an abnormal functional response to exercise. Such patients would exhibit no discrete focal defects with stress perfusion imaging.

Despite these limitations, the prognostic utility of exercise radionuclide angiography for risk stratification has clearly been demonstrated. High-risk CAD patients have a greater degree of LV functional impairment than their counterparts at low risk in response to exercise stress manifested by a lower exercise EF. Such patients should be considered for invasive evaluation even in the absence of inducible ischemia. Patients in the highest-risk category whose EF falls below 30% with exercise are presumably the same patients who exhibit an increased lung-heart Tl-201 ratio on stress myocardial perfusion imaging. Results of the perfusion imaging studies and the radionuclide angiographic studies are quite consistent. The physiologic assessment of either perfusion or function adds significant prognostic information to clinical data and ECG exercise stress testing. Patients with a depressed resting EF who exhibit a further fall in EF during exercise are in the highest-risk subgroup. When associated with poor exercise tolerance and ST-segment depression, the subsequent cardiac event rate may exceed 50% over 5 years' follow-up.

EXERCISE ECHOCARDIOGRAPHY FOR ASSESSING PROGNOSIS

Exercise echocardiography is increasingly being performed for detection of CAD (see Chap. 3) and for risk stratification. There are scant published data pertaining to the prognostic value of exercise echocardiography in patients with known or suspected CAD.[76–80] Sawada et al.[76] evaluated the prognostic worth of a normal exercise echocardiogram in 148 consecutive patients whose mean age was 53 years and who had a pretest likelihood for CAD of 39%. Follow-up was for a period of 28 ± 8 months. There were no deaths during follow-up in this group, and there were two nonfatal MIs. Interestingly, the exercise ECG was abnormal in 47% of patients. The event rate in this study is not too dissimilar from the event rate observed in patients with either a normal exercise Tl-201 scintigram or a normal exercise radionuclide angiogram. Hecht et al.[77] found that digital supine bicycle stress echocardiography was 88% correct in predicting multivessel CAD in 180 patients who underwent coronary angiography. Krivokapich et al.[78] reported that cardiac events occurred in 34% of patients with a positive exercise echocardiogram as compared with 9% of patients with a negative one. Roger et al.[80] examined the ability of exercise echocardiography to identify patients with multivessel CAD. The criterion for a positive test for this identification was the presence of more than one abnormal vascular region at rest or after exercise. Using an angiographic criterion for a significant stenosis as 50% or greater narrowing, the overall sensitivity and specificity of exercise echocardiography for the identification of multivessel CAD were 73% and 70%, respectively. The number of abnormal regions on the postexercise images was the strongest independent predictor of multivessel disease. Thus, these studies demonstrate that a normal left ventricular functional response to exercise stress portends a good short-term prognosis, whereas extensive regional wall motion abnormalities occurring with exercise suggest multivessel CAD. Well-designed clinical research studies comparing the prognostic value of exercise radionuclide imaging with exercise echocardiography have not been carried out in institutions possessing comparable expertise in both noninvasive modalities.

SUMMARY

Using exercise ECG stress testing in conjunction with either myocardial perfusion imaging or radionuclide angiography, patients with either undiagnosed chest pain or stable CAD can initially be risk stratified by clinical and physiologic evaluation. Figure 4–34 shows a decision tree for separating low-risk patients from high-risk ones by exercise radionuclide imaging. A low-risk group can be identified as having minimal or no ischemia and good exercise capacity. The lowest-risk group is comprised of patients who achieve more than 85% of maximum predicted heart rate for age, have no inducible ischemic ST-segment depression, and have a normal or minimally abnormal myocardial perfusion scan. Using radionuclide angiography, patients at low risk should exhibit an increase in exercise EF to greater than 55% without ischemic ST depression at an adequate exercise workload. A low-risk exercise echocardiogram is one that exhibits no inducible wall motion abnormalities with stress. Low-risk patients may not require coronary angiography as long as symptoms are minimal.

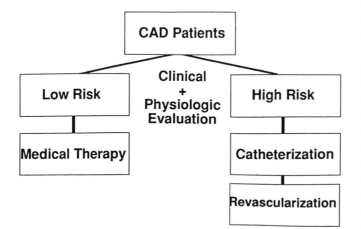

Figure 4–34. Decision tree outline for separating low- and high-risk subsets of CAD patients by clinical and physiologic evaluation using exercise perfusion imaging, radionuclide angiography, or echocardiography. See text for criteria for low-risk and high-risk subgroups.

Interrelated Prognostic Variables

LV Dysfunction	Ischemia
CHF	Multivessel CAD
Prior MI	Exercise ↓ BP
↓ rest LVEF	Exercise angina
Wall motion abnormality	ST depression
↓ exercise tolerance	↓ exercise HR
↑ lung Tl-201	Tl-201 Rd defects
Persistent Tl-201 defects	↓ exercise LVEF
Ventricular ectopy	↑ lung Tl-201

Figure 4–35. Interrelated prognostic variables reflecting either LV dysfunction (left column) or inducible ischemia (right column). Some variables are reflective of both resting LV dysfunction and extensive ischemia (e.g., increased lung Tl-201 uptake). (Key: ↓, decreased; CHF, congestive heart failure; MI, myocardial infarction; BP, blood pressure; HR, heart rate; Rd, redistribution; LVEF, left ventricular ejection fraction.)

Medical therapy would be a prudent initial plan of management. Progression of disease can be monitored by periodic repeat stress imaging. This may be most useful in patients who manifest predominantly silent ischemic responses to stress.

High-risk patients exhibit extensive ischemia at low exercise heart rates or workloads and should benefit from early catheterization. If anatomy is suitable, subsequent revascularization should be performed. Patients with a diminution in resting LV function in association with stress-induced ischemia and impaired exercise capacity are the subset at highest risk. An increased lung-heart Tl-201 ratio, even when just a few segments demonstrate hypoperfusion, identifies patients at high risk for premature cardiac death if they are managed by medical therapy. Figure 4–35 depicts the interrelationship between prognostic variables that reflect LV dysfunction extensive inducible ischemia, or both. Some variables such as diminished exercise tolerance and increased lung Tl-201 uptake reflect the combination of resting LV dysfunction and ischemia. High-risk patients with single-vessel CAD also can be well identified by assessment of defect severity on quantitative exercise SPECT Tl-201 imaging. Matzer et al.[81] found that the Tl-201 defect severity score was significantly related to the maximal percentage of luminal stenosis diameter ($r = 0.93$), percentage of area narrowing ($r = 0.89$), absolute stenotic area ($r = 0.79$), and absolute stenotic diameter ($r = 0.81$). The authors concluded that Tl-201 defect severity on SPECT imaging could be useful for noninvasive characterization of the functional severity of coronary artery stenosis and may complement coronary angioplasty in predicting functionally significant stenosis.

A potential limitation of technetium-99m–methoxyisobutyl isonitrile (Tc-99m sestamibi) imaging for prognosis is the absence of lung tracer uptake as a variable for risk stratification. Nevertheless, SPECT Tc-99m–sestamibi imaging is highly sensitive for individual stenosis detection in patients undergoing stress imaging for assessment of known or suspected CAD (see Chap. 3). Perhaps the extent of hypoperfusion on Tc-99m–sestamibi images, as quantified on polar bull's-eye maps, may substitute for the increased lung-heart Tl-201 ratio for risk stratification. As discussed in Chapter 3, some investigators have advocated combining first-pass radionuclide angiography and perfusion imaging with a single intravenous dose of Tc-99m sestamibi. The exercise EF, coupled with the determination of the perfusion pattern, could provide the same prognostic information presently derived from combining the lung-heart Tl-201 ratio with the number of hypoperfused scan segments. Undoubtedly, patients with increased lung Tl-201 uptake would demonstrate a subnormal EF response to exercise consequent to significant stress-induced ischemia.

The data from the literature summarized in this chapter suggest that exercise ECG stress testing alone may not be as good at separating high- and low-risk subgroups as the combination of exercise ECG stress testing and radionuclide imaging (whether myocardial perfusion imaging or radionuclide angiography).

In conclusion, one of the most useful clinical applications of nuclear cardiology testing is the assessment of prognosis for patients with suspected or documented CAD. Further technical advances in the field of radionuclide imaging should afford the clinician the capability of better quantifying the extent of abnormal perfusion so that patients with functionally significant CAD can be identified and referred for further invasive workup.

REFERENCES

1. Cerqueira M, Ritchie JL: Thallium-201 scintigraphy in risk assessment for ambulatory patients with chest pain: Does everyone need catheterization? J Am Coll Cardiol 1988;12:35–36.
2. Hammermeister KE, DeRouen TA, Dodge HT: Variables predictive of survival in patients with coronary disease. Selection by univariate and multivariate analyses from the clinical, electrocardiographic, exercise, arteriographic, and quantitative angiographic evaluations. Circulation 1979;59:421–430.
3. Harris PJ, Harrell FE Jr, Lee KL, Behar VS, Rosati RA: Survival in medically treated coronary artery disease. Circulation 1979;60:1259–1269.
4. Mock MB, Ringqvist I, Fisher LD, Davis KB, Chaitman BR, Kouchoukos NT, Kaiser GC, Alderman E, Ryan TJ, Russell RO Jr, Mullin S, Fray D, Killip T: Survival of medically treated patients in the coronary artery surgery study (CASS) registry. Circulation 1982;66:562–568.
5. Proudfit WJ, Bruschke AV, MacMillan JP, Williams GW, Sones FM Jr: Fifteen year survival study of patients with obstructive coronary artery disease. Circulation 1983;68:986–997.
6. Alderman EL, Fisher LD, Litwin P, Kaiser GC, Myers WO, Maynard C, Levine F, Schloss M: Results of coronary artery surgery in patients with poor left ventricular function (CASS). Circulation 1983;68:785–795.
7. Rahimtoola S: Clinical overview of management of chronic ischemic heart disease. Circulation 1991;84[suppl I]:I-81–I-84.
8. Weiner DA, Ryan TJ, McCabe CH, Chaitman BR, Sheffield LT, Fisher LD, Tristani F: Value of exercise testing in determining the risk classification and the response to coronary artery bypass grafting in three-vessel coronary artery disease: A report from the Coronary

Artery Surgery Study (CASS) registry. Am J Cardiol 1987;60:262–266.
9. European Coronary Study Group: Long-term results of prospective randomized study of coronary artery bypass surgery in stable angina pectoris. Lancet 1982;2:1173–1180.
10. Morris CK, Morrow K, Froelicher VF, Hideg A, Hunter D, Kawaguchi T, Ribisl PM, Ueshima K, Wallis J: Prediction of cardiovascular death by means of clinical and exercise test variables in patients selected for cardiac catheterization. Am Heart J 1993;125:1717–1726.
11. Weiner D, McCabe C, Ryan T: Identification of patients with left main and three-vessel coronary disease with clinical and exercise test variables. Am J Cardiol 1980;46:21–27.
12. Weiner DA, Ryan TJ, McCabe CH, Chaitman BR, Sheffield LT, Ferguson JC, Fisher LD, Tristani F: Prognostic importance of a clinical profile and exercise test in medically treated patients with coronary artery disease. J Am Coll Cardiol 1984;3:772–779.
13. Weiner DA, McCabe CH, Cutler SS, Ryan TJ: Decrease in systolic blood pressure during exercise testing: Reproducibility, response to coronary bypass surgery and prognostic significance. Am J Cardiol 1982;49:1627–1631.
14. Weiner DA, Levine SR, Klein MD, Ryan TJ: Ventricular arrhythmias during exercise testing: Mechanism, response to coronary bypass surgery and prognostic significance. Am J Cardiol 1984;53:1553–1557.
14a. Weiner DA, Ryan T, McCabe CH, Chaitman BR, Sheffield T, Ferguson JC, Fisher LD, Tristani F: Prognostic importance of a clinical profile and exercise test in medically treated patients with coronary artery disease. J Am Coll Cardiol 1984;3:772–779.
15. McNeer JF, Margolis JR, Lee KL, Kisslo JA, Peter RH, Kong Y, Behar VS, Wallace AG, McCants CB, Rosati RA: The role of the exercise test in the evaluation of patients for ischemic heart disease. Circulation 1978;57:64–70.
16. Mark DB, Shaw L, Harrell FE Jr, Hlatky MA, Lee KL, Bengtson JR, McCants CB, Califf RM, Pryor DB: Prognostic value of a treadmill exercise score in outpatients with suspected coronary artery disease. N Engl J Med 1991;325:849–853.
17. Morrow K, Morris CK, Froelicher VF, Hideg A, Hunter D, Johnson E, Kawaguchi T, Lehmann K, Ribisl PM, Thomas R, et al.: Prediction of cardiovascular death in men undergoing noninvasive evaluation for coronary artery disease. Ann Intern Med 1993;118:689–695.
18. Beller GA: Current status of nuclear cardiology techniques. Curr Probl Cardiol 1991;16:451–535.
19. Brown KA: Prognostic value of thallium-201 myocardial perfusion imaging. A diagnostic tool comes of age. Circulation 1991;83:363–381.
19a. Beller GA: Myocardial perfusion imaging with thallium-201. J Nucl Med 1994;35:674–680.
20. Esquivel L, Pollock SG, Beller GA, Gibson RS, Watson DD, Kaul S: Effect of the degree of effort on the sensitivity of the exercise thallium-201 stress test in symptomatic coronary artery disease. Am J Cardiol 1989;63:160–165.
21. Brown KA, Boucher CA, Okada RD, Guiney TE, Newell JB, Strauss HW, Pohost GM: Prognostic value of exercise thallium-201 imaging in patients presenting for evaluation of chest pain. J Am Coll Cardiol 1983;1:994–1001.
22. Ladenheim ML, Pollock BH, Rozanski A, Berman DS, Staniloff HM, Forrester JS, Diamond GA: Extent and severity of myocardial hypoperfusion as predictors of prognosis in patients with suspected coronary artery disease. J Am Coll Cardiol 1986;7:464–471.
23. Iskandrian AS, Hakki AH, Kane-Marsch S: Prognostic implications of exercise thallium-201 scintigraphy in patients with suspected or known coronary artery disease. Am Heart J 1985;110:135–143.
24. Kaul S, Lilly DR, Gascho JA, Watson DD, Gibson RS, Oliner CA, Ryan JM, Beller GA: Prognostic utility of the exercise thallium-201 test in ambulatory patients with chest pain: Comparison with cardiac catheterization. Circulation 1988;77:745–758.
25. Kaul S, Finkelstein DM, Homma S, Leavitt M, Okada RD, Boucher CA: Superiority of quantitative exercise thallium-201 variables in determining long-term prognosis in ambulatory patients with chest pain: A comparison with cardiac catheterization. J Am Coll Cardiol 1988;12:25–34.
25a. Travin MI, Boucher CA, Newell JB, LaRaia PJ, Flores AR, Eagle KA: Variables associated with a poor prognosis in patients with an ischemic thallium-201 exercise test. Am Heart J 1993;125:335–344.
26. Melin JA, Robert A, Luwaert R, Beckers C, Detry JM: Additional prognostic value of exercise testing and thallium-201 scintigraphy in

catheterized patients without previous myocardial infarction. Int J Cardiol 1990;27:235–243.

26a. Machecourt J, Longère P, Fagret D, Vanzetto G, Wolf JE, Polidori C, Comet M, Denis B: Prognostic value of thallium-201 single-photon emission computed tomographic myocardial perfusion imaging according to extent of myocardial defect. Study in 1,926 patients with a follow-up at 33 months. J Am Coll Cardiol 1994;23:1090–1106.

27. Taylor A, Beller G: Correlation of resting electrocardiographic ST-T wave abnormalities with exercise thallium-201 stress testing in patients with known or suspected coronary artery disease. Am J Cardiol 1994;74:211–215.

28. Weiss AT, Berman DS, Lew AS, Nielsen J, Potkin B, Swan HJ, Waxman A, Maddahi J: Transient ischemic dilation of the left ventricle on stress thallium-201 scintigraphy: A marker of severe and extensive coronary artery disease. J Am Coll Cardiol 1987;9:752–729.

28a. Roberti RR, Van Tosh A, Baruchin MA, Gallagher R, Friedman P, Ventura B, Horowitz SF: Left ventricular cavity-to-myocardial count ratio: A new parameter for detecting resting left ventricular dysfunction directly from tomographic thallium perfusion scintigraphy. J Nucl Med 1993;34:193–198.

29. Boucher CA, Zir LM, Beller GA, Okada RD, McKusick KA, Strauss HW, Pohost GM: Increased lung uptake of thallium-201 during exercise myocardial imaging: Clinical, hemodynamic and angiographic implications in patients with coronary artery disease. Am J Cardiol 1980;46:189–196.

30. Mannting F: Pulmonary thallium uptake: Correlation with systolic and diastolic left ventricular function at rest and during exercise. Am Heart J 1990;119:1137–1146.

31. Ilmer B, Reijs AE, Reiber JH, Bakker W, Fioretti P: Relationships between the lung-heart ratio assessed from post-exercise thallium-201 myocardial tomograms, myocardial ischemia and the extent of coronary artery disease. Int J Cardiac Imaging 1990;6:135–141.

32. Kurata C, Tawarahara K, Taguchi T, Sakata K, Yamazaki N, Naitoh Y: Lung thallium-201 uptake during exercise emission computed tomography. J Nucl Med 1991;32:417–423.

33. Homma S, Kaul S, Boucher CA: Correlates of lung/heart ratio of thallium-201 in coronary artery disease. J Nucl Med 1987;28:1531–1535.

34. Kushner FG, Okada RD, Kirshenbaum HD, Boucher CA, Strauss HW, Pohost GM: Lung thallium-201 uptake after stress testing in patients with coronary artery disease. Circulation 1981;63:341–347.

35. Lahiri A, O'Hara MJ, Bowles MJ, Crawley JC, Raftery EB: Influence of left ventricular function and severity of coronary artery disease on exercise-induced pulmonary thallium-201 uptake. Int J Cardiol 1984;5:475–490.

36. Jain D, Lahiri A, Raftery EB: Clinical and prognostic significance of lung thallium uptake on rest imaging in acute myocardial infarction. Am J Cardiol 1990;65:154–159.

37. Califf RM, Harrell FE Jr, Lee KL, Rankin JS, Hlatky MA, Mark DB, Jones RH, Muhlbaier LH, Oldham HN Jr, Pryor DB: The evolution of medical and surgical therapy for coronary artery disease. A 15-year perspective. JAMA 1989;261:2077–2086.

38. Nygaard TW, Gibson RS, Ryan JM, Gascho JA, Watson DD, Beller GA: Prevalence of high-risk thallium-201 scintigraphic findings in left main coronary artery stenosis: Comparison with patients with multiple- and single-vessel coronary artery disease. Am J Cardiol 1984;53:462–469.

39. Rehn T, Griffith LS, Achuff SC, Bailey IK, Bulkley BH, Burow R, Pitt B, Becker LC: Exercise thallium-201 myocardial imaging in left main coronary artery disease: Sensitive but not specific. Am J Cardiol 1981;48:217–223.

40. Pollock SG, Abbott RD, Boucher CA, Watson DD, Kaul S: A model to predict multivessel coronary artery disease from the exercise thallium-201 stress test. Am J Med 1991;90:345–352.

41. Christian TF, Miller TD, Bailey KR, Gibbons RJ: Noninvasive identification of severe coronary artery disease using exercise tomographic thallium-201 imaging. Am J Cardiol 1992;70:14–20.

41a. Iskandrian AS, Heo J, Lemlek J, Ogilby JD: Identification of high-risk patients with left main and three-vessel coronary artery disease using stepwise discriminant analysis of clinical, exercise, and tomographic thallium data. Am Heart J 1993;125:221–225.

42. Gill JB, Ruddy TD, Newell JB, Finkelstein DM, Strauss HW, Boucher CA: Prognostic importance of thallium uptake by the lungs during exercise in coronary artery disease. N Engl J Med 1987;317:1486–1489.

43. Iskandrian AS, Heo J, Decoskey D, Askenase A, Segal BL: Use of exercise thallium-201 imaging for risk stratification of elderly patients with coronary artery disease. Am J Cardiol 1988;61:269–272.

44. Hilton TC, Shaw LJ, Chaitman BR, Stocke KS, Goodgold HM, Miller DD: Prognostic significance of exercise thallium-201 testing in patients aged greater than or equal to 70 years with known or suspected coronary artery disease. Am J Cardiol 1992;69:45–50.

45. Iskandrian AS, Hakki AH, Kane-Marsch S: Exercise thallium-201 scintigraphy in men with nondiagnostic exercise electrocardiograms. Prognostic implications. Arch Intern Med 1986;146:2189–2193.

46. Fagan LF Jr, Shaw L, Kong BA, Caralis DG, Wiens RD, Chaitman BR: Prognostic value of exercise thallium scintigraphy in patients with good exercise tolerance and a normal or abnormal exercise electrocardiogram and suspected or confirmed coronary artery disease. Am J Cardiol 1992;69:607–611.

47. Wackers FJ, Russo DJ, Russo D, Clements JP: Prognostic significance of normal quantitative planar thallium-201 stress scintigraphy in patients with chest pain. J Am Coll Cardiol 1985;6:27–30.

48. Staniloff HM, Forrester JS, Berman DS, Swan HJ: Prediction of death, myocardial infarction, and worsening chest pain using thallium scintigraphy and exercise electrocardiography. J Nucl Med 1986;27:1842–1848.

49. Pamelia FX, Gibson RS, Watson DD, Craddock GB, Sirowatka J, Beller GA: Prognosis with chest pain and normal thallium-201 exercise scintigrams. Am J Cardiol 1985;55:920–926.

49a. Brown K, Rowen M: Impact of antianginal medications, peak heart rate and stress level on the prognostic value of a normal exercise myocardial perfusion imaging study. J Nucl Med 1993;34:1467–1471.

49b. Steinberg EH, Koss JH, Lee M, Grunwald A, Bodenheimer MM: Prognostic significance from a 10-year follow-up of a qualitatively normal planar exercise thallium test in suspected coronary artery disease. Am J Cardiol 1993;71:1270–1273.

49c. Fattah AA, Kamal AM, Pancholy S, Ghods M, Russell J, Cassel D, Wasserleben V, Heo J, Iskandrian AS: Prognostic implications of normal exercise tomographic thallium images in patients with angiographic evidence of significant coronary artery disease. Am J Cardiol 1994;74:769–771.

49d. Wahl JM, Hakki AH, Iskandrian AS: Prognostic implications of normal exercise thalllium-201 images. Arch Intern Med 1985;145:253–256.

50. Bairey CN, Rozanski A, Maddahi J, Resser KJ, Berman DS: Exercise thallium-201 scintigraphy and prognosis in typical angina pectoris and negative exercise electrocardiography. Am J Cardiol 1989;64:282–287.

50a. Morise AP, Detrano R, Bobbio M, Diamond GA: Development and validation of a logistic regression-derived algorithm for estimating the incremental probability of coronary artery disease before and after exercise testing. J Am Coll Cardiol 1992;20:1187–1196.

50b. Petretta M, Cuocolo A, Carpinelli A, Nicolai E, Valva G, Bianchi V, Salemme L, Salvatore M, Bonaduce D: Prognostic value of myocardial hypoperfusion indexes in patients with suspected or known coronary artery disease. J Nucl Cardiol 1994;1:325–337.

51. Pollock SG, Abbott RD, Boucher CA, Beller GA, Kaul S: Independent and incremental prognostic value of tests performed in hierarchical order to evaluate patients with suspected coronary artery disease. Validation of models based on these tests. Circulation 1992;85:237–248.

52. Vita N, Allam A, Jain D, Maniawski P, Wackers F, Zaret B: Prognostic significance of negative exercise thallium imaging in the presence of a positive electrocardiogram. Circulation 1990;82(S3):357.

52a. Brown K: Critical assessment of prognostic applications of thallium-201 myocardial perfusion imaging. In Zaret B, Beller G (eds): Nuclear Cardiology: State of the Art and Future Directions. St. Louis, CV Mosby, 1993, pp 155–169.

52b. Iskandrian A, Chae S, Hea J, Stanberry C, Wasserleben V, Cave V: Independent and incremental prognostic value of exercise in single-photon emission computed tomography (SPECT) thallium imaging in coronary artery disease. J Am Coll Cardiol 1993;22:665–670.

52c. Brown KA, Rowen M: Prognostic value of a normal exercise myocardial perfusion imaging study in patients with angiographically significant coronary artery disease. Am J Cardiol 1993;71:865–867.

52d. Iskandrian AS, Johnson J, Le TT, Wasserleben V, Care V, Heo J: Comparison of the treadmill exercise score and single-photon emission computed tomographic thallium imaging in risk assessment. J Nucl Cardiol 1994;1:144–149.

53. Wackers F: Artifacts in planar and SPECT myocardial perfusion imaging. Am J Cardiac Imaging 1992;6:42–58.

54. DePuey EG, Garcia EV: Optimal specificity of thallium-201 SPECT through recognition of imaging artifacts. J Nucl Med 1989;30:441–449.

54a. Stratmann HG, Williams GA, Wittry MD, Chaitman BR, Miller DD: Exercise technetium-99m sestamibi tomography for cardiac risk stratification of patients with stable chest pain. Circulation 1994;89:615–622.

54b. Brown KA, Altland E, Rowen M: Prognostic value of normal technetium-99m sestamibi cardiac imaging. J Nucl Med 1994;35:554–557.

54c. Saha M, Farrand TF, Brown KA: Lung uptake of technetium 99m sestamibi: Relation to clinical, exercise, hemodynamic, and left ventricular function variables. J Nucl Cardiol 1994;1:52–56.

54d. Raiker K, Sinusas AJ, Wackers FJ Th, Zaret BL: One-year prognosis of patients with normal planar or single-photon emission computed tomographic technetium-99m–labeled sestamibi exercise imaging. J Nucl Cardiol 1994;1:449–456.

55. Gibbons RJ: The use of radionuclide techniques for identification of severe coronary disease. Curr Probl Cardiol 1990;15:301–352.

56. Gibbons RJ, Fyke FE, Clements IP, Lapeyre AC, Zinsmeister AR, Brown ML: Noninvasive identification of severe coronary artery disease using exercise radionuclide angiography. J Am Coll Cardiol 1988;11:28–34.

57. Leong K, Jones RH: Influence of the location of left anterior descending coronary artery stenosis on left ventricular function during exercise. Circulation 1982;65:109–114.

58. Bonow RO, Kent KM, Rosing DR, Lan KK, Lakatos E, Borer JS, Bacharach SL, Green MV, Epstein SE: Exercise-induced ischemia in mildly symptomatic patients with coronary-artery disease and preserved left ventricular function. Identification of subgroups at risk of death during medical therapy. N Engl J Med 1984;311:1339–1345.

59. Pryor DB, Harrell FE Jr, Lee KL, Rosati RA, Coleman RE, Cobb FR, Califf RM, Jones RH: Prognostic indicators from radionuclide angiography in medically treated patients with coronary artery disease. Am J Cardiol 1984;53:18–22.

60. Iskandrian AS, Hakki AH, Schwartz JS, Kay H, Mattleman S, Kane S: Prognostic implications of rest and exercise radionuclide ventriculography in patients with suspected or proven coronary heart disease. Int J Cardiol 1984;6:707–718.

61. DePace NL, Iskandrian AS, Hakki AH, Kane SA, Segal BL: Value of left ventricular ejection fraction during exercise in predicting the extent of coronary artery disease. J Am Coll Cardiol 1983;1:1002–1010.

62. Mazzotta G, Bonow RO, Pace L, Brittain E, Epstein SE: Relation between exertional ischemia and prognosis in mildly symptomatic patients with single or double vessel coronary artery disease and left ventricular dysfunction at rest. J Am Coll Cardiol 1989;13:567–573.

63. Lee KL, Pryor DB, Pieper KS, Harrell FE Jr, Califf RM, Mark DB, Hlatky MA, Coleman RE, Cobb FR, Jones RH: Prognostic value of radionuclide angiography in medically treated patients with coronary artery disease. A comparison with clinical and catheterization variables. Circulation 1990;82:1705–1717.

64. Taliercio CP, Clements IP, Zinsmeister AR, Gibbons RJ: Prognostic value and limitations of exercise radionuclide angiography in medically treated coronary artery disease. Mayo Clin Proc 1988;63:573–582.

65. Simari RD, Miller TD, Zinsmeister AR, Gibbons RJ: Capabilities of supine exercise electrocardiography versus exercise radionuclide angiography in predicting coronary events. Am J Cardiol 1991;67:573–577.

66. Jones RH, Johnson SH, Bigelow C, Pieper KS, Coleman RE, Cobb FR, Pryor DB, Lee KL: Exercise radionuclide angiocardiography predicts cardiac death in patients with coronary artery disease. Circulation 1991;84:I52–I58.

67. Miller TD, Taliercio CP, Zinsmeister AR, Gibbons RJ: Risk stratifi-

cation of single or double vessel coronary artery disease and impaired left ventricular function using exercise radionuclide angiography. Am J Cardiol 1990;65:1317–1321.

68. Johnson LL, McCarthy DM, Sciacca RR, Cannon PJ: Right ventricular ejection fraction during exercise in patients with coronary artery disease. Circulation 1979;60:1284–1291.

68a. Igbal A, Gibbons RJ, Zinsmeister AR, Mock MB, Ballard DJ: Prognostic value of exercise radionuclide angiography in a population-based cohort of patients with known or suspected coronary artery disease. Am J Cardiol 1994;74:119–124.

69. Gibbons RJ: Rest and exercise radionuclide angiography for diagnosis in chronic ischemic heart disease. Circulation 1991;84:I93–I99.

70. Weintraub WS, Schneider RM, Seelaus PA, Wiener DH, Agarwal JB, Helfant RH: Prospective evaluation of the severity of coronary artery disease with exercise radionuclide angiography and electrocardiography. Am Heart J 1986;111:537–542.

71. Campos CT, Chu HW, D'Agostino HJ Jr, Jones RH: Comparison of rest and exercise radionuclide angiocardiography and exercise treadmill testing for diagnosis of anatomically extensive coronary artery disease. Circulation 1983;67:1204–1210.

72. DePace NL, Hakki AH, Weinreich DJ, Iskandrian AS: Noninvasive assessment of coronary artery disease. Am J Cardiol 1983;52:714–720.

73. Bonow RO, Bacharach SL, Green MV, LaFreniere RL, Epstein SE: Prognostic implications of symptomatic versus asymptomatic (silent) myocardial ischemia induced by exercise in mildly symptomatic and in asymptomatic patients with angiographically documented coronary artery disease. Am J Cardiol 1987;60:778–783.

74. Gibbons RJ, Zinsmeister AR, Miller TD, Clements IP: Supine exercise electrocardiography compared with exercise radionuclide angiography in noninvasive identification of severe coronary artery disease. Ann Intern Med 1990;112:743–749.

74a. Miller TD, Christian TF, Taliercio CP, Zinsmeister AR, Gibbons RJ: Severe exercise-induced ischemia does not identify high risk patients with normal left ventricular function and one- or two-vessel coronary artery disease. J Am Coll Cardiol 1994;23:219–224.

74b. Port SC: The role of radionuclide ventriculography in the assessment of prognosis in patients with CAD. J Nucl Med 1994;35:721–725.

74c. Bonow RO: Prognostic assessment in coronary artery disease: Role of radionuclide angiography. J Nucl Cardiol 1994;1:280–291.

75. Jones EL, Craver JM, Hurst JW, Bradford JA, Bone DK, Robinson PH, Cobbs BW, Thompkins TR, Hatcher CR Jr: Influence of left ventricular aneurysm on survival following the coronary bypass operation. Ann Surg 1981;193:733–742.

76. Sawada SG, Ryan T, Conley MJ, Corya BC, Feigenbaum H, Armstrong WF: Prognostic value of a normal exercise echocardiogram. Am Heart J 1990;120:49–55.

77. Hecht HS, DeBord L, Shaw R, Dunlap R, Ryan C, Stertzer SH, Myler RK: Digital supine bicycle stress echocardiography: A new technique for evaluating coronary artery disease. J Am Coll Cardiol 1993;21:950–956.

78. Krivokapich J, Child JS, Gerber RS, Lem V, Moser D: Prognostic usefulness of positive or negative exercise stress echocardiography for predicting coronary events in ensuing twelve months. Am J Cardiol 1993;71:646–651.

79. Mertes H, Erbel R, Nixdorff U, Mohr-Kahaly S, Kruger S, Meyer J: Exercise echocardiography for the evaluation of patients after nonsurgical coronary artery revascularization. J Am Coll Cardiol 1993;21:1087–1093.

80. Roger V, Pellika PA, Oh JK, Bailey KR, Tajik AJ: Identification of multivessel coronary artery disease by exercise echocardiography. J Am Coll Cardiol 1994;24:109–114.

81. Matzer L, Kiat H, VanTrain K, Germano G, Papinicalaou M, Silagan G, Eigler N, Maddahi J, Berman D: Quantitative severity of stress thallium-201 myocardial perfusion single-photon emission computed tomography defects in one-vessel coronary artery disease. Am J Cardiol 1993;72:273–279.

Chapter 5

Noninvasive Evaluation of Silent Myocardial Ischemia

Silent myocardial ischemia is defined as objective evidence of myocardial ischemia by direct or indirect measurements of left ventricular (LV) function, perfusion, metabolism, or electrical activity in a patient who has no chest pain or other angina equivalents. Objective manifestations of myocardial ischemia, at rest or during stress, without associated angina have increasingly been recognized in totally asymptomatic subjects, in patients with suspected coronary artery disease (CAD), chronic stable angina or unstable angina, and after myocardial infarction (MI), coronary angioplasty, or bypass surgery.[1–6] Cohn has proposed a classification scheme for silent ischemia that has been useful for categorizing asymptomatic and symptomatic populations for epidemiologic retrospective or prospective studies.[5] Type I silent ischemia is totally asymptomatic; type II is silent ischemia that is detected after an MI, and type III describes manifestations of both angina and silent ischemia at different periods or events during the course of several hours or days.

PATHOPHYSIOLOGY OF SILENT ISCHEMIA

The mechanism and pathogenesis of silent myocardial ischemia are currently unresolved. Some proposed mechanisms include a high pain threshold; varying concentration of endogenous opiates in response to stress; insufficient ischemia to reach anginal threshold; and destruction of neural pathways from the heart by infarction, diabetes, surgical intervention with bypass surgery, or cardiac transplantation.[1]

Various "triggers" of silent ischemia have been identified.[7] These include a sudden increase in heart rate or systemic pressure during daily activities or at rest, transient diminution in blood flow due to exaggerated vasomotor sensitivity to such mediators as norepinephrine, histamine, serotonin, and acetylcholine. Mental stress and cigarette smoking are other triggers of silent ischemia. A pathogenic mechanism for transient diminutions in blood flow is platelet aggregation, which can occur as a consequence of many of the triggers cited above.

A primary reduction in myocardial blood flow appears to be an important factor in precipitating episodes of silent ischemia. Silent ischemia precipitated by mental arithmetic and a cold pressor test was shown to decrease regional myocardial blood flow as assessed by rubidium-82 (Rb-82) positron emission tomography (PET).[8] Rozanski et al.[9] suggested that increased myocardial oxygen demand may be an important factor in silent myocardial ischemia provoked by mental stress. This group of investigators reported that silent ischemia precipitated by mental stress was associated with an increase in systolic and diastolic blood pressures comparable to that associated with exercise-induced ischemia in the same patients. Figure 5–1 shows the deterioration in LV segmental wall motion on radionuclide angiography during mental stress in one of the patients in this study. Langer et al.[10] also noted that the rate-pressure product increased significantly before and during asymptomatic episodes of ischemia in 196 patients with unstable angina.

REST

SPEECH

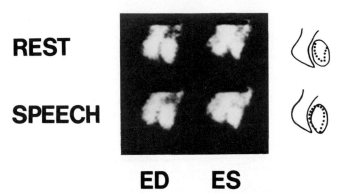

ED   ES

Figure 5–1. End-diastolic (ED) and end-systolic (ES) radionuclide angiographic images obtained at rest and after mental stress (SPEECH) in the left anterior oblique projection. Note the worsening of left ventricular segmental wall motion when the patient spoke about his feelings of personal stress. The diagrams on the right of the images show superimposed end-diastolic and end-systolic contours. During stress, dyskinesis was observed in the septum. (Reprinted by permission of *The New England Journal of Medicine* from Rozanski A, et al.: Mental stress and induction of silent myocardial ischemia in patients with coronary artery disease. N Engl J Med 318:1005–1012, Copyright 1988, Massachusetts Medical Society.)

The heart rate at the onset of ischemia that is silent and recorded during daily activities is lower than the peak heart rate associated with ischemia on a maximal exercise test. McLenachan et al.[11] found that the heart rate at onset of ischemia by ambulatory electrocardiographic (ECG) monitoring in 21 patients averaged 95 bpm, whereas the heart rate at onset of ischemia during a Bruce exercise test averaged 117 bpm in the same patients. Thus, it is possible that the combination of a primary decrease in regional flow and an increase in oxygen demand is the important pathophysiologic factor associated with silent ischemia during daily life.

Frequency of Silent Ischemia and Circadian Pattern

There appears to be a circadian variation in the timing of transient myocardial ischemia.[7, 12–14] With the improved

techniques of ambulatory ECG monitoring, several groups have firmly established that, in the absence of antiischemic therapy, most patients with chronic CAD exhibit frequent episodes of transient ischemia manifested by ST-segment depression during routine out-of-hospital activities. As many as 70% to 90% of these episodes of ST-segment depression are clinically silent.[15] The continuous ambulatory ECG monitoring surveys have consistently shown a peak incidence of episodes of ischemia between the hours of 6:00 A.M. and noon. Interestingly, many of the triggers of transient ischemia cited previously are most prominent during the early morning hours. Heart rate, blood pressure, and contractility rate are increased in the morning hours, which support the hypothesis that increases in myocardial oxygen demand contribute to increased prevalence of ischemia in the morning. However, increased coronary vascular tone may contribute to increased ischemia in the morning hours. Quyyumi et al.[14] recently reported that, in patients with stable angina, exercise performance was most limited in the morning and at night at times when forearm vascular resistance, and presumably coronary vascular resistance, was highest. They observed a circadian variation in vascular tone, basal forearm vascular resistance being significantly higher, and the blood flow significantly lower, in the morning than in the afternoon or evening. Figure 5–2 shows the hourly variation in transient episodes of ST-segment depression and mean hourly heart rate on 24-hour ambulatory ECG monitoring in patients with stable CAD studied by Quyyumi et al.[14] Eighty-eight percent of the transient episodes of ST depression were silent. The frequency of ST depression had a strong correlation with postischemic forearm vascular resistance.

DETECTION OF SILENT MYOCARDIAL ISCHEMIA

Four noninvasive approaches to detection of silent myocardial ischemia have gained significant clinical use: (1) conventional exercise ECG symptom-limited submaximal stress tests; (2) stress radionuclide imaging using an agent

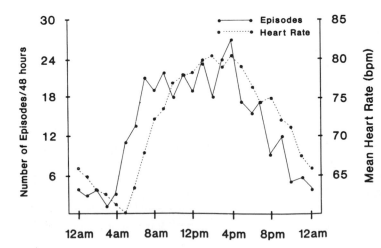

Figure 5–2. Graph shows hourly variation in transient episodes of ST-segment depression *(solid line)* and mean hourly heart rate in beats per minute (bpm). Episodes of ST depression were most likely to occur around 7:00 A.M., whereas episodes were least likely to occur between 7:00 P.M. and 7:00 A.M. (Quyyumi AA, et al.: Circulation 1992;86:22–28.)

either to assess myocardial perfusion or to evaluate global and regional function; (3) ambulatory ECG (Holter monitoring); and (4) ambulatory assessment of global LV function employing a portable scintillation probe applied on the chest wall over the LV chamber or using the VEST device (see Chap. 1). The latter technique can measure LV ejection fraction (LVEF) on line during ambulatory activities.

In the sections to follow, the prevalence and prognostic significance of silent myocardial ischemia in various patient subgroups are discussed. In each of these sections, the clinical utility of the noninvasive approaches cited above is examined.

DETECTION OF SILENT MYOCARDIAL ISCHEMIA IN TOTALLY ASYMPTOMATIC SUBJECTS

Exercise Electrocardiographic Stress Testing

Screening asymptomatic subjects for occult CAD has been undertaken principally with exercise ECG stress testing. Bertolet and Pepine[1] determined the prevalence of silent ischemia in totally asymptomatic populations employing more than 1.0 mm of ST-segment depression as evidence of stress-induced ischemia. When such populations have been screened, the prevalence of a positive stress test averaged 9% in the pooled analysis of 23,688 people. Most of the studies from which this pooled analysis was derived included middle-aged men. When coronary angiography was employed to confirm the presence or absence of CAD in patients with a positive ECG response, only 3% of patients with abnormal ST-segment depression had significant coronary stenosis. This implies that, for every three patients screened who manifested a positive ST-segment response for ischemia, only one demonstrates significant CAD by angiography. This illustrates that the false-positive rate for the silent ST-depression response is high in this group of asymptomatic persons.

Nevertheless, when asymptomatic subjects with a positive ST-segment response are followed over the long term, the subsequent cardiac event rate is significantly higher than that for subjects who exhibit a normal response to exercise stress testing.[1] The event rate is substantially higher among patients who have underlying cardiac risk factors for CAD in addition to a positive ECG response to stress. McHenry et al.[16] followed 916 healthy men for 8 to 15 years with serial exercise testing. Of 61 with ST-segment depression, 29% developed angina, one died suddenly, and one had a subsequent infarction. Of the remaining 833, 25 had a subsequent infarction, seven experienced sudden death, and 12 developed angina. Thus, an abnormal ST-segment response is more predictive of the subsequent appearance of angina but not of MI or sudden death as an initial coronary event.

Bruce and coworkers studied 2365 clinically healthy men. Only 2% had a primary cardiac event at 5.6 ± 1.4 years after exercise testing.[17] One percent of the study population had at least one risk factor for CAD and two or more exercise predictors, and their risk for a subsequent cardiac event was 33%. Certain findings on clinical evaluation and an exercise stress test were shown to improve the predictive value for detecting significant CAD in asymptomatic men.[18] High-risk CAD was seen with greater frequency if a patient had a conventional risk factor and two of three of the following exercise test abnormalities: (1) more than 3.0 mm ST-segment depression by stage 2 of the Bruce protocol; (2) 1.0 mm of ST depression persisting for 6 minutes after exercise; (3) total exercise duration less than 10 minutes. Of 225 asymptomatic men evaluated, 13 had multivessel disease. Sixteen of the 33 could be classified as being at high risk by the presence of a CAD risk factor and of two of the three variables described above. This yielded an 84% predictive value for detection of multivessel CAD.

Other patient populations described in the Multiple Risk Factor Intervention Trial (MRFIT)[19] and the Lipid Research Clinics Trial[20] have demonstrated that positive exercise test responders had a severalfold greater change of developing subsequent cardiac events than negative responders.

Limitations of Exercise Electrocardiographic Stress Testing

Significant limitations exist for utilizing ST depression alone on exercise testing for silent myocardial ischemia. First, sensitivity for CAD detection utilizing exercise electrocardiography is only in the range of 60% to 75% (see Chap. 3). The false-positive rate of the ST-segment response is high in low-prevalence CAD populations. Diamond and Forrester have indicated that the exercise ECG alone generally is not useful when applied to a patient population with a low pretest likelihood of CAD.[21] The predictive accuracy of any test for CAD detection, such as the exercise ECG, is based not only on sensitivity and specificity values but also on the prevalence of the disease in the population under study. This is recognized as Bayes' theorem (see Chap. 3). For example, in a subject with only a 10% pretest likelihood of CAD, 1.0 mm ST-segment depression at peak exercise increases the likelihood of CAD after testing to only 35%. This is because the false-positive rate is quite high for the mildly positive exercise ST response in this type of patient.

The exercise ECG is also limited when resting ST-segment abnormalities are present such as those induced by hyperventilation or those present because of underlying LV hypertrophy. Non–coronary artery disease entities such as mitral valve prolapse or Wolff-Parkinson-White syndrome can be associated with resting ST-segment abnormalities that can be associated with a false-positive ST response during exercise stress.

Exercise radionuclide imaging can enhance both sensitivity and specificity for detecting silent myocardial ischemia in totally asymptomatic subjects. The rationale for using exercise radionuclide imaging to detect ischemia in symptomatic populations is based on the following facts: (1) Perfusion imaging is more sensitive and specific than exercise ST-segment depression in identifying patients with ischemia. (2) Patients at high risk for CAD can be identified by the combination of imaging and exercise ECG stress test variables better than by exercise ECG stress tests alone. (3) Ischemia-induced perfusion abnormalities tend to occur before the onset of angina in patients who undergo treadmill testing. Exercise thallium-201 (Tl-201) imaging has proven to be very useful in distinguishing between true-positive and false-positive ECG responses, thereby reducing the requirement for coronary angiography to determine whether an abnormal exercise ECG stress test response indicates underlying CAD or is a false-positive result.[22]

Myocardial Perfusion Imaging and Detection of Silent Ischemia

Myocardial perfusion imaging in conjunction with exercise ECG stress testing has been employed to identify patients who manifest silent ischemia due to occult CAD and who are totally asymptomatic. An interesting study involved 130 asymptomatic Air Force pilots who were referred for cardiac catheterization because of coronary risk factors or a positive stress ECG.[23] Of the 22 who had significant CAD characterized by at least 50% stenosis, all had an abnormal Tl-201 scan. Of all 130 patients, 12 were deemed by angiography to have nonsignificant disease (lesions ranging between 25% and 50% reduction in luminal diameter). Of these, eight also had abnormal Tl-201 scans. These data suggested that exercise scintigraphy can be useful for identifying or confirming silent ischemia in an asymptomatic patient demonstrating painless ST depression on a screening exercise ECG.

Asymptomatic patients at increased risk for occult CAD include siblings of patients with premature-onset CAD. In one study by Rissanen et al.,[24] when a male had a myocardial infarction before age 46, his unaffected brothers had a 55% chance of developing CAD by age 55. Becker et al.[25] initiated the Johns Hopkins Sibling Screening Project in 1982, in which exercise ECG and tomographic Tl-201 imaging were utilized to detect asymptomatic CAD in siblings of patients who manifested premature CAD. In a preliminary report, they enrolled 83 sibling participants whose average age was 46 years; 79 underwent planar Tl-201 imaging and 65 had tomographic studies. The tomographic Tl-201 study demonstrated an abnormality in 23% of siblings; 6% had abnormal planar Tl-201 scan, and 11% demonstrated exercise-induced ischemic ST-segment depression. When borderline scintigraphic results were included, 28% of the tomographic Tl-201 scans revealed perfusion abnormalities, 20% of the planar Tl-201 studies were abnormal, and the exercise ECG was abnormal in 12% of siblings. Interestingly, only 4% of these subjects had chest pain on the treadmill suggestive of angina pectoris. As expected, the frequency of a scan abnormality increased with decade of age in men and increased in relation to the number of coronary risk factors (Fig. 5–3). The single-photon emission computed tomography (SPECT) Tl-201 studies were abnormal or borderline in only 16% of siblings who had no CAD risk factors but were abnormal in 50% of those who had two or three risk factors. These results suggest that exercise SPECT Tl-201 imaging may be useful for detecting occult symptomatic CAD in a high-risk population with CAD risk factors and a strong family history of premature CAD. A conclusion derived from this study was that the sensitivity of exercise ECG alone is insufficient for screening this type of population.

Fleg et al. examined whether detection of abnormal myocardial perfusion with exercise Tl-201 scintigraphy could identify occult CAD in an asymptomatic population.[26] They performed maximal treadmill ECG exercise testing with Tl-201 scintigraphy in 407 asymptomatic volunteers aged 40 to 96 years (mean, 60 years) from the Baltimore Longitudinal Study on Aging. The prevalence of exercise-induced silent ischemia, which was defined by the concordant presence of ST-segment depression and a Tl-201 perfusion defect, increased more than sevenfold, from 2% in the fifth and sixth decades of life to 15% in the ninth decade. Over

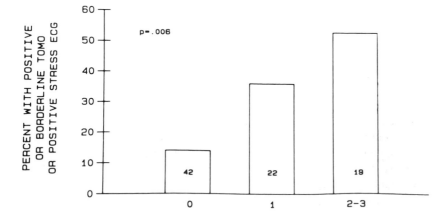

Figure 5–3. Frequency of SPECT Tl-201 scan abnormality relative to number of coronary risk factors (hypertension, classifiable lipid disorder, or low HDL cholesterol) in asymptomatic subjects. Numbers in bars represent number of participants in each risk factor group. (Becker LC, et al.: Circulation 1987;75:II-14–II-17.)

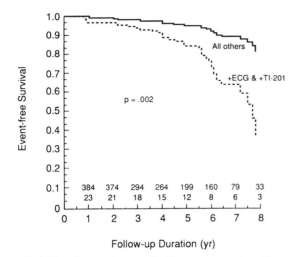

Figure 5–4. Plot of event-free survival in asymptomatic subjects with concordant positive ECG and Tl-201 results for ischemia versus all other patient subgroups. A concordant positive result predicted a 3.6-fold risk for a coronary event, independent of conventional risk factors. Numbers along the *x* axis indicate the number of persons at risk for each year in the All-others *(top)* and the positive ECG and positive Tl-201 *(bottom)* groups, respectively. (Fleg J, et al.: Circulation 1990;81:428–436.)

a mean follow-up period of 4.6 years, cardiac events developed in 9.8% of subjects: 20 patients experienced new-onset angina pectoris, 13 had nonfatal myocardial infarctions, and seven died. Cardiac events were observed in 7% of subjects who had both a negative Tl-201 scan and a negative ECG, 8% of those who had one positive test result, and 48% of those whose tests were both positive ($P <$ 0.001). By proportional hazards analysis, age, hypertension, exercise duration, and a concordant positive ECG and Tl-201 perfusion scan were independent predictors of coronary events. Patients with a concordantly positive exercise ECG for ischemia and an abnormal Tl-201 scan had a 3.6-fold relative risk for subsequent coronary events, independent of conventional risk factors. Figure 5–4 illustrates a worse rate

of event-free survival during an 8-year follow-up for subjects with a positive exercise ST response and an abnormal Tl-201 scan, as compared with other subgroups followed in this study. Thus, in an asymptomatic population, occult CAD was detected with a high degree of accuracy when the criteria for a positive test included the proviso that both the exercise ECG and Tl-201 scan be abnormal. Exercise-induced silent ischemia increases progressively with age and does identify a small group of subjects who subsequently have an almost 50% cardiac event rate. It should be pointed out, however, that, of the 20 patients who died ($N = 7$) or experienced a nonfatal infarction ($N = 13$) during the study, 13 had two negative results on initial screening and two had only a positive exercise ECG. Thus, 65% of the patients who experienced a "hard event" had a negative Tl-201 scan on initial testing. Even though the event-free survival rate was better for patients with a negative than with a positive ischemic response to stress, more than 50% of the patients who experienced events had negative responses.

Approach to Detecting Silent Ischemia in Asymptomatic Subjects

Some basic guidelines, derived from clinical experience, can improve the efficiency and accuracy of diagnosing silent MI in asymptomatic patients. Figure 5–5 provides an approach to stress testing in totally asymptomatic subjects referred for stress testing for a variety of reasons,[26a] including a strong family history of CAD, multiple CAD risk factors, or consideration for a large amount of life insurance. The exercise ECG stress test is cost effective as the initial test to be performed. If the exercise ECG shows no ST-segment depression or no angina at a very high workload (at least 85% or more of maximum predicted heart rate for age) with a normal exercise blood pressure response,

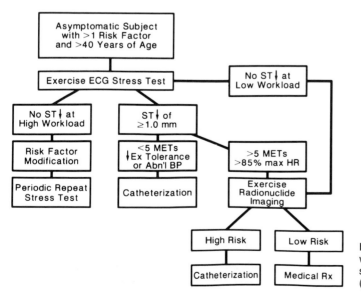

Figure 5–5. Approach to stress testing in an asymptomatic subject with >1 risk factor and >40 years of age. (Key: ST ↓, ST depression; Ex, exercise; Abn'l BP, abnormal blood pressure response.) (Beller GA: Am J Cardiol 1987;59:31C–38C.)

then risk-factor modification would be appropriate since the patient would have a low probability of having significant functionally important CAD. If the patient exhibits a positive ischemic ST-segment response (1 mm or more of horizontal or downsloping depression) that occurs at less than 5 MET and is associated with either diminished exercise tolerance or abnormal blood pressure response, the test probably represents a true-positive ischemic response. A positive test in response to a light workload or slow exercise heart rate response suggests a strong possibility of silent ischemia. The patient could then be referred directly to cardiac catheterization without performing a repeat exercise stress test with a radionuclide study.

A normal ST-segment response to a light exercise workload may represent a false-negative response and should lead to repeat exercise testing in association with a myocardial perfusion scan. If the perfusion scan suggests high risk, catheterization is appropriate. If the scan is positive for ischemia but shows defects confined to one myocardial segment, suggestive of one-vessel CAD, medical therapy and risk factor modification could be a reasonable first-line therapeutic step. Finally, certain asymptomatic patients develop transient ST-segment depression at a high heart rate or heavy workload without accompanying angina or hemodynamic alterations. This often proves to be a false-positive ST-segment response. Repeat testing with myocardial perfusion imaging should be used to distinguish a true-positive response from a false-positive one, thereby avoiding unnecessary cardiac catheterization. If a transient regional perfusion abnormality was observed on repeat testing, the diagnosis of CAD would be firmly established. If the scan was negative, particularly by quantitative criteria, then the ST-segment depression would be deemed a false-positive response. Figure 5–6 shows the SPECT perfusion tomograms acquired in a patient with silent ST depression with no evidence for stress-induced perfusion abnormalities. This represents a false-positive ST-segment depression response rather than silent myocardial ischemia.

DETECTION OF SILENT MYOCARDIAL ISCHEMIA IN SYMPTOMATIC PATIENTS SUSPECTED OR KNOWN TO HAVE CORONARY ARTERY DISEASE

Ambulatory (Holter) Electrocardiographic Monitoring

Ambulatory ECG recording has enjoyed increased use for detection of silent ischemia in patients with known CAD, which may at times be symptomatic (e.g., stable exertional angina).[6, 27–35a] In a recent review of the literature, Bertolet and Pepine[1] determined from a pooled analysis of published studies that 63% of patients with stable angina pectoris demonstrated silent ischemia on ambulatory ECG monitoring. Of all episodes of ST-segment depression re-

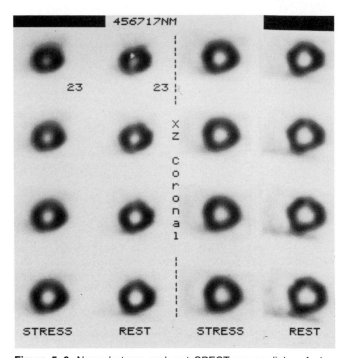

Figure 5–6. Normal stress and rest SPECT myocardial perfusion scan in a patient with a false-positive ST-segment depression response.

corded in these patients during daily activities, 81% were silent. Of interest is that most symptomatic episodes of ischemia are preceded by prolonged periods of silent ischemia before the patient is cognizant of symptoms. In one of the largest studies undertaken to assess the efficacy of various treatment strategies for suppressing silent myocardial ischemia, Pepine et al.[35a] found that 982 (49%) of 1959 patients with angiographic CAD had asymptomatic ischemia on ambulatory ECG monitoring. Most patients were men, were older than 60 years of age, and had multivessel CAD. The majority (81%) had two or more ischemic episodes per 48 hours and many had ST-segment depression early during an exercise test. Review of the published literature suggests that the number of episodes of silent ischemia ranges from approximately 4 to 5 per 24 hours' monitoring. As mentioned previously, the frequency of episodes of silent as well as symptomatic ST-segment depression peaks in the first 1 to 4 hours after awakening, and perhaps as much as 40% of ischemic activity is detected between 6 A.M. and noon.

There are some distinct advantages to the ambulatory ECG monitoring technique for detecting and quantitating episodes of silent ischemia. They include the ability to correlate episodes of ischemia with triggers such as mental stress or cigarette smoking, and the ability to provide a relatively long period of survey, permitting assessment of responses to antiischemic therapy when posttreatment and pretreatment recordings are compared. The continuous monitoring can determine whether or not ischemic episodes are preceded by an increase in heart rate or blood pressure

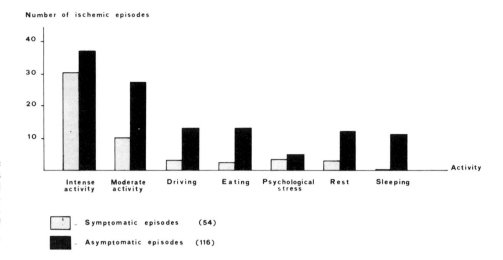

Number of ischemic episodes

Figure 5–7. Frequency of symptomatic or asymptomatic ischemic episodes relative to different activity levels and relative to various daily tasks. (Reprinted with permission from the American College of Cardiology (Journal of the American College of Cardiology, 1983, Vol. 1, pp. 934–939).)

or are precipitated by a primary diminution in coronary blood flow, as with vasoconstrictor stimuli. Figure 5–7 shows the number of symptomatic and asymptomatic episodes of ischemia on ambulatory ECG monitoring with various activities such as driving, eating, sleeping, and psychological stress in the study by Cecchi et al.[36] Episodes of ST depression on ambulatory ECG monitoring can last as long as 100 minutes.[37]

Currently, most of the equipment used for recording the ambulatory ECG provides an accurate reproduction of the ischemic ST-segment response, but great quality control and meticulous attention to detail are required. Conscientious skin preparation is mandatory. One significant technical factor is the required frequency response in the recording and playback system. The ST-segment response is a low-frequency event compared with the QRS signal, so frequency-modulated (FM) recorders with extended low-frequency responses should be used. Selection of at least two leads, one of which is V_4 or V_5, provides the greatest extent of cardiac electrical sampling of the left ventricle. Performance of a Valsalva maneuver and hyperventilation should be done before each monitoring period, for baseline sampling. Sophisticated computers have been used to assist in the analysis of long recordings, and caution should be exercised when digitization and storage of the ECG is undertaken. Compression of data may cause loss of the ability to play back some or all of the original recording. Operator interaction permits interpretation of questionable signals and artifact. Patients must be encouraged to keep an accurate diary of events during monitoring.

The precise duration of ambulatory monitoring to obtain maximum sensitivity has not yet been determined, but some have advocated at least 48 hours of recording. Despite some potential technical factors that can contribute to false-positive ST-segment responses on ambulatory ECG monitoring, the technique has proven useful for identifying patients who have frequent episodes of silent ischemia during daily activities and, thus, are at higher risk for subsequent ischemic events than are patients with known stable CAD who do

not routinely manifest frequent episodes of asymptomatic ST-segment depression. Because of its low sensitivity and specificity, ambulatory ECG ST-segment analysis is not as accurate as other modalities for establishing or excluding CAD. Its use should be limited to patients whose coronary disease status is already known.[38]

Exercise Electrocardiographic Stress Testing

Exercise ECG testing, with or without radionuclide imaging, has been widely employed for detection of ischemia, whether silent or associated with angina, in patients suspected or known to have CAD. As many as 50% of patients with CAD who undergo symptom-limited exercise testing exhibit ischemic ST-segment depression without accompanying angina.[39] Mark et al. from Duke evaluated the exercise tests of 1698 consecutive symptomatic patients with CAD.[40] Of these, 856 had no exercise ST deviation, 242 had painless exercise ST deviation, and 600 had ST-segment deviation accompanied by angina during stress testing. Of all 842 patients who had a positive ST-segment response during exercise, 29% had silent ischemia on testing, as evidenced by painless ST depression. This prevalence is slightly lower than that reported by the CASS investigators.[41] Patients with exercise-induced angina had a history of a longer and more aggressive clinical course with more anginal episodes and a higher prevalence of a progressive anginal pattern than patients without angina on testing. In this study, those who exhibited angina with ST depression had more severe anatomic CAD than patients who demonstrated only silent ST-segment depression. In the report by Miranda et al.,[42] 41% of patients who had no clinical or ECG evidence of MI had silent ST depression on treadmill testing. Thus, many patients with stable symptomatic CAD have a positive ischemic response on exercise ECG stress testing without accompanying angina. The prognostic implications of painless ST depression on treadmill testing are discussed later in this chapter.

The limitations of the exercise ECG stress test in patients with a low pretest likelihood of CAD have already been discussed in some detail (see Chap. 3). It suffices to say that the predictive value of an asymptomatic ST-segment depression response in a patient with a low pretest likelihood of CAD (atypical chest pain in a middle-aged woman) is low. The principle of Bayes' theorem is that, as the prevalence of a disease in a population diminishes, false-positive results comprise a larger proportion of all abnormal results. The pretest likelihood of CAD would be approximately 20% in a 50-year-old woman with atypical chest pain.[43] Even for a man with atypical chest pain, the pretest likelihood of coronary disease is still only about 40%. The probability increases to 90% for the hypothetical 50-year-old man who presents with symptoms typical of angina pectoris. The sensitivity of the exercise ECG stress test for detection of CAD is also suboptimal (see Chap. 3). Results of studies published in the literature have demonstrated that the sensitivity of more than 1.0 mm of horizontal or down-sloping ST-segment depression for CAD detection is only in the range of 65%. Because of limited sensitivity and specificity of the exercise ECG for detecting ischemia, myocardial perfusion imaging or exercise radionuclide angiography has been performed in association with treadmill or bicycle ECG stress testing to enhance both sensitivity and specificity for CAD in patients suspected to have silent myocardial ischemia. Identification of such patients, even though asymptomatic on antianginal medications, may be of significant prognostic importance (see Chap. 4).

Myocardial Perfusion Imaging and Radionuclide Angiography

Tl-201 imaging may yield important supplementary information in assessing patients with possible silent myocardial ischemia. Perfusion imaging with Tl-201 is (1) more sensitive and specific for the ischemic response than ST-segment depression analysis; (2) can define the anatomic site of ischemia; and (3) detects ischemia even in the presence of baseline ECG abnormalities. Enhanced sensitivity of Tl-201 scintigraphy over that of the ST-segment response is observed at all levels of exercise.[44] The prognostic value of Tl-201 redistribution defects in patients with known or suspected coronary disease has been reported to be superior to that of the exercise stress test variables alone.[45]

Gasperetti et al.[46] sought to prospectively determine the prevalence of silent ischemic responses in a group of patients who underwent symptom-limited exercise Tl-201 testing. The clinical, exercise test, and angiographic variables that best correlated with painless ischemia as determined by exercise Tl-201 scintigraphic criteria were also determined. There were 103 consecutive patients who manifested exercise-induced Tl-201 redistribution (criteria for ischemia) on symptom-limited exercise scintigraphy. Of

these, 59 (57%) had no angina accompanying this ischemic response on serial Tl-201 images. A significantly greater percentage of patients with silent ischemia than of those with angina had recently had an MI (31% vs. 7%), had no prior angina (91% vs. 64%), had dyspnea as an exercise test endpoint (56% vs. 35%), and exhibited redistribution defects in the supply regions of the right and circumflex coronary arteries (50% vs. 35%). The group with exercise angina and Tl-201 redistribution had more ST depression (64% vs. 41%) than did patients with silent Tl-201 redistribution.

In the study of Gasperetti et al,[46] no difference was observed between the silent ischemia and angina groups with respect to the mean total Tl-201 perfusion score, number of redistribution defects per patient, multivessel Tl-201 redistribution pattern, or extent of angiographic CAD. Figure 5-8 compares the extent of ischemia on quantitative Tl-201 scintigrams for the 59 patients with silent ischemia and the 44 patients with angina in this study. There was no significant difference in the number of Tl-201 redistribution defects per patient between those with silent ischemia (2.3 ± 1.1) and those with angina (2.5 ± 1.4) subgroups. There was no difference between silent ischemia and angina groups with respect to antiangina drug use, prevalence of diabetes mellitus, exercise duration, peak exercise heart rate, peak workload, peak double product, and percentage of patients who achieved at least 85% of maximal predicted heart rate for age. Thus, in this study group of consecutive patients who manifested a positive Tl-201 scan for ischemia, there was a rather high prevalence of silent ischemia (57%) by exercise Tl-201 criteria. Patients with silent ischemia and those with exercise angina had comparable (1) exercise tolerance and hemodynamics, (2) extent of angiographic CAD, and (3) extent of exercise-induced perfusion abnormalities. Table 5-1 compares angina and silent ischemia groups in this study with respect to extent of angiographic CAD, prevalence of ischemic ST-segment depression, and presence of a multivessel CAD scan pattern.

Hecht et al.[47] compared the amount of ischemic myocardium, utilizing SPECT Tl-201 exercise and redistribution imaging in patients experiencing angina during exercise treadmill testing and in those who had silent ischemia on

Table 5-1. **Comparison of Angina and Silent Ischemia Groups Who Had Exercise Tl-201 Redistribution**

	Angina (N = 44)	Silent Ischemia (N = 59)
Multivessel coronary artery disease (%)	79	70
Jeopardy score	7.5 ± 3.5	7.3 ± 3.7
ST ↓ ≥1.0 mm (%)	64	41*
Multiple redistribution defects (%)	25	25

*$P < 0.05$.
(Reprinted with permission from the American College of Cardiology (Journal of the American College of Cardiology, 1990, Vol. 16, pp. 115–123).)

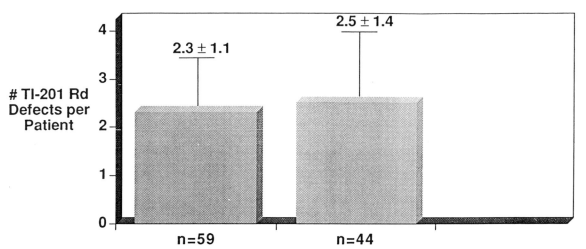

Figure 5–8. Comparison of silent ischemia *(left bar)* and angina *(right bar)* groups with respect to extent of Tl-201 redistribution. The number of Tl-201 redistribution (Rd) defects per patient was similar in the group who manifested silent Tl-201 redistribution on exercise scintigraphy and in those who exhibited exercise-induced angina in association with Tl-201 redistribution. (Adapted from Gasperetti CM, et al.: J Am Coll Cardiol 1990;16:115–123.)

testing. In 112 consecutive patients who demonstrated Tl-201 redistribution defects on tomographic imaging, only 28 had associated pain with stress. The number of ischemic scan segments was comparable in silent ischemia (7.4 segments) and painful ischemia (7.6 segments) groups (Fig. 5–9). As shown in the study by Gasperetti et al.,[46] no difference was observed in the incidence of single-, double-, or triple-vessel disease between silent and painful ischemia groups. Those with chest pain accompanying an ischemic scintigraphic response had a higher incidence of positive ECGs (70%) than did patients with silent ischemia (32%). Thus, these two studies[46, 47] found that patients who exhibit silent or painful ischemia have similar amounts of ischemic myocardium on Tl-201 imaging and a similar extent of CAD on angiography.

Mahmarian et al.[48] found that the extent of quantified SPECT perfusion defects was comparable in patients with (20.9% ± 15.9%) and without (20.5% ± 15.6%) exertional chest pain, which confirms the findings of Gasperetti et al.[46] and Hecht et al.[47] Furthermore, silent ischemia was five times more common than symptomatic ischemic (83% vs. 17%) in patients with significant CAD. Figure 5–10 shows that the perfusion defect size (% left ventricle) was comparable in patients with or without chest pain in this study.

Travin et al.[49] compared 134 patients with Tl-201 redistribution and no angina on exercise Tl-201 scintigraphy with 134 patients who demonstrated redistribution and had angina during testing. In contrast to the findings just described,[46–48] these investigators found that patients with si-

Figure 5–9. Comparison of silent versus painful ischemia in patients undergoing SPECT Tl-201 scintigraphy with respect to number of ischemic segments showing total or partial Tl-201 redistribution *(left panel)* and number of segments showing total redistribution *(right panel)*. (Adapted from Hecht HS, et al.: J Am Coll Cardiol 1989;14:895–900.)

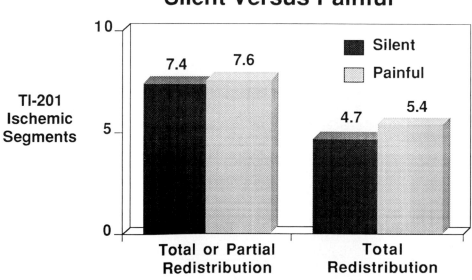

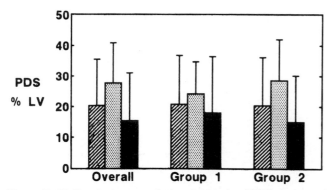

Figure 5–10. Graph shows perfusion defect size (PDS) expressed as a percentage of the left ventricle (%LV) in the overall patient population who have significant CAD and in patients with (group 1) and without (group 2) chest pain. Patients with myocardial infarction are depicted by the dotted bars, and patients without myocardial infarction by the solid bars. The striped bars represent all patients in each group. (Mahmarian JJ, et al.: Circulation 1990;82:1305–1315.)

lent ischemia by Tl-201 scan criteria had fewer redistribution defects and less severity of the worst redistribution defect and a lower ischemic index (both extent and severity of perfusion abnormalities), and that the worst of their redistribution defects was less severe. Nevertheless, the prevalence of adverse events was comparable in silent ischemia and angina groups (21% vs. 29%). In the silent ischemia group, the lung-heart Tl-201 ratio correlated best with subsequent nonfatal MI or cardiac death. Klein et al.[49a] evaluated a population of patients who manifested ischemic ST-segment depression during treadmill testing. Of these, 75% had silent ischemia. Compared with those with silent ischemia, patients with exercise-induced chest pain had a shorter exercise duration, a lower peak exercise heart rate and double product, earlier ST-segment depression, a higher prevalence of ischemic defects on SPECT Tl-201 images, and a higher summed reversibility score. However, when the population was restricted to represent a cohort with a high likelihood of CAD, the extent of ischemia was more comparable in those with and those without chest pain accompanying exercise. This latter observation is consistent with the findings of Gasperetti et al.[46] in which all patients had reversible Tl-201 defects indicative of a high prevalence of CAD and definite inducible ischemia during stress. Figure 5–11 depicts the frequency of Tl-201 scan abnormalities in patients with a positive exercise test with or without chest pain in the study of Klein et al.[49a]

The intensity of exercise achieved may play a role in determining whether or not a patient develops angina with an ischemic scintigraphic response on exercise Tl-201 stress testing.[50] Heller et al.[50] studied 19 CAD patients at two different levels of exercise. A symptom-limited exercise test according to the Bruce protocol was followed within 2 weeks by a submaximal, steady-state exercise test performed at 70% of the maximal heart rate achieved on the first test. Incremental exercise resulted in angina symptoms

in 84% of patients and ECG changes and Tl-201 redistribution in all patients. In contrast, submaximal exercise produced angina symptoms in only 26% of patients, ischemic ECG changes in 47%, but Tl-201 defects in 89%. The authors concluded that their findings supported the concept of the "ischemic cascade," where blood flow alterations precede the appearance of ECG abnormalities and angina as myocardial oxygen demand is increased. A similar study using exercise radionuclide angiography was performed by Upton et al.[51] The LVEF response was measured at submaximal and maximal levels of exercise. Eighteen of 25 patients with CAD had an abnormal ejection response in the absence of chest pain and ST-segment depression at the first level of exercise. All patients had hemodynamic abnormalities and ST-segment depression at the second higher level of exercise. Thus, these observations suggest that hypoperfusion and ventricular dysfunction occur early in the course of graded exercise stress testing, before the onset of ST-segment depression and angina. Angina is least likely to occur at submaximal effort.

PROGNOSTIC IMPLICATIONS OF SILENT MYOCARDIAL ISCHEMIA IN PATIENTS SUSPECTED OR KNOWN TO HAVE CORONARY ARTERY DISEASE

Ambulatory Electrocardiographic Monitoring and Prognosis

In patients with chronic CAD and stable angina, silent myocardial ischemia identifies a subgroup whose prognosis is worse than that of patients with chronic stable angina who do not manifest episodes of silent ischemia. Bertolet

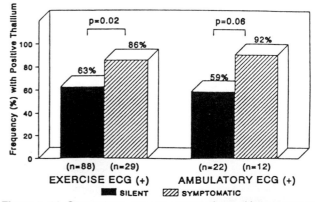

Figure 5–11. Comparison of the frequency of a positive exercise Tl-201 study in patients with ischemic ST segment depression on exercise testing *(left)* and a positive ambulatory ECG response *(right)*. The groups are divided into those with presence or absence of chest pain with exercise. (Klein J, Choo SY, Berman DS, Rozanski A: Is "silent" myocardial ischemia really as severe as symptomatic ischemia? The analytical effect of patient selection biases. Circulation 1994;89:1958–1966.)

and Pepine[1] reviewed five studies in the literature comprising 644 patients; 36% had silent ischemia. This group experienced a 54% cardiac event rate, as compared with a 30% event rate for the 410 patients without silent ischemia. Thus, silent ischemia appears to provide significant prognostic information.

Deedwania et al.[52] prospectively examined the prognostic significance of silent myocardial ischemia detected by the ambulatory ECG during daily life in 107 patients with chronic stable angina who were symptomatically controlled on conventional antianginal agents. Approximately 45% of this group demonstrated one or more episodes of silent ischemia on monitoring, whereas the remaining patients had no ischemic ST-segment changes. Survival analysis between the two groups confirmed that patients with silent ischemia had a worse prognosis during the follow-up period. By stepwise Cox regression multivariate analysis of multiple clinical and exercise variables, detection of silent myocardial ischemia was the most powerful and independent predictor of cardiac mortality during follow-up. When examined in comparison to the prognostic significance in patients who had a positive exercise test, silent ischemia during ambulatory ECG monitoring was a better predictor of outcome than exercise duration, exercise time to ischemia, peak heart rate during exercise, or peak blood pressure during exercise.

In a subsequent study, Deedwania and Carbazal reported that, in patients with chronic stable angina and positive exercise tests, silent ischemia during daily life was the most powerful predictor of cardiac mortality.[53] These authors concluded that ambulatory ischemia by Holter monitoring provides significant additional prognostic information to that obtained from exercise test variables alone. Figure 5–12 shows the survival curves for patients with and without silent ischemia from this study.

Yeung et al.[54] confirmed the observations of Deedwania et al. in 138 patients with chronic stable angina and positive exercise tests who underwent ambulatory ECG monitoring after stopping antianginal medications. Cox survival analysis during an average 37 months' follow-up showed that

the finding of ischemia on ambulatory ECG monitoring was the most significant predictor of death and MI in the subsequent 2 years and of all adverse events for 5 years. Mody et al.[55] found that though evidence of prolonged ischemia on ambulatory ECG monitoring increases the likelihood of multivessel CAD, its absence has little predictive value. In their study of 102 patients with stable angina and 42 volunteers, Holter recordings were 92% specific and 80% positively predictive, but their sensitivity was only 37% and their negative predictive value for CAD was 27%. There was no significant correlation between cumulative duration of ischemia on Holter monitoring and exercise duration or time-to-segment depression on treadmill exercise. Klein et al.[55a] performed ambulatory ECG monitoring in 244 patients referred for stress Tl-201 scintigraphy and found that 50% of those with negative ambulatory ECG responses had Tl-201 redistribution that was sometimes prominent. A positive ambulatory ECG response, however, was associated with a greater frequency of ischemic Tl-201 responses ($P = 0.07$), a greater number of reversible defects ($P < 0.05$), and a greater summed Tl-201 "reversibility score" ($P < 0.05$) than was a positive stress ECG response but a negative ambulatory ECG. Thus, this study also shows that a negative ambulatory ECG response for ischemia does not exclude functionally important CAD. Quyyumi et al.[55b] prospectively assessed the incidence and prognostic significance of ST segment changes recorded on ambulatory ECG monitoring in 116 asymptomatic or minimally symptomatic low-risk patients with CAD followed for 29 ± 13 months. Forty-five patients (39%) had transient ST-segment depression during 48-hour monitoring; in 82% this finding was "silent." Of the eight acute cardiac events (seven infarctions, one unstable angina), seven occurred in patients without silent ischemia during monitoring. No differences in event-free survival from either acute events or elective revascularization (nine patients) during follow-up were observed in patient subgroups with or without silent ischemia on ambulatory ECG monitoring. The authors concluded that, in patients categorized as low risk (i.e., those who do not have (1) left main CAD, (2) three-vessel CAD and LV

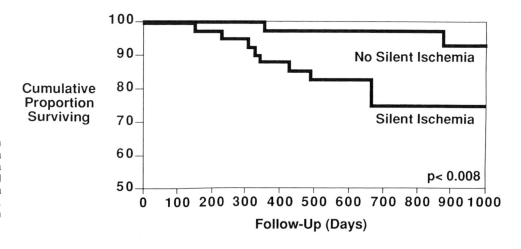

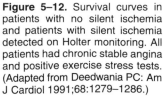

Figure 5–12. Survival curves in patients with no silent ischemia and patients with silent ischemia detected on Holter monitoring. All patients had chronic stable angina and positive exercise stress tests. (Adapted from Deedwania PC: Am J Cardiol 1991;68:1279–1286.)

dysfunction, (3) three-vessel CAD and inducible ischemia, or (4) two-vessel CAD, LV dysfunction, and inducible ischemia), silent ischemia on ambulatory monitoring failed to predict subsequent coronary events.

Thus, these studies show that prolonged and frequent episodes of silent ST-segment depression observed on 24-hour ambulatory ECG monitoring identify patients at high risk for a future cardiac event. Silent ST-segment depression is not prognostically significant in low-risk CAD patients as categorized by angiography and stress testing. None of the studies cited compared the prognostic value of Holter monitoring with stress radionuclide variables considered to be indices of high risk.

Exercise Electrocardiographic Stress Testing

The exercise ECG response in patients with CAD provides useful prognostic information, even in the absence of angina. Mark et al.[40] evaluated the clinical correlates and long-term prognostic significance of silent ischemia during exercise ECG testing in 1698 consecutive symptomatic patients with CAD who underwent both treadmill testing and cardiac catheterization. Patients who had angina in response to exercise testing had more extensive angiographic CAD than patients who experienced painless ST-segment depression on testing. The 5-year survival rate was 73% for those with exercise-limiting angina, which was worse than the 86% survival rate for patients with painless exercise ST-segment depression. Thus, in this study using treadmill testing for detection of ischemia, patients who demonstrated angina as a symptom-limited endpoint during exercise testing did have a worse prognosis than patients with an ECG ischemic response but no associated angina. Miranda et al.[42] also showed that patients with symptomatic exercise-induced ischemia and no history of infarction had a higher prevalence of severe CAD than those who had only silent ischemia (30% vs. 25%, P = 0.005). No follow-up data

were reported for this patient cohort, who were all men referred for exercise testing for evaluation of symptoms.

In the study by Callaham et al.,[56] the mortality rate was significantly greater (P = 0.02) among patients with an abnormal ST-segment response than in patients without ST-segment depression in a retrospective analysis of 1747 consecutive predominantly male inpatients and outpatients referred for exercise testing. In this survey, the presence or absence of angina pectoris during exercise testing was not significantly related to death. These findings are in contrast to those reported by Mark et al.,[40] cited earlier. The prevalence of silent ischemia was directly related to age. Event-free survival for 1019 patients in the CASS registry was analyzed in relation to exercise ECG stress test responses.[39] As shown in Figure 5–13, patients with ST-segment depression and no angina had a survival rate comparable to that for patients who experienced angina *and* manifested ischemic ST-segment depression on treadmill testing. In a subsequent study, Weiner et al.[57] reported that patients with silent ischemia during exercise testing who were at the highest risk were those with three-vessel CAD and abnormal LV function. In that group, the 7-year survival was only 37% for those treated medically; for the surgically treated group it was 90%.

Silent ischemia carries an adverse prognosis for patients who have undergone initially beneficial coronary bypass graft or surgery. Weiner et al.[58] showed that, though the prevalence of symptomatic ischemia significantly decreased postoperatively in 174 patients from the Coronary Artery Surgery Study (CASS) randomized surgical population who underwent exercise testing before and 6 months after coronary bypass surgery, the frequency of silent ischemia did not change (30% vs. 29%). Survival 12 years after bypass surgery based on the postoperative exercise test results was significantly better for the patients with no postoperative silent ischemia (80%) than for those with persistent silent ischemia (68%) or those with symptomatic ischemia (45%).

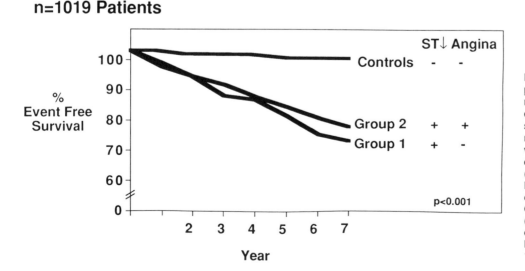

Figure 5–13. Cumulative 7-year probability of remaining free of myocardial infarction and sudden death among patients with ST-segment depression (ST↓) and no angina (Group 1) and patients with ST↓ and angina (Group 2) compared with control patients (Controls) with no ST↓ or angina. No differences were observed in event rates between Group 1 and Group 2 patients. Control patients (P<0.001) had significantly fewer events. (Adapted from Weiner DA, et al.: Am J Cardiol 1988;62:1155–1158.)

Thus, except for one study,[40] it appears that silent ST depression provoked on exercise ECG testing has the same adverse prognostic implications as ST depression associated with exercise-induced angina.

Thallium-201 Scintigraphy

The prognostic significance of silent myocardial ischemia detected on exercise Tl-201 scintigraphy has also been examined.[59, 59a] Heller et al.[59] determined whether the presence or absence of angina during a positive Tl-201 stress test for ischemia was independently predictive of an adverse outcome. Of 234 consecutive patients who had an ischemic response to Tl-201 scintigraphy, 105 had no angina. There was no significant difference between the angina and the silent ischemia groups with respect to gender, previous infarction, prevalence of multivessel disease, or incidence of diabetes mellitus. There was no difference in cardiac events (defined as MI, angioplasty, or bypass surgery) between the two groups during follow-up. Similarly, survival analysis revealed no significant difference in mortality (Fig. 5–14). Thus, in this study where Tl-201 redistribution was used as the endpoint for an ischemic response, the prognosis for patients with silent ischemia was similar to that for those who developed angina during testing. These findings are not surprising in light of the data summarized previously from Gasperetti et al.[46] and Hecht et al.,[47] who showed that extent of stress-induced hypoperfusion and extent of angiographic CAD were comparable in patients with silent Tl-201 redistribution and in patients with angina and Tl-201 redistribution.

Reisman et al.[60] determined the 1-year cardiac event rate in asymptomatic and typical angina patients with an abnormal Tl-201 perfusion scan on testing. The overall cardiac event rate was 8% in the 83 asymptomatic patients and 18% in the 77 patients who exhibited typical angina on testing. On the postexercise images the number of redistribution segments for asymptomatic patients was comparable (1.9) to that for those with angina (1.4). These investigators

further subdivided their two groups based on whether or not at least 85% of maximum predicted heart rate was achieved on testing. The subgroup with silent ischemia who failed to achieve at least 85% of maximum predicted heart rate had a 16% rate of subsequent cardiac events and 2.0 redistribution segments per patient. This contrasted to a 5% event rate and 1.1 redistribution segments per patient in those who had silent ischemia but did achieve at least 85% of maximum predicted heart rate. The subgroup with typical angina on testing who failed to reach 85% of maximum predicted heart rate had a similar event rate (19%) to the silent ischemia subgroup who failed to reach this exercise endpoint. Patients with typical angina who achieved more than 85% of maximum predicted heart rate, however, had a higher event rate (17%) than the silent ischemia subgroup that achieved at least 85% of maximum predicted heart rate. The investigators concluded that silent ischemia has a worse prognosis when it occurs at suboptimal exercise heart rates, than when it occurs at fast exercise heart rates. Travin et al.[48] found that patients with Tl-201 redistribution but no angina on exercise testing, less frequently had ST-segment depression and had "less ischemic" Tl-201 images (in terms of number of redistribution defects, severity of the worst redistributing defect, and an ischemic index) than patients with Tl-201 redistribution and angina on testing. Nevertheless, the cardiac event rate was similar (21% vs. 29%).

Stress Tl-201 imaging has been shown to be of benefit in detecting the presence of ischemia in asymptomatic young adults with familial hypercholesterolemia.[61] Of 54 patients screened, 11 heterozygotes and three homozygotes had abnormal Tl-201 scans. Those who had positive scans could not be distinguished from those who had negative scans by age, sex, or cholesterol level.

Stress Radionuclide Angiography

Stress radionuclide angiography has also been employed to detect asymptomatic myocardial ischemia in patients

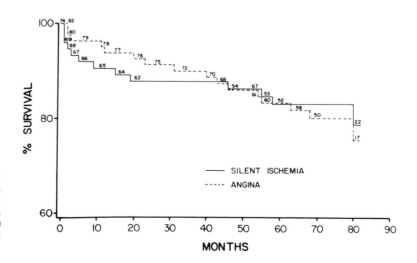

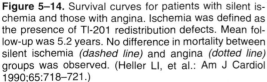

Figure 5–14. Survival curves for patients with silent ischemia and those with angina. Ischemia was defined as the presence of Tl-201 redistribution defects. Mean follow-up was 5.2 years. No difference in mortality between silent ischemia *(dashed line)* and angina *(dotted line)* groups was observed. (Heller LI, et al.: Am J Cardiol 1990;65:718–721.)

PATIENTS WITH BOTH ↓EF AND +ST RESPONSES TO EXERCISE

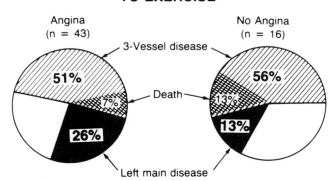

Figure 5–15. Prevalence of left main and three-vessel disease among patients with both a decrease (↓) in EF and a positive (+) ST-segment response. Patients are subdivided on the basis of angina and no angina during exercise. As shown, patients with these ischemic responses had similar prevalences of high-risk coronary anatomy and death during medical therapy. (Reprinted from American Journal of Cardiology: 60:10; October 1, 1987, 778–783.)

with chronic ischemic heart disease and to assess prognosis. Bonow et al.[62] examined the prognostic implications of asymptomatic exercise-induced ischemia as assessed by radionuclide angiography in 131 consecutive patients with CAD. In this study, once inducible ischemia was demonstrated, the risk stratification and prognostic implications of silent ischemia and asymptomatic ischemia were similar. In patients who during exercise developed both EF and ST-segment abnormalities the likelihood of three-vessel left main coronary artery disease—and the risk of death during subsequent medical management—were comparable, regardless of whether they had exercise-induced angina (Fig. 5–15). The prevalence of three-vessel disease in patients who demonstrated a drop in EF, a positive ST-segment response, and chest pain during exercise was 51%. The prevalence of three-vessel CAD was 56% in patients who had an abnormal EF response and ischemic ST depression but no exercise-induced angina. Thus, as demonstrated in studies utilizing Tl-201 scintigraphy, the presence or absence of angina did not influence prognosis in patients who had an abnormal exercise EF response as measured on radionuclide angiographic imaging.

Breitenbucher et al.[63] reported a 5-year follow-up study of 140 patients who had an unequivocal ischemic response during exercise radionuclide angiography (at least 10% decrease from LVEF or at least 5% decrease in EF together with a distinct regional wall motion abnormality). In 60% of this patient cohort, ischemia during radionuclide angiography was silent. Table 5–2 compares angina and silent ischemia groups with an abnormal exercise radionuclide angiographic response in this study. The workload was similar for the silent and symptomatic groups, a finding comparable to the observations of Gasperetti et al.[46] using Tl-201 redistribution as the criterion for detection of ischemia. The event-free survival rate was comparable whether patients had symptomatic or silent ischemia (Fig. 5–16). Cardiac events (unstable angina, MI, cardiac death) occurred in 27% of patients in the silent ischemia group and in 16% of patients in the symptomatic group (*P* = NS). Interestingly, death or MI during follow-up was significantly more frequent in patients with silent ischemia (22%

vs. 9%). These findings are not unexpected since Cohn et al.[64] reported previously that patients with silent ischemia and patients with angina have a comparable decrease in LVEF during exercise and a comparable percentage of regions with normal EF at rest that showed a decrease during exercise. In their study,[64] the prevalence of multivessel CAD was similar in patients with and in those without angina. Upton et al.[51] reported that abnormalities in LV function frequently develop before angina and ischemic ST-segment depression.

Mental stress has been employed with radionuclide angiography to elicit an ischemic response. In a group of patients with CAD studied by Rozanski et al.,[9] 59% had wall motion abnormalities during mental stress and 36% had a fall in EF of more than 5 percentage points. The ischemia induced by mental stress was silent in 83% of the patients who exhibited wall motion abnormalities consequent to mental stress. The heart rate at which wall motion abnormalities were observed was slower than the heart rate associated with exercise-induced ischemia. Antiischemic medical therapy can abolish the painless drop in LVEF during exercise in some patients who have CAD and silent ischemia.[65] This was seen in 35% of patients and was associated with an 8% event rate at 9 months' follow-up. Patients whose ischemic response on radionuclide angiog-

Table 5–2. Comparison of Angina and Silent Ischemia Groups Who Had an Abnormal Exercise Radionuclide Angiogram

	Angina (N = 56)	Silent Ischemia (N = 84)
History of myocardial infarction (%)	41	51
↓ Ejection fraction during exercise	−13 ± 8	−11 ± 6
Three-vessel CAD (%)	34	38
Maximum workload	63 ± 18	75 ± 27
Sudden death	1 (2%)	7 (8%) *
Myocardial infarction	4 (7%)	12 (14%)*
Unstable angina	5 (7%)	4 (5%)

*P < 0.05 for death and myocardial infarction, combined.
(Reprinted with permission from the American College of Cardiology (Journal of the American College of Cardiology, 1990, Vol. 15, pp. 999–1003).)

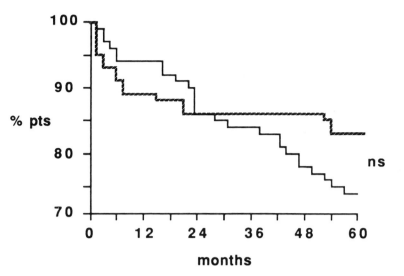

Figure 5–16. Event-free survival for 56 patients (pts) with symptomatic *(dotted line)* and 84 patients with silent *(solid line)* ischemia during exercise radionuclide angiography. (Reprinted with permission from the American College of Cardiology (Journal of the American College of Cardiology, 1990, Vol. 15, pp. 999–1003).)

raphy was not abolished had a 45% event rate at follow-up ($P < 0.025$). Lim et al.[65] concluded that therapeutic efficacy should be assessed by titration against ischemia, not against angina.

Silent ischemia has been well identified by exercise stress echocardiography.[65a] The authors found the incidence of silent exercise-induced ischemic LV dysfunction to be 43%. The patients had no chest pain or ST-segment depression and were considered to have "truly silent ischemia." As observed in the Tl-201 studies cited previously, extent of angiographic CAD was comparable for silent and painful ischemia groups.

Summary

Several conclusions can be drawn from the results of the prognostic studies summarized above. First, silent myocardial ischemia is quite prevalent in patients with chronic ischemic heart disease, no matter which technique is employed for detection of ischemia. It stands to reason, however, that more patients with silent ischemia will be detected when either myocardial Tl-201 scintigraphy or radionuclide angiography is performed in association with standard exercise ECG stress testing. This is because the detection rate for either symptomatic or asymptomatic ischemia is greater when the radionuclide techniques are used than when the exercise ECG tests alone are given. Nevertheless, a positive ischemic response on any of these noninvasive tests identifies patients whose prognosis is worse than that of patients with chronic ischemic heart disease without silent ischemia. Prognosis for patients with silent ischemia on either exercise ECG testing, exercise myocardial perfusion imaging, exercise radionuclide angiography, or ambulatory ECG monitoring is similar to the prognosis for those who experience angina during testing. Whether information from ambulatory ECG recordings of CAD patients can add to the prognostic information derived solely

from an exercise radionuclide study performed in conjunction with ECG testing is still unclear. Patients with chronic stable angina who manifest frequent episodes of asymptomatic ST-segment depression on ambulatory ECG monitoring certainly have a worse outcome than patients with stable angina who do not exhibit such episodes. It remains to be shown, however, whether or not such high-risk patients can be identified with equal accuracy by radionuclide stress testing alone.

DETECTION OF SILENT ISCHEMIA IN PATIENTS WITH UNSTABLE ANGINA PECTORIS

Ambulatory Electrocardiographic Monitoring and Exercise Electrocardiographic Stress Testing

Several groups have examined the prevalence and prognostic significance of silent ischemia detected by continuous ECG monitoring in patients with unstable angina. Gottlieb et al.[66] examined the prognostic value of continuous ECG recording during the first 48 hours in the coronary care unit for 70 patients hospitalized with unstable angina. By multivariate analysis, silent ischemia during the monitoring period was the best predictor of subsequent death, nonfatal MI, and bypass surgery or angioplasty, among 15 variables tested. Patients who exhibited silent ischemia for 60 minutes or more in 24 hours had a worse prognosis than those who had ischemia less than 60 minutes per 24 hours. Of interest, silent ischemia was seen in more than 50% of patients with unstable angina, despite intensive medical therapy. Figure 5–17 depicts the Kaplan-Meier curves for not experiencing a subsequent ischemic event in those who did and those who did not exhibit silent ischemia in this study. In a subsequent study, Gottlieb and coworkers showed that presence of silent ischemia was the best predic-

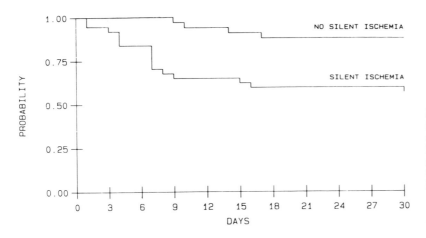

Figure 5–17. Kaplan-Meier survival curves comparing the cumulative probability of not experiencing myocardial infarction or revascularization or recurrent angina in patients with no silent ischemia and silent ischemia as detected by continuous ECG monitoring. All patients had a diagnosis of unstable angina. (Reprinted by permission of *The New England Journal of Medicine* from Gottlieb SO, et al.: N Engl J Med 314:1214–1219, Copyright 1986, Massachusetts Medical Society.)

tor of outcome over the ensuing two years after discharge.[67] Nademanee et al.[68] confirmed these findings and found that when silent ischemia persists after medical therapy of unstable angina, the short-term prognosis is adversely affected. Only 6% of patients in this group whose ischemia lasted more than 60 minutes in 24 hours had a favorable clinical outcome. In contrast, 70% of patients with an ischemia that lasted less than 60 minutes in 24 hours had a favorable outcome. Figure 5–18 shows the relationship between the presence and duration of transient myocardial ischemia on Holter monitoring and the number of diseased vessels seen on angiography. Note that ischemia that persisted longer than 60 minutes was more prevalent in patients with multivessel CAD than with single-vessel CAD.

Bertolet and Pepine[1] undertook a pooled analysis of five studies in the literature concerning the risk of future coronary events in patients with unstable angina with and without silent myocardial ischemia. Fifty percent of the pooled patient cohort manifested silent ischemia on monitoring. The event rate was 55% for the unstable angina patients who manifested silent ischemia and only 14% for those patients without evidence of silent myocardial ischemia. Nyman et al.[69] determined the prognostic value of silent ischemia during symptom-limited predischarge exercise

testing in 740 men with unstable angina or non–Q wave infarction. As expected, patients with ST-segment depression had a higher rate of cardiac death on infarction (18%) than those without ST-segment depression (9%) at 1 year. The event rate was similar in those with silent (18.1%) and those with painful (18.3%) ischemia, but patients with both ST-segment depression and angina had a higher incidence of class 3 or 4 angina at follow-up (44% vs. 17%).

Amanullah et al.[69a] found that 90% of episodes of transient ischemia and ECG monitoring early after admission for unstable angina were silent. The results of monitoring did not add significant long-term prognostic information to the results of the exercise test and Tl-201 imaging; however, patients who experienced subsequent events had a longer duration of ischemia overall than did ''nonevent'' patients.

Exercise Radionuclide Imaging

Data are scant on the application of exercise radionuclide imaging performed soon after stabilization of unstable angina for the purpose of separating high- and low-risk subgroups. The utility for detecting silent ischemia on sub-

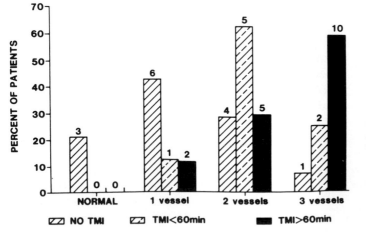

Figure 5–18. Relation between presence and duration of transient myocardial ischemia (TMI) shown on Holter monitoring and the number of diseased coronary vessels found at angiography. Numbers on top of each bar refer to the number of patients. Severity of transient myocardial ischemia, as indicated by its duration, increases as a function of the number of diseased vessels. (Reprinted with permission from the American College of Cardiology (Journal of the American College of Cardiology, 1987, Vol. 10, pp. 1–9).)

maximal exercise radionuclide imaging 4 to 7 days after hospitalization in patients with unstable angina who are stabilized with medical therapy should be similar to that reported for patients with uncomplicated MI. The goal of such testing would be to (1) determine noninvasively the extent of underlying CAD; (2) derive information related to the area at risk distal to the culprit stenosis involved with the unstable syndrome; and (3) determine the response to medical therapy. Patients whose condition stabilizes with medical therapy and who have during exercise only a small localized perfusion abnormality, with or without angina, might be spared early coronary angiography and be managed medically until symptoms recur. Patients who exhibit high-risk radionuclide test findings, such as multiple redistribution defects in more than one vascular region or increased lung Tl-201 uptake, would be candidates for early aggressive intervention with angiography and coronary revascularization. Marmur et al.[70] assessed the relative value of invasive and noninvasive predictors of outcome in patients after unstable angina. When patients with a favorable outcome at 6 months' follow-up were compared with patients with an unfavorable outcome, no statistical difference was found in duration of ST-segment depression of at least 1.0 mm on ambulatory ECG monitoring, exercise duration on treadmill testing, magnitude of exercise-induced ST-segment depression, or LVEF measured on contrast ventriculography. Patients with a good prognosis were distinguished from those with an unfavorable outcome by a higher maximum rate-pressure product, a small redistribution Tl-201 defect size, expressed as percentage of the total myocardium imaged, and a small number of vessels with at least 50% stenosis. By multiple logistic regression analysis, reversible exercise Tl-201 defect size was the only predictor for patients without myocardial infarction. This study showed the superiority of exercise Tl-201 scintigraphy over ambulatory ECG monitoring for risk stratification after unstable angina.

Many clinicians seem more comfortable with performing early coronary angiography in patients admitted to the hospital with unstable angina. The goal of angiography is to rapidly assess extent of CAD and refer patients with left main or proximal three-vessel disease for coronary bypass surgery. Patients with one- or two-vessel CAD can either be treated medically or undergo coronary angioplasty. Angioplasty would not be an appropriate option in patients with diffuse distal disease or poor left ventricular function. With the emergence of highly effective medical therapy for unstable angina using aspirin, intravenous heparin, and intravenous nitroglycerin, most patients can be stabilized and do not require urgent invasive evaluation. Low-level exercise radionuclide imaging could be quite effective as the first step in the risk-stratification process in these stabilized patients, and angiography could be recommended only for those with high-risk ECG or radionuclide stress test variables. Certainly, patients with continuing ischemic symptoms should promptly undergo cardiac catheterization rather than noninvasive evaluation. (The approach to the radionuclide assessment of patients with unstable angina is discussed in more detail in Chap. 7.) Also, practice guidelines for the use of noninvasive and invasive testing in patients with unstable angina have recently been published by the Agency for Health Care Policy and Research of the U.S. Department of Health and Human Services.[70a]

DETECTION OF SILENT MYOCARDIAL ISCHEMIA IN PATIENTS WITH ACUTE MYOCARDIAL INFARCTION

Ambulatory Electrocardiographic Monitoring

Survivors of acute MI have a high prevalence of silent myocardial ischemia, whether it is detected by exercise ECG alone or by predischarge radionuclide stress testing (Chap. 6).[71-83] Silent ischemia can develop quite soon after MI, during the hospital stay. Gottlieb et al.[71] investigated the relative prognostic significance of ischemic ST-segment changes on continuous ECG monitoring in the coronary care unit in 103 high-risk hospitalized postinfarction patients. Ischemic ST depression on monitoring was detected in approximately 30%. Only a third of these patients reported any postinfarction angina during hospitalization. Furthermore, most of the episodes of ischemic ST depression were silent. By 1-year follow-up, 30% of the patients with ischemic ST changes on Holter monitoring died, as compared with only 11% of the postinfarction patients who showed no evidence of ischemia on Holter monitoring. By multivariate Cox's hazard function analysis, the presence of ST changes on Holter monitoring was a significant predictive variable for 1-year mortality and had particular prognostic significance for the patients who were not able to undergo early exercise treadmill testing.

Tzivoni et al.[72] examined the prognostic significance of ischemic changes recorded on ambulatory ECG monitoring during daily activity after uncomplicated MI. He found that 33% of postinfarction patients had transient ischemic episodes on prolonged ECG monitoring. During an average 28 months' follow-up, the cardiac event rate among those with ischemic episodes on Holter monitoring was 51%, as compared with 12% for those without such changes ($P < 0.0001$). Similar cardiac event rates were observed for patients with silent ischemic episodes and for those who had symptomatic episodes. In that study, ST-segment depression on ambulatory monitoring identified a high-risk subset among patients whose LVEF at rest was below 40%. The event rate was 62.5% for patients with ambulatory ECG evidence of ST depression and an EF below 40%, as compared with a 19.5% event rate for patients with a similarly depressed EF but no manifestations of ST depression during monitoring. Figure 5–19 shows the event-free survival for the 224 patients in this study with a positive or negative Holter monitor recording for detection of ischemia after an acute MI.

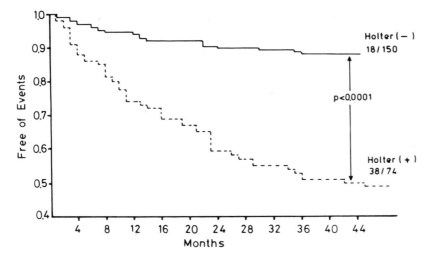

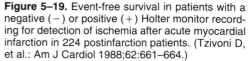

Figure 5–19. Event-free survival in patients with a negative (−) or positive (+) Holter monitor recording for detection of ischemia after acute myocardial infarction in 224 postinfarction patients. (Tzivoni D, et al.: Am J Cardiol 1988;62:661–664.)

A similar study was undertaken by Petretta et al.,[73] who monitored 270 consecutive postinfarction patients. At 2-year follow-up, patients who showed ST-segment changes had higher incidences of cardiac death and reinfarction. By multivariate analysis, Killip class and ST-segment changes were the variables most predictive of outcome. In the subset of patients who could not perform an exercise stress test, ST-segment depression on ambulatory ECG monitoring was the most important prognostic variable, followed by Killip class. Ruberman et al.[74] determined the contribution of intermittent ST-segment depression to subsequent mortality in patients undergoing ambulatory ECG monitoring in the Beta Blocker Heart Attack Trial. In a model that included relative covariates, ST-segment depression on Holter monitoring had a relative risk of 1.73, but the relative risk was 2.56 for untreated patients and 0.98 for propranolol-treated patients.

Currie et al.[79] determined the prognostic value of both early (6 days) and late (38 days) ambulatory ECG monitoring in 203 postinfarction patients. Early ST-segment depression was significantly associated with increased mortality (24% vs. 8%; $P < 0.05$) and increased reinfarction or coronary revascularization (45% vs. 17%; $P < 0.001$) and had independent value after allowance was made for clinical factors and coronary prognostic indices. ST-segment depression on late monitoring was associated with increased cardiac events only when it was frequent (at least three episodes per day), prolonged (at least 20 minutes per day), or severe (maximum of at least 1.5 mm). Mickley et al.[80] found that patients with ST-segment depression during 36 hours of ambulatory monitoring at 11 ± 5 days after acute infarction had a 52% cardiac event rate, as compared with 22% ($P < 0.01$) for patients with no demonstrable ischemia. In this study, ambulatory ECG monitoring was superior to exercise ECG testing alone for predicting future events; however, more of the 5 patients who died had ischemia on either ambulatory monitoring or exercise testing. Interestingly, 98% of ischemic episodes on ambulatory monitoring were silent.

Solimene et al.[81] reported that patients with silent ischemia on 48-hour ambulatory ECG monitoring conducted between 2 and 8 weeks postinfarction had significantly more extensive CAD (45% multivessel disease) when compared with those without ischemia (14.8% multivessel disease; $P < 0.05$). At 2 years' follow-up, 36.4% of patients who had a silent ischemia and 3.4% of patients who did not experienced a cardiac event ($P < 0.05$). Figure 5–20 shows the Kaplan-Meier curves illustrating event-free survival for patients with and without silent ischemia in this study. Vaagenilsen et al.[83] found that patients with acute infarction

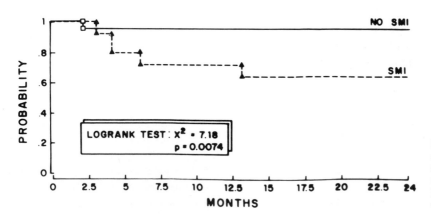

Figure 5–20. Kaplan-Meier curves show probability of not experiencing coronary events over 24 months of follow-up for patients with (SMI) and without silent myocardial ischemia (no SMI) after uncomplicated MI. (Solimene MC, et al.: Int J Cardiol 1993;38:41–47.)

who received thrombolytic therapy had a greater prevalence of ischemia on ambulatory ECG monitoring 6 months postinfarction than patients treated with placebo in the Anglo-Scandinavian Study of Early Thrombolysis (ASSET) trial. All events by 1 year occurred in the group who had an ischemic response.

Thus, as observed in patients with chronic stable angina and unstable angina, post–myocardial infarction patients with silent ST-segment depression on Holter monitoring have a worse prognosis than those who show no evidence of silent ischemia when surveyed. Treatment with antiischemia drugs appears to improve prognosis in this population. Again, the question can be raised about the added prognostic value of ambulatory ECG monitoring over the prognostic information obtained from a predischarge exercise test (with or without associated perfusion imaging).

Thallium-201 Scintigraphy

The addition of myocardial Tl-201 scintigraphy to predischarge exercise testing enhances the detection rate of silent myocardial ischemia in patients with uncomplicated MI. Assey et al.[75] compared the clinical outcome in patients with proven CAD who did or did not manifest angina with Tl-201 scintigraphic manifestations of ischemia on exercise testing. Of 27 patients who exhibited silent ischemia on Tl-201 imaging, six had a subsequent infarction and three of those died during at least 30 months' follow-up. This contrasted with only one nonfatal infarction among the 28 patients with Tl-201 redistribution and associated angina on testing.

Of 190 postinfarction patients reported by Gibson et al.,[76] 100 had neither angina nor ST depression on predischarge submaximal exercise testing. Of these, half had Tl-201 redistribution and subsequently experienced a 24% rate of death or recurrent infarction at 27 months' follow-up. This compared to only a 2% event rate for patients with no Tl-201 redistribution, ST depression, or angina. A group of 43 patients in this study had painless ST depression on predischarge exercise Tl-201 imaging. The event rate was 20%

for those who had silent ST depression associated with Tl-201 redistribution, as compared with 9% for those with ST depression and no scintigraphic evidence of ischemia. Finally, there was a third group of 47 patients who experienced angina as the endpoint in the stress test. The event rate for patients with exercise-induced angina and Tl-201 redistribution was 24%, a rate identical to that for patients with Tl-201 redistribution and no angina or ST depression. The findings of this study are summarized in Table 5–3. Thus, the prognosis for postinfarction patients was not related to whether or not angina was observed as an endpoint during exercise testing. An interesting observation of this study related to the specificity of the ST-segment response in certain subgroups of postinfarction patients. Some patients with circumflex or right coronary infarct–related vessels had significant precordial ST-segment depression in leads V_2 and V_3 during exercise stress but no evidence of left anterior descending disease on either angiography or Tl-201 scintigraphy (no redistribution defects in the anterior wall or septum). Some patients had increasing ST-segment elevation in inferior posterior leads during exercise. The ST depression seen in the anterior precordial leads in these patients who had a posterior transmural infarction presumably represented "reciprocal changes" induced during exercise rather than true anterior wall ischemia. This may account for the good prognosis in the group of patients who had silent ST depression without Tl-201 redistribution. To conclude, silent ischemia often occurs after uncomplicated MI, and it identifies a subset of patients who are at higher risk for recurrent cardiac events. Tl-201 scintigraphy is both more sensitive and more specific for identifying these high-risk postinfarction patients than is exercise ECG alone.

Pharmacologic stress imaging can be substituted for exercise stress for identifying patients with silent postinfarction ischemia. Bolognese et al.[77] prospectively assessed the prognostic significance of silent ischemia on predischarge dipyridamole echocardiography after an uncomplicated infarction. Ninety-four of 128 patients with dipyridamole-induced wall motion abnormalities had silent ischemia. Life table analysis showed no difference between silent and symptomatic ischemia, and a positive echocardiogram was

Table 5–3. Cardiac Event Rates for 190 Patients Based on Predischarge Exercise Tl-201 Results

| | Group Assignment | | | | | |
| | No ST ↓ or Angina | | Painless ST ↓ | | Angina with or Without ST ↓ | |
	No Rd (%)	*Rd (%)*	*No Rd (%)*	*Rd (%)*	*No Rd (%)*	*Rd (%)*
Death (N = 15)	0	10*	4	15	10	14
MI (N = 17)	2	18†	4	5	0	14
Death or MI (N = 30)	2	24†	9	20	10	24
Death, MI, or USAP (N = 69)	16	43†	22	55*	20	57‡

*$P < 0.05$.
†$P < 0.01$ compared with no redistribution.
‡$P \leq 0.09$.
Key: Rd, Tl-201 redistribution by quantitative criteria; MI, myocardial infarction; USAP, unstable angina pectoris.
(Gibson RS, et al.: Circulation 1987; 75(suppl II):II-36–II-39.)

the best predictor of cardiac events. Chapter 6 contains an extensive discussion of the role of stress radionuclide imaging in patients with a recent uncomplicated MI.

Summary

There is probably little value in routinely performing ambulatory ECG monitoring in the predischarge phase of acute MI to identify patients with residual silent myocardial ischemia. An exception may be those who are unable to exercise, though in postinfarction patients pharmacologic stress perfusion imaging may yield prognostic information comparable to that from exercise imaging. For those who can exercise, high-risk findings suggesting underlying multivessel disease or residual ischemia within the zone of infarction are best identified by exercise testing associated with myocardial perfusion imaging. As summarized in Chapter 6, low-risk postinfarction patients would merely manifest persistent defects within the zone of infarction without redistribution provoked either within or remote from the infarct zone. Even if exercise-induced ST-segment depression was observed without concomitant Tl-201 redistribution, such patients may not be at increased risk for subsequent events since the ST-segment depression could represent a false-positive response.

Recently, a method for monitoring changes in global LV function in the ambulatory state has become available using the "cardiac VEST." As described in Chapter 1, this device consists of a scintillation detector that is placed over the cardiac blood pool while a second detector is positioned over a background region. This technique has been applied successfully in the postinfarction setting in patients who previously received thrombolytic therapy during the acute phase of hospitalization. Patients with evidence for transient decreases of LVEF during ambulation have a significantly higher cardiac event rate than those who exhibit no asymptomatic diminution in global LV function.[84] In that study, 12 of 33 patients monitored demonstrated 19 episodes of transient LV dysfunction (defined as a greater than 0.05 decrease in EF lasting at least 1 minute). Only two episodes were accompanied by chest pain and ST-segment depression on ambulatory ECG monitoring.

DETECTION OF SILENT MYOCARDIAL ISCHEMIA AFTER CORONARY ANGIOPLASTY

Many patients who have initially successful balloon dilatation of coronary stenoses manifest silent ischemia on routine testing some 2 weeks to 6 months after the procedure. The clinical application of stress radionuclide imaging for detection of silent restenosis is discussed in detail in Chapter 10. It suffices to say, silent ischemia by radionuclide criteria is associated with a high prevalence of re-stenosis on coronary angiography and is a predictor of recurrent angina pectoris.[85]

SUMMARY AND CONCLUSIONS

Radionuclide imaging has been proven to be a valuable adjunct to exercise stress testing for identification of patients with CAD who manifest silent myocardial ischemia. Detection of asymptomatic ischemia is clinically important, because it identifies a subgroup of patients who appear to be at high risk for subsequent cardiac events. Silent ischemia is detected with greater sensitivity and specificity with stress radionuclide imaging than by exercise ECG stress testing alone—in totally asymptomatic subjects, in patients with chronic stable angina, in patients who have recovered from unstable angina, in patients who have survived an uncomplicated MI, and in patients who have undergone revascularization surgery or coronary angioplasty. There is no good evidence, from review of the literature, that prolonged ambulatory ECG monitoring for detection of asymptomatic episodes of ST-segment depression during daily life has supplementary prognostic value to the assessment of clinical, exercise ECG stress test and radionuclide imaging variables. Similarly, important prognostic information is obtained from pharmacologic stress imaging in patients who cannot exercise. Ambulatory ECG monitoring during daily life, however, could provide useful information on the efficacy of antiischemia medical therapy. For example, Knatterud et al.[86] reported that ambulatory ECG ischemia was no longer present at 12 weeks after instituting ischemia-guided pharmacologic therapy in 41% of patients with documented CAD. Also, continuous ECG monitoring could have prognostic value for detection of silent resting ischemia in the first 72 hours after hospital admission for unstable angina or acute infarction.

More prospective studies are warranted to fairly evaluate the relative additional prognostic value of variables derived from ambulatory ECG monitoring to the radionuclide stress test variables in different patient populations. In any event, silent ischemia detected by any noninvasive method is quite prevalent among patients who present with various clinical syndromes of acute and chronic CAD, and is an important prognostic variable in the risk stratification process. Most studies have shown that the extent of myocardium at jeopardy in the distribution of coronary artery stenosis is the same whether or not angina accompanies ECG or radionuclide evidence of ischemia.

REFERENCES

1. Bertolet B, Pepine C: Silent myocardial ischemia. Baylor Cardiol Ser 1989;12:5–31.
2. Epstein SE, Quyyumi AA, Bonow RO: Myocardial ischemia—silent or symptomatic. N Engl J Med 1988;318:1038–1043.
3. Cohn PF: Silent myocardial ischemia. Ann Intern Med 1988;109:312–317.

4. Cohn PF: Clinical importance of silent myocardial ischemia in asymptomatic subjects. Circulation 1990;81:691–693.

5. Cohn PF: Prognosis for patients with different types of silent coronary artery disease. Circulation 1987;75:II33–II35.

6. Deanfield JE: Holter monitoring in assessment of angina pectoris. Am J Cardiol 1987;59:18C–22C.

7. Muller JE, Tofler GH, Stone PH: Circadian variation and triggers of onset of acute cardiovascular disease. Circulation 1989;79:733–743.

8. Deanfield JE, Shea M, Kensett M, Horlock P, Wilson RA, De Landsheere CM, Selwyn AP: Silent myocardial ischaemia due to mental stress. Lancet 1984;2:1001–1005.

9. Rozanski A, Bairey CN, Krantz DS, Friedman J, Resser KJ, Morell M, Hilton-Chalfen S, Hestrin L, Bietendorf J, Berman DS: Mental stress and the induction of silent myocardial ischemia in patients with coronary artery disease. N Engl J Med 1988;318:1005–1012.

10. Langer A, Freeman M, Armstrong P: Ischemic ST changes on admission ECG and 24 hour Holter monitor predict unfavourable outcome, multivessel disease, and left main stenosis in unstable angina. J Am Coll Cardiol 1988;11:233A.

11. McLenachan JM, Weidinger FF, Barry J, Yeung A, Nabel EG, Rocco MB, Selwyn AP: Relations between heart rate, ischemia, and drug therapy during daily life in patients with coronary artery disease. Circulation 1991;83:1263–1270.

12. Rocco MB, Barry J, Campbell S, Nabel E, Cook EF, Goldman L, Selwyn AP: Circadian variation of transient myocardial ischemia in patients with coronary artery disease. Circulation 1987;75:395–400.

13. Muller JE, Stone PH, Turi ZG, Rutherford JD, Czeisler CA, Parker C, Poole WK, Passamani E, Roberts R, Robertson T, et al.: Circadian variation in the frequency of onset of acute myocardial infarction. N Engl J Med 1985;313:1315–1322.

14. Quyyumi AA, Panza JA, Diodati JG, Lakatos E, Epstein SE: Circadian variation in ischemic threshold. A mechanism underlying the circadian variation in ischemic events. Circulation 1992;86:22–28.

15. Deanfield JE, Shea M, Ribiero P, De Landsheere CM, Wilson RA, Horlock P, Selwyn AP: Transient ST-segment depression as a marker of myocardial ischemia during daily life. Am J Cardiol 1984;54:1195–1200.

16. McHenry PL, O'Donnell J, Morris SN, Jordan JJ: The abnormal exercise electrocardiogram in apparently healthy men: A predictor of angina pectoris as an initial coronary event during long-term follow-up. Circulation 1984;70:547–551.

17. Bruce RA, Hossack KF, DeRouen TA, Hofer V: Enhanced risk assessment for primary coronary heart disease events by maximal exercise testing: 10 years' experience of Seattle Heart Watch. J Am Coll Cardiol 1983;2:565–573.

18. Hopkirk JA, Uhl GS, Hickman JR Jr, Fischer J, Medina A: Discriminant value of clinical and exercise variables in detecting significant coronary artery disease in asymptomatic men. J Am Coll Cardiol 1984;3:887–894.

19. Multiple Risk Facto Intervention Trial Research Group: Exercise electrocardiogram and coronary heart disease mortality in the Multiple Risk Factor Intervention Trial. Am J Cardiol 1985;55:16–24.

20. Gordon DJ, Ekelund LG, Karon JM, Probstfield JL, Rubenstein C, Sheffield LT, Weissfeld L: Predictive value of the exercise tolerance test for mortality in North American men: The Lipid Research Clinics Mortality Follow-up Study. Circulation 1986;74:252–261.

21. Diamond GA, Forrester JS, Hirsch M, Staniloff HM, Vas R, Berman DS, Swan HJ: Application of conditional probability analysis to the clinical diagnosis of coronary artery disease. J Clin Invest 1980;65:1210–1221.

22. Guiney TE, Pohost GM, McKusick KA, Beller GA: Differentiation of false- from true-positive ECG responses to exercise stress by thallium 201 perfusion imaging. Chest 1981;80:4–10.

23. Uhl GS, Kay TN, Hickman JR Jr: Computer-enhanced thallium scintigrams in asymptomatic men with abnormal exercise tests. Am J Cardiol 1981;48:1037–1043.

24. Rissanen AM: Familial occurrence of coronary heart disease: Effect of age at diagnosis. Am J Cardiol 1979;44:60–66.

25. Becker LC, Becker DM, Pearson TA, Fintel DJ, Links J, Frank TL: Screening of asymptomatic siblings of patients with premature coronary artery disease. Circulation 1987;75:II14–II17.

26. Fleg J, Gestenblith G, Zanderman A, Becker L, Weisfeldt M, Costa P, Lakatta E: Prevalence and prognostic significance of exercise-induced myocardial ischemia detected by thallium scintigraphy and electrocardiograph in asymptomatic volunteers. Circulation 1990;81:428–436.

26a. Beller GA: Role of nuclear cardiology in evaluating the total ischemic burden in coronary artery disease. Am J Cardiol 1987;59:31C–38C.

27. Rocco MB, Campbell S, Barry J, Rebecca G, Nabel E, Deanfield J, Selwyn AP: Activity of transient myocardial ischemia out of hospital in coronary artery disease and implications for management. Am J Cardiol 1985;56:19I–22I.

28. Tzivoni D, Gavish A, Benhorin J, Banai S, Keren A, Stern S: Day-to-day variability of myocardial ischemic episodes in coronary artery disease. Am J Cardiol 1987;60:1003–1005.

29. Barry J, Campbell S, Nabel EG, Mead K, Selwyn AP: Ambulatory monitoring of the digitized electrocardiogram for detection and early warning of transient myocardial ischemia in angina pectoris. Am J Cardiol 1987;60:483–488.

30. Barry J, Selwyn AP, Nabel EG, Rocco MB, Mead K, Campbell S, Rebecca G: Frequency of ST-segment depression produced by mental stress in stable angina pectoris from coronary artery disease. Am J Cardiol 1988;61:989–993.

31. Nabel EG, Rocco MB, Selwyn AB: Characteristics and significance of ischemia detected by ambulatory electrocardiographic monitoring. Circulation 1987;75:V74–V83.

32. Pepine CJ, Imperi GA, Lambert CR Jr: Detection of silent myocardial ischemia in patients with angina using continuous electrocardiographic monitoring. Cardiol Clin 1986;4:627–633.

33. Stern S, Gavish A, Weisz G, Benhorin J, Keren A, Tzivoni D: Characteristics of silent and symptomatic myocardial ischemia during daily activities. Am J Cardiol 1988;61:1223–1228.

34. Hausmann D, Nikutta P, Daniel WG, Wenzlaff P, Lichtlen PR: Anginal symptoms without ischemic electrocardiographic changes during ambulatory monitoring in men with coronary artery disease. Am J Cardiol 1991;67:465–469.

35. Panza JA, Quyyumi AA, Diodati JG, Callahan TS, Bonow RO, Epstein SE: Long-term variation in myocardial ischemia during daily life in patients with stable coronary artery disease: Its relation to changes in the ischemic threshold. J Am Coll Cardiol 1992;19:500–506.

35a. Pepine CJ, Geller NL, Knatterud GL, et al.: The asymptomatic cardiac ischemia pilot (ACIP) study: Design of a randomized clinical trial, baseline data and implications for a long-term outcome trial. J Am Coll Cardiol 1994;24:1–10.

36. Cecchi AC, Dovellini EV, Marchi F, Pucci P, Santoro GM, Fazzini PF: Silent myocardial ischemia during ambulatory electrocardiographic monitoring in patients with effort angina. J Am Coll Cardiol 1983;1:934–939.

37. Campbell S, Barry J, Rebecca GS, Rocco MB, Nabel EG, Wayne RR, Selwyn AP: Active transient myocardial ischemia during daily life in asymptomatic patients with positive exercise tests and coronary artery disease. Am J Cardiol 1986;57:1010–1016.

38. American College of Physicians (position paper): Ambulatory ECG (Holter) monitoring. J Am Coll Cardiol 1989;14:885.

39. Weiner DA, Ryan TJ, McCabe CH, Ng G, Chaitman BR, Sheffield LT, Tristani FE, Fisher LD: Risk of developing an acute myocardial infarction or sudden coronary death in patients with exercise-induced silent myocardial ischemia. A report from the Coronary Artery Surgery Study (CASS) registry. Am J Cardiol 1988;62:1155–1158.

40. Mark DB, Hlatky MA, Califf RM, Morris JJ Jr, Sisson SD, McCants CB, Lee KL, Harrell FE Jr, Pryor DB: Painless exercise ST deviation on the treadmill: long-term prognosis. J Am Coll Cardiol 1989;14:885–892.

41. Weiner DA, Ryan TJ, McCabe CH, Luk S, Chaitman BR, Sheffield LT, Tristani F, Fisher LD: Significance of silent myocardial ischemia during exercise testing in patients with coronary artery disease. Am J Cardiol 1987;59:725–729.

42. Miranda CP, Lehmann KG, Lachterman B, Coodley EM, Froelicher VF: Comparison of silent and symptomatic ischemia during exercise testing in men. Ann Intern Med 1991;114:649–656.

43. Schulman P: Bayes' theorem—a review. Cardiol Clinics 1984;2:319–328.

44. Esquivel L, Pollock SG, Beller GA, Gibson RS, Watson DD, Kaul S: Effect of the degree of effort on the sensitivity of the exercise thallium-201 stress test in symptomatic coronary artery disease. Am J Cardiol 1989;63:160–165.

45. Kaul S, Lilly DR, Gascho JA, Watson DD, Gibson RS, Oliner CA,

Ryan JM, Beller GA: Prognostic utility of the exercise thallium-201 test in ambulatory patients with chest pain: Comparison with cardiac catheterization. Circulation 1988;77:745–758.

46. Gasperetti CM, Burwell LR, Beller GA: Prevalence of and variables associated with silent myocardial ischemia on exercise thallium-201 stress testing. J Am Coll Cardiol 1990;16:115–123.

47. Hecht HS, Shaw RE, Bruce T, Myler RK: Silent ischemia: Evaluation by exercise and redistribution tomographic thallium-201 myocardial imaging. J Am Coll Cardiol 1989;14:895–900.

48. Mahmarian JJ, Pratt CM, Cocanougher MK, Verani MS: Altered myocardial perfusion in patients with angina pectoris or silent ischemia during exercise or assessed by quantitative thallium-201 single-photon emission tomography. Circ 1990;82:1305–1315.

49. Travin MI, Flores AR, Boucher CA, Newell JB, LaRaia PJ: Silent versus symptomatic ischemia during a thallium-201 exercise test. Am J Cardiol 1991;68:1600–1608.

49a. Klein J, Chao SY, Berman DS, Rozanski A: Is "silent" myocardial ischemia really as severe as symptomatic ischemia? The analytical effect of patient selection biases. Circulation 1994;89:1958–1966.

50. Heller GV, Ahmed I, Tilkemeier PL, Barbour MM, Garber CE: Comparison of chest pain, electrocardiographic changes and thallium-201 scintigraphy during varying exercise intensities in men with stable angina pectoris. Am J Cardiol 1991;68:569–574.

51. Upton MT, Rerych SK, Newman GE, Port S, Cobb FR, Jones RH: Detecting abnormalities in left ventricular function during exercise before angina and ST-segment depression. Circulation 1980;62:341–349.

52. Deedwania PC, Carbajal EV: Silent ischemia during daily life is an independent predictor of mortality in stable angina. Circulation 1990;81:748–756.

53. Deedwania PC, Carbajal EV: Usefulness of ambulatory silent myocardial ischemia added to the prognostic value of exercise test parameters in predicting risk of cardiac death in patients with stable angina pectoris and exercise-induced myocardial ischemia. Am J Cardiol 1991;68:1279–1286.

54. Yeung AC, Barry J, Orav J, Bonassin E, Raby KE, Selwyn AP: Effects of asymptomatic ischemia on long-term prognosis in chronic stable coronary disease. Circulation 1991;83:1598–1604.

55. Mody FV, Nademanee K, Intarachot V, Josephson MA, Robertson HA, Singh BN: Severity of silent myocardial ischemia on ambulatory electrocardiographic monitoring in patients with stable angina pectoris: Relation to prognostic determinants during exercise stress testing and coronary angiography. J Am Coll Cardiol 1988;12:1169–1176.

55a. Klein J, Rodrigues EA, Berman DS, Prigent F, Chao SY, Maryon T, Rozanski A: Prevalence and functional significance of transient ST-segment depression during daily life activity: Comparisons of ambulatory ECG with stress redistribution thallium 201 single-photon emission computed tomographic imaging. Am Heart J 1993;125:1247–1257.

55b. Quyyumi AA, Panza JA, Diodati JG, Callahan TS, Bonow RO, Epstien SE: Prognostic implications of myocardial ischemia during daily life. J Am Coll Cardiol 1993;21:700–708.

56. Callaham PR, Froelicher VF, Klein J, Risch M, Dubach P, Friis R: Exercise-induced silent ischemia: Age, diabetes mellitus, previous myocardial infarction and prognosis. J Am Coll Cardiol 1989;14:1175–1180.

57. Weiner DA, Ryan TJ, McCabe CH, Chaitman BR, Sheffield LT, Ng G, Fisher LD, Tristini FE: Comparison of coronary artery bypass surgery and medical therapy in patients with exercised-induced silent myocardial ischemia: A report from the Coronary Artery Surgery Study (CASS) registry. J Am Coll Cardiol 1988;12:595–599.

58. Weiner DA, Ryan TJ, Parsons L, Fisher LD, Chaitman BR, Sheffield LT, Tristani FE: Prevalence and prognostic significance of silent and symptomatic ischemia after coronary bypass surgery: A report from the Coronary Artery Surgery Study (CASS) randomized population. J Am Coll Cardiol 1991;18:343–348.

59. Heller LI, Tresgallo M, Sciacca RR, Blood DK, Seldin DW, Johnson LL: Prognostic significance of silent myocardial ischemia on a thallium stress test. Am J Cardiol 1990;65:718–721.

59a. Pancholy SB, Scholet B, Kuhlmeier V, Cave V, Heo J, Iskandrian AS: Prognostic significance of silent ischemia. J Nucl Cardiol 1994;1:434–440.

60. Reisman S, Berman D, Maddahi J: Silent myocardial ischemia during treadmill exercise: Thallium scintigraphic and angiographic correlates (Abstract). J Am Coll Cardiol 1985;5:406.

61. Mouratidis B, Vaughan-Neil EF, Gilday DL, Ash JM, Cullen-Dean G, McIntyre S, MacMillan JH, Rose V: Detection of silent coronary artery disease in adolescents and young adults with familial hypercholesterolemia by single-photon emission computed tomography thallium-201 scanning. Am J Cardiol 1992;70:1109–1112.

62. Bonow RO, Bacharach SL, Green MV, LaFreniere RL, Epstein SE: Prognostic implications of symptomatic versus asymptomatic (silent) myocardial ischemia induced by exercise in mildly symptomatic and in asymptomatic patients with angiographically documented coronary artery disease. Am J Cardiol 1987;60:778–783.

63. Breitenbucher A, Pfisterer M, Hoffmann A, Burckhardt D: Long-term follow-up of patients with silent ischemia during exercise radionuclide angiography. J Am Coll Cardiol 1990;15:999–1003.

64. Cohn PF, Brown EJ Jr, Wynne J, Holman BL, Atkins HL: Global and regional left ventricular ejection fraction abnormalities during exercise in patients with silent myocardial ischemia. J Am Coll Cardiol 1983;1:931–933.

65. Lim R, Dyke L, Dymond DS: Effect on prognosis of abolition of exercise-induced painless myocardial ischemia by medical therapy. Am J Cardiol 1992;69:733–735.

65a. Hecht HS, DeBord L, Sotomayor N, Shaw R, Ryan C: Truly silent ischemia and the relationship of chest pain and ST segment changes to the amount of ischemic myocardium: Evaluation by supine bicycle stress echocardiography. J Am Coll Cardiol 1994;23:369–376.

66. Gottlieb SO, Weisfeldt ML, Ouyang P, Mellits ED, Gerstenblith G: Silent ischemia as a marker for early unfavorable outcomes in patients with unstable angina. N Engl J Med 1986;314:1214–1219.

67. Gottlieb SO, Weisfeldt ML, Ouyang P, Mellits ED, Gerstenblith G: Silent ischemia predicts infarction and death during 2 year follow-up of unstable angina. J Am Coll Cardiol 1987;10:756–760.

68. Nademanee K, Intarachot V, Josephson MA, Rieders D, Vaghaiwalla Mody F, Singh BN: Prognostic significance of silent myocardial ischemia in patients with unstable angina. J Am Coll Cardiol 1987;10:1–9.

69. Nyman I, Larsson H, Areskog M, Areskog NH, Wallentin L: The predictive value of silent ischemia at an exercise test before discharge after an episode of unstable coronary artery disease. RISC Study Group. Am Heart J 1992;123:324–331.

69a. Amanullah AM, Lindvall K: Prevalence and significance of transient—predominantly asymptomatic—myocardial ischemia on Holter monitoring in unstable angina pectoris and correlation with exercise test and thallium-201 myocardial perfusion imaging. Am J Cardiol 1993;72:144–148.

70. Marmur JD, Freeman MR, Langer A, Armstrong PW: Prognosis in medically stabilized unstable angina: Early Holter ST-segment monitoring compared with predischarge exercise thallium tomography. Ann Intern Med 1990;113:575–579.

70a. Clinical Practice Guideline Number 10. Unstable angina: Diagnosis and management. AHCPR Publication No. 94-0602, U.S. Department of Health and Human Services, Rockville, MD, March 1994, pp. 1–154.

71. Gottlieb SO, Gottlieb SH, Achuff SC, Baumgardner R, Mellits ED, Weisfeldt ML, Gerstenblith G: Silent ischemia on Holter monitoring predicts mortality in high-risk postinfarction patients. JAMA 1988;259:1030–1035.

72. Tzivoni D, Gavish A, Zin D, Gottlieb S, Moriel M, Keren A, Banai S, Stern S: Prognostic significance of ischemic episodes in patients with previous myocardial infarction. Am J Cardiol 1988;62:661–664.

73. Petretta M, Bonaduce D, Bianchi V, Vitagliano G, Conforti G, Rotundi F, Themistoclakis S, Morano G: Characterizations and prognostic significance of silent myocardial ischemia on predischarge ECG monitoring in unselected patients with myocardial infarction. Am J Cardiol 1992;69:579.

74. Ruberman W, Crow R, Rosenberg CR, Rautaharju PM, Shore RE, Pasternack BS: Intermittent ST depression and mortality after myocardial infarction. Circulation 1992;85:1440–1446.

75. Assey ME, Walters GL, Hendrix GH, Carabello BA, Usher BW, Spann JF Jr: Incidence of acute myocardial infarction in patients with exercise-induced silent myocardial ischemia. Am J Cardiol 1987;59:497–500.

76. Gibson RS, Beller GA, Kaiser DL: Prevalence and clinical significance of painless ST segment depression during early postinfarction exercise testing. Circulation 1987;75:II36–II39.

77. Bolognese L, Rossi L, Sarasso G, Prando MD, Bongo AS, Dellavesa P, Rossi P: Silent versus symptomatic dipyridamole-induced ischemia after myocardial infarction: clinical and prognostic significance. J Am Coll Cardiol 1992;19:953–959.

78. Kayden DS, Wackers FJ, Zaret BL: Silent left ventricular dysfunction during routine activity after thrombolytic therapy for acute myocardial infarction. J Am Coll Cardiol 1990;15:1500–1507.

79. Currie P, Ashby D, Saltissi S: Prognostic significance of transient myocardial ischemia on ambulatory monitoring after acute myocardial infarction. Am J Cardiol 1993;71:773–777.

80. Mickley H, Pless P, Nielson JR, Berning J, Moller M: Transient myocardial ischemia after a first acute myocardial infarction and its relation to clinical characteristics, predischarge exercise testing and cardiac events at one year follow-up. Am J Cardiol 1993;71:139–144.

81. Solimene MC, Ramires JA, Gruppi CJ, Alfieri RG, de Oliveira SF, da Luz PL, Pileggi F: Prognostic significance of silent myocardial ischemia after a first uncomplicated myocardial infarction. Int J Cardiol 1993;38:41–47.

82. Jereczek M, Andresen D, Schroder J, Voller H, Bruggemann T, Duetschmann C, Schroder R: Prognostic value of ischemia during Holter monitoring and exercise testing after acute myocardial infarction. Am J Cardiol 1993;72:8–13.

83. Vaagenilsen M, Aurup P, Hoegolm A, Eioemark I, Rasmussen V, Jensen G: The prevalence of myocardial ischemia six months after thrombolytic treatment of acute coronary episodes—a subset of a placebo-controlled, randomized trial, the ASSET study. Int J Cardiol 1993;39:187–193.

84. Kayden DS, Wackers FJ, Zaret BL: Silent left ventricular dysfunction during routine activity after thrombolytic therapy for acute myocardial infarction. J Am Coll Cardiol 1990;15:1500–1507.

85. Stuckey TD, Burwell LR, Nygaard TW, Gibson RS, Watson DD, Beller GA: Quantitive exercise thallium-201 scintigraphy for predicting angina recurrence after percutaneous transluminal coronary angioplasty. Am J Cardiol 1989;63:517–521.

86. Knatterud GL, Bourassa MG, Pepine CJ, et al.: Effects of treatment strategies to suppress ischemia in patients with coronary artery disease: 12-week results of the asymptomatic cardiac ischemia pilot (ACIP) study. J Am Coll Cardiol 1994;24:11–20.

Chapter 6

Radionuclide Imaging in Acute Myocardial Infarction

Radionuclide imaging techniques are being utilized increasingly for assessment of global and cardiac function, regional myocardial perfusion, and myocardial cellular viability in patients who present with acute myocardial infarction (MI). Not only can imaging techniques be employed for detecting and localizing areas of infarction and sizing the extent of irreversible injury, they can also be used in combination with exercise or pharmacologic stress in the risk stratification process for evaluating prognosis. Selection of postinfarction patients who would benefit from further invasive evaluation and subsequent revascularization to reduce their risk of death has been aided by nuclear cardiology approaches to imaging of perfusion, function, and metabolism.

Positron emission tomography (PET) with short-lived radionuclides may permit high accuracy in distinguishing viable myocardium from necrotic tissue in patients with MI and in identifying areas of stunned myocardium that remain viable. In an era of cost-effective decision making for management of postinfarction patients, it is important to be aware of the role of noninvasive testing in separating high- and low-risk subsets of myocardial infarct survivors. A group judged at low risk by clinical and functional assessment would be spared more costly invasive testing since knowledge of coronary anatomy would have little supplemental prognostic value for risk stratification. Conversely, patients identified as high risk would be identified based on clinical and physiologic parameters, thus providing a sound basis for further invasive evaluation with a view toward coronary bypass surgery or coronary angioplasty, anatomy permitting. Recognition of prognostic factors derived from the clinical history, physical examination, and the routine chest x-ray is, indeed, important and provides vital information for the overall process of risk assessment. These clinical variables include symptoms and signs of heart failure, peak creatine kinase (CK) level, history of previous infarction, resting ST and T-wave abnormalities, diabetes mellitus, history of angina pectoris, pulmonary congestion on admission chest x-ray, x-ray cardiothoracic ratio, digoxin use, history of diastolic hypertension, and age. Table 6–1 summarizes the various clinical applications of radionuclide imaging techniques in patients with acute MI.

DETECTION, LOCALIZATION, AND SIZING OF ACUTE MYOCARDIAL INFARCTION

Detection of Infarction with Resting Thallium-201 Scintigraphy

Planar or single-photon emission computed tomography (SPECT) resting thallium-201 (Tl-201) imaging may be useful in the acute phase of a suspected MI to confirm the clinical suspicion of myocardial damage. However, whether or not an apparent Tl-201 defect is new and attributable to acute myocardial necrosis or old and due to prior scar cannot be determined when an earlier Tl-201 imaging study is available for comparison. Van der Wieken et al.[1] demonstrated that resting Tl-201 imaging could be undertaken in the emergency room setting to diagnose acute infarction in patients who present with chest pain and a nondiagnostic electrocardiogram (ECG). These investigators reported that

Table 6–1. Clinical Applications of Radionuclide Imaging Techniques in Patients with Acute Myocardial Infarction

Myocardial perfusion imaging (planar or SPECT)
    Diagnosis and location of infarction
    Determination of "area at risk"
    Assessment of myocardial salvage after reperfusion
    Determination of final infarct size
    Assessment of viability in asynergic infarct zone
    Stress imaging for detection of infarct zone ischemia
    Stress imaging for identification of multivessel
      disease
Radionuclide angiography
    Determination of LVEF and RVEF
    Diagnosis of RV infarction
    Assessment of regional wall motion
    Serial imaging for identifying myocardial stunning
    Diagnosis of LV aneurysm
    Exercise imaging to identify zones of inducible
      ischemia
Infarct-avid Imaging
    Diagnosis of infarction
    Infarct size determination
Positron imaging
    Assessment of regional blood flow
    Distinguishing viable from necrotic myocardium

if the scintigram was unequivocally normal, the probability of an infarction's being confirmed by other testing was in the range of 1%. Of 57 patients in this study who exhibited a Tl-201 defect on acute-phase scintigraphy, 35 were confirmed to have experienced an infarction within 24 hours, four developed an infarction within 1 to 7 days, and three had an infarction within 7 and 55 days. Ten patients had proven coronary artery disease (CAD) but no infarction. This left five patients with probable noncardiac causes of chest pain, whose defects were probably false positive. Not all patients who present with chest pain and an abnormal resting Tl-201 perfusion scan subsequently show evidence of acute infarction by enzymatic criteria. Some may have a history of MI and residual scar formation. Certain patients with unstable angina who receive Tl-201 in the midst of an episode of rest angina may also exhibit Tl-201 perfusion abnormalities when scanned soon afterward (see Chap. 7).[2–5] Nevertheless, even if such patients do not rule in for infarction, they would certainly benefit from admission to a cardiac inpatient unit for further observation and management.

The earlier a patient is scanned, the greater is the sensitivity of rest Tl-201 scintigraphy for detection of MI. Wackers et al.[6] showed that the prevalence of positive scans in patients who present with symptoms and signs of acute infarction was significantly higher (94%) for patients imaged within 24 hours of onset of symptoms than for those studied later during the course of hospitalization (72%). Table 6–2 summarizes the major findings of this study. Patients in this study who were serially imaged exhibited decreased Tl-201 defect size, most likely related to resolution of periinfarction ischemia with enhanced antegrade coronary flow or development of coronary collaterals. Improvement in regional wall motion over time would also have contributed to an apparent decrease in resting Tl-201 defect size, because of the partial volume effect. Thus, sensitivity of Tl-201 imaging for detecting perfusion abnormalities consequent to acute coronary occlusion decreases with the interval after presentation.

Right ventricular (RV) infarction can also be identified in patients presenting with ECG evidence of an inferior MI on Tl-201 scintigrams.[7, 7a] Absent or markedly diminished RV Tl-201 or Tc-99m sestamibi uptake would be observed predominantly on the 45-degree left anterior oblique (LAO) scintigram. Figure 6–1 shows an LAO Tl-201 scintigram in a patient with an RV infarction.

SPECT Tl-201 scintigraphy may prove superior to planar Tl-201 imaging for detection of acute MI. Tamaki et al.[8] performed SPECT and planar imaging at rest in 160 patients who had had a first MI and whose infarct size was estimated by peak CK activity. Tomography was significantly more sensitive than planar imaging for detecting anterior (87% vs. 96%), inferior (73% vs. 97%), and nontransmural (47% vs. 87%) infarctions. The enhanced sensitivity was restricted to detecting smaller infarcts when the peak CK activity was no more than 1000 IU/L (Table 6–3). For infarcts of that severity, planar techniques were positive in 44% of patients, as compared with an 89% detection rate for SPECT. It should be mentioned that specificity in this study was similar (92%) with the two techniques. Similar findings were reported by Ritchie et al.,[9] who found an 87% detection rate for Tl-201 tomographic imaging, as compared with 63% for planar imaging for detection of infarction. In that study, improvement of the SPECT method occurred only in the combined subset of transmural inferior

Table 6–2. Results of Thallium-201 Scintigraphy in 200 Patients with Acute Myocardial Infarction

Time of Scintigraphy After Onset of Symptoms (hr)	Patients (No.)	Scintiscan Findings		
		Defect	Questionable	Negative
<6	44	44	—	—
6–24	52	46	5	1
24–48	36	21	13	2
>48	68	54	8	6

(Reprinted by permission of *The New England Journal of Medicine* from Wackers FJT, et al.: N Engl J Med 1976;295:1–5. Copyright 1976, Massachusetts Medical Society.)

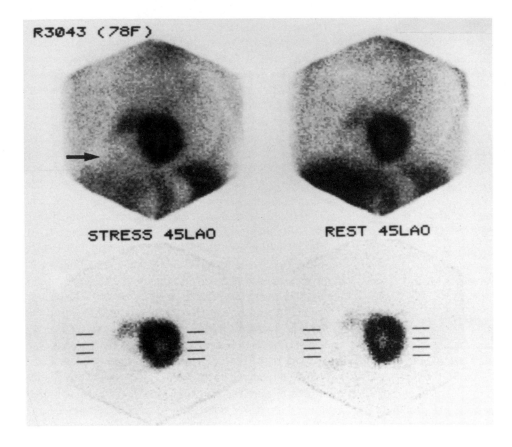

R3043 (78F)

STRESS 45LAO   REST 45LAO

Figure 6–1. Unprocessed *(top)* and background-subtracted *(bottom)* stress and delayed rest myocardial Tl-201 scintigrams in the 45-degree LAO projection in a patient with RV infarction. Note the diminished tracer uptake in the RV wall *(arrow)*. There is marked LV hypertrophy, and a defect in the LV myocardium is not apparent.

and subendocardial infarctions and not in transmural anterior infarctions. As reported in the Tamaki study,[8] the peak CK level was lower in patients whose disease was detectable only by SPECT than in those whose disease was detectable by both planar and SPECT techniques. The specificity for infarct detection was 93% for both techniques in the study by Ritchie et al.[9] The increased sensitivity of SPECT Tl-201 imaging for detection of small infarcts is not surprising, considering the technical advantages of the SPECT technique over conventional planar imaging (Chap. 1).

Localization of Myocardial Infarction by Rest Thallium-201 Scintigraphy

Rest Tl-201 scintigraphy can localize the zone of infarction to the vascular region supplied by the involved infarct-related vessel. A defect involving the middle and upper septal region seen on the 45-degree LAO planar view or on the SPECT short-axis images is nearly 100% specific for a left anterior descending (LAD) artery obstruction. Similarly, defects noted in the middle and upper posterolateral wall are highly specific for left circumflex (LCx) coronary artery occlusion. Approximately 90% of inferior wall defects are associated with narrowing of the right coronary artery. Perfusion defects localized to the left ventricular (LV) apex may represent infarction in the vascular risk region of any of the three major coronary arteries; however,

when a large area of the apex is involved that extends to the distal anterolateral wall, LAD artery obstruction is almost always the underlying event. Circumflex-related MI may be quite difficult to identify by conventional 12-lead ECG. In a study by Hucy et al.,[10] only 48% of patients with a circumflex infarction had acute ST-segment elevation in any ECG leads on admission. The size of the perfusion defect in patients with a circumflex infarct–related vessel was substantially larger than could be predicted from the ECG. In fact, Tl-201 defect size in patients with a circumflex infarction in that study was comparable to the defect size seen in patients with infarction related to an LAD

Table 6–3. **Results of Planar Imaging and Tomography with Thallium-201 in 63 Patients Whose Peak Creatine Kinase Value Was ≤1000 IU/L**

Peak CK Value (IU/L)	Patients No. (%)	
	Planar Imaging	*Tomography*
≤200	0/6 (0)	3/6 (50)
201–400	1/10 (10)	7/10 (70)
401–600	7/16 (44)	15/16 (94)
601–800	8/15 (53)	15/15 (100)
801–1000	12/16 (75)	16/16 (100)
Total	28/63 (44)	56/63 (89)

(Tamaki S, et al.: Br Heart J 1984;52:621–627.)

coronary artery occlusion. However, the LV ejection fraction (LVEF) was significantly higher in association with circumflex-related infarction than with LAD-related infarction (Fig. 6–2). Figure 6–3 shows SPECT tomographic images from representative patients with acute myocardial infarctions demonstrating the typical locations of infarctions related to the left anterior descending, left circumflex, and right coronary arteries.

Non–Q-wave MI is less easily localized and detected than is Q-wave infarction. Wahl et al.[11] reported that patients with acute Q-wave infarction had, on average, 5.6 Tl-201 defects per patient, as compared with 2.9 defects per "non–Q-wave infarction patient." In that study, Q-wave infarct patients demonstrated a 92% prevalence of persistent Tl-201 defects on serial images, as compared with a 50% prevalence of persistent defects for non–Q-wave patients. This finding supports the notion that non–Q-wave patients have less extensive necrosis than do Q-wave infarct patients.

In patients with a totally occluded infarct vessel, Imamura[12] reported that the Tl-201 defect was smaller in patients whose coronary collaterals could be demonstrated on angiography than in those whose occluded vessels had no angiographically demonstrable collaterals. Christian et al.[13] also showed that final defect size on rest technetium-99m–methoxyisobutyl isonitrile (Tc-99m sestamibi) images in patients with acute infarction was much influenced by angiographic demonstrability of collaterals (Fig. 6–4). Myocardium at risk was also significantly associated with infarct size. Patients exhibiting the "no reflow" phenomenon after reperfusion reflected by a progressive decrease in great cardiac vein flow had significantly larger SPECT Tl-201 defects compared to patients without such a decrease.[13a]

Rest Tl-201 scintigraphy in the acute phase of MI may also yield information about the status of resting perfusion of myocardial zones remote from the infarct. Such remote defects may represent either previous scar or resting "ischemia at a distance." Gibson et al.[14] reported that 52% of patients with acute inferior MI had concomitant anterior defects on rest Tl-201 imaging.

Sizing of Myocardial Infarction with Rest Thallium-201 Scintigraphy

The subject of infarct sizing with Tl-201 scintigraphy is extensively reviewed by Kirchner.[15] Sizing of MI by radionuclide techniques can provide useful prognostic information. Prognosis is related, in part, to the size of infarction, and when infarct size exceeds 40% of the left ventricle, the incidence of cardiogenic shock is great.

Several experimental studies have indicated that extent of myocardial hypoperfusion on Tl-201 scintigrams accurately reflects MI size. In a 24-hour closed-chest canine infarct model, DiCola et al.[16] reported that the diminution in regional Tl-201 uptake at postmortem examination correlated well with depletion of CK and alterations in regional myocardial blood flow. In a similar canine model, Okada et al.[17] showed that planar Tl-201 infarct size correlated closely ($r = 0.89$) with infarct size as assessed histologically. Nelson et al.[18] also found excellent correlation ($r = 0.88$) between Tl-201 infarct size and pathologic infarct volume. Kaul et al.[19] reported that the myocardial area at risk, as determined by SPECT Tl-201 defect size, correlated well ($r = 0.98$) with postmortem Tl-201 autoradiography findings. Prigent et al.[20] measured SPECT Tl-201 infarct size in closed-chest dogs and found that it correlated well ($r = 0.93$) with pathologic infarct size. Figure 6–5 depicts the relationship between tomographic and pathologic infarct size in another study by Prigent et al.[21] SPECT infarct size was defined as the percentage of the maximum-count dif-

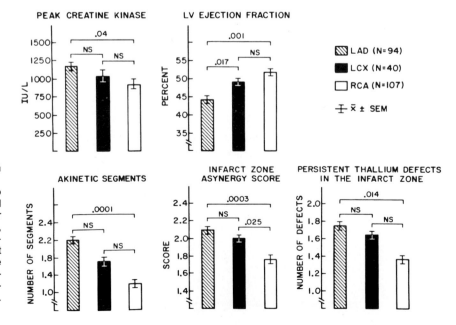

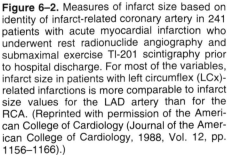

Figure 6–2. Measures of infarct size based on identity of infarct-related coronary artery in 241 patients with acute myocardial infarction who underwent rest radionuclide angiography and submaximal exercise Tl-201 scintigraphy prior to hospital discharge. For most of the variables, infarct size in patients with left circumflex (LCx)-related infarctions is more comparable to infarct size values for the LAD artery than for the RCA. (Reprinted with permission of the American College of Cardiology (Journal of the American College of Cardiology, 1988, Vol. 12, pp. 1156–1166).)

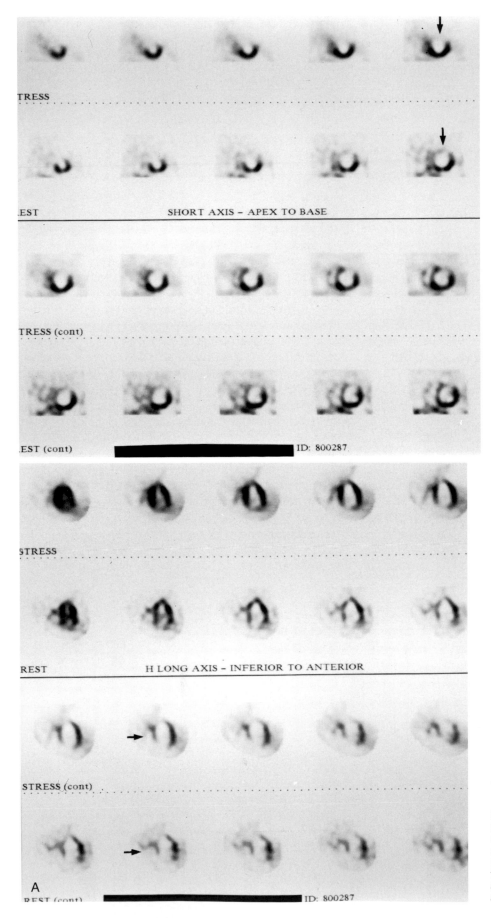

Figure 6–3. A. SPECT Tc-99m sesta-mibi images in a patient with an anterior myocardial infarction. *Top:* Stress and rest short-axis tomograms showing non-reversible apical, anterior, and septal defects *(arrows). Bottom:* Horizontal long-axis tomograms showing nonreversible anterior and septal defects *(arrows).*

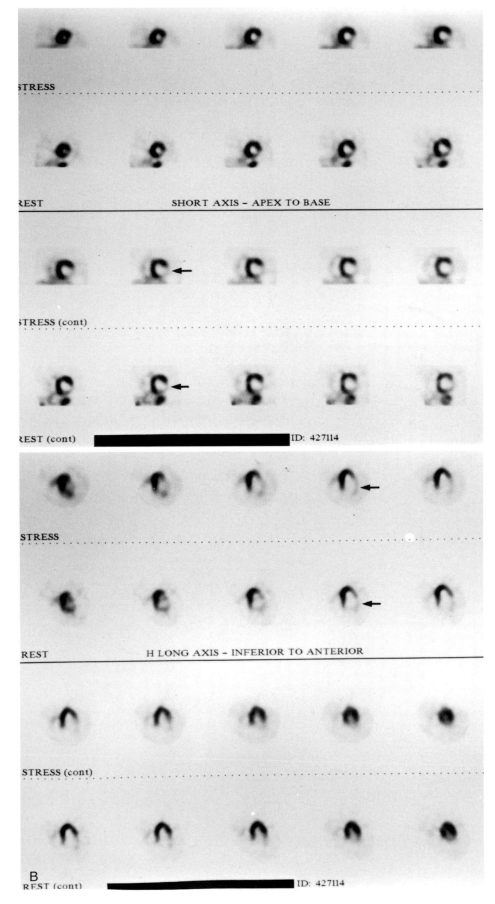

Figure 6–3 *Continued* **B.** SPECT Tc-99m sestamibi images in a patient with a posterolateral wall infarction secondary to left circumflex coronary artery occlusion. *Top:* Stress and rest short-axis tomograms showing a nonreversible posterolateral defect *(arrow). Bottom:* Horizontal long-axis tomograms showing the defect, which is more prominent in midventricular compared to basal images *(arrow).*

Illustration continued on following page

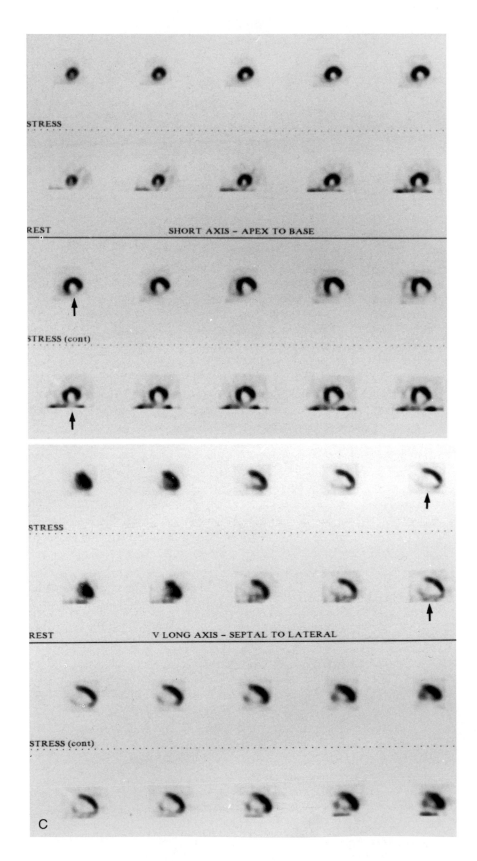

STRESS

REST   SHORT AXIS – APEX TO BASE

STRESS (cont)

STRESS

REST   V LONG AXIS – SEPTAL TO LATERAL

STRESS (cont)

C

Figure 6–3 *Continued* **C.** SPECT Tc-99m sestamibi images in a patient with an inferior myocardial infarction secondary to a right coronary artery occlusion. *Top:* Short-axis tomograms during stress and at rest showing a nonreversible inferior defect *(arrow)* extending from the apex to the base. *Bottom:* Vertical long-axis tomograms showing the inferior defect *(arrow)* with a slight amount of reversibility.

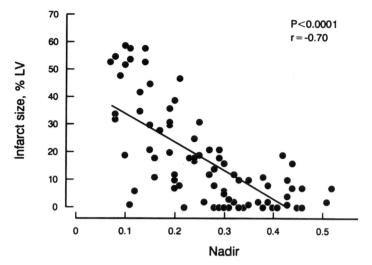

Figure 6–4. Scatter plot shows final infarct size compared with the radionuclide Tc-99m–sestamibi estimate of collateral flow (nadir). The nadir is defined as the lowest ratio of minimal counts per pixel over maximum counts per pixel on the short-axis slices. (Christian TF, et al.: Circulation 1992;86:81–90.)

ferential profile points that fall below normal. Total LV infarct size is calculated by adding together infarct sizes of each slice multiplied by a coefficient k that reflected the contribution of that slice to total LV mass. Weiss et al.[22] also demonstrated that SPECT Tl-201 defect mass correlated well with histologic perfusion mass in their canine model. Keyes et al.[23] calculated the extent of infarcted myocardial mass, using SPECT Tl-201 scintigraphy in an isolated heart model. The correlation between scintigraphic infarct size and histologic infarct size was excellent ($r = 0.87$). Gerber and Higgins[24] reported that Tl-201 images of transverse slices of hearts that previously underwent infarction, systematically underestimated the true infarct size as determined histochemically. Nevertheless, there was an excellent linear relationship ($r = 0.94$) between the scintigrams of the myocardial slices and the infarct size measured by nitro blue tetrazolium (NBT).

Clinical pathologic studies have been performed in pa-tients who died from an acute MI and who had previously undergone rest Tl-201 scintigraphy during the acute phase. Wackers et al.[25] correlated the scintigraphic location and estimated size of infarction in vivo with postmortem findings. There was a good agreement (91%) between scintigraphic and postmortem location of infarction. The size of infarction determined from computer-processed drawings of postmortem sections of the heart correlated well with infarct size determined from scintigrams. The size of the scintigraphically abnormal area reflected the extent of necrosis. The correlation between scintigraphically and pathologically measured infarct size was linear ($r = 0.72$) for all patients: $r = 0.91$ for anterior infarctions and $r = 0.97$ for inferior infarctions.

Tamaki et al.[26] evaluated the ability of SPECT Tl-201 imaging to estimate infarct size in 18 patients studied within 4 weeks of their first MI. Infarct volume determined by SPECT Tl-201 imaging correlated closely with accu-

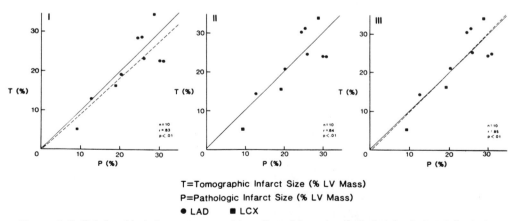

T=Tomographic Infarct Size (% LV Mass)
P=Pathologic Infarct Size (% LV Mass)
● LAD   ■ LCX

Figure 6–5. Relationship between tomographic radionuclide and pathologic infarct size. Infarct size was quantitated in dogs with an acute closed-chest coronary occlusion using circumferential profile analysis of Tl-201 SPECT images. Pathologic infarct size was determined by triphenyl tetrazolium chloride staining. SPECT infarct size was defined as the percentage of the maximum-count circumferential profile points that fall below normal. Three different methods were employed, and all showed a linear relationship between SPECT infarct size and pathologic infarct size. (Reprinted by permission of the Society of Nuclear Medicine from Prigent F, et al.: J Nucl Med 1987;28:325–333.)

mulated CK release ($r = 0.89$). As expected, infarct area measured from planar images correlated less well with enzymatic infarct size ($r = 0.73$).

Mahmarian et al.[27] prospectively investigated whether SPECT Tl-201 scintigraphy could accurately quantify the extent of MI when compared with infarct size determined by plasma MB-CK activity. Infarct size was quantified with computer-generated polar maps of the myocardial Tl-201 activity and expressed as a percentage of a total LV volume. Scintigraphy and enzymatic estimates of infarct size correlated well for the group as a whole ($r = 0.78$) but particularly for patients with anterior infarction ($r = 0.91$; Fig. 6–6). The poor correlation seen in patients with inferior infarction was thought probably to be related to the frequent RV involvement.

Taken together, the results of the experimental and human studies suggest that the size of an acute MI can, indeed, be accurately estimated by quantitation of perfusion defects on rest myocardial Tl-201 scintigraphy. SPECT techniques appear to be more accurate than planar imaging for estimating Tl-201 infarct size. An obvious limitation of Tl-201 imaging for infarct size determination is that recent infarction cannot be distinguished from old scar. Also, there can be an overestimation of infarct size if periinfarction "resting ischemia" is present. In such an instance, the perfusion abnormality would represent a combination of irreversible myocardial injury and ischemic but viable myocardium. Because of this possibility, delayed rest Tl-201 imaging should be performed. Zones of resting hypoperfusion that are viable should show redistribution on these delayed images, whereas regions of irreversibly injured myocardium would correspond to persistent Tl-201 defects.

Resting Thallium-201 Imaging and Prognostication in Acute Myocardial Infarction

Based on the experimental and clinical data described in the previous section with respect to infarct size determination by Tl-201 scintigraphy, it is not surprising that clinical

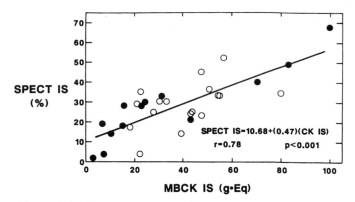

Figure 6–6. Linear regression analysis comparing SPECT and enzymatic estimates of infarct size (IS) for patients with enzymatic evidence of infarction who were imaged within 12 to 36 hours of chest pain. IS by SPECT was quantified with computer-generated polar maps of the myocardial radioactivity and is expressed as a percentage of the total left ventricular volume. (Mahmarian JJ, et al.: Circulation 1988;78:831–839.)

experience has shown prognostic value in determining Tl-201 defect size in patients with an acute MI. The extent of the perfusion abnormality on the acute-phase Tl-201 scintigram has significant prognostic value in patients with suspected or documented acute infarction. Perez-Gonzalez et al.[28] related the extent of Tl-201 defect size with prognosis at 16 months in patients undergoing imaging during the acute phase of hospitalization. Sixty-one percent of the postinfarction patients for the scintigraphic infarct size greater than 25 cm[2] and a perfusion abnormality of more than 35% of the ventricular area died during follow-up. This was compared to a 93% survival rate for patients with less severe abnormalities. Scintigraphic parameters were more accurate than any other clinical or laboratory indicator for determining late prognosis. Figure 6–7 depicts the scintigraphic data for survivors and nonsurvivors in that study. As shown, the perfusion abnormality expressed as percent of the LV and average perfusion abnormality values were significantly greater for nonsurvivors, whereas their LVEF was lower. In a subsequent study from the same group by

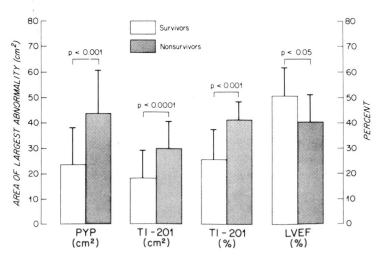

Figure 6–7. Quantitative Tl-201 and Tc-99m pyrophosphate (PYP) scan data from survivors and nonsurvivors of acute MI. Nonsurvivors had significantly larger PYP and Tl-201 scan abnormalities and a lower LVEF than survivors. (Perez-Gonzalez J, et al.: Circulation 1982;66:960–971.)

Botvinick et al.,[29] Tl-201 defect size was twice as large in infarct patients who experienced a subsequent cardiac event than in patients who remained asymptomatic after discharge. Early scintigraphic measurement of myocardial Tl-201 defect size was a better variable than even the resting EF for differentiating between event and nonevent groups.

Using a qualitative scoring system, Becker et al.[30] reported that a Tl-201 defect score of 7.0 or greater (corresponding to a defect of 40% of the LV circumference) identified a subset of patients whose subsequent 6-month mortality rate was 64%. An LVEF of 35% or less identified a high-risk subgroup of patients whose 6-month mortality was 60%. In that study, the mortality rate was 83% for patients who had both a Tl-201 defect score of 7.0 or greater and an LVEF of no more than 35%. This was compared with an 8% mortality rate for patients with low-risk perfusion and functional measurements. Figure 6–8 provides a summary of these findings.

Hakki et al.[31] reported that the Tl-201 perfusion score at rest provided discriminating power for survival similar to that of combining the LVEF and Holter monitor findings of complex arrhythmias. Patients with an LVEF of at least 40%, a relatively low Tl-201 perfusion score, and no complex ventricular ectopy had a 100% 1-year survival rate. The survival rate for patients who had a combination of a large perfusion defect score and an LVEF of less than 40%, and who exhibited complex ventricular arrhythmias on ambulatory ECG monitoring, was only 44% (Fig. 6–9).

Gibson et al.[14] found that the event rate during follow-up was 77% for patients with inferior MI who had defects both in the inferior zones and anteroseptal regions on rest redistribution imaging, as compared with a 33% event rate for inferior infarct patients whose defects were confined solely to the risk region of the right coronary artery. Thus, total defect size, which includes the area of necrosis and the zone of remote hypoperfusion, provides important prognostic information and enhances noninvasive detection of severe multivessel CAD in postinfarction patients.

Assessment of RV Tl-201 uptake on resting Tl-201 scin-

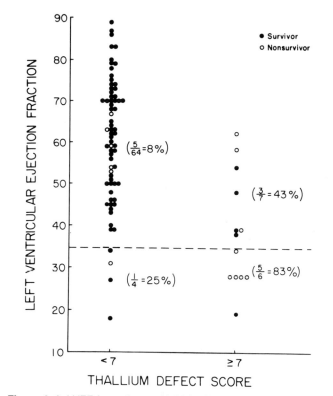

Figure 6–8. LVEF for patients with high- (thallium defect score ≥7) and low-risk (thallium defect score <7) scintigraphic studies. A Tl-201 (thallium) defect score of ≥7 corresponds to involvement of 40% of the LV circumference. Values indicate 6-month mortality for each quadrant of the figure. Concordant high- and low-risk studies were associated with very high and low mortality rates, respectively, whereas discordant results had an intermediate rate of mortality. Note that the patients with the lowest mortality (8%) had ejection fraction values >40% and low-risk (<7) Tl-201 defect scores. (Becker LC, et al.: Circulation 1983;67:1272–1282.)

tigraphy also may provide useful prognostic information. Nestico et al.[32] reported that patients who show enhanced RV Tl-201 uptake had a lower mean LVEF, more extensive myocardial perfusion abnormalities, a higher incidence of complex ventricular arrhythmias, a greater prevalence of

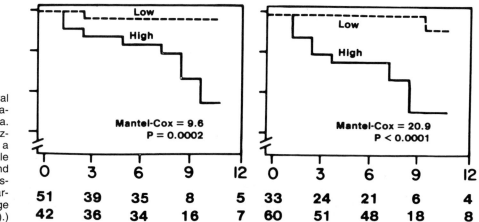

Figure 6–9. Life table analysis of survival in low- and high-risk postinfarction patients by LVEF and Tl-201 score criteria. The Tl-201 score was derived by analyzing the extent of diminished uptake in a total of 15 segments, graded on a scale of 0 to 4, where 4 is normal uptake and 0 is no uptake. (Reprinted with permission from the American College of Cardiology (Journal of the American College of Cardiology, 1987, Vol. 10, pp. 25–32).)

abnormal lung Tl-201 uptake, and a higher mortality rate than patients with normal RV Tl-201 uptake after infarction. It appears that increased RV Tl-201 uptake is a reflection of RV failure with increased blood flow to the RV myocardium required for increased work of that ventricle. The higher the pulmonary artery pressure, the greater should be the uptake of Tl-201 in RV myocardium.

A subsequent improvement in LV function after MI can be predicted by serial rest Tl-201 scintigraphy. Hirsowitz et al.[33] showed that improved Tl-201 uptake observed when comparing images acquired at 9 days and approximately 24 hours after admission predicted ultimate improvement in LV function. The reduction in Tl-201 defect size may be related to enhanced flow to viable myocardium with uptake of Tl-201 in viable zones of asynergy. Tl-201 uptake in the presence of severe regional dysfunction is a marker of viability and implies intact cell membrane function and presence of residual flow, albeit via collateral channels (see Chap. 9).

Rest Thallium-201 Imaging for Predicting Viability After Acute Myocardial Infarction

Viability detection by rest Tl-201 imaging is discussed in Chapter 9. Briefly, evidence for Tl-201 uptake at rest in the risk area of the infarct-related artery implies myocardial viability. Some patients show significant rest redistribution over time on serial resting Tl-201 images. This finding implies that there is a persistent diminution in regional blood flow but intact cells that are capable of extracting Tl-201 from the blood pool between the early and delayed images. Tl-201 uptake is preserved in stunned myocardium following reperfusion as long as myocardial membrane integrity is intact.

Conclusions

The results of the radionuclide studies in acute MI cited above suggest that resting Tl-201 imaging in the acute phase of infarction is useful in detecting, localizing, and sizing regions of myocardial necrosis. Additionally, a high-risk subset of postinfarction patients can be identified who exhibit extensive perfusion abnormalities that are the result of acute necrosis or acute necrosis superimposed on a previous myocardial scar. The extent of Tl-201 defect abnormalities may be a better predictor of high risk than resting EF or presence of complex ventricular arrhythmias on ECG monitoring. This is because depression of global and regional LV function early after infarction may represent both "stunned" and irreversibly injured myocardium.

When resting Tl-201 imaging is undertaken in patients with acute infarction, it is important to obtain a set of delayed images at 3 to 4 hours to evaluate for "rest redistribution," which is suggestive of resting ischemia and preserved viability. Defect size observed on initial images after resting injection is often a combination of irreversible myocardial injury and periinfarction resting ischemia. A reduction of defect size from early to delayed rest images suggests presence of viable but underperfused myocardium in the distribution of the infarct related vessel. A patient who exhibits this scintigraphic finding may be a candidate for early angiography with a view toward revascularization. This would certainly be indicated if postinfarction angina or silent ischemia is evident.

Few large-scale studies in the literature have directly compared the prognostic value of resting Tl-201 defect size with other noninvasive and clinical variables for identifying patients at high risk. Rest Tl-201 imaging performed in patients with markedly depressed LV function, with or without heart failure, certainly would be useful for determining how much of the EF depression is due to necrosis and how much to a combination of necrosis and stunned or hibernating myocardium (see Chap. 9). Tl-201 uptake in zones of akinesis or dyskinesis certainly suggests viability. Marked reduction of Tl-201 uptake in an area of infarction with no delayed redistribution portends a poor prognosis and may predict subsequent remodeling with progressive LV dilatation and heart failure. The larger the irreversible defect, the greater is the infarct and the worse the long-term prognosis. No studies have been undertaken to determine whether early Tl-201 scintigraphy could be useful in identifying which patients may benefit from early angiotensin-converting enzyme (ACE) inhibitor therapy.

MYOCARDIAL REPERFUSION IMAGING WITH THALLIUM-201 AFTER ACUTE MYOCARDIAL INFARCTION

Myocardial perfusion imaging techniques can certainly provide useful information for early and late assessment of MI patients who have received thrombolytic agents.[34] In addition, quantitative perfusion imaging approaches can be incorporated into clinical trials of thrombolytic therapy when defect size is recognized as an endpoint for ultimate myocardial salvage.[35] Rest Tl-201 imaging in patients with markedly depressed LV function after thrombolytic therapy could prove useful in the selection of patients who might benefit from early angiography to further enhance antegrade blood flow and achieve greater subsequent myocardial salvage. Certain patients may have very high-grade infarct-related stenosis after successful reperfusion. In such a patient, the defect size may be quite large on initial resting Tl-201 images but show substantial delayed redistribution on rest images repeated 4 hours later. This implies resting ischemia with a substantial degree of residual myocardial viability. The basic principles and clinical applications of myocardial reperfusion imaging with radionuclide agents are summarized in a review by Beller.[35a]

Experimental Validation of Rest Thallium-201 Imaging to Assess Reperfusion

As cited earlier, myocardial uptake of Tl-201 is directly proportional to myocardial blood flow and the ability of myocardial cells to extract the tracer.[36] When regional flow is restored early following acute coronary occlusion, myocardial salvage is reflected by improved survival and enhanced LV function.[37] Since Tl-201 uptake requires intact nutrient flow and a viable sarcolemmal membrane (see Chap. 2), one may hypothesize that the demonstration of Tl-201 uptake on postreperfusion scintigrams in the distribution of the previously occluded and reperfused vessel would reflect salvage and viability. Granato et al. performed experiments in which Tl-201 was administered intravenously to anesthetized dogs during either 1 hour or 3 hours of LAD coronary artery occlusion.[38, 39] Serial myocardial biopsy specimens were obtained before and after coronary reperfusion to assess the degree of delayed Tl-201 redistribution following reflow. The degree of Tl-201 redistribu-

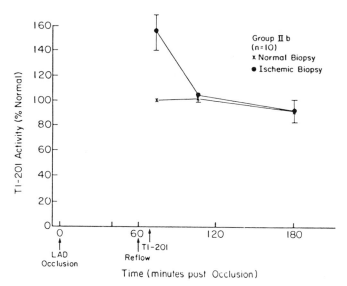

Figure 6–11. Myocardial Tl-201 time-activity curves in dogs subjected to 1 hour of coronary occlusion followed by total and rapid reperfusion through a patent LAD coronary artery. Tl-201 was administered immediately after reflow. Note the "excess" Tl-201 uptake in the previously ischemic zone, suggesting that uptake reflected hyperemic flow rather than viability. (Granato JE, et al.: Circulation 1986;73:150–160.)

tion in the reperfused zone correlated well with the degree of salvage as assessed by microsphere-determined regional flow values and histochemical staining. Figure 6–10 shows myocardial Tl-201 time-activity curves in dogs undergoing either 3 hours of sustained LAD occlusion or 1 hour of LAD occlusion followed by 2 hours of reflow through a residual critical stenosis. Dogs reperfused after 1 hour of LAD occlusion showed significantly more delayed redistribution on serial biopsy measurements of Tl-201 activity than the group of dogs with sustained LAD occlusion. Final defect size in that study correlated well with histologic area of necrosis. In another group of dogs, Tl-201 was administered intravenously for the first time immediately after reperfusion during the hyperemic phase of reflow. With this method of Tl-201 administration, the degree of salvage was overestimated, perhaps because "excess" Tl-201 uptake was measured in the infarct zone, presumably owing to hyperemia at the time of Tl-201 administration (Fig. 6–11). Weinstein et al[47a] also demonstrated that when Tl-201 is given soon after reflow, the initial uptake pattern is more reflective of flow than of viability.

Tl-201 given immediately after reflow could become "trapped" in the noncellular compartments of the infarct zone, initially yielding a smaller defect than would be expected when compared with the ultimate extent of necrosis as assessed histologically. Forman and Kirk[40] showed that when Tl-201 is given early after reperfusion to dogs undergoing experimental coronary occlusion, the immediate Tl-201 uptake pattern was also related more to hyperemic flow than to cellular viability. These investigators found when Tl-201 was administered 24 hours after reperfusion, uptake of the radionuclide relative to flow was significantly

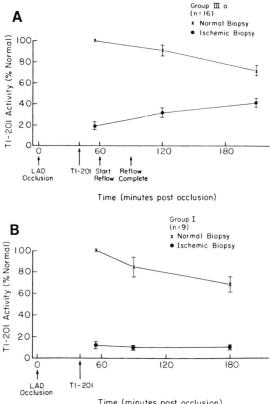

Figure 6–10. A. Myocardial Tl-201 time-activity curves in dogs subjected to 1 hour of coronary occlusion followed by reperfusion through a residual critical stenosis. Tl-201 was administered during occlusion, and the degree of delayed redistribution was monitored. Note the slow clearance of Tl-201 from the normal zone (x) as compared with delayed accumulation of Tl-201 after reperfusion in the previously ischemic (●) zone. **B.** Myocardial Tl-201 time-activity curves in dogs undergoing 3 hours of sustained occlusion of the LAD coronary artery. Note that there is no delayed Tl-201 accumulation in the ischemic zone. (Granato JE, et al.: Circulation 1986;73:150–160.)

less than what was observed when the radionuclide was given early after reperfusion. Another potential explanation for higher Tl-201 uptake when the tracer is given soon after reflow is the influence of reperfusion injury. That is, there may be viable cells that are able to concentrate Tl-201 when the tracer is given immediately upon flow restoration that ultimately becomes injured in the reperfusion process. That would make defects larger after reperfusion when Tl-201 is given 6 hours or more after flow restoration.

Melin et al.[41] assessed both Tl-201 redistribution and glucose uptake as predictors of myocardial salvage after experimental coronary occlusion and reperfusion in a canine model. Tl-201 was injected intravenously 20 minutes before reperfusion, and fluorine-18 2-deoxyglucose (FDG) was injected 3 hours after reperfusion. Coronary occlusion was sustained for 2 hours, and reperfusion lasted 4 hours. The results of this study confirm the observations of Granato et al.[38] in that the final degree of Tl-201 uptake in the ischemic region correlated with the extent of necrosis. The metabolic rate for glucose was low in the endocardial and epicardial necrotic samples as compared with that in the ischemic and normal samples. These investigators concluded that delayed redistribution of Tl-201 during reflow when the tracer is injected before reperfusion is an indicator of viable myocardium. Diminished Tl-201 activity in association with depressed glucose uptake indicates irreversible cell injury, whereas normal FDG uptake is predictive of viable tissue. Okada and Boucher[42] also administered Tl-201 early (5 minutes) after reperfusion preceded by 2 hours of LAD coronary occlusion in anesthetized dogs. These investigators observed faster clearance for Tl-201 that was taken up early in the reperfused zone (Fig. 6–12). This implies that much of the Tl-201 uptake early after reflow was not extracted in viable myocytes but was predominantly trapped in extracellular compartments (e.g., interstitial fluid) and subsequently washed out rapidly.

Rest Thallium-201 Scintigraphy in Acute Myocardial Infarction Patients Receiving Thrombolytic Therapy

In the clinical setting, Tl-201 can be administered intravenously before administration of a thrombolytic agent and serial images can be obtained both during the occlusion phase and after reperfusion.[43] As would have been predicted from the experimental studies described in the previous section, patients who exhibit successful thrombolysis have more Tl-201 redistribution and smaller final Tl-201 defects than patients with persistently occluded, infarct-related vessels. In a study by De Coster et al.,[44] patients who demonstrated Tl-201 redistribution 4 hours after institution of thrombolytic therapy (when Tl-201 was injected before the thrombolytic drug was administered) showed even further improvement in myocardial Tl-201 uptake when imaging was repeated 4 days and 6 weeks later. This continued

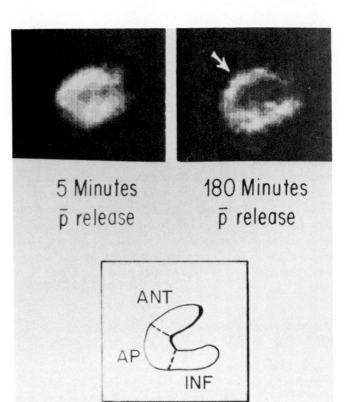

Figure 6–12. Five- and 180-minute postrelease ($\bar{p}$) Tl-201 images from a dog with an experimental MI that received Tl-201 5 minutes after reflow, plus another image obtained 3 hours later. Note the normal Tl-201 activity initially, whereas the 180-minute image shows appearance of an anterolateral wall defect *(arrow)* in this animal with MI. The explanation for the normal Tl-201 uptake in the infarct region is that the tracer was given during the hyperemic phase of reflow. (Okada RD, Boucher CA: Am Heart J 1987;113:241–250.)

reduction in Tl-201 defect size after reperfusion could be related to further enhancement of nutrient blood flow, reversal of postischemic metabolic abnormalities in Tl-201 cellular transport, or improvement in wall motion, reducing the influence of the partial volume effect on measuring Tl-201 defect size. Figure 6–13 shows the mean values for Tl-201 defect scores obtained before and serially after reperfusion in 18 nonreperfused and 26 reperfused patients. The latter group showed a substantial reduction in defect scores over 6 weeks after thrombolytic therapy.

There are some limitations to the use of serial rest Tl-201 redistribution in the early evaluation of patients receiving thrombolytic therapy. It may take as long as 30 to 40 minutes to obtain pretreatment images, particularly with SPECT acquisition, which delays the administration of a thrombolytic agent. Also, if, as described in the experimental studies, Tl-201 is administered for the very first time immediately after reperfusion, the degree of salvage could be overestimated because Tl-201 would be taken up more in proportion to hyperemic flow and not necessarily in proportion to the extent of viable myocardial tissue that was salvaged.

Another approach to rest Tl-201 scintigraphy for assessment of myocardial salvage in patients undergoing throm-

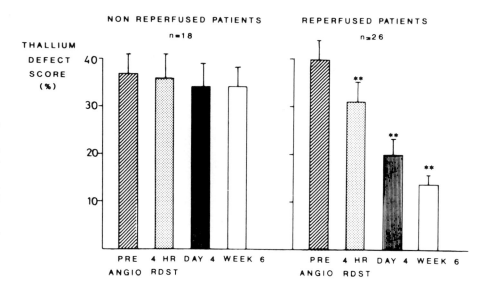

Figure 6–13. Mean values (± SEM) of sequential Tl-201 defect scores in patients with acute MI before intracoronary streptokinase (preangio), 4 hours after streptokinase (4-hr redistribution, RDST), and 4 days and 6 weeks later in nonreperfused patients *(left)* and reperfused patients *(right)*. A serial improvement in Tl-201 defect score is noted from the 4-hour redistribution images to the 4-day and 6-week images *(right)*. (Reprinted from American Journal of Cardiology: 58:8; April 11, 1985; 889–895.)

bolytic therapy is to administer Tl-201 for the first time 24 hours or more after thrombolysis. By delaying the imaging procedure to this time, trapping of Tl-201 in the infarct region during the hyperemic flow phase that immediately follows reflow is avoided. Schwarz et al.[45] performed resting Tl-201 scintigraphy before and 24 hours after streptokinase therapy. The regional EF was serially assessed up to 4 weeks after treatment. The improvement in Tl-201 defect size was greatest in the patients who demonstrated successful reperfusion. The regional EF was improved only in the patients with the greatest improvement in Tl-201 defect size who experienced successful reflow as determined by angiography.

Schuler et al.[46] studied 21 patients undergoing thrombolytic therapy using Tl-201 tomography before and 1 hour and 24 hours after treatment. The size of the perfusion defect decreased from 36% to 19% of LV circumference at 24 hours in patients whose vessels were successfully recanalized. Tl-201 defect size was decreased most in patients who had collateral vessels supplying the infarct region. Figure 6–14 shows resolution of a large perfusion defect in

the inferior aspect of the LV circumference from a patient in this study.

In the Western Washington Intracoronary Streptokinase in Myocardial Infarction Trial, Ritchie et al. undertook quantitative rest SPECT Tl-201 imaging for the first time at 8 weeks after infarction.[47] No difference was observed in Tl-201 defect size between controls and streptokinase-treated patients. This result suggested no substantial influence on infarct size with intracoronary streptokinase therapy. This conclusion was supported by the observation of no difference in global or regional EF between streptokinase and placebo groups. The explanation given for these negative findings was that the time to reperfusion was about 5 hours, perhaps too long to afford significant myocardial salvage. In a subsequent thrombolytic trial by the same collaborative research group employing intravenous streptokinase, SPECT Tl-201 defect size was significantly smaller in the streptokinase-treated patients than in the placebo-treated controls.[35] The patients who received intravenous streptokinase were treated sooner after the onset of symptoms than those who were treated in the intracoronary

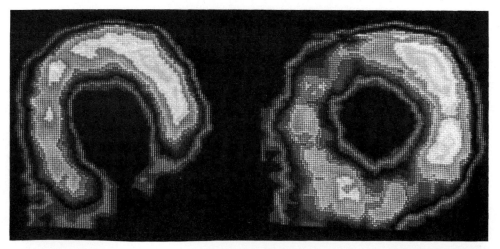

Figure 6–14. Tl-201 scintigram obtained in a patient before *(left)* and 24 hours after *(right)* successful coronary recanalization. Note the resolution of a large perfusion defect in the inferior segment of the left ventricle (see color Figure 6–14). (Schuler G, et al.: Circulation 1982;66:658–664.)

See Color Figure 6–14.

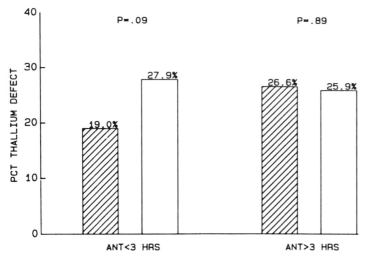

Figure 6–15. Infarct size by quantitative Tl-201 tomography expressed as a percentage (PCT) of the left ventricle for patients with anterior (ANT) infarction and stratified by time to treatment. Note the 32% limitation in size for the treatment group of <3 hours *(left bars)*. No difference was seen in patients treated after 3 hours *(right bars)*. (Key: hatched bars, streptokinase; open bars, control patients.) (Reprinted with permission from the American College of Cardiology (Journal of the American College of Cardiology, 1988, Vol. 11, pp. 689–697).)

trial. Patients with anterior infarcts given intravenous streptokinase within 3 hours after the onset of symptoms had a 32% reduction in infarct size, as compared with patients treated after 3 hours who had only a minimal decrease in infarct size. A long-term follow-up of this patient population showed that patients with large Tl-201 defects had a significantly higher 5-year mortality rate compared to those patients with small defects after thrombolytic therapy[35b] (Fig. 6–15).

Krause et al.[47b] performed both Tl-201 and technetium-99m (Tc-99m) pyrophosphate (PYP) imaging in patients receiving anisoylated plasminogen streptokinase activator complex (APSAC) for acute MI. Patients with an inhomogeneous Tc-99m PYP pattern within the Tl-201 defect, characterized by the maximal activity localized in the infarct periphery and relatively less or no central uptake, had a higher incidence of in-hospital complications and a lower incidence of patent infarct vessels than patients with a homogeneous Tc-99m accumulation pattern. The Tl-201 defect size by itself was significantly larger in patients who experienced cardiogenic shock or heart failure. It is unclear whether or not the combined imaging technique provides any greater prognostic information than rest-redistribution Tl-201 imaging alone to separate high- and low-risk subgroups.

The results of the experimental and clinical studies discussed above indicate that rest Tl-201 imaging performed after administration of a thrombolytic agent can provide information about the degree of myocardial salvage and a final estimate of myocardial infarct size. The point should be made again here that delayed rest images should always be obtained in these infarction patients receiving thrombolytic therapy, to determine the degree of periinfarction ischemia. Acquisition of images before institution of thrombolytic therapy is not practical, as therapy would be substantially delayed. Acquisition of pretreatment Tl-201 images may not be necessary, since the final defect size dictates ultimate prognosis and final status of LV global

function. As will be discussed later in this chapter, Tc-99m sestamibi is quite suited for serial assessment of risk area during occlusion and infarct size after reperfusion, respectively, in patients with acute MI.

ASSESSMENT OF VENTRICULAR FUNCTION AFTER ACUTE MYOCARDIAL INFARCTION

Resting Radionuclide Angiography in Acute Myocardial Infarction

Many of the clinical uses of resting radionuclide angiography (RNA) in the setting of acute infarction can also be achieved well with two-dimensional (2-D) echocardiography; the exception is a highly accurate quantitative determination of global LVEF and RVEF. Table 6–4 summarizes the clinical application of RNA after acute MI. As described in Chapter 1, quantitation of EF by either first-pass or gated-equilibrium RNA technique is count based and not dependent on ventricular geometry. No edge detection techniques are required, and tracing of the borders of the heart is not required to calculate end-diastolic and end-systolic volumes for EF determination. Regional wall motion abnormalities detected by RNA (or 2-D echocardiog-

Table 6–4. Clinical Applications of Radionuclide Angiography after Acute Myocardial Infarction

Diagnosis of acute infarction
Measurement of global LV function
Prognostication using extent of asynergy
Demonstrating viability by virtue of preserved systolic function
RV function assessment in inferior infarction
Detection of LV aneurysm
Qualitative determination of degree of ischemic mitral regurgitation
   with exercise to detect residual ischemia

raphy) are not specific for acute myocardial necrosis in patients who present with chest pain. Patients with acute infarction, old infarction, or acute regional ischemia without necrosis may exhibit regional systolic wall motion abnormalities. For as long as 1 week after reperfusion therapy myocardial stunning can be observed, which is characterized by systolic wall motion abnormalities secondary to postischemic dysfunction. RNA performed in the acute phase of an inferior infarction may demonstrate a reduced RVEF and RV asynergy. RV systolic function usually recovers over time in such patients.

Resting Radionuclide Angiography and Complications of Acute Myocardial Infarction

Resting RNA can help determine the presence or absence of certain complications of acute MI such as LV aneurysm, RV infarction, pseudoaneurysm, mitral regurgitation, ventricular septal rupture, and resting remote ischemia. The RNA is particularly well-suited for recognition of aneurysmal LV dilatation, which most often can be distinguished from pseudoaneurysms or akinetic myocardial segments. Volume overload patterns resulting from mitral regurgitation caused by papillary muscle dysfunction or acute cardiac dilatation after infarction can be identified as a cause of congestive heart failure by RNA techniques. Patients with valvular regurgitation have an enlarged LV end-diastolic volume but relatively preserved LVEF, as long as there has not been extensive myocardial damage. Semiquantitative assessment of valvular regurgitation can be determined with RNA techniques by measuring the ratio of LV stroke volume to RV stroke volume (see Chap. 1 for further details). In patients with no valvular regurgitation, this ratio is approximately 1.15, whereas in patients with mitral regurgitation it usually exceeds 1.30.[48] Echocardiog-

raphy and Doppler echocardiography are probably better suited than RNA to the identification of mechanical complications of MI such as ventricular septal defect and mitral regurgitation. Similarly, for overall assessment of regional myocardial dysfunction in acute infarction, 2-D echocardiography permits more complete evaluation of a larger number of segments than RNA. Rest RNA and 2-D echocardiography may be complementary in the noninvasive evaluation of patients with suspected LV aneurysm.[49] In that study, use of both techniques identified 100% of patients with LV aneurysm confirmed at operation. Berger et al.[49a] found a 5% prevalence of RV dysfunction on predischarge RNA in 1110 patients with inferior infarction enrolled in the Thrombolysis in Myocardial Infarction (TIMI) II trial. Figure 6–16 shows the radionuclide angiogram from a patient in this study. Patients with RV dysfunction had a lower mean LVEF ($51\% \pm 1\%$) than patients without RV dysfunction ($55\% \pm 0.3\%$; $P < 0.001$) and a greater frequency of in-hospital complications. Angiographic data obtained 18 to 48 hours after admission demonstrated that the infarct-related artery was more likely to be occluded in those with RV dysfunction (48% vs. 14%; $P < 0.001$). One year after discharge mortality was comparable for those with and without RV dysfunction, and by 6 weeks postdischarge RV wall motion abnormalities persisted in only 18% of patients who showed such abnormalities before discharge.

Rest RNA may also be complementary to rest Tl-201 imaging in the identification of patients with acute MI and congestive heart failure who might benefit from early angiography with a view toward revascularization. Evidence of extensive myocardial asynergy with preserved Tl-201 uptake would suggest that there is viable but stunned or hibernating myocardium (see Chap. 9). Similarly, demonstration of wall motion abnormalities outside the zone of infarction associated with remote Tl-201 defects would suggest the

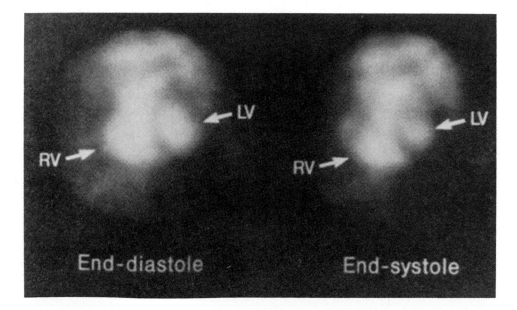

Figure 6–16. Predischarge end-diastolic and end-systolic frames from a 45-degree left anterior oblique radionuclide ventriculogram in a patient with an acute inferior infarction. The images reveal RV dilatation and hypokinesis. The left ventricle (LV) is of normal size and demonstrates normal systolic function. (Reprinted from American Journal of Cardiology: 71:3; May 15, 1993; 1148–1152.)

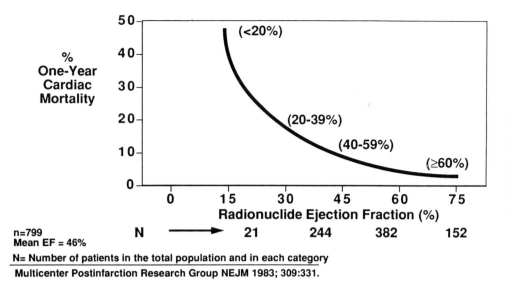

% One-Year Cardiac Mortality

n=799
Mean EF = 46%
N= Number of patients in the total population and in each category
Multicenter Postinfarction Research Group NEJM 1983; 309:331.

Figure 6–17. One-year cardiac mortality related to the predischarge radionuclide ejection fraction after acute MI. Note the marked increase in cardiac mortality when the ejection fraction falls below 40%. The mean ejection fraction was 46%. (Reprinted by permission of *The New England Journal of Medicine* from Multicenter Postinfarction Research Group: N Engl J Med 1983; 309:331–336. Copyright 1983, Massachusetts Medical Society.)

presence of extensive multivessel disease where the global LV dysfunction was contributed to by both necrosis in the infarct region and ischemic dysfunction in the distribution of another stenotic coronary vessel. Undoubtedly, such patients would benefit from revascularization, since multicenter randomized trials have shown that patients with multivessel disease and depressed LV function are more likely to survive when treated with surgery than when given medical therapy.[50]

Rest Radionuclide Angiography and Prognostication After Acute Myocardial Infarction

One of the best prognostic measurements that can be derived by RNA in patients experiencing an acute MI is LVEF.[51] In this setting, the depression of EF reflects both new damage and previous myocardial scar rather than being secondary to acute necrosis alone. Many postinfarction patients show depressed LVEF without manifesting signs or symptoms of congestive heart failure. A postinfarct patient who presents in Killip class I or II with an LVEF below 30% has a high likelihood of cardiac death in the first year after admission.[52] Patients with a non–Q-wave MI tend to have a higher resting LVEF than patients with Q-wave infarction and have more hypokinesis in the infarct zone than akinesis or dyskinesis.[53] This is expected, since postmortem studies of these patients have demonstrated a smaller degree of myocardial necrosis. Patients with anterior infarction have greater depression of LVEF than inferior infarction patients.[54]

Norris et al.[55] examined factors associated with total cardiac mortality, sudden death, and reinfarction after a first MI in 325 male survivors younger than 60 years. Total cardiac mortality was best predicted by the LVEF and by a coronary prognostic index. In this study, neither the severity of coronary artery lesions measured with a scoring system nor the results of the exercise tests were a significant

predictor of mortality. Sudden death not associated with reinfarction was significantly more common when EF was 40% or less than when it was greater.

Perhaps the most often-cited study relating to the resting radionuclide EF obtained before discharge in MI patients and subsequent mortality is the report from the Multicenter Postinfarction Research Group.[56] In that study composed of 866 patients, univariate analysis showed a progressive increase in cardiac mortality during 1 year as the EF fell below 40% (Fig. 6–17). Only four risk factors were independent predictors of mortality: a radionuclide EF below 0.40, ventricular ectopy of 10 or more depolarizations per hour, advanced New York Heart Association (NYHA) functional class before infarction, and rales in the upper two-thirds of the lung fields while the patient was in the

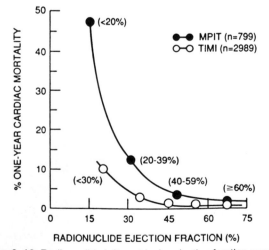

Figure 6–18. Radionuclide left ventricular ejection fraction versus 1-year cardiac mortality from the Multicenter Postinfarction Research Group (MPIT) (see Fig. 6–17) and the 1-year mortality from the TIMI-IIB (TIMI) trial in which all patients received thrombolytic therapy. (Bonow R: J Nucl Cardiol 1994;1:280–291.)

Table 6–5. **Regional and Global Left Ventricular Ejection Fraction Exercise Data at Hospital Discharge and 6-Week Follow-Up Obtained at Comparable Workloads**

	Hospital Discharge			6-Week Follow-Up		
	Invasive (N = 796)	*Conservative (N = 778)*	*P Value*	*Invasive (N = 796)*	*Conservative (N = 778)*	*P Value*
Baseline LVEF (%)	51.3 ± 12.0	50.5 ± 12.1	NS	51.4 ± 12.2	50.4 ± 12.0	NS
Peak exercise LVEF (%)	55.2 ± 13.4	53.4 ± 13.7	0.01	54.3 ± 13.9	52.6 ± 13.5	0.02
Δ Peak exercise LVEF (%)	4.0 ± 6.6	2.9 ± 7.1	0.002	2.9 ± 7.1	2.2 ± 6.6	0.04
Peak exercise infarct zone regional LVEF* (%)	53.2 ± 30.4	50.2 ± 31.5	0.001	51.6 ± 30.5	50.2 ± 31.5	NS

*Adjusted for distribution of infarct artery in each treatment group.
Key: NS, not significant; Δ, mean change.
(Reprinted from American Journal of Cardiology: 69:1; January 1, 1992; 1–9.)

coronary care unit. Various combinations of these four factors identified five risk subgroups whose 2-year mortality rates ranged from 3% (no factors) to 60% (all four factors).

In patients who have received thrombolytic therapy for acute MI, the LVEF is still an important predictor of subsequent outcome. However, it appears that postinfarction patients who have been treated with a thrombolytic agent may have a better chance of survival at any level of LVEF than infarction patients treated in the prethrombolytic era.[57] This improved survival at any level of LVEF in thrombolytic patients is illustrated in Figure 6–18, where the mortality rate at 1 year is plotted against the LVEF in the Multicenter Postinfarction Research Group study from the prethrombolytic era and against the LVEF in the TIMI-IIB trial performed in patients receiving thrombolytic therapy.[57a] Simoons et al.[57b] showed that global left ventricular function was an important determinant of survival in the thrombolytic era. Mortality exceeded 50% at 5 years in patients who received thrombolytic therapy but were discharged with an LVEF of less than 30%. In contrast, patients with an LVEF of greater than 40% experienced an annual mortality of only about 2% per year. Left ventricular end-systolic volume may be a more important prognostic variable than the LVEF.[57c] Resting LVEF at discharge and at 6 weeks was comparable in MI patients receiving thrombolytic therapy on admission who were randomized to a "conservative" strategy and those randomized to an "invasive" strategy in the TIMI study.[58] Table 6–5 summarizes the baseline rest and exercise LVEF values in patients randomized to either the invasive or noninvasive strategy after thrombolytic therapy for acute MI in this study.

There is a significant interaction between age and LVEF in determining prognosis after an acute MI.[59] Patients who had a first MI before age 50 years and an LVEF greater than 40% and patients between 51 and 70 years of age whose LVEF was over 50% had a 1.2% ± 1.1% 1-year mortality rate. Mortality for the remaining patients younger than 70 years was 7.4% ± 3.5%. Mortality for patients older than 70 years was high at 22.2% ± 6.6%. Figure 6–19 summarizes these data.

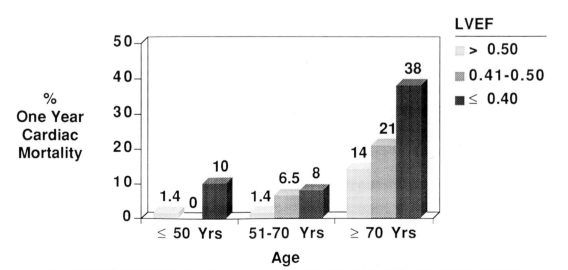

Figure 6–19. One-year cardiac mortality rate related to age and resting LVEF after acute MI. Note that for patients ≥70 years of age, mortality is higher for every LVEF range. (From Ahnve S, et al.: Am Heart J 1988;116:925–932.)

Table 6–6. Number of Diseased Vessels Compared with Outcome Variables after Acute Myocardial Infarction

Involved Vessels* (No.)	Total Patients	Dead† No. (%)	New MI† No. (%)	Proximal LCA Stenosis ≥ 50%‡ No. (%)	EF < 40% No. (%)
1	28	1/28 (4)	2/28 (7)	7 (25)	6 (21)
2	22	1/18 (6)	4/18 (22)	9 (41)	2 (9)
3	56	11/41 (27)	6/41 (15)	44 (79)	21 (38)
		$P < 0.025$§	NS	$P < 0.001$	$P < 0.05$

*At least 50% obstruction.
†Excluding 19 patients who had coronary artery bypass graft surgery.
‡Includes 12 patients who had left main coronary artery stenosis ≥50% and 48 with LAD stenosis ≥50%. (Taylor GJ, et al.: Circulation 1980; 62:960–970.)
§P values for columns above the solid line (contingency table analysis, 2 by 3 matrix).

NONINVASIVE RISK STRATIFICATION USING EXERCISE STRESS AND PERFUSION IMAGING

Exercise Electrocardiographic Stress Testing for Prognostication

Prognosis after uncomplicated MI is related to (1) the degree of LV dysfunction as described above, (2) the presence of complex ventricular arrhythmias, and (3) the presence of inducible residual myocardial ischemia. These risk variables are prognostically more important for patients with underlying multivessel CAD than for those who have experienced an acute infarction with single-vessel disease.[60] Table 6–6 summarizes event rates related to number of diseased vessels, presence or absence of proximal left coronary artery stenosis, and LVEF less than 40% in the 106 patients who comprised this study cohort.

Exercise testing after MI may be useful in separating these high- and low-risk subsets on the basis of hemodynamic, exercise, and ECG endpoints. Table 6–7 summarizes exercise test variables associated with high risk after acute MI. Postinfarction patients who are unable to attain a target heart rate of 120 bpm or a workload of 4 METs are at greater risk for subsequent cardiac events than those who can exceed these endpoints. Patients who exhibit an inappropriate blood pressure response to exercise or develop exercise-induced ventricular tachycardia are also at increased risk for subsequent cardiac events after discharge. If ST-segment depression greater than 1.0 mm occurs, particularly at a slow exercise heart rate or light workload, this is also associated with a significant increase in mortality during follow-up. In one recent review of the literature,[61] 29% of 3776 patients pooled from 17 series in the literature from the prethrombolytic era exhibited exercise-induced ST-segment depression on submaximal predischarge exercise testing. The subsequent cardiac mortality rate was 15.6% for patients who manifested exercise-induced ST-segment depression, as compared with 4.8% for those who did not manifest ischemic ST-segment changes during exercise. In a study reported by Gibson et al.[62] from the University of Virginia in a group of 241 postinfarction

patients who did not receive thrombolytic therapy, 29% of 154 Q-wave infarct patients and 36% of 87 non–Q-wave infarct patients exhibited ST-segment depression on predischarge submaximal treadmill exercise testing. As expected, those who demonstrated exercise-induced ST depression had a greater cardiac event rate during follow-up than those without ST depression.

The incidence of exercise-induced ST depression on predischarge stress testing is less for patients treated with thrombolytic therapy. In the TIMI-IIB Multicenter Trial, the prevalence of exercise ST depression at discharge in the 1626 patients in the conservative arm of the trial was 17.7%.[63, 63a] Six weeks after discharge, the incidence of ST depression was slightly higher, 19.4%. This value is certainly lower than the approximate 30% prevalence of inducible ST depression reported in postinfarction patients in the prethrombolytic era, as cited previously. Similarly, the incidence of an ischemic response on exercise testing in myocardial infarction patients undergoing immediate angioplasty is lower than the incidence of a positive response in patients not undergoing angioplasty, and is even lower than in patients receiving only thrombolytic therapy.[63b, 63c] The prognostic implications of a positive ST-segment response to exercise testing, as compared with a negative one, in patients receiving thrombolytic therapy who are then treated medically are unknown, because when ST depression is induced in such patients, the usual modus operandi is referral for coronary angiography and subsequent revascularization. In the GISSI-2 trial, in which the rate of revascularization after MI treated with thrombolytic therapy was low, patients with a negative exercise ECG stress test had only a 1.1% mortality rate by 6 months, but patients with a positive test had a 1.7% mortality rate at 6 months' follow-

Table 6–7. High-Risk Exercise ECG Test Variables after Acute Myocardial Infarction

Horizontal or down-sloping ST depression greater than 1.0 mm at submaximal heart rate or workload
Workload achieved ≤4 MET
Exercise-induced drop in systolic blood pressure
Nonsustained ventricular tachycardia
Limiting angina as test endpoint

up. Interestingly, patients deemed ineligible for predischarge exercise testing had the highest mortality rate, 9.8%.[63a] White et al.[63d] sought to determine the prognostic value of exercise testing in postinfarction patients who received thrombolytic therapy on admission. At 39 ± 13 months of follow-up, cardiac death had occurred in 5.8% of the 305 patients. No difference was seen between patients who died and patients who survived with respect to exercise duration, percent with angina during exercise, and the time to development of angina. It should be pointed out that revascularization was performed in 11.5% of patients, mean LVEF was 58%, and 77% had one- or two-vessel CAD on angiography suggesting that this was a "low-risk" cohort of MI patients at baseline.

Tilkemeier et al.[64] compared the incidence of ST-segment depression in postinfarction patients receiving thrombolytic therapy or angioplasty with that for those receiving no intervention during a comparable period of survey. In 64 patients receiving thrombolytic therapy, 15% had exercise-induced ST-segment depression. The postinfarction patients who were treated medically and did not undergo any intervention had a 35% incidence of predischarge exercise-induced ST depression. Similarly, Haber et al.[65] reported that only 14% of 67 patients treated with a thrombolytic agent exhibited exercise-induced ST-segment depression on submaximal predischarge exercise testing. This value is comparable to the incidence of ST depression reported from the TIMI-IIB trial (17%)[63] and the Massachusetts General Hospital study[64] (15%) in comparable patient cohorts.

An increase in the magnitude of ST-segment elevation in leads with Q waves during peak exercise is a marker of LV dysfunction and identifies a subgroup of patients at increased risk for subsequent cardiac death. Haines et al.[66] found that patients with increasing ST-segment elevation during exercise had larger persistent Tl-201 defects but no redistribution defects and more extensive wall motion abnormalities at rest than patients who did not demonstrate further ST-segment elevation during stress (Figs. 6–20, 6–21). Thus, exercise ST elevation after uncomplicated infarction is a marker of greater impairment of global and regional LV function due to more extensive myocardial necrosis rather than of more extensive ischemia.

Froelicher et al.[67] described limitations to the use of exercise ECG alone for determining prognosis following MI. In a metaanalysis of various studies that looked at exercise test responses after MI, they found that only 11 institutions of 24 reported that exercise-induced ST-segment shifts predicted high risk. These authors found from their review of the literature that patients with an abnormal blood pressure response and those with poor exercise capacity are at a higher risk after MI than those who have only 1.0 mm of ST-segment depression. Specificity of the ST-segment depression response in postinfarction patients may also present a problem. Exercise-induced ST-segment depression appears to be predictive of increased risk only in patients with inferior posterior Q-wave infarction, not in those with anterior Q-wave infarction. This is because ST depression in the presence of anterior precordial Q waves after anterior infarction is not predictive of increased ischemic event rate. In contrast, ST depression in leads without Q waves is highly predictive of an increased cardiac event rate. Patients with ST depression are more likely to have multivessel than single-vessel CAD, and the greater the magnitude of ST depression, the greater is the likelihood of severe CAD.[68] A 10-year follow-up of 258 patients who underwent predischarge exercise testing following acute MI revealed that 3 exercise test variables—hypotensive blood pressure response (hazard ratio: 5.1), ST-segment depression (hazard ratio: 1.8), and ST-segment elevation (hazard ratio: 2.4)—were strong independent predictors of cardiovascular death

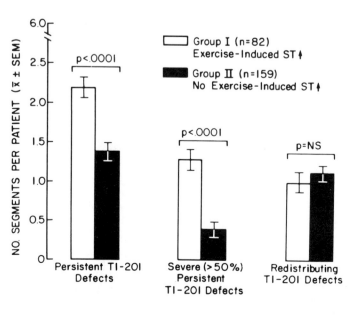

Figure 6–20. Exercise Tl-201 perfusion imaging data for 241 patients undergoing predischarge submaximal exercise scintigraphy after uncomplicated MI. The patients are grouped by presence or absence of exercise-induced ST-segment elevation (ST ↑). Patients with exercise-induced ST elevation had more persistent Tl-201 defects but a similar prevalence of redistribution defects compared to patients without increased ST ↑ . (Reprinted with permission from the American College of Cardiology (Journal of the American College of Cardiology, 1987, Vol. 9, pp. 996–1003).)

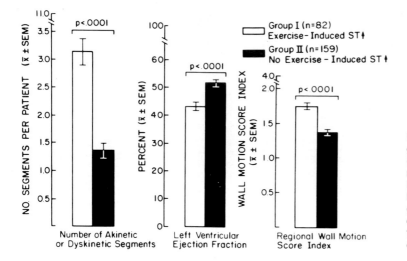

Figure 6–21. Resting gated equilibrium radionuclide angiographic data on 241 patients with (group I) and without (group II) exercise-induced ST-segment elevation on submaximal exercise stress testing after uncomplicated acute MI. Patients with exercise-induced ST-segment elevation had more segmental wall motion abnormalities and worse global and regional LV function than patients without exercise-induced ST elevation. (Reprinted with permission from the American College of Cardiology (Journal of the American College of Cardiology, 1987, Vol. 9, pp. 996–1003).)

after controlling for age, sex, and clinical variables.[67a] These patients underwent testing between 1977 and 1980, preceding the thrombolytic era.

Controversy persists with respect to whether or not symptom-limited exercise testing is preferable to submaximal testing for detection of residual ischemia and for identifying high-risk patients who may need further invasive evaluation. Juneau et al.[68a] performed both low-level and symptom-limited exercise tests in 200 patients with uncomplicated infarction, of whom 115 had received thrombolytic therapy. The symptom-limited test was associated with a greater exercise duration (554 vs. 389 seconds), a higher peak work load (5.7 vs. 4.2 METS), and a higher peak heart rate (121 vs. 108 bpm), as compared with the low-level stress test. The number of patients who developed ST depression significantly increased (56 to 89) from the low level to the symptom-limited test ($P < 0.0001$). There was an 86% increase in the number of patients who exhibited at least 2.0 minutes of ST depression. Exercise duration was longer and exercise-induced ST depression less frequent in patients who had received thrombolytic therapy. In contrast, Wilson et al.[68b] observed no change in the prevalence of ST depression from the predischarge submaximal treadmill exercise test to the symptom-limited test performed 3 months postdischarge. Similarly, there was no net change in prevalence of exercise-induced angina or Tl-201 redistribution from predischarge to the 3-month test. In neither of these studies was the prognostic value for future events of the two tests compared.

Stress Thallium-201 Scintigraphy for Risk Stratification After Infarction

Although clinical and ECG variables are perhaps useful in separating high-risk from low-risk subsets of patients after MI, stress perfusion imaging provides additional prog-

nostic information, and when utilized appropriately it can better separate high- and low-risk patients than these other variables.[68c] The factors that render exercise perfusion imaging superior to ECG stress testing alone for risk stratification after uncomplicated MI are summarized in Table 6–8. Myocardial perfusion imaging is more sensitive for simply detecting ischemia, particularly when exercise stress is undertaken with a submaximal protocol (see Chap. 3). Also, perfusion imaging can better identify patients with underlying multivessel CAD than exercise ECG alone (see Chap. 4) because of the better localizing capability of myocardial perfusion imaging. For example, stress-induced defects seen in anterior and posterior territories suggest ischemia in the distribution of at least two of the three major coronary arteries. The location of ST-segment depression does not precisely reflect the region of myocardium rendered ischemic during stress. ST depression is identified in a similar number of ECG leads, whether the patient has single- or multivessel CAD.

One of the first studies investigating the prognostic value of exercise Tl-201 imaging was undertaken by Smeets et al.[69] The investigators performed exercise stress ECG and planar Tl-201 scintigraphy in 224 patients 3 months after MI. By a scintigraphic criterion, 59% of them demonstrated a multivessel disease scan pattern. Those who exhibited this

Table 6–8. **Advantages of Exercise Perfusion Imaging Over Exercise ECG Testing Alone for Risk Stratification After Acute Myocardial Infarction**

Greater sensitivity for detecting residual ischemia at submaximal exercise heart rates
Better identification of multivessel CAD and ischemia remote from region of infarction
Can identify inducible ischemia within zone of infarction
Defect size related to MI size, which has prognostic significance
Increased lung Tl-201 uptake excellent marker of high risk

pattern experienced a 28% subsequent cardiac event rate, as compared with an 8% event rate for patients without a multivessel scintigraphic ischemic pattern. When both ST-segment depression and a multivessel scan pattern were combined as one variable, a subset of patients was identified whose subsequent cardiac event rate was 43%.

In the study reported by Gibson et al.[62] approximately 50% of patients with an uncomplicated MI who were younger than 65 years and who demonstrated multiple Tl-201 defects in more than one vascular region (multivessel disease scan pattern), delayed Tl-201 redistribution within or outside the infarct zone, or abnormal lung Tl-201 uptake on predischarge submaximal imaging subsequently experienced a cardiac event (7 deaths, 9 fatal infarctions, and 34 hospitalizations for class III to IV angina). In contrast, the cardiac event rate was only 6% for postinfarction patients who had either a normal scan or only persistent defects and no associated redistribution (Fig. 6–22). There was a subset of 21 of these 140 patients who demonstrated multiple Tl-201 defects in more than one vascular region, increased lung Tl-201 uptake, and redistribution in at least one segment on their scans. This subgroup's subsequent event rate was 86% at a mean of 15 months' follow-up (see Fig. 6–22). As expected, exercise Tl-201 scintigraphic variables were superior to exercise-induced ST-segment depression or angina in separating the high- and low-risk subgroups (Fig. 6–23). Twenty-six per cent of patients with a normal

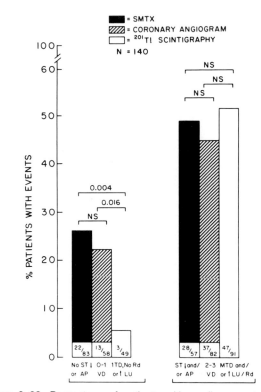

Figure 6–23. Percentage of patients with cardiac events (death, nonfatal infarction, class III–IV angina based on either high-risk or low-risk findings on submaximal electrocardiographic exercise testing *(black bars)*, coronary angiography *(crosshatched bars)*, and quantitative Tl-201 scintigraphy *(open bars)*. Note that the low-risk group was better identified by Tl-201 scintigraphy than by coronary angiography. Abbreviations are the same as in Figure 6–22, and VD, vessel disease; ST ↓ , ST-segment depression.) (Gibson RS, et al.: Circulation 1983;68:321–336.)

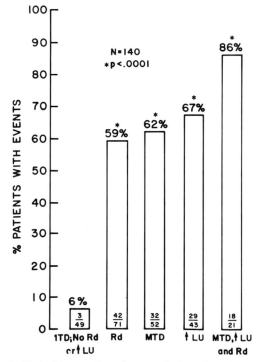

Figure 6–22. Incidence of cardiac events based on Tl-201 scintigraphic findings from predischarge exercise testing. (Key: 1TD, Tl-201 defect in one vascular region; Rd, redistribution; MTD, Tl-201 defects observed in >1 coronary vascular supply region; ↑ LU, increased lung Tl-201 uptake.) (Gibson RS, et al.: Circulation 1983;68:321–336.)

exercise ECG response still experienced a cardiac event during follow-up. On the other hand, 49% of patients who exhibited ischemic ST-segment depression experienced a cardiac event during follow-up. This event rate was comparable to that for patients who had redistribution defects on the predischarge scintigram. Figure 6–24 shows the cumulative probability of cardiac events as a function of time for patients with high- and low-risk findings on submaximal ECG stress testing, Tl-201 scintigraphy, or coronary angiography in this study. Note that the Tl-201 scintigram best separated high- and low-risk groups. Figure 6–25 is an example of a postinfarction patient with a high risk predischarge exercise myocardial perfusion scan showing multiple perfusion defects. Defects are observed in inferior, posterior, and posterolateral segments with partial reversibility observed in the posterolateral wall, best seen on the horizontal long axis tomograms.

Patterson et al.[70] also found that multiple defects extending throughout more than one coronary supply region were 65% sensitive and 96% specific for detection of left main or multivessel disease in postinfarction patients. Tl-201 scintigraphic data were also superior to exercise ECG data in distinguishing patients with underlying high-risk CAD.

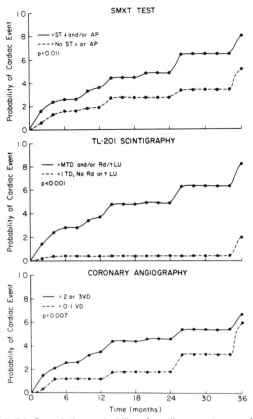

Figure 6–24. Cumulative probability of cardiac events as a function of time for different subgroups formed by the exercise test response *(top)*, Tl-201 scintigraphic findings *(middle)*, or angiographic findings *(bottom)*. The solid and dashed lines represent high-risk and low-risk cumulative probability, respectively. Note that the separation of high- and low-risk subgroups was best achieved by Tl-201 scintigraphy. (Key: ST↓, ST-segment depression; AP, angina pectoris; MTD, multiple Tl-201 defects >1 coronary supply region; Rd, redistribution; ↑LU, lung uptake; TD, thallium defect; VD, vessel disease.) (Gibson RS, et al.: Circulation 1983;68:321–336.)

Dunn et al.[71] also reported high specificity for planar Tl-201 scintigraphy for detecting multivessel CAD. They found that 92% of patients who demonstrated Tl-201 defects in more than one coronary supply region had angiographic evidence of multivessel disease, as compared with 72% of patients who had a positive exercise ECG. Multivessel disease was better differentiated from single-vessel disease by Tl-201 scintigraphy than by exercise ECG. A review of reports in the literature in the prethrombolytic era would conclude that Tl-201 scintigraphy possesses greater sensitivity than exercise ECG for identifying patients with multivessel disease after MI. In a pooled analysis of 508 patients,[53, 70–73] there was 72% sensitivity for multiple Tl-201 defects in more than one vascular region for detecting multivessel disease, and 86% specificity. In these earlier series, 59% of patients with multivessel disease had ischemic ST-segment depression. The positive predictive value of multiple Tl-201 defects in more than one coronary supply region for identifying multivessel disease was significantly higher than the positive predictive value of ST-segment depression.

Exercise Tl-201 Imaging in Patients Receiving Thrombolytic Therapy

In the thrombolytic era, the detection rate for multivessel disease in postinfarction patients by Tl-201 scintigraphy is less than that reported above for patients studied in the prethrombolytic era. In a study by Haber et al.,[65] 35% of patients in the thrombolytic patient cohort had angiographic multivessel disease. Twenty-two per cent had two-vessel, and 13% had three-vessel disease. Multiple Tl-201 defects in more than one vascular supply region were observed in 35% of these patients, with 87% specificity. This sensitivity rate of 35% for detection of multivessel disease was slightly, but not significantly, higher than that of exercise-

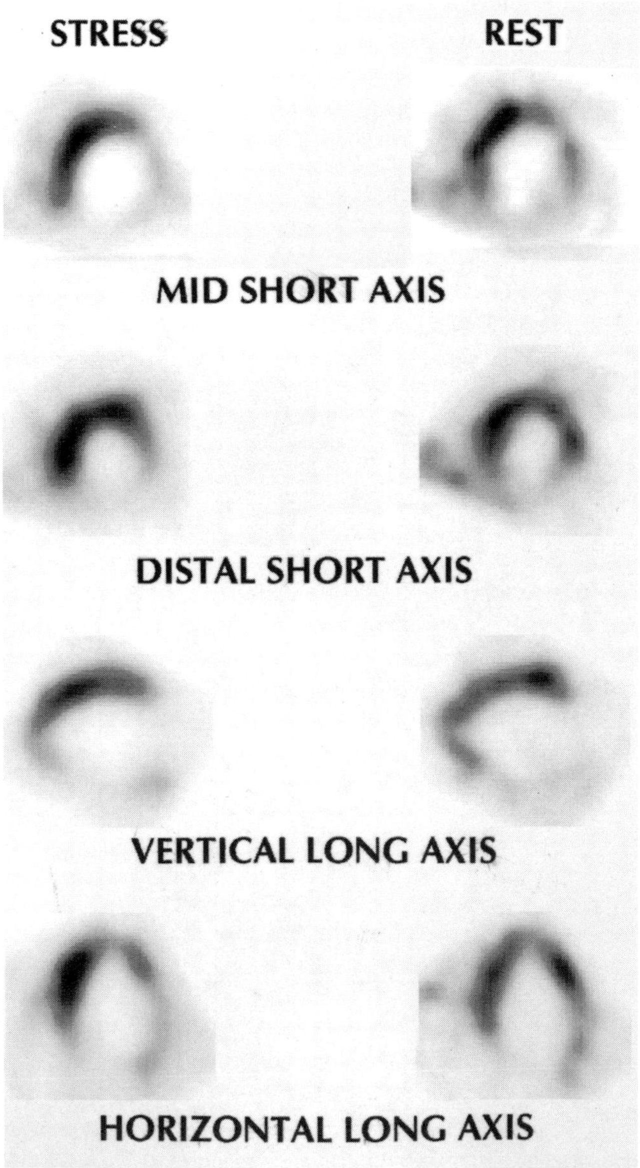

STRESS **REST**

MID SHORT AXIS

DISTAL SHORT AXIS

VERTICAL LONG AXIS

HORIZONTAL LONG AXIS

Figure 6–25. Exercise and rest Tc-99m sestamibi tomograms in a patient with an inferior myocardial infarction. Note extensive inferior, posterior, and posterolateral defects on stress images with partial reversibility in the posterolateral region, best seen in the mid short-axis and the horizontal long-axis tomograms.

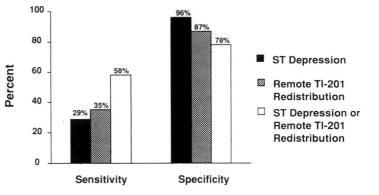

Figure 6–26. Sensitivity and specificity of exercise ST-segment depression *(solid bars)*, a remote Tl-201 redistribution defect *(crosshatched bars)*, and either ST depression or an inducible remote Tl-201 defect considered as a single variable for the detection of multivessel CAD in 88 consecutive postinfarction patients who received thrombolytic therapy and underwent both predischarge exercise Tl-201 scintigraphy and coronary angiography. (Haber HL, et al.: Am J Cardiol 1993;71:1257–1261.)

induced ST-segment depression (29%). Interestingly, if multiple Tl-201 defects in more than one vascular region or ischemic ST depression had been considered as a single variable for multivessel disease detection, then 58% of the patients with angiographic multivessel disease would have been identified (Fig. 6–26). Using either ST-segment depression or multiple Tl-201 defects in more than one vascular region as a single variable, the specificity for angiographic multivessel disease detection was reduced to 78%.

Using SPECT Tl-201 imaging, Sutton et al.[74] also reported a sensitivity of 35% for detection of multivessel disease in MI patients receiving thrombolytic therapy. This was identical to that reported by Haber et al. from the University of Virginia.[65]

There are several possible explanations for diminished sensitivity of a remote defect for identification of multivessel disease in the thrombolytic era. First, the prevalence of previous infarction is lower in patients who are included in series where thrombolytic therapy is given than in series reported before the thrombolytic era. In one study undertaken in the prethrombolytic era,[53] 17% of patients had a history of infarction, as compared with 7% in the cohort studied in the thrombolytic era from the same institution by Haber et al.[65] A prior infarction at a site remote from the zone of new myocardial necrosis would be associated with a high prevalence of a remote defect on Tl-201 scintigraphy. Second, non–Q-wave infarct patients comprised a substantial percentage of postinfarction cohorts reported in the prethrombolytic era, whereas patients with ST-segment elevation, most of whom evolve Q waves, are included solely in series of infarct patients who receive thrombolytic agents. In the present study, 81% of patients evolved Q waves on serial ECG evaluation, compared with 64% who had Q waves in the prethrombolytic infarction group cited previously.[53] Patients with non–Q-wave infarction have an extent of angiographic CAD comparable to that of patients with Q-wave infarction but have a higher prevalence of stress-induced ischemia.[53] With less myocardial damage in the infarct zone, non–Q-wave patients with multivessel CAD can exercise to higher peak heart rates or workloads, so the chance is greater that a remote Tl-201 defect in the supply region of a stenotic coronary artery will be induced. Third, in the prethrombolytic era, 50% to 60% of patients had two- or three-vessel disease.[75] In contrast, approximately 10% of infarction patients treated with thrombolytic therapy have three-vessel disease. In the TIMI-II trial, the prevalence of three-vessel disease was 5% in the "routine catheterization" subgroup and 11% in the "selective catheterization" subgroup.[76] In the Global Utilization of Streptokinase and Tissue Plasminogen Activator for Occluded Coronary Arteries (GUSTO) trial, only 14% of patients had three-vessel CAD; 24% had two-vessel CAD, and 62% had single-vessel CAD (Fig. 6–27).[76a] As seen in the prethrom-

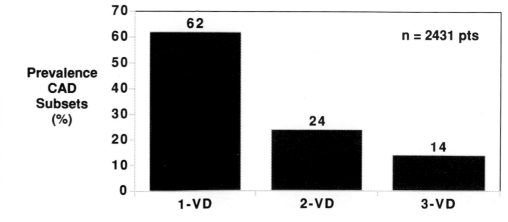

Figure 6–27. Prevalence of one-vessel disease (1-VD), two-vessel disease (2-VD), and three-vessel disease (3-VD) in the angiographic arm of the GUSTO trial. (Adapted from the GUSTO Angiographic Investigators: N Engl J Med 1993;329:1615–1622. Copyright 1993, Massachusetts Medical Society.)

bolytic era, more elderly patients with acute MI receiving thrombolytic therapy have a greater prevalence of multivessel CAD.[76b] On the other hand, only 12% of patients from 65 to 75 years of age had three-vessel CAD compared with 8% for patients whose ages were 50 to 64 years and 4% for patients less than 50 years old. This again supports the notion that thrombolytic patients are a lower risk group than nonthrombolytic patients by dint of the criteria for eligibility for thrombolysis. In the thrombolytic postinfarction cohort of Haber et al.,[65] 35% of patients treated with thrombolytic therapy had multivessel disease and only 13% had three-vessel disease.

Since a defect remote from the infarct zone is more likely to be induced by exercise stress in the presence of three-vessel than two-vessel disease,[77] it is not surprising that in the thrombolytic era the detection rate of remote defects in patients with multivessel disease is decreasing. Patients with three-vessel disease have more stress-induced perfusion abnormalities than patients with either single- or two-vessel disease. Thus, it should be emphasized that patient populations with acute infarction reported in the literature in the thrombolytic era are perhaps a lower-risk group, in general, than infarct populations of patients included in reports in the prethrombolytic era, fewer having a history of infarction, non–Q-wave infarction, and three-vessel CAD. Thus, fewer will manifest both residual ischemia and a multivessel disease scintigraphic pattern.

Detecting Residual Ischemia in the Infarct Zone

Brown et al.[72] compared the prognostic implications of Tl-201 redistribution defects within the territory of an acute infarction to those of stress-induced defects outside the infarct region. In a cohort of consecutive patients who underwent both exercise Tl-201 imaging and cardiac catheterization for evaluation of chest pain that developed after

hospital discharge after an acute MI, nearly 50% had Tl-201 redistribution confined within the infarct zone, and approximately 26% had redistribution defects outside the infarct zone. Stepwise multivariate logistic regression analysis revealed that the presence of a Tl-201 redistribution defect anywhere and multivessel CAD on angiography were the only significant predictors of cardiac events during average 10-month follow-up. When coronary bypass surgery was excluded as an endpoint, Tl-201 redistribution within the infarct zone was the only significant predictor of cardiac events. Wilson et al.[78] reported that Tl-201 redistribution within the zone of infarction was the best predictor of recurrent infarction and unstable angina in patients with single-vessel disease and otherwise uncomplicated MI. Figure 6–28 shows the event-free survival, comparing patients with and without infarct zone redistribution on submaximal exercise Tl-201 scintigraphy. Figure 6–29 shows stress and rest short-axis SPECT images in a patient who underwent predischarge TC-99m sestamibi submaximal exercise testing. The scan demonstrates a reversible defect in the infarct zone in the distribution of the right coronary artery.

Timing of Exercise Perfusion Imaging after Acute Myocardial Infarction

The prognostic value of exercise Tl-201 scintigraphy diminishes the longer the interval between the acute event and the noninvasive evaluation. In such situations the highest-risk patients may already have been referred for invasive testing or have experienced early events.[78a, 78b] Moss et al.[78a] determined the clinical significance of myocardial ischemia detected by noninvasive testing in stable patients 1 to 6 months after hospitalization for acute infarction or unstable angina. This was a low-risk group of survivors of an acute ischemic event, since 91% performed 6 minutes or more of treadmill exercise and 78% achieved a heart rate

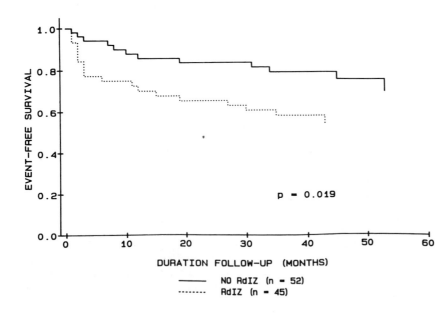

Figure 6–28. Event-free survival comparing patients with no redistribution in the infarct zone (No RdIZ) to patients with redistribution in the infarct zone (RdIZ) following acute MI. All patients had angiographic single-vessel CAD, and none received thrombolytic therapy. (Reprinted with permission from the American College of Cardiology (Journal of the American College of Cardiology, 1988, Vol. 11, pp. 223–234.)

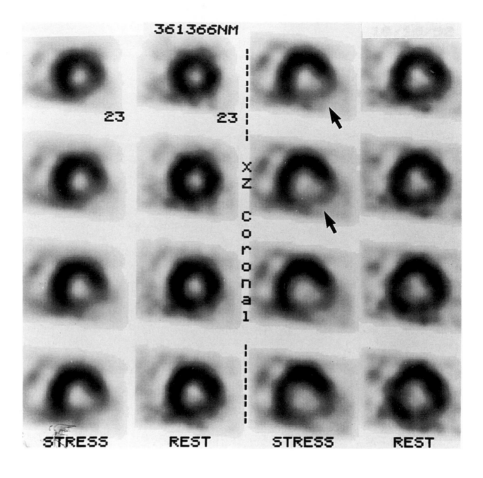

Figure 6–29. Stress and rest short-axis tomograms from a SPECT Tc-99m–sestamibi perfusion scan performed prior to hospital discharge in a patient with a right coronary–related MI. Apical slices are shown at upper left and basilar slices at lower right. Note a reversible defect in the low posterolateral and inferior segments *(arrows)* consistent with residual ischemia in the infarct zone.

of 120 bpm or more. ST-segment depression on the rest ECG and reversible defects by stress Tl-201 imaging were each associated with an increased incidence of primary cardiac events ($P < 0.05$). By multivariate Cox analyses, ST depression on the resting ECG was the only noninvasive ischemic test variable that identified a significantly increased risk ($P = 0.05$) for recurrent events. Reversible Tl-201 defects made a borderline contribution ($P = 0.09$) to primary events. Neither ST segment depression on the ambulatory ECG nor exercise-induced ST depression made a significant additional prognostic contribution. Significantly increased risk ($P < 0.05$) was noted when exercise-induced ST depression occurred in patients who also had reduced exercise duration (hazard ratio, 3.4) or when reversible Tl-201 defects occurred in patients who also had increased lung uptake (hazard ratio, 2.8). It should be pointed out that the cardiac death rate was only 2.6% at 2 years' follow-up in this patient population, suggesting that many high-risk postinfarction patients were not enrolled in the study.

Stress Thallium-201 Scintigraphy for Prognostication in Non–Q-Wave Infarction

Not all patients who evolve a non–Q-wave infarction require urgent cardiac catheterization. Certainly, patients with non–Q-wave infarction who experience recurrent an-

gina at rest or with low-level activity require urgent coronary angiography, particularly when transient ECG changes are documented during spontaneous pain episodes. Some non–Q-wave patients actually have circumflex-related transmural infarction with little myocardium still jeopardized.[10] These patients may show minimal ST elevation on admission in inferolateral leads and subsequently exhibit only diminished R waves in ECG leads I, AVL, V_5, and V_6. Many patients with "non-Q" Cx-related infarctions can develop an increased R-S ratio in lead V_2. This finding is indicative of posterior wall involvement.

High-risk non–Q-wave infarct patients can be identified by demonstrating Tl-201 redistribution within the zone of infarction on predischarge exercise scintigraphy. The prevalence and extent of Tl-201 redistribution within the infarct zone is greater with non–Q-wave than with Q-wave infarctions (Fig. 6–30).[53] Patients with non–Q-wave infarction who subsequently experience cardiac events have a higher incidence of infarct zone redistribution than those whose course was event free. This finding is not surprising, since, as a group, patients with non–Q-wave infarction have less myocardial necrosis than Q-wave infarct patients, a higher prevalence of infarct vessel patency, and more coronary collaterals, resulting in more myocardium still at risk for recurrent ischemia or reinfarction. In the 1990s, the prevalence of a high-risk exercise ECG stress test or high-risk Tl-201 perfusion scan in patients with unstable angina or

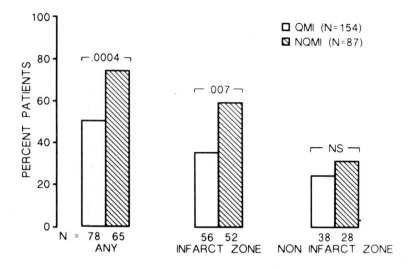

Figure 6–30. Prevalence and location of exercise-induced Tl-201 redistribution by quantitative submaximal exercise Tl-201 scintigraphy performed at 10 ±3 days in patients with a Q-wave myocardial infarction (QMI) and non–Q-wave myocardial infarction (NQMI). Note the significant increase in Tl-201 redistribution in the infarct zone in NQMI patients. (Gibson RS, et al.: Circulation 1986;73:1186–1198.)

non–Q-wave infarction is rather low, suggesting perhaps a change in this patient population. Results of the TIMI IIIB study showed patients with non–Q-wave MI or unstable angina receiving tPA or placebo had only an 8.6% (for both groups) prevalence of either two or more Tl-201 scan regions with reversible defects or increased lung Tl-201 uptake with one region of hypoperfusion.[78c]

Reverse Tl-201 Redistribution on Serial Images in Postinfarction Patients

Reverse redistribution, in which initial images are normal or show a minimal perfusion abnormality but delayed images show a significant defect, can be seen in the infarct zone of patients who have undergone reperfusion therapy. This scan pattern is a sign of nontransmural infarction, most often with a patent infarct-related coronary artery. In a study by Weiss et al.,[79] a reverse redistribution pattern in patients who initially underwent streptokinase therapy was associated with patency of the infarct-related artery in 100%, improvement in Tl-201 defect size from day 1 to day 10 in 94%, and normal or nearly normal 10-day RNA in 80% of segments with marked, and 54% of segments with mild, reverse redistribution. Tl-201 washout was more rapid in regions with reverse redistribution (49% ±15%) than in the contralateral normal zone. Touchstone et al.[80] also found that reverse Tl-201 redistribution was associated with improvement in infarct zone wall motion in the week following thrombolytic therapy. Thus, reverse redistribution is a marker of myocardial salvage and preservation of viability in MI treated with reperfusion therapy.

Summary

Thus, as observed in patients with chronic coronary disease, exercise Tl-201 scintigraphy in a patient with a recent MI has important prognostic value for noninvasive risk stratification. Figure 6–31 illustrates a proposed decision-making algorithm for risk assessment in patients who survive an acute MI. Patients who are clinically at high risk (e.g., because of recurrent angina, prior infarction, heart failure) could be referred directly for an invasive strategy. This would be applied to patients who did or did not receive thrombolytic therapy on admission. Patients evaluated using the noninvasive strategy who exhibit high-risk Tl-201 scintigraphic findings of residual ischemia (redistribution), a multivessel CAD defect pattern, or increased lung Tl-201 uptake would be candidates for an invasive evaluation and perhaps revascularization, anatomy permitting. This would be the case even in the absence of exercise-induced angina. If multivessel CAD is demonstrated on angiography, coronary revascularization or multivessel angioplasty should be strongly considered.

For patients with single-vessel CAD and residual Tl-201 redistribution within the zone of infarction on exercise scintigraphy, angioplasty is probably the procedure of choice. This may be particularly indicated in patients who exhibit a large area of redistribution at a slow exercise heart rate or a workload of 4 METs or less. This strategy may also be appropriate for patients with LAD-related infarction and anterior non–Q-wave MI. Many patients with anterior non-Q infarction would be referred directly for angiography, particularly if widespread ST-segment depression or T-wave inversion persisted on serial ECGs after hospital admission. Since Tl-201 scintigraphy is both more sensitive and more specific than exercise ST-segment depression for detecting residual infarct zone ischemia after MI, it should be employed whenever possible in conjunction with exercise testing in the process of predischarge risk stratification. Many patients exhibit Tl-201 redistribution on predischarge stress scintigraphy after MI who have no associated chest pain or even ST-segment depression (see Chap. 5). The cardiac event rate for such patients is comparable to that for those who have postinfarction Tl-201 redistribution in association with ST-segment depression or angina.

The approach to risk stratification for identifying high-

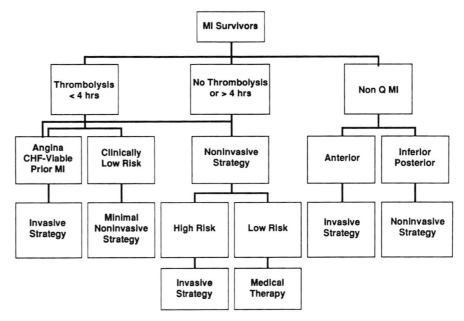

Figure 6–31. Proposed decision-making algorithm for predischarge risk stratification in patients with acute MI. (Key: CHF, congestive heart failure.)

risk patients who received thrombolytic therapy less than 4 hours or more than 4 hours after onset of symptoms is also shown in Figure 6–31. Since the cardiac mortality rate is so low (less than 2%) in the first year after discharge in clinically low-risk patients who received thrombolytic therapy within 4 hours, no test is probably very cost effective for prognostication in this subgroup. Nevertheless, exercise ECG testing alone could identify patients with significant ischemia or LV dysfunction by demonstration of inducible ST depression or poor exercise tolerance, respectively. Patients who received thrombolytic therapy more than 4 hours after onset of symptoms should undergo stress perfusion imaging, as in the prethrombolytic era. Haber et al.[65] reported that the detection rate for residual ischemia with exercise Tl-201 scintigraphy is still higher than the detection rate for ischemia with exercise ECG alone. There was a 48% prevalence of Tl-201 redistribution in a group of patients with uncomplicated MI who were treated with thrombolytic therapy, which was significantly higher than the 14% prevalence of ST-segment depression. Tilkemeier et al.[64] reported a 42% incidence of exercise-induced Tl-201 redistribution in postinfarction patients who received a thrombolytic agent on admission, as compared with an incidence of 15% for ischemic ST-segment depression in the same patient population. Employing SPECT Tl-201 scintigraphy, Sutton et al.[74] evaluated postinfarction patients receiving thrombolytic therapy who had at least 70% residual stenosis of the infarct vessel by angiography. Of these patients, 51% had inducible ischemia on SPECT Tl-201 scintigrams. Thus, it is clear that more patients with residual ischemia will be identified by exercise Tl-201 scintigraphy than by exercise ST-segment shifts alone when thrombolytic therapy is administered in the course of hospitalization.

For asymptomatic patients with no scintigraphic evidence of ischemia on stress imaging after thrombolytic therapy for acute infarction, medical therapy would be the most prudent approach. The TIMI-IIB study[63] found that routine angiography and prophylactic angioplasty did not reduce the cardiac event rate below that associated with initially employing a conservative strategy. With the conservative strategy, angiography and angioplasty are undertaken only when spontaneous ischemia or exercise-induced ischemia is evident. Table 6–9 summarizes mortality rates for patients randomized to invasive or conservative strategies. Even after 3 years, the mortality rate is similar for the two groups.[80a]

In patients with a markedly depressed LVEF, with or without congestive heart failure, resting Tl-201 imaging may be useful in deciding which patients with LV dysfunction might benefit from coronary arteriography. Patients with severe wall motion abnormalities and global LV dysfunction who manifest Tl-201 uptake in these asynergic regions have considerable myocardium that is viable (see Chap. 9). With revascularization, asynergic segments that show preserved Tl-201 uptake (at least 50% of normal zone uptake) on rest scintigraphy show improved systolic function after revascularization. In contrast, asynergic segments with severely reduced viability are unlikely to show im-

Table 6–9. Event Rate (%) in TIMI-II Trial at 3-Year Follow-Up

Follow-up Period	Invasive (% Mortality)	Conservative (% Mortality)
6 wk	6.3	5.0
1 yr	8.2	8.3
2 yr	9.7	9.3
3 yr	11.5	11.0

(Reprinted with permission from the American College of Cardiology (Journal of the American College of Cardiology, 1993, Vol. 22, pp. 1763–1772).)

provement in regional function postoperatively. Patients with a markedly reduced LVEF with an acute infarction often have multivessel CAD and have a history of a previous MI. Asynergy can be a manifestation of both stunned (in the infarct zone) and hibernating (remote asynergy) myocardium. Rest Tl-201 imaging may be useful for distinguishing such patients from those whose asynergy is a result of irreversible cell injury. The use of pharmacologic stress in patients who cannot exercise and the use of Tc-99m sestamibi as the imaging agent for exercise testing after infarction is discussed later in this chapter.

EXERCISE RADIONUCLIDE ANGIOGRAPHY FOR RISK STRATIFICATION AFTER ACUTE MYOCARDIAL INFARCTION

Exercise Left Ventricular Ejection Fraction and Prognosis

Exercise RNA has been employed for risk stratification in patients following an uncomplicated MI, though this technique is not widely performed in this setting. (The technique for using RNA in conjunction with exercise stress is described in Chap. 3.) Clinicians seem to favor stress perfusion imaging performed in conjunction with submaximal exercise testing for predischarge risk assessment of postinfarction patients. Whether or not the exercise EF provides additional prognostic data to the resting EF is still unsettled. Patients who subsequently experience a fatal or nonfatal cardiac event have a higher prevalence of abnormal EF or end-systolic volume response to exercise on predischarge stress testing. Wasserman et al.[81] reported that patients with inferior infarction and single-vessel CAD tend to show an increase in LVEF with exercise whereas inferior infarction patients with multivessel disease most often show a flat response or a decrease in EF with exercise. In another study,[82] peak treadmill workload and the change in LVEF

during exercise were significant predictors of cardiac events as assessed by multivariate analysis in men tested 3 weeks postinfarction. A treadmill workload of 4 METS or less, or a decrease in EF of 5% or more below the value at rest during submaximal effort, distinguished high- from low-risk subgroups with 23% and 2% event rates, respectively.

Morris et al.[83] reported that the rest and exercise LVEF were correlated inversely with subsequent mortality in 106 consecutive survivors of acute MI (Fig. 6–32). Using the Cox regression model, they showed that, as the EF fell below 45%, mortality increased dramatically. The expected mortality in 2 years was 11% with an exercise EF of 50%, 29% with an exercise EF of 30%, and 56% with an exercise EF of 15%. Corbett et al.[84] observed that the change in EF from rest to exercise in postinfarction patients was the most important prognostic variable in predicting the combined events of death, recurrent infarction, refractory angina, and heart failure. Abraham et al.[85] reported that when the exercise EF was below 50%, the 2-year survival rate free of medical complications was 42%, as compared with 83% for patients whose EF exceeded this value. Figure 6–33 shows event-free survival curves for 45 patients with an exercise EF of at least 50% and 30 patients with an exercise EF below 50% in this study. Dewhurst and Muir[86] determined the prognostic value of RNA performed at rest and during exercise in 100 patients experiencing their first MI. A resting EF below 35% identified a high-risk subgroup of patients destined for a poor outcome. Of interest, the exercise EF did not add prognostic value to this group. In contrast, a decrease in EF of 5% or more in patients whose resting EF was at least 35% identified a subset of patients at high risk for postinfarction angina.

The results of these RNA studies indicate that the exercise EF response to submaximal exercise after uncomplicated MI can adequately separate high- and low-risk subgroups. One limitation of some of these studies is that death represented a small percentage of all the cardiac events.[84] The majority of events were recurrent infarction, unstable angina, and the development of angina or heart

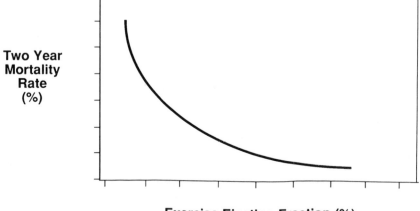

Figure 6–32. Exercise LVEF versus 2-year mortality rate in patients undergoing predischarge testing after acute MI. (Morris KG, et al.: Am J Cardiol 1985;55:318–324.)

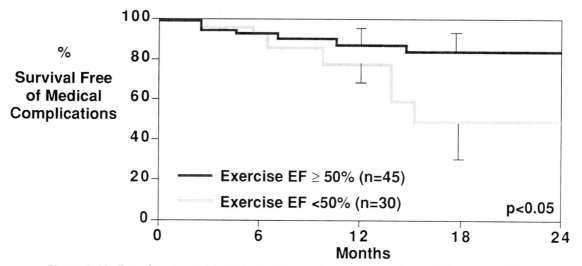

Figure 6–33. Event-free survival in patients with exercise ejection fraction ≥50% versus <50%. (Abraham RD, et al.: Am J Cardiol 1987;60:225–230.)

failure. No large follow-up studies have been performed to determine the true supplemental value of the exercise EF over the resting EF for mortality prediction.

Wallis et al.[87] sought to determine the impact of exercise EF on prognosis in patients whose resting EF was severely depressed (below 30%). Among the entire group of 265 patients studied, stepwise Cox regression analysis identified NYHA class as the strongest survival predictor; resting EF, systolic blood pressure, sex, age, and LV end-diastolic pressure were other significant predictive variables. Among the 194 patients who underwent exercise testing, the exercise EF, heart failure class, age, and sex were significant predictors. Exercise EF of at least 20% separated survivors from those who died during follow-up and significantly modified the prognostic conclusions based on heart failure class alone. Exercise EF of at least 20% identified operated patients with excellent late postoperative survival despite a resting EF below 30%. Resting EF and the change in EF from rest to exercise added no prognostic information to that supplied by the exercise EF.

Borer et al.[88] from the same group found that the LVEF determined during exercise testing before hospital discharge appears to be additive to the prognostic information derived from the resting EF. An LVEF below 40% during peak exercise, and a drop in EF of at least 5% from rest to exercise, were identified as the most potent descriptors of high risk. This group found that the radionuclide-based risk variables were superior in accuracy for prognosis to variables derived from exercise ECG, Holter rhythm analysis, and a host of clinical variables previously shown to provide prognostic information. Mazzotta et al.[88a] found that exercise-induced angina, ST-segment depression, decrease in LVEF on exercise radionuclide angiography, or inadequate increase in systolic blood pressure and low exercise tolerance were significantly associated with 4-year incidence of ischemic events. Only the onset of both ST-segment depression and a decrease in LVEF with exercise was an independent predictor. Figure 6–34 shows the survival curves.

Few studies deal with the clinical application of exercise RNA for risk stratification in postinfarction patients who were treated with thrombolytic agents.[58, 89, 89b] In the TIMI-II study,[58] patients randomized to the invasive strategy more

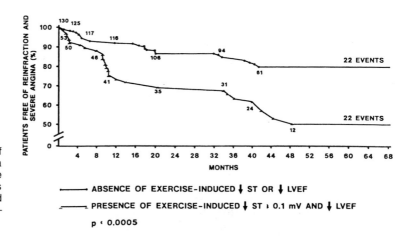

Figure 6–34. Event curves in patients with absence of both exercise-induced ST segment depression (↓) and a decrease (↓) in exercise LVFF *(upper curve)* or presence of both variables *(lower curve)*. Numbers along the curves represent patients still entering follow-up at the indicated timepoints. (Mazzotta G, et al: J Nucl Cardiol 1994;1:246–253.)

frequently had normal exercise EF responses (29.7% vs. 25.8%; $P = 0.01$) than patients assigned to the conservative strategy. Peak exercise LVEF and peak infarct zone regional EF were also greater in the patients randomized to the invasive strategy (see Table 6–5). However, at 6 weeks' follow-up, the differences between treatment groups were no longer evident. In another report from the TIMI-II study, the peak-exercise LVEF was 55% in patients randomized to angioplasty 18 to 48 hours after thrombolytic therapy compared with 58% in patients who did not undergo angioplasty.[89a] This finding suggests that routine angioplasty after thrombolytic therapy did enhance LV functional reserve under stress conditions.

Relative Prognostic Role of Thallium-201 Scintigraphy as Compared with Other Noninvasive Tests

Only one study has sought to evaluate the relative value of multiple noninvasive tests for risk stratification after MI. Candell-Riera et al.[90] performed all the tests cited above in 115 consecutive patients who had had a first acute MI without in-hospital complications and who were younger than 65 years. All studies were performed before hospital discharge, and follow-up was performed for 12 months. Logistic regression analysis revealed that the combination of studies with the highest predictive power for future cardiac events was the association of the exercise test, stress Tl-201 scintigraphy, and the resting echocardiogram. The variables in the three tests were presence of aneurysm on echo, greater than one redistribution segment on Tl-201 scintigraphy, and a resting EF of less than 45%. The probability of any complications in the presence of these variables was 99%. The combination of the exercise test plus Tl-201 scintigraphy plus 2-D echocardiography also provided the greatest probability of severe complications (95%). The variables included for this latter analysis were a resting EF below 45%, maximal systolic blood pressure below 150 mm Hg, and pulmonary Tl-201 uptake. Comparing the predictive value of the different individual studies, Tl-201 variables showed the highest predictive power for severe complications (88%), followed by 2-D echocardiography (68%), cardiac catheterization (66%), RNA (61%), and exercise testing alone (54%).

PHARMACOLOGIC STRESS PERFUSION IMAGING FOR PROGNOSTICATION AFTER ACUTE MYOCARDIAL INFARCTION

The clinical application of dipyridamole and adenosine Tl-201 imaging for risk stratification after acute MI in patients unable to exercise is discussed at length in Chapter 8.

The subject was also recently reviewed in detail by Verani.[90a] Patients who demonstrate redistribution in regions within or remote from the infarct zone have a higher risk of future cardiac events than those who do not.[91] In this latter study, there were 12 deaths among 51 postinfarction patients followed for an average of 19 months after hospital discharge. Eleven of the 12 patients who died showed redistribution defects on predischarge scintigraphy. In a subsequent study from this group, Gimple et al.[92] showed that redistribution outside the infarct zone was more specific for events than infarct zone redistribution (75% vs. 29%) and just as sensitive, (63%). Brown et al.[93] showed that dipyridamole Tl-201 imaging could be performed early in the course of infarction, and redistribution within the infarct zone was the best and only statistically significant predictor of in-hospital ischemic events. Of 20 patients with infarct zone redistribution, 45% developed in-hospital ischemic events, as compared with no events in patients without infarct zone redistribution. Pirelli et al.[94] also performed early dipyridamole Tl-201 imaging in 35 patients with uncomplicated infarction. Seven of eleven patients who showed redistribution defects developed subsequent angina, and five required bypass surgery for severe angina that was refractory to medical therapy. Six of the seven patients who developed angina had multivessel CAD. In both the study by Brown et al.[93] and the study by Pirelli et al.,[94] dipyridamole infusion was found to be safe when administered 3 to 5 days after admission.

Adenosine Tl-201 SPECT imaging has been shown to be useful for risk stratification when performed at a mean of 5 ±3 days after infarction.[94a] Defect size was 45% ± 18% in patients who experienced in-hospital cardiac events as compared with 22% +15% in those without events. The positive predictive value for events was 70% when the defect size was larger than 30%. Figure 6–35 depicts the sensitivity for detective multivessel disease by adenosine SPECT in this study. Ten of eleven patients with three-vessel CAD had remote defects on adenosine images.

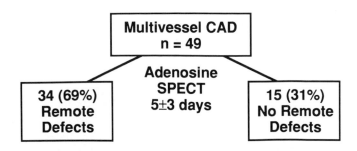

10/11 pts with 3-VD had remote defects

Figure 6–35. Detection of multivessel disease by adenosine SPECT imaging after uncomplicated MI. Note that of 49 patients with multivessel CAD by angiography, 34 (69%) had defects remote from the infarct zone. (Adapted from Mahmarian JJ, et al.: Circulation 1993;87:1197–1210.)

AMBULATORY RADIONUCLIDE MONITORING OF LEFT VENTRICULAR FUNCTION AFTER ACUTE MYOCARDIAL INFARCTION

The methods available for continuous radionuclide monitoring of LV function are described in Chapter 1. Breisblatt et al.[95] used the nuclear device known as the VEST early after MI in 35 patients. There were 56 responses suggestive of ischemia in 23 patients, 75% being silent and only 39% having associated ECG changes. In that study, mental stress identified 13 patients who had significant decreases in EF, 11 of whom subsequently had abnormal exercise Tl-201 scans. Long-term follow-up of these patients was not reported. In a subsequent study by this group, Kayden et al.[96] continuously monitored a group of 33 patients who had received thrombolytic therapy. Twelve demonstrated a transient decrease in LVEF (greater than 0.05 unit lasting at least 1 minute). At 19 ±5 months' follow-up, cardiac events had been recorded for 8 of the 12 patients with transient LV dysfunction by the VEST but in only 3 of the 21 patients without this finding. Interestingly, of the 9 patients who experienced events who also had undergone exercise Tl-201 scintigraphy, 8 had no Tl-201 scintigraphic evidence of ischemia. Again, the majority of episodes of diminished EF on ambulatory radionuclide monitoring were not associated with angina. The authors propose that this technique may be useful for risk stratification after thrombolytic therapy.

MYOCARDIAL INFARCT-AVID IMAGING IN ACUTE MYOCARDIAL INFARCTION

As described in Chapter 2, infarct-avid scintigraphy can be used to identify regions of myocardial necrosis in patients with acute infarction. The principle behind this approach is that the radiopharmaceutical administered is sequestered in zones of recently-infarcted myocardium and can be localized on gamma camera images as "hot spots." Formerly, the most commonly used infarct-avid imaging agent was Tc-99m stannous pyrophosphate, which reached maximal intensity in the necrotic region 48 to 72 hours after onset of infarction.[97] This technique was shown to be most useful clinically when patients presented later than 24 hours after the onset of chest pain, when enzymes and ECG may be nondiagnostic. The presumed mechanism for cellular sequestration of this agent is described in Chapter 2.

A new infarct-avid imaging technique presently under investigation involves scintigraphic detection and quantification of myocardial necrosis after intravenous injection of radiolabeled myosin-specific antibodies.[97a–100] It is based on the principle that myosin-specific antibodies bind to intracellular myosin when sarcolemmal membrane integrity has been altered by ischemic damage. Studies have shown that the location of radiolabeled antimyosin antibody corresponds precisely to histochemically delineated zones of MI (see Chap. 2). As with Tc-99m PYP, 24 hours must elapse after tracer administration before imaging can commence, permitting blood pool clearance of the agent. Indium-111 (In-111) is the radioisotope that is currently employed with Fab segments of antimyosin antibody for clinical imaging. Discrete, as opposed to diffuse, myocardial uptake of either In-111 antimyosin or Tc-99m PYP is specific for necrosis. Both techniques are less sensitive for detecting nontransmural infarction than transmural infarction. Figure 6–36 shows the ECG and planar antimyosin scars of a patient with an acute Q-wave anterior infarction from the study of Johnson et al.[100] A large area of In-111 antimyosin uptake can be seen. More recently, smaller labeled fragments of antimyosin such as recombinant single-chain Fv (sFv) antimyosin protein, have been tested in the experimental laboratory for their feasibility as infarct-imaging agents.[100a] This agent is labeled with Tc-99m and is half the size of the Fab fragment. It clears significantly faster from the blood pool without compromising infarct localization.

Antimyosin antibody imaging has yielded 92% sensitivity for acute transmural MI. Focal myocardial uptake of antimyosin corresponds to the ECG infarct location.[100] Patients with an inferior posterior infarction have a more "faint" uptake pattern than those with infarcts at other sites. "Faint" tracer uptake is more likely to be seen in patients with a persistently occluded infarct-related vessel with no collateral flow. The size of the antimyosin uptake pattern has been shown to correlate well with the computer-derived hypokinetic segment length ($r = 0.79$) and peak CK ($r = 0.90$).[98] Interestingly, when antimyosin antibody imaging was compared to Tc-99m PYP imaging in the same patients, the infarct size was 1.7 times larger with PYP than with antimyosin SPECT. This may be related to the finding that myocardial zones of severe ischemia without necrosis can take up Tc-99m PYP.[100b] Volpini et al.[101] showed that "old" infarction did not take up antimyosin. Similarly, no uptake was observed in healthy volunteers.

Dual Imaging with Indium-111 Antimyosin and Thallium-201

In-111–antimyosin and Tl-201 imaging can be undertaken simultaneously to separate regions of necrosis from zones of periinfarction ischemia. This dual-imaging approach may be useful for identifying patients with acute MI who have additional regions of myocardium at risk, particularly in the distribution of vessels reperfused by thrombolytic agents but where there is residual high-grade stenosis. Johnson et al.[102] reported the results of dual-isotope Tl-201 and In-111–antimyosin SPECT imaging to identify infarct patients who might be at risk for subsequent ischemic events. There was a significant correlation between subsequent ischemic events and "mismatching" Tl-201 and In-111–antimyosin findings (i.e., presence of Tl-201 defects

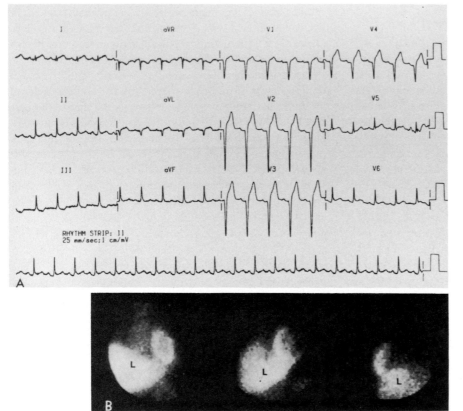

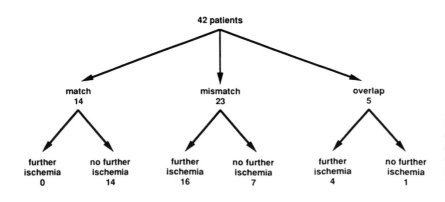

Figure 6–36. A. ECG from a patient with an anterior Q-wave MI. **B**. Planar anterior, 45-degree left anterior oblique and left lateral antimyosin images in the same patient showing tracer uptake in anterior, septal, and apical regions. Liver (L) uptake is also seen. (Reprinted with permission from the American College of Cardiology (Journal of the American College of Cardiology, 1989, Vol. 13, pp. 27–35).)

without corresponding antimyosin uptake). As shown in Figure 6–37, 16 of 23 patients with a mismatch pattern had further evidence of ischemia (infarct extension, recurrent angina, positive stress test). Thus, identifying reduced perfusion in myocardial regions adjacent to or remote from the area of necrosis from simultaneously recorded dual-isotope In-111 and Tl-201 SPECT scans could be useful for risk assessment. The results of all studies published to date show that administration of Fab fragments of antimyosin antibody to humans is also safe; no important adverse reactions have been noted.

Indium-111–Antimyosin Uptake as a Prognostic Indicator

Myocardial infarct size is a critical measurement in the determination of mortality risk following MI. Because In-111–antimyosin imaging permits assessment of infarct size in vivo during the early period after MI, it may prove to be an important indicator of future cardiac events. This role for In-111–antimyosin imaging was investigated in a multicenter study[103] at 25 sites that included 497 patients. Antimyosin antibody injection was given within 48 hours of the onset of chest pain and imaging was performed 24 to 48 hours after injection. Preliminary results of this trial showed sensitivity of 94% (190 of 202) in the subgroup of patients with transmural MI and of 84% (48 of 57) in the subgroup with nontransmural infarction. Specificity for chest pain without infarction was 93% (38 of 41). The infarct size determined by antimyosin antibody uptake was a significant predictor of subsequent cardiac events during follow-up. There was a linear relationship between extent of antimyosin uptake and the incidence of major cardiac events. The slope of the relationship relating the incidence

Figure 6–37. Correlation between further ischemic events and mismatched Tl-201–In-111 antimyosin activity. A mismatch pattern is defined as the presence of Tl-201 defects without corresponding antimyosin uptake. (Johnson LL, et al.: Circulation 1990;81:37–45.)

of cardiac death and the extent of myocardial uptake was steep; the cumulative event rate ranged from 4% in patients with negative images to more than 30% in patients with 18 positive myocardial segments. This finding is not surprising since infarct size by antimyosin antibody measurements correlates closely with EF in patients after a first MI.[104] Figure 6–38 depicts the event-free survival in this multicenter trial for patients with extensive antimyosin uptake (in more than 10 segments) versus those with less than 10-segments uptake. The event rate was 25% in the former group and 5% in the latter group ($p < 0.05$).[104a]

Early In-111–antimyosin imaging with quantitation of count density of the radionuclide can predict improvement in regional systolic function in patients receiving thrombolytic therapy. The degree of antimyosin uptake is predictive of regional function at the time of discharge. The count density index was lower in patients with mild regional asynergy on discharge than in patients with severe regional asynergy.

To date, few patients are undergoing infarct-avid imaging in the acute or subacute phase of myocardial infarction. The detection of acute myocardial necrosis can more easily be performed by inspection of serial ECGs and quantification of the MB isoenzyme of creatine kinase. Infarct sizing and localization can be achieved with a high degree of accuracy using myocardial perfusion imaging techniques or echocardiographic assessment of regional myocardial asynergy. Prognostication can be achieved by evaluation of clinical variables, the resting LVEF, and determination of the amount of residual ischemic myocardium by stress perfusion imaging.

TECHNETIUM-99m–ISONITRILE IMAGING IN ACUTE MYOCARDIAL INFARCTION

Detection of Acute Infarction

Like Tl-201, Tc-99m sestamibi can be employed for assessment of risk area, infarct size, and identifying viable but ischemic myocardium after MI. The basic mechanism of myocardial uptake of Tc-99m sestamibi and experimental data describing its uptake and clearance characteristics in animal models are described in Chapter 2. The precise mechanism of cellular uptake and myocardial sequestration of Tc-99m sestamibi is unknown, but it appears that viable mitochondria are required for intracellular binding. Ischemic or stunned myocardium can take up Tc-99m sestamibi in proportion to blood flow, even when severe ischemic systolic dysfunction is present.[105] The results of a multicenter trial have shown that Tc-99m–sestamibi imaging at rest is associated with an extraordinarily high sensitivity for detection of MI.[106] Boucher et al.[106] found that the resting Tc-99m–sestamibi scan was abnormal in 104 of 111 patients (94%) who on RNA exhibited both a Q-wave and a wall motion abnormality and was normal in 23 of 25 patients (92%) in whom both findings were normal. In that study, the "gold standard" for infarction was the combination of new Q waves on the ECG and abnormal regional wall motion on radionuclide ventriculography. Tc-99m–sestamibi imaging is also very sensitive for detection of myocardium at risk in patients with chest pain without ST elevation who subsequently develop enzymatic evidence of acute infarction.[107] In nearly 50% of these patients, the LCx was the infarct-related artery.

Technetium-99m–Isonitrile Imaging for Assessment of Thrombolytic Therapy

A promising alternative to Tl-201 scintigraphy for assessment of thrombolytic therapy is the administration of Tc-99m sestamibi. The experimental validation for this use is described in Chapter 2. Since Tc-99m sestamibi is not redistributed, the agent can be administered just before thrombolytic therapy, and imaging is then postponed several hours, until drug administration is complete. This is undertaken to obtain pretreatment assessment of myocardial perfusion. By postponing imaging until after treatment, the institution of thrombolysis is not delayed. A "snapshot" of the perfusion pattern of the time of administration is obtained with this initial injection of Tc-99m sestamibi. These images reflect the "area at risk" in the supply region of the infarct-related vessel. Even images obtained 6 hours after

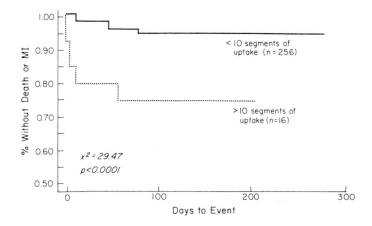

Figure 6–38. Event-free survival in postinfarction patients with >10 segments showing In-111 antimyosin uptake compared to that for patients with <10 segments of uptake. (Maddahi J, Di Carli M: Am J Cardiac Imaging 1993;7:45–52.)

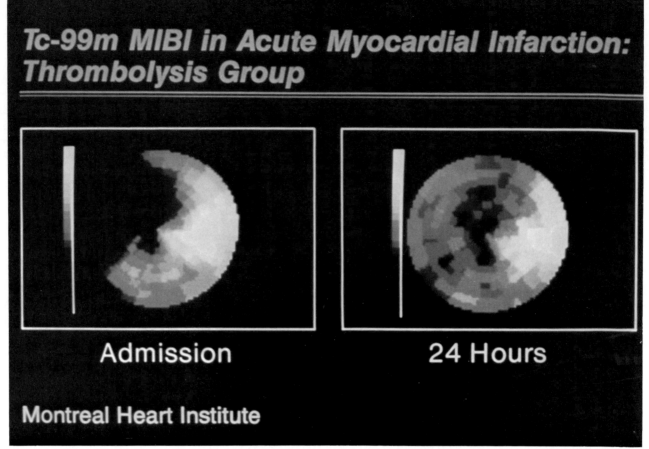

See Color Figure 6–39.

Figure 6–39. Bulls-eye SPECT images performed on admission before thrombolytic therapy and 24 hours later in a patient with an acute anteroseptal MI study at the Montreal Heart Institute. Note the marked improvement in Tc-99m–sestamibi uptake in the anteroseptal region indicative of substantial salvage (see Color Figure 6–39). (Kindly provided by Dr. Pierre Theroux, Montreal Heart Institute.)

injection show the perfusion pattern that existed at the time of tracer administration before thrombolytic therapy. A second injection of Tc-99m sestamibi is given sometime after thrombolytic therapy and after acquisition of the "pretreatment" images. The second set of images delineate the degree of improvement in regional flow and extent of salvage. Figure 6–39 shows the prethrombolysis bull's-eye SPECT image and the repeat study performed 24 hours after thrombolysis, showing marked improvement in sestamibi uptake in the apex and anteroseptal region, suggesting substantial salvage.

Wackers et al.[108] and Gibbons et al.,[109] with assistance of several collaborating institutions, successfully applied serial Tc-99m–sestamibi imaging to patients with acute MI undergoing thrombolytic therapy. Patients with a patent infarct artery had a significantly greater decrease in defect size on repeat images performed 18 to 48 hours after thrombolytic therapy than did patients with persistently occluded vessels (Fig. 6–40). Wackers et al.[108] found that a relative decrease of more than 30% in the size of the Tc-99m–sestamibi perfusion defect on planar images predicted pa-

tency of the infarct-related artery. Plots of the initial and final defect regions, expressed as a percentage of the LV for individual patients in the thrombolysis group and in the conventionally treated group, are shown in Figure 6–41 from the study by Gibbons et al. in which serial SPECT Tc-99m–sestamibi imaging was performed.[109] Gibson et al.[109a] from the same group subsequently reported that the change in defect area varied significantly with both infarct location ($P = 0.0001$) and infarct vessel patency ($P = 0.002$). Defect extent and severity were significantly greater for anterior infarctions than for lateral or inferior ones. Thus, the studies indicate that Tc-99m–sestamibi imaging can be utilized to assess risk area at the time of hospital admission and infarct size after therapy in acute infarction patients.

Pellikka et al.[110] reported that, in patients with acute MI, the Tc-99m–sestamibi defect size continued to shrink at 6 to 14 days after thrombolytic therapy in nearly 50% of patients. Thus, failure to show a significant reduction in defect size 18 to 48 hours after reperfusion does not rule out the possibility that salvage has occurred. There may be

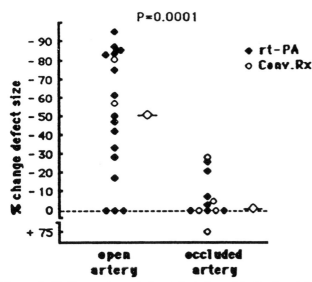

Figure 6–40. Change in perfusion defect size related to the status of the infarct-related artery in patients receiving Tc-99m–sestamibi before and after thrombolytic therapy or after conventional treatment (conv Rx). The percentage of change in defect size in individual patients prior to thrombolytic therapy and afterward is shown. The open diamonds represent mean values. (Reprinted with permission from the American College of Cardiology (Journal of the American College of Cardiology, 1989, Vol. 14, pp. 861–873).)

a temporary reversible disturbance of Tc-99m–sestamibi transport in the early postreperfusion period that resolves within a week after treatment. Antegrade flow or collateral flow could increase over time, resulting in better nutrient perfusion, which would be associated with a reduction in Tc-99m defect size.

As reported by Christian et al.,[111] Tc-99m defect size prior to reperfusion is significantly greater with anterior infarction than with inferior infarction ($52\% \pm 9\%$ vs. $18\% \pm 10\%$ of the left ventricle, $P = 0.0001$). The final defect size after thrombolytic therapy or angioplasty was also significantly larger with anterior infarction ($30\% \pm 20\%$ vs. $9\% \pm 8\%$, $P < 0.01$). Of interest, the proportion of jeopardized myocardium salvaged was not significantly different

for patients with anterior and inferior infarction (0.49 vs. 0.59). As expected, patients who had an occluded infarct-related artery showed no change in defect size. Figure 6–42 shows the acute and final defect size in patients with anterior and inferior infarction in this study who had patent infarct vessels. In four patients who received Tc-99m sestamibi before suffering fatal cardiogenic shock, the extent of infarction by pathologic inspection was smaller than the perfusion defect.[112] This finding emphasizes the point that perfusion defects in acute MI patients represent the combination of necrosis and ischemia, particularly when such patients are imaged early. Finally, if wall motion in the infarct zone improved, the Tc-99m defect size would diminish even without enhanced tracer uptake, owing to the partial volume effect.

Tc-99m–sestamibi imaging can be used to determine the efficacy of primary angioplasty in salvaging myocardium in acute MI.[113–113b] Behrenbeck et al. reported a significant reduction in defect size after primary angioplasty in 17 consecutive patients with a first transmural MI. The initial acute defect size with angioplasty was $48\% \pm 17\%$ of the left ventricle, and it decreased significantly, to $29\% \pm 19\%$ on images obtained 6 to 10 days after balloon dilatation of the infarct-related artery. Interestingly, they found no correlation between the time to therapy and the reduction in defect size. Gibbons et al.[113b] found that myocardial salvage, reflected by per cent of the LV showing a reduction in defect size on SPECT Tc-99m sestamibi images, was similar in patients randomized to immediate primary angioplasty and patients randomized to thrombolytic therapy. In another study by Clements et al.,[113a] antegrade flow prior to direct angioplasty and collateral flow resulted in a significantly smaller final SPECT sestamibi defect and more myocardial salvage after angioplasty. Both antegrade infarct artery flow and collateral flow to the infarct zone had significant independent ability to predict infarct size (assessed by Tc-99m sestamibi) after angioplasty.

Tc-99m–sestamibi imaging after reperfusion therapy is predictive of the LVEF at 1 year ($r = -0.78$).[114] It is also

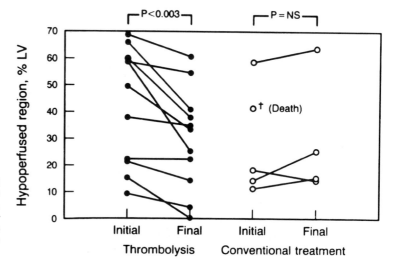

Figure 6–41. Plot of the initial and final hypoperfused region as a percentage of the LV volume for each MI patient in the thrombolysis group and in the conventional treatment group. A significant decrease between initial and final Tc-99m–sestamibi SPECT studies is shown for the thrombolysis group and not for the conventional treatment group. (Gibbons RJ, et al.: Circulation 1989;80:1277–1286.)

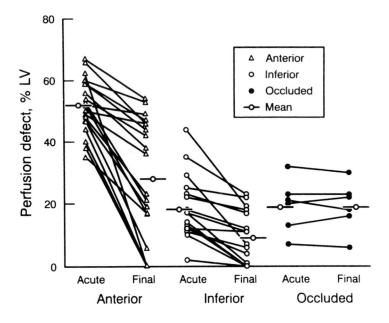

Figure 6–42. Perfusion defect size by infarct location and arterial patency, as determined before reperfusion therapy (Acute) and at discharge (Final) with Tc-99m isonitrile SPECT imaging. Both anterior and inferior infarct locations showed a significant decrease in perfusion defect size after reperfusion therapy ($P < 0.001$ for both). (Reprinted with permission from the American College of Cardiology (Journal of the American College of Cardiology, 1991, Vol. 17, pp. 1303–1308).)

predictive of end-diastolic and end-systolic volume indices. The LVEF at the time of discharge may not accurately reflect perfusion defect size because of effects of stunning and compensatory hyperkinesia;[115] however, the relationship between the Tc-99m–sestamibi defect as a percentage of the LV correlated well with global LVEF in this study at 6 weeks ($r = 0.81$).

Determination of Infarct Size from Resting Technetium-99m–Sestamibi Imaging

Verani et al.,[116] in an experimental canine model, reported that the scintigraphic perfusion defect size correlated well with pathologic infarct size ($r = 0.95$ for tomographic imaging, $r = 0.85$ for planar imaging). Sinusas et al.[117] confirmed these findings and found that the final Tc-99m–sestamibi defect area defined by autoradiography correlated closely with post mortem infarct area ($r = 0.98$) as assessed by histologic methods. In this study, among dogs injected with Tc-99m sestamibi after 90 minutes' reperfusion preceded by 3 hours' coronary occlusion, myocardial Tc-99m–sestamibi uptake did not correlate with reperfusion flow in either endocardial or transmural segments. Tc-99m–sestamibi activity was significantly less than reperfusion flow at the time of injection in the central ischemic zone (sestamibi, 25% ±5% of normal; flow, 74% ±24% of normal). This indicates that Tc-99m–sestamibi uptake after reperfusion does not simply reflect efficacy of reflow but represents myocardial salvage and residual viable myocardium. Christian et al.[118] found that the important determinants of final infarct size as assessed by Tc-99m–sestamibi imaging were myocardium at risk, angiographic collateral grade, time to reperfusion, and infarct site. These investigators found that collateral flow could be accurately deter-

mined noninvasively from the acute Tc-99m–sestamibi short-axis profile curve by methods that assess the severity of the perfusion defect. An infarct larger than 40% of the left ventricle as quantitated by Tc-99m–sestamibi SPECT imaging was seen in 16 of 166 patients with acute infarction prospectively studied.[118a] The LAD coronary artery was the infarct-related artery in 14 of the 15 patients who underwent angiography. All had open infarct-related arteries. Only 1 patient died and the remaining 15 patients were asymptomatic at 13 ±9 months' follow-up.

Technetium-99m–Sestamibi Imaging and Clinical Decision Making

With the advent of a same-day imaging technique that enables serial Tc-99m–sestamibi images to be obtained at intervals of several hours rather than 24 hours, decision making with respect to who might benefit from "rescue" angioplasty during an acute MI might be assisted. If the prethrombolysis Tc-99m–sestamibi defect is small and the posttreatment defect remains small (even if not reduced), emergency angiography would not be considered, because the area at risk is not substantial, and even if vessel patency were not restored, the prognosis would be excellent. If the pretreatment defect was large and the posttreatment defect was significantly reduced, it could be assumed that thrombolysis had been successful in restoring nutrient blood flow. Emergent angiography would not be required, since reflow was accomplished and myocardium salvaged. In contrast, if the initial Tc-99m–sestamibi defect was large and remained large after thrombolytic therapy, it might be assumed that the infarct-related vessel was still occluded. A patient with this defect pattern would be assumed to be at high risk for extensive myocardial damage. Emergent angiography, with a view toward rescue angioplasty (if the vessel was still occluded), would then be of benefit. Further clinical research is required to evaluate this potential decision-making process. A potential limitation of Tc-99m sestamibi in patients with acute infarction is accurate assessment of viability in asynergic infarct zones supplied by a persistently severe stenotic coronary artery. Since Tc-99m sestamibi is not redistributed much, the uptake pattern in this situation may reflect residual flow more than viability. Nevertheless preliminary data from clinical research studies suggest that Tc-99m sestamibi imaging may provide information concerning myocardial viability with an accuracy comparable to that achieved with Tl-201 scintigraphy.[118b] The use of this agent for evaluating regional viability is discussed in Chapter 9.

POSITRON EMISSION TOMOGRAPHY IN ACUTE MYOCARDIAL INFARCTION

Imaging of Perfusion and Metabolism

The role of PET imaging in assessment of myocardial viability after MI and in chronic CAD and remote infarction is discussed in Chapter 9. There is a large amount of data in the literature that indicate that markedly decreased FDG uptake in areas of myocardium with reduced regional blood flow indicates irreversible myocardial damage (match pattern). FDG uptake in the presence of diminished perfusion has been proposed as a marker of myocardial viability. Thus, PET imaging of myocardial viability with such tracers as nitrogen-13 (N-13) ammonia and rubidium-82 (Rb-82) may be useful in distinguishing viable from irreversibly injured myocardium in patients with acute MI. Metabolic imaging with PET may be most useful in detecting residual myocardial viability in regions of reversibly depressed systolic dysfunction (myocardial stunning). The identification of viable myocardium still at risk may improve decision making about further invasive evaluation with an aim toward aggressive interventions such as angioplasty or coronary bypass surgery.

PET imaging is not much utilized for very early evaluation of acute MI because of logistic considerations. Few PET scanners are located adjacent to emergency rooms or acute care units; however, it can be employed in the subacute phase to assess perfusion and viability.

Schwaiger et al.[119] performed FDG PET imaging in patients within 72 hours of acute MI. Diminished FDG uptake in the infarct zone was highly predictive of no subsequent change in myocardial function. Maintained FDG uptake was associated with a variable functional outcome. These investigators showed that FDG uptake was significantly greater in patients with residual antegrade flow in the infarct-related vessel than in patients with an occluded artery. Postinfarction patients with an increase in FDG uptake have an increased cardiac event rate during follow-up.[119a] Figure 6–43 shows survival curves for 8 uncomplicated infarction patients who had an increase in FDG in at least one myocardial segment and those without increased FDG uptake in this study. This PET finding was the best predictor of future events among all clinical, angiographic and radionuclide variables.

Metabolic PET imaging with carbon-11 (C-11) acetate can be used to identify residual myocardial metabolic activity after reperfusion therapy in acute MI. Walsh et al.[120] found that reduction in C-11–acetate clearance rate from the infarct zone reflected impaired oxidative metabolism. Periinfarction zones with reduced blood flow showed only a mild decrease of C-11–acetate clearance.

Myocardial blood flow has been measured in MI patients receiving thrombolytic therapy utilizing oxygen-15 (O-15)–labeled water and PET imaging. In a study by Hanes et al.,[121] postinfarction patients who had received rt-PA were imaged by 24 hours after thrombolytic therapy, 24 to 48 hours after treatment, and before hospital discharge. These investigators found that myocardial blood flow was restored

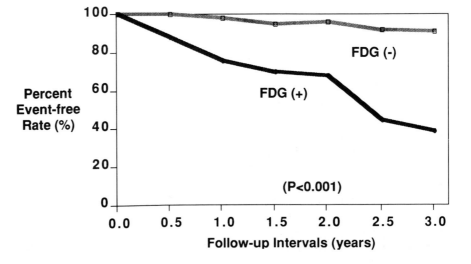

Figure 6–43. Event-free survival rates for patients with uncomplicated MI who had an increase in FDG uptake (+) in at least one myocardial segment and those without increased FDG uptake (–). (Reprinted with permission from the American College of Cardiology (Journal of the American College of Cardiology, 1993, Vol. 22, pp. 1621–1627).)

toward normal levels in most patients at the time of the first scan without a subsequent decrement in flow. They concluded that the "no reflow" phenomenon was not observed in patients undergoing reperfusion therapy in this study.

Planar Rb-82 imaging has been shown to correlate well with extent of regional wall motion abnormalities and Tl-201 defect size in patients with acute infarction.[122]

OVERALL SUMMARY

In an era of cost containment, it is vitally important for the practicing clinician to understand when to order tests for either diagnostic or prognostic purposes.[123] This is most relevant for suspected or known acute MI. Radionuclide imaging techniques are rarely required to make a diagnosis of acute infarction in patients who present with chest pain. MI can be accurately diagnosed in nearly all patients by serial determination of CK levels with quantitation of the MB fraction, which is specific for cardiac muscle. The standard 12-lead ECG shows typical alterations in the ST segment in the majority, and some patients exhibit changes only in the T wave. In situations of uncertainty, the 2-D echocardiogram will be helpful by demonstrating regional wall motion abnormality, although patients with a remote MI or unstable angina also manifest regional asynergy. Rarely is In-111–antimyosin or Tc-99m–PYP imaging necessary to diagnose an infarction, though there may be an occasional patient with a nondiagnostic ECG, such as left bundle branch block, whose infarct may have occurred more than 3 days before admission and whose CK level may be back to normal. In such an instance the infarct-avid scan will still be abnormal, showing focal uptake of antimyosin or Tc-99m PYP in the zone of necrosis.

Myocardial perfusion imaging can provide information on the degree of myocardial salvage after reperfusion therapy and the amount of viable but still jeopardized myocardium in the subacute phase of infarction. As discussed in this chapter, knowing how much myocardium is still at risk for future ischemic injury can be useful for identifying patients who might benefit from early angiography with an intent to revascularize myocardium distal to persistently stenotic vessels. Rest Tl-201 imaging appears to be the noninvasive method of choice for detecting residual viability in regions of akinesis or dyskinesis. Defects remote from the infarct zone that demonstrate delayed rest redistribution are indicative of physiologically significant multivessel CAD and should prompt a decision for early coronary angiography. Echocardiography is, indeed, a competing noninvasive technique for the assessment of residual viability in zones of asynergy when used in conjunction with intravenous infusion of small-dose dobutamine (see Chap. 9). Gated Tc-99m–sestamibi imaging may also prove to be a valid approach for viability detection after acute infarction. Areas of diminished Tc-99m–sestamibi uptake that show preserved systolic thickening when images are viewed in the gated mode would indicate that the infarct segment in

question was viable. Preliminary experimental data suggest that though there is less redistribution with Tc-99m sestamibi than with Tl-201, myocardial zones supplied by severely stenotic coronary vessels take up almost as much Tc-99m sestamibi in the resting state as Tl-201.

Perhaps the most useful and cost-effective clinical application of nuclear cardiology techniques in the setting of acute MI is stress imaging to identify high- and low-risk patients at the time of hospital discharge. As summarized in this chapter, stress perfusion imaging is more sensitive than exercise ECG testing alone for prognosis. Stress echocardiography has been advocated for the same purpose but is limited by lower sensitivity for residual ischemia in an infarct zone that already shows a severe wall motion abnormality at rest. Stress echocardiography cannot be adequately performed in all patients because of technical limitations; however, when wall motion abnormalities are induced remote from the infarct zone, multivessel CAD is likely, and this finding is associated with increased risk of future cardiac events.

Ambulatory ECG monitoring has been used to detect residual ischemia in postinfarction patients by documenting ST-segment depression during daily activities. There is no evidence that this approach is more likely than exercise testing to separate high- and low-risk subsets, and it may yield more false-positive results. Some patients who have recovered from an acute infarction have persistent resting ST- and T-wave abnormalities, which may preclude accurate interpretation of changes recorded with physical activity. Ambulatory ECG monitoring can play a role in the evaluation of antiischemia therapy by noting whether certain pharmacologic regimens can eliminate episodes of transient ST depression associated with physical or mental stress. Certain nonimaging variables on exercise testing— workload achieved, systolic blood pressure response, peak exercise heart rate—provide independent prognostic information. Ambulatory ECG monitoring documents ST-segment deviation and heart rate at the time of the ischemic response.

As we enter the era of health care system reform, attention must be paid to the cost-effectiveness of diagnostic testing in the risk stratification process after acute myocardial infarction.[124, 125] No justification exists from studies in the literature for routine coronary angiography in uncomplicated myocardial infarction patients. A noninvasive strategy can be successfully employed for prognostication only if the data from nuclear cardiology (or echocardiography) procedures are of high quality and the interpreters of test results are well trained to distinguish true perfusion defects or regional wall motion abnormalities from artifacts or noncoronary abnormalities.

REFERENCES

1. van der Wieken LR, Kan G, Belfer AJ, Visser CA, Jaarsma W, Lie KI, Busemann-Sokole E, van der Schoot J, Durrer D: Thallium-201 scanning to decide CCU admission in patients with non-diagnostic electrocardiograms. Int J Cardiol 1983;4:285–299.

2. Berger BC, Watson DD, Burwell LR, Crosby IK, Wellons HA, Teates CD, Beller GA: Redistribution of thallium at rest in patients with stable and unstable angina and the effect of coronary artery bypass surgery. Circulation 1979;60:1114–1125.

3. Gewirtz H, Beller GA, Strauss HW, Dinsmore RE, Zir LM, McKusick KA, Pohost GM: Transient defects of resting thallium scans in patients with coronary artery disease. Circulation 1979;59:707–713.

4. Wackers FJ, Lie KI, Liem KL, Sokole EB, Samson G, van der Schoot JB, Durrer D: Thallium-201 scintigraphy in unstable angina pectoris. Circulation 1978;57:738–742.

5. Parodi O, Uthurralt N, Severi S, Bencivelli W, Michelassi C, L'Abbate A, Maseri A: Transient reduction of regional myocardial perfusion during angina at rest with ST-segment depression or normalization of negative T waves. Circulation 1981;63:1238–1247.

6. Wackers FJ, Sokole EB, Samson G, Schoot JB, Lie KI, Liem KL, Wellens HJ: Value and limitations of thallium-201 scintigraphy in the acute phase of myocardial infarction. N Engl J Med 1976;295:1–5.

7. Wackers FJ, Lie KI, Sokole EB, Res J, van der Schoot JB, Durrer D: Prevalence of right ventricular involvement in inferior wall infarction assessed with myocardial imaging with thallium-201 and technetium-99m pyrophosphate. Am J Cardiol 1978;42:358–362.

7a. Travin MI, Malkin RD, Garber CE, Messinger DE, Cloutier DJ, Heller GV: Prevalence of right ventricular perfusion defects after inferior myocardial infarction assessed by low-level exercise with Technetium 99m sestamibi tomographic myocardial imaging. Am Heart J 1994;127:797–804.

8. Tamaki S, Kambara H, Kadota K, Suzuki Y, Nohara R, Kawai C, Tamaki N, Torizuka K: Improved detection of myocardial infarction by emission computed tomography with thallium-201. Relation to infarct size. Br Heart J 1984;52:621–627.

9. Ritchie JL, Williams DL, Harp G, Stratton JL, Caldwell JH: Transaxial tomography with thallium-201 for detecting remote myocardial infarction. Comparison with planar imaging. Am J Cardiol 1982;50:1236–1241.

10. Huey BL, Beller GA, Kaiser DL, Gibson RS: A comprehensive analysis of myocardial infarction due to left circumflex artery occlusion: Comparison with infarction due to right coronary artery and left anterior descending artery occlusion. J Am Coll Cardiol 1988;12:1156–1166.

11. Wahl JM, Hakki AH, Iskandrian AS, Yacone L: Scintigraphic characterization of Q wave and non–Q-wave acute myocardial infarction. Am Heart J 1985;109:769–775.

12. Imamura T, Araki H, Fukuyama T, Maruoka Y, Ootsubo H, Nakamura M, Koiwaya Y, Tanaka K: Significance of collateral circulation on peri-infarct zone: Assessment with stress thallium-201 scintigraphy. Clin Cardiol 1986;9:137–144.

13. Christian TF, Schwartz RS, Gibbons RJ: Determinants of infarct size in reperfusion therapy for acute myocardial infarction. Circulation 1992;86:81–90.

13a. Komamura K, Kitakaze M, Nishida K, Naka M, Tamai J, Uematsu M, Koretsune Y, Nanto S, Hori M, Inoue M, Kamada T, Kodama K: Progressive decreases in coronary vein flow during reperfusion in acute myocardial infarction: Clinical documentation of the no reflow phenomenon after successful thrombolysis. J Am Coll Cardiol 1994;24:370–377.

14. Gibson RS, Taylor GJ, Watson DD, Berger BC, Crampton RS, Martin RP, Beller GA: Prognostic significance of resting anterior thallium-201 defects in patients with inferior myocardial infarction. J Nucl Med 1980;21:1015–1021.

15. Kirchner P: Infarct size with thallium 201 scintigraphy. Am J Cardiac Imaging 1990;4:46–58.

16. DiCola VC, Downing SE, Donabedian RK, Zaret BL: Pathophysiological correlates of thallium-201 myocardial uptake in experimental infarction. Cardiovasc Res 1977;11:141–146.

17. Okada RD, Lim YL, Chesler DA, Kaul S, Pohost GM: Quantitation of myocardial infarct size from thallium-201 images: Validation of a new approach in an experimental model. J Am Coll Cardiol 1984;3:948–955.

18. Nelson AD, Khullar S, Leighton RF, Budd GC, Gohara A, Ross JN Jr, Andrews LT, Windham J: Quantification of thallium-201 scintigrams in acute myocardial infarction. Am J Cardiol 1979;44:664–669.

19. Kaul S, Okada RD, Pandian NG, Pohost GM, Weyman AE, Strauss HW: Determination of left ventricular "area at risk" with high-resolution single photon emission computerized tomography in experimental coronary occlusion. Am Heart J 1985;109:1369–1374.

20. Prigent F, Maddahi J, Garcia EV, Satoh Y, Van Train K, Berman DS: Quantification of myocardial infarct size by thallium-201 single-photon emission computed tomography: Experimental validation in the dog. Circulation 1986;74:852–861.

21. Prigent F, Maddahi J, Garcia EV, Resser K, Lew AS, Berman DS: Comparative methods for quantifying myocardial infarct size by thallium-201 SPECT. J Nucl Med 1987;28:325–333.

22. Weiss RJ, Buda AJ, Pasyk S, O'Neill WW, Keyes JW Jr, Pitt B: Noninvasive quantification of jeopardized myocardial mass in dogs using 2-dimensional echocardiography and thallium-201 tomography. Am J Cardiol 1983;52:1340–1344.

23. Keyes JW Jr, Brady TJ, Leonard PF, Svetkoff DB, Winter SM, Rogers WL, Rose EA: Calculation of viable and infarcted myocardial mass from thallium-201 tomograms. J Nucl Med 1981;22:339–343.

24. Gerber KH, Higgins CB: Quantitation of size of myocardial infarctions by computerized transmission tomography. Comparison with hot-spot and cold-spot radionuclide scans. Invest Radiol 1983;18:238–244.

25. Wackers FJ, Becker AE, Samson G, Sokole EB, van der Schoot JB, Vet AJ, Lie KI, Durrer D, Wellens II: Location and size of acute transmural myocardial infarction estimated from thallium-201 scintiscans. A clinicopathological study. Circulation 1977;56:72–78.

26. Tamaki S, Nakajima H, Murakami T, Yui Y, Kambara H, Kadota K, Yoshida A, Kawai C, Tamaki N, Mukai T, Ishii Y, Torizuka K: Estimation of infarct size by myocardial emission computed tomography with thallium-201 and its relation to creatine kinase–MB release after myocardial infarction in man. Circulation 1982;66:994–1001.

27. Mahmarian JJ, Pratt CM, Borges-Neto S, Cashion WR, Roberts R, Verani MS: Quantification of infarct size by ^{201}Tl single-photon emission computed tomography during acute myocardial infarction in humans. Comparison with enzymatic estimates. Circulation 1988;78:831–839.

28. Perez-Gonzalez J, Botvinick E, Dunn R, Rahimtoola S, Ports T, Chatterjee K, Parmley W: The late prognostic value of acute scintigraphic measurement of myocardial infarct size. Circulation 1982;66:960–971.

29. Botvinick EH, Perez-Gonzalez JF, Dunn R, Ports T, Chatterjee K, Parmley W: Late prognostic value of scintigraphic parameters of acute myocardial infarction size in complicated myocardial infarction without heart failure. Am J Cardiol 1983;51:1045–1051.

30. Becker LC, Silverman KJ, Bulkley BH, Kallman CH, Mellits ED, Weisfeldt M: Comparison of early thallium-201 scintigraphy and gated blood pool imaging for predicting mortality in patients with acute myocardial infarction. Circulation 1983;67:1272–1282.

31. Hakki AH, Nestico PF, Heo J, Unwala AA, Iskandrian AS: Relative prognostic value of rest thallium-201 imaging, radionuclide ventriculography and 24 hour ambulatory electrocardiographic monitoring after acute myocardial infarction. J Am Coll Cardiol 1987;10:25–32.

32. Nestico PF, Hakki AH, Felsher J, Heo J, Iskandrian AS: Implications of abnormal right ventricular thallium uptake in acute myocardial infarction. Am J Cardiol 1986;58:230–234.

33. Hirsowitz GS, Lakier JB, Marks DS, Lee TG, Goldberg AD, Goldstein S: Sequential radionuclide angiographic assessment of left and right ventricular performance and quantitative thallium-201 scintigraphy following acute myocardial infarction. Am Heart J 1984;107:934–939.

34. Beller GA: Role of myocardial perfusion imaging in evaluating thrombolytic therapy for acute myocardial infarction. J Am Coll Cardiol 1987;9:661–668.

35. Ritchie JL, Cerqueira M, Maynard C, Davis K, Kennedy JW: Ventricular function and infarct size: The Western Washington Intravenous Streptokinase in Myocardial Infarction Trial. J Am Coll Cardiol 1988;11:689–697.

35a. Beller GA: Myocardial reperfusion imaging: Basic principles and clinical applications. Am J Cardiac Imaging 1993;7:11–23.

35b. Cerqueira MD, Maynard C, Ritchie JL, Davis KB, Kennedy JW: Long-term survival in 618 patients from the Western Washington Streptokinase in Myocardial Infarction trials. J Am Coll Cardiol 1992;20:1452–1459.

36. Strauss HW, Harrison K, Langan JK, Lebowitz E, Pitt B: Thallium-201 for myocardial imaging. Relation of thallium-201 to regional myocardial perfusion. Circulation 1975;51:641–645.

37. GISSI The Italian Group for the Study of Streptokinase in Myocardial Infarction: Effectiveness of intravenous thrombolytic treatment in acute myocardial infarction. Lancet 1986;1:397–402.

38. Granato JE, Watson DD, Flanagan TL, Gascho JA, Beller GA: Myocardial thallium-201 kinetics during coronary occlusion and reperfusion: Influence of method of reflow and timing of thallium-201 administration. Circulation 1986;73:150–160.

39. Granato JE, Watson DD, Flanagan TL, Beller GA: Myocardial thallium-201 kinetics and regional flow alterations with 3 hours of coronary occlusion and either rapid reperfusion through a totally patent vessel or slow reperfusion through a critical stenosis. J Am Coll Cardiol 1987;9:109–118.

40. Forman R, Kirk ES: Thallium-201 accumulation during reperfusion of ischemic myocardium: Dependence on regional blood flow rather than viability. Am J Cardiol 1984;54:659–663.

41. Melin JA, Wijns W, Keyeux A, Gurne O, Cogneau M, Michel C, Bol A, Robert A, Charlier A, Pouleur H: Assessment of thallium-201 redistribution versus glucose uptake as predictors of viability after coronary occlusion and reperfusion. Circulation 1988;77:927–934.

42. Okada RD, Boucher CA: Differentiation of viable and nonviable myocardium after acute reperfusion using serial thallium-201 imaging. Am Heart J 1987;113:241–250.

43. Reduto LA, Freund GC, Gaeta JM, Smalling RW, Lewis B, Gould KL: Coronary artery reperfusion in acute myocardial infarction: Beneficial effects of intracoronary streptokinase on left ventricular salvage and performance. Am Heart J 1981;102:1168–1177.

44. De Coster PM, Melin JA, Detry JM, Brasseur LA, Beckers C, Col J: Coronary artery reperfusion in acute myocardial infarction: Assessment by pre- and postintervention thallium-201 myocardial perfusion imaging. Am J Cardiol 1985;55:889–895.

45. Schwarz F, Hofmann M, Schuler G, von Olshausen K, Zimmermann R, Kubler W: Thrombolysis in acute myocardial infarction: Effect of intravenous followed by intracoronary streptokinase application on estimates of infarct size. Am J Cardiol 1984;53:1505–1510.

46. Schuler G, Schwarz F, Hofmann M, Mehmel H, Manthey J, Maurer W, Rauch B, Herrmann HJ, Kubler W: Thrombolysis in acute myocardial infarction using intracoronary streptokinase: Assessment by thallium-201 scintigraphy. Circulation 1982;66:658–664.

47. Ritchie JL, Davis KB, Williams DL, Caldwell J, Kennedy JW: Global and regional left ventricular function and tomographic radionuclide perfusion: The Western Washington Intracoronary Streptokinase in Myocardial Infarction Trial. Circulation 1984;70:867–875.

47a. Weinstein H, Reinhardt CP, Wironen JF, Leppo JA: Myocardial uptake of thallium-201 and technetium-99m labeled sestamibi after ischemia and reperfusion: Comparison by quantitative dual-tracer autoradiography in rabbits. J Nucl Cardiol 1994;1:351–364.

47b. Krause T, Kasper W, Meinertz T, Schnitzler M, Just H, Schumichen C, Moser E: Comparison in acute myocardial infarction of anisoylated plasminogen streptokinase activator complex versus heparin evaluated by simultaneous thallium-201/technetium-99m pyrophosphate tomography. Am J Cardiol 1993;71:8–13.

48. Rigo P, Alderson PO, Robertson RM, Becker LC, Wagner HN Jr.: Measurement of aortic and mitral regurgitation by gated cardiac blood pool scans. Circulation 1979;60:306–312.

49. Sorensen SG, Crawford MH, Richards KL, Chaudhuri TK, O'Rourke RA: Noninvasive detection of ventricular aneurysm by combined two-dimensional echocardiography and equilibrium radionuclide angiography. Am Heart J 1982;104:145–152.

49a. Berger PB, Ruocco NA Jr, Ryan TJ, Jacobs AK, Zaret BL, Wackers FJ, Frederick MM, Faxon DP: Frequency and significance of right ventricular dysfunction during inferior wall left ventricular myocardial infarction treated with thrombolytic therapy (results from the thrombolysis in myocardial infarction [TIMI] II trial). The TIMI Research Group. Am J Cardiol 1993;71:1148–1152.

50. CASS: Myocardial infarction and mortality in the coronary artery surgery study (CASS) randomized trial. N Engl J Med 1984;310:750–758.

51. Multicenter Postinfarction Research Group: Risk stratification and survival after myocardial infarction. N Engl J Med 1983;303:331–336.

52. Ong L, Green S, Reiser P, Morrison J: Early prediction of mortality in patients with acute myocardial infarction: A prospective study of clinical and radionuclide risk factors. Am J Cardiol 1986;57:33–38.

53. Gibson RS, Beller GA, Gheorghiade M, Nygaard TW, Watson DD, Huey BL, Sayre SL, Kaiser DL: The prevalence and clinical signifi-cance of residual myocardial ischemia 2 weeks after uncomplicated non-Q wave infarction: A prospective natural history study. Circulation 1986;73:1186–1198.

54. Reduto LA, Berger HJ, Cohen LS, Gottschalk A, Zaret BL: Sequential radionuclide assessment of left and right ventricular performance after acute transmural myocardial infarction. Ann Intern Med 1978;89:441–447.

55. Norris RM, Barnaby PF, Brandt PW, Geary GG, Whitlock RM, Wild CJ, Barratt-Boyes BG: Prognosis after recovery from first acute myocardial infarction: Determinants of reinfarction and sudden death. Am J Cardiol 1984;53:408–413.

56. Multicenter Postinfarction Research Group: Risk stratification and survival after myocardial infarction cooperative study. N Engl J Med 1983;303:331–336.

57. Califf RM, Topol EJ, Gersh BJ: From myocardial salvage to patient salvage in acute myocardial infarction: The role of reperfusion therapy. J Am Coll Cardiol 1989;14:1382–1388.

57a. Bonow RO: Prognostic assessment in coronary artery disease. Role of radionuclide angiography. J Nucl Cardiol 1994;1:280–291.

57b. Simoons ML, Vos J, Tijssen JGB, Vermeer F, Verheugt FWA, Krauss XH, Manger-Cats V: Long-term benefit of early thrombolytic therapy in patients with acute myocardial infarction: 5-year follow-up of a trial conducted by the Interuniversity Cardiology Institute of the Netherlands. J Am Coll Cardiol 1989;14:1609–1615.

57c. White HD, Norris RM, Brown MA, Brandt PWT, Whitlock RML, Wild CJ: Left ventricular end-systolic volume as the major determinant of survival after recovery from myocardial infarction. Circulation 1987;76:44–51.

58. Zaret BL, Wackers FJ, Terrin ML, Ross R, Weiss M, Slater J, Morrison J, Bourge RC, Passamani E, Knatterud G, Braunwald E, for the TIMI Investigators: Assessment of global and regional left ventricular performance at rest and during exercise after thrombolytic therapy for acute myocardial infarction: Results of the Thrombolysis in Myocardial Infarction (TIMI) II Study. Am J Cardiol 1992;69:1–9.

59. Ahnve S, Gilpin E, Dittrich H, Nicod P, Henning H, Carlisle J, Ross J Jr: First myocardial infarction: Age and ejection fraction identify a low-risk group. Am Heart J 1988;116:925–932.

60. Taylor G, Humphries J, Mellits D, Pitt B, Schulze R, Griffith L, Achuff S: Prediction of clinical course, coronary anatomy and left ventricular function after recovery from acute myocardial infarction. Circulation 1980;62:960–970.

61. Froelicher VF, Perdue ST, Atwood JE, Des Pois P, Sivarajan ES: Exercise testing of patients recovering from myocardial infarction. Curr Probl Cardiol 1986;11:369–444.

62. Gibson RS, Watson DD, Craddock GB, Crampton RS, Kaiser DL, Denny MJ, Beller GA: Prediction of cardiac events after uncomplicated myocardial infarction: A prospective study comparing predischarge exercise thallium-201 scintigraphy and coronary angiography. Circulation 1983;68:321–336.

63. TIMI Research Group: Comparison of invasive and conservative strategies after treatment with intravenous tissue plasminogen activation in acute myocardial infarction. N Engl J Med 1989;320:612–627.

63a. Volpi A, DeVita C, Franzusi MG, Geraci E, Maggioni AP, Mauri F, Negri E, Santoro E, Tavazzi L, Tognoni G, the Ad hoc Working Group of the Gruppo Italiano per lo Studio della Sopravvivenza nele'Infarto Miocardico (GISSI)-2 Data Base: Determinants of 6-month mortality in survivors of myocardial infarction after thrombolysis. Results of the GISSI-2 data base. Circulation 1993;88:416–429.

63b. Grines CL, Browne KF, Marco J, Rothbaum D, Stone GW, O'Keefe J, Overlie P, Donohue B, Chelliah N, Timmis GC, Vliestra RE, Strzelecki M, Puchrowicz KK, Ochocki S, O'Neill WW, for the Primary Angioplasty in Myocardial Infarction Study Group: A comparison of immediate angioplasty with thrombolytic therapy for acute myocardial infarction. N Engl J Med 1993;328:673–679.

63c. DeBoer MJ, Hoorntje JCA, Ottervanger JP, Reiffers S, Suryapranata H, Zijlstra F: Immediate coronary angioplasty versus intravenous streptokinase in acute myocardial infarction: Left ventricular ejection fraction, hospital mortality and reinfarction. J Am Coll Cardiol 1994;23:1004–1008.

63d. White HD, Cross DB, Elliott JM, Norris RM, Yee TW: Long-term prognostic importance of patency of the infarct-related coronary artery after thrombolytic therapy for acute myocardial infarction. Circulation 1994;89:61–67.

64. Tilkemeier PL, Guiney TE, LaRaia PJ, Boucher CA: Prognostic value of predischarge low-level exercise thallium testing after thrombolytic treatment of acute myocardial infarction. Am J Cardiol 1990;66:1203–1207.

65. Haber HL, Beller GA, Watson DD, Gimple LW: Exercise thallium-201 scintigraphy after thrombolytic therapy with or without angioplasty for acute myocardial infarction. Am J Cardiol 1993;71:1257–1261.

66. Haines DE, Beller GA, Watson DD, Kaiser DL, Sayre SL, Gibson RS: Exercise-induced ST segment elevation 2 weeks after uncomplicated myocardial infarction: Contributing factors and prognostic significance. J Am Coll Cardiol 1987;9:996–1003.

67. Froelicher VF, Perdue S, Pewen W, Risch M: Application of meta-analysis using an electronic spread sheet to exercise testing in patients after myocardial infarction. Am J Med 1987;83:1045–1054.

67a. Froelicher ES: Usefulness of exercise testing shortly after acute myocardial infarction for predicting 10-year mortality. Am J Cardiol 1994;74:318–323.

68. Miranda CP, Herbert WG, Dubach P, Lehmann KG, Froelicher VF: Post-myocardial infarction exercise testing. Non–Q wave versus Q wave correlation with coronary angiography and long-term prognosis. Circulation 1991;84:2357–2365.

68a. Juneau M, Colles P, Theroux P, de Guise P, Pelletier G, Lam J, Waters D: Symptom-limited versus low level exercise testing before hospital discharge after myocardial infarction. J Am Coll Cardiol 1992;20:927–933.

68b. Wilson W, Beller G, Watson D, Sayre S, Kaiser D, Nygaard T, Gibson R: Symptom-limited thallium-201 exercise testing at three months after myocardial infarction: A comparison with submaximal predischarge testing (Abstract). J Am Coll Cardiol 1986;7:198A.

68c. Gimple LW, Beller GA: Assessing prognosis after acute myocardial infarction in the thrombolytic era. J Nucl Cardiol 1994;1:198–209.

69. Smeets JP, Rigo P, Legrand V, Chevigne M, Hastir F, Kulbertus HE: Prognostic value of thallium-201 stress myocardial scintigraphy with exercise ECG after myocardial infarction. Cardiology 1981;68(suppl 2):67–70.

70. Patterson RE, Horowitz SF, Eng C, Meller J, Goldsmith SJ, Pichard AD, Halgash DA, Herman MV, Gorlin R: Can noninvasive exercise test criteria identify patients with left main or 3-vessel coronary disease after a first myocardial infarction? Am J Cardiol 1983;51:361–372.

71. Dunn RF, Freedman B, Bailey IK, Uren R, Kelly DT: Noninvasive prediction of multivessel disease after myocardial infarction. Circulation 1980;62:726–734.

72. Brown KA, Weiss RM, Clements JP, Wackers FJ: Usefulness of residual ischemic myocardium within prior infarct zone for identifying patients at high risk late after acute myocardial infarction. Am J Cardiol 1987;60:15–19.

73. Abraham RD, Freedman SB, Dunn RF, Newman H, Roubin GS, Harris PJ, Kelly DT: Prediction of multivessel coronary artery disease and prognosis early after acute myocardial infarction by exercise electrocardiography and thallium-201 myocardial perfusion scanning. Am J Cardiol 1986;58:423–427.

74. Sutton JM, Topol EJ: Significance of a negative exercise thallium test in the presence of a critical residual stenosis after thrombolysis for acute myocardial infarction. Circulation 1991;83:1278–1286.

75. Topol EJ, Holmes DR, Rogers WJ: Coronary angiography after thrombolytic therapy for acute myocardial infarction. Ann Intern Med 1991;114:877–885.

76. Rogers WJ, Babb JD, Baim DS, Chesebro JH, Gore JM, Roberts R, Williams DO, Frederick M, Passamani ER, Braunwald E: Selective versus routine predischarge coronary arteriography after therapy with recombinant tissue-type plasminogen activator, heparin and aspirin for acute myocardial infarction. TIMI II Investigators. J Am Coll Cardiol 1991;17:1007–1016.

76a. The GUSTO Angiographic Investigators: The effects of tissue plasminogen activator, streptokinase or both on coronary-artery patency, ventricular function, and survival after acute myocardial infarction. N Engl J Med 1993;329:1615–1622.

76b. Aguirre FV, McMahon RP, Mueller H, Kleiman NS, Kerin MJ, Desvigne-Nickens P, Hamilton WP, Chaitman BR, for the TIMI Investigators: Impact of age on clinical outcome and postlytic management strategies in patients treated with intravenous thrombolytic therapy. Results from the TIMI II study. Circulation 1994;90:78–86.

77. Nygaard TW, Gibson RS, Ryan JM, Gascho JA, Watson DD, Beller GA: Prevalence of high-risk thallium-201 scintigraphic findings in left main coronary artery stenosis: Comparison with patients with multiple- and single-vessel coronary artery disease. Am J Cardiol 1984;53:462–469.

78. Wilson WW, Gibson RS, Nygaard TW, Craddock GB Jr, Watson DD, Crampton RS, Beller GA: Acute myocardial infarction associated with single vessel coronary artery disease: An analysis of clinical outcome and the prognostic importance of vessel patency and residual ischemic myocardium. J Am Coll Cardiol 1988;11:223–234.

78a. Moss AJ, Goldstein RE, Hall WJ, Bigger JT Jr, Fleiss JL, Greenberg H, Bodenheimer M, Krone RJ, Marcus FI, Wackers FJ, et al: Detection and significance of myocardial ischemia in stable patients after recovery from an acute coronary event. Multicenter Myocardial Ischemia Research Group. JAMA 1993;269:2379–2385.

78b. Krone RJ, Gregory JJ, Freedland KE, Kleiger RE, Wackers FJ Th, Bodenheimer MM, Benhorin J, Schwartz RG, Parker JO, Vorhees LV, Moss AJ, for the Multicenter Myocardial Ischemia Research Group: J Am Coll Cardiol 1994;24:1274–1281.

78c. The TIMI IIIB Investigators: Effects of tissue plasminogen activator and a comparison of early invasive and conservative strategies in unstable angina and non–Q-wave myocardial infarction. Results of the TIMI IIB trial. Circulation 1994;89:1545–1556.

79. Weiss AT, Maddahi J, Lew AS, Shah PK, Ganz W, Swan HJ, Berman DS: Reverse redistribution of thallium-201: A sign of non-transmural myocardial infarction with patency of the infarct-related coronary artery. J Am Coll Cardiol 1986;7:61–67.

80. Touchstone DA, Beller GA, Nygaard TW, Watson DD, Tedesco C, Kaul S: Functional significance of predischarge exercise thallium-201 findings following intravenous streptokinase therapy during acute myocardial infarction. Am Heart J 1988;116:1500–1507.

80a. Terrin ML, Williams DO, Kleiman NS, et al.: Two and three-year results of the thrombolysis in myocardial infarction (TIMI) phase II clinical trial. J Am Coll Cardiol 1993;22:1763–1772.

81. Wasserman AG, Katz RJ, Cleary P, Varma VM, Reba RC, Ross AM: Noninvasive detection of multivessel disease after myocardial infarction by exercise radionuclide ventriculography. Am J Cardiol 1982;50:1242–1247.

82. Hung J, Goris ML, Nash E, Kraemer HC, DeBusk RF, Berger WE, Lew H: Comparative value of maximal treadmill testing, exercise thallium myocardial perfusion scintigraphy and exercise radionuclide ventriculography for distinguishing high- and low-risk patients soon after acute myocardial infarction. Am J Cardiol 1984;53:1221–1227.

83. Morris KG, Palmeri ST, Califf RM, McKinnis RA, Higginbotham MB, Coleman RE, Cobb FR: Value of radionuclide angiography for predicting specific cardiac events after acute myocardial infarction. Am J Cardiol 1985;55:318–324.

84. Corbett JR, Dehmer GJ, Lewis SE, Woodward W, Henderson E, Parkey RW, Blomqvist CG, Willerson JT: The prognostic value of submaximal exercise testing with radionuclide ventriculography before hospital discharge in patients with recent myocardial infarction. Circulation 1981;64:535–544.

85. Abraham RD, Harris PJ, Roubin GS, Shen WF, Sadick N, Morris J, Kelly DT: Usefulness of ejection fraction response to exercise one month after acute myocardial infarction in predicting coronary anatomy and prognosis. Am J Cardiol 1987;60:225–230.

86. Dewhurst NG, Muir AL: Comparative prognostic value of radionuclide ventriculography at rest and during exercise in 100 patients after first myocardial infarction. Br Heart J 1983;49:111–121.

87. Wallis JB, Holmes JR, Borer JS: Prognosis in patients with coronary artery disease and low ejection fraction at rest: Impact of the exercise ejection fraction. Am J Cardiac Imag 1990;4:1–10.

88. Borer JS, Miller D, Schreiber T, Charash B, Gerling B: Radionuclide cineangiography in acute myocardial infarction: Role in prognostication. Semin Nucl Med 1987;17:89–94.

88a. Mazzotta G, Camerini A, Scopinarô G, Villavecchiâ G, Lionetto R, Vecchio C: Predicting severe ischemic events after uncomplicated myocardial infarction by exercise testing and rest and exercise radionuclide ventriculography. J Nucl Cardiol 1994;1:246–253.

89. Wackers FJ, Terrin ML, Kayden DS, Knatterud G, Forman S, Braunwald E, Zaret BL: Quantitative radionuclide assessment of regional ventricular function after thrombolytic therapy for acute myocardial infarction: Results of phase I Thrombolysis in Myocardial Infarction (TIMI) trial. J Am Coll Cardiol 1989;13:998–1005.

89a. Rogers WJ, Bourge RC, Papapietro SE, Wackers FJ Th, Zaret BL, Forman S, Dodge HT, Robertson TL, Passamani ER, Braunwald E, for the TIMI Investigators: Variables predictive of good functional outcome following thrombolytic therapy in the thrombolysis in myocardial infarction phase II (TIMI II) pilot study. Am J Cardiol 1989;63:503–512.

89b. Zhu W-X, Gibbons RJ, Bailey KR, Gersh BJ: Predischarge exericse radionuclide angiography in predicting multivessel coronary artery disease and subsequent cardiac events after thrombolytic therapy for acute myocardial infarction. Am J Cardiol 1994;74:554–559.

90. Candell-Riera J, Permanyer-Miralda G, Castell J, Rius-Davi A, Domingo E, Alvarez-Aunon E, Olona M, Rossello J, Ortega D, Domenech-Torne FM, et al.: Uncomplicated first myocardial infarction: Strategy for comprehensive prognostic studies. J Am Coll Cardiol 1991;18:1207–1219.

90a. Verani MS: Exercise and pharmacologic stress testing for prognosis after acute myocardial infarction. J Nucl Med 1994;35:716–720.

91. Leppo JA, O'Brien J, Rothendler JA, Getchell JD, Lee VW: Dipyridamole-thallium-201 scintigraphy in the prediction of future cardiac events after acute myocardial infarction. N Engl J Med 1984;310:1014–1018.

92. Gimple LW, Hutter AM Jr, Guiney TE, Boucher CA: Prognostic utility of predischarge dipyridamole-thallium imaging compared to predischarge submaximal exercise electrocardiography and maximal exercise thallium imaging after uncomplicated acute myocardial infarction. Am J Cardiol 1989;64:1243–1248.

93. Brown KA, O'Meara J, Chambers CE, Plante DA: Ability of dipyridamole-thallium-201 imaging one to four days after acute myocardial infarction to predict in-hospital and late recurrent myocardial ischemic events. Am J Cardiol 1990;65:160–167.

94. Pirelli S, Inglese E, Suppa M, Corrada E, Campolo L: Dipyridamole-thallium 201 scintigraphy in the early post-infarction period. (Safety and accuracy in predicting the extent of coronary disease and future recurrence of angina in patients suffering from their first myocardial infarction). Eur Heart J 1988;9:1324–1331.

94a. Mahmarian JJ, Pratt CM, Nishimura S, Abreu A, Verani MS: Quantitative adenosine ^{201}Tl single-photon emission computed tomography for the early assessment of patients surviving acute myocardial infarction. Circulation 1993;87:1197–1210.

95. Breisblatt WM, Weiland FL, McLain JR, Tomlinson GC, Burns MJ, Spaccavento LJ: Usefulness of ambulatory radionuclide monitoring of left ventricular function early after acute myocardial infarction for predicting residual myocardial ischemia. Am J Cardiol 1988;62:1005–1010.

96. Kayden DS, Wackers FJ, Zaret BL: Silent left ventricular dysfunction during routine activity after thrombolytic therapy for acute myocardial infarction. J Am Coll Cardiol 1990;15:1500–1507.

97. Willerson JT, Parkey RW, Bonte FJ, Meyer SL, Atkins JM, Stokely EM: Technetium stannous pyrophosphate myocardial scintigrams in patients with chest pain of varying etiology. Circulation 1975;51:1046–1052.

97a. Corbett J, Quaife R, Parkey R: Current state of infarct-avid imaging—advantages of SPECT evaluations: Promise of antimyosin antibodies. Am J Cardiac Imaging 1992;6:59.

98. Khaw BA, Gold HK, Yasuda T, Leinbach RC, Kanke M, Fallon JT, Barlai-Kovach M, Strauss HW, Sheehan F, Haber E: Scintigraphic quantification of myocardial necrosis in patients after intravenous injection of myosin-specific antibody. Circulation 1986;74:501–508.

99. Khaw BA, Yasuda T, Gold HK, Leinbach RC, Johns JA, Kanke M, Barlai-Kovach M, Strauss HW, Haber E: Acute myocardial infarct imaging with indium-111–labeled monoclonal antimyosin Fab. J Nucl Med 1987;28:1671–1678.

100. Johnson LL, Seldin DW, Becker LC, LaFrance ND, Liberman HA, James C, Mattis JA, Dean RT, Brown J, Reiter A, et al.: Antimyosin imaging in acute transmural myocardial infarctions: Results of a multicenter clinical trial. J Am Coll Cardiol 1989;13:27–35.

100a. Nedelman MA, Shealy DJ, Boulin R, Brunt E, Seasholtz JI, Allen IE, McCartney JE, Warren FD, Oppermann H, Pang RH, et al.: Rapid infarct imaging with a technetium-99m–labeled antimyosin recombinant single-chain Fv: Evaluation in a canine model of acute myocardial infarction. J Nucl Med 1993;34:234–241.

100b. Okuda K, Nohara R, Fujita M, Tamaki N, Konishi J, Sasayama S: Technetium-99m-pyrophosphate uptake as an indicator of myocardial injury without infarct. J Nucl Med 1994;35:1366–1370.

101. Volpini M, Giubbini R, Gei P, Cuccia C, Franzoni P, Riva S, Terzi A, Metra M, Bestagno M, Visioli O: Diagnosis of acute myocardial infarction by indium-111 antimyosin antibodies and correlation with the traditional techniques for the evaluation of extent and localization. Am J Cardiol 1989;63:7–13.

102. Johnson LL, Seldin DW, Keller AM, Wall RM, Bhatia K, Bingham CO, Tresgallo ME: Dual isotope thallium and indium antimyosin SPECT imaging to identify acute infarct patients at further ischemic risk. Circulation 1990;81:37–45.

103. Berger H, Lahiri A, Leppo J, et al.: Risk stratification and myocardial infarct sizing with quantification antimyosin in patients suspected of acute myocardial infarction. Submitted for Publication.

104. Antunes ML, Seldin DW, Wall RM, Johnson LL: Measurement of acute Q-wave myocardial infarct size with single photon emission computed tomography imaging of indium-111 antimyosin. Am J Cardiol 1989;63:777–783.

104a. Maddahi J, Di Carli M: Antimyosin monoclonal antibody imaging to assess myocardial viability in the setting of thrombolysis. Am J Cardiac Imaging 1993;7:45–52.

105. Sinusas AJ, Watson DD, Cannon JM Jr, Beller GA: Effect of ischemia and postischemic dysfunction on myocardial uptake of technetium-99m–labeled methoxyisobutyl isonitrile and thallium-201. J Am Coll Cardiol 1989;14:1785–1793.

106. Boucher CA, Wackers FJ, Zaret BL, Mena IG: Technetium-99m sestamibi myocardial imaging at rest for assessment of myocardial infarction and first-pass ejection fraction. Multicenter Cardiolite Study Group. Am J Cardiol 1992;69:22–27.

107. Christian TF, Clements IP, Gibbons RJ: Noninvasive identification of myocardium at risk in patients with acute myocardial infarction and nondiagnostic electrocardiograms with technetium-99m sestamibi. Circulation 1991;83:1615–1620.

108. Wackers FJ, Gibbons RJ, Verani MS, Kayden DS, Pellikka PA, Behrenbeck T, Mahmarian JJ, Zaret BL: Serial quantitative planar technetium-99m isonitrile imaging in acute myocardial infarction: Efficacy for noninvasive assessment of thrombolytic therapy. J Am Coll Cardiol 1989;14:861–873.

109. Gibbons RJ, Verani MS, Behrenbeck T, Pellikka PA, O'Connor MK, Mahmarian JJ, Chesebro JH, Wackers FJ: Feasibility of tomographic ^{99m}Tc-hexakis-2-methoxy-2-methylpropyl-isonitrile imaging for the assessment of myocardial area at risk and the effect of treatment in acute myocardial infarction. Circulation 1989;80:1277–1286.

109a. Gibson WS, Christian TF, Pellikka PA, Behrenbeck T, Gibbons RJ: Serial tomographic imaging with technetium-99m sestamibi for the assessment of infarct-related arterial patency following reperfusion therapy. J Nucl Med 1992;33:2080–2085.

110. Pellikka PA, Behrenbeck T, Verani MS, Mahmarian JJ, Wackers FJ, Gibbons RJ: Serial changes in myocardial perfusion using tomographic technetium-99m-hexakis-2-methoxy-2-methylpropyl-isonitrile imaging following reperfusion therapy of myocardial infarction. J Nucl Med 1990;31:1269–1275.

111. Christian TF, Gibbons RJ, Gersh BJ: Effect of infarct location on myocardial salvage assessed by technetium-99m isonitrile. J Am Coll Cardiol 1991;17:1303–1308.

112. Hvid-Jacobsen K, Moller JT, Kjoller E, Nielsen SL, Engel U, Duus S, Kanstrup IL, Jensen PF, Carlsen J, Nielsen F, et al.: Myocardial perfusion at fatal infarction: Location and size of scintigraphic defects. J Nucl Med 1992;33:251–253.

113. Biersack HJ, Grunwald F, Kropp J: Single photon emission computed tomography imaging of brain tumors. Semin Nucl Med 1991;21:2–10.

113a. Clements IP, Christian TF, Higano ST, Gibbons RJ, Gersh BJ: Residual flow to the infarct zone as a determinant of infarct size after direct angioplasty. Circulation 1993;88:1527–1533.

113b. Gibbons RJ, Holmes DR, Reeder GS, Bailey KR, Hopfenspirger MR, Gersh BJ, for the Mayo Coronary Care Unit and Catheterization Laboratory Groups: Immediate angioplasty compared with the administration of a thrombolytic agent followed by conservative treatment for myocardial infarction. N Engl J Med 1993;328:685–691.

114. Christian TF, Behrenbeck T, Gersh BJ, Gibbons RJ: Relation of left ventricular volume and function over one year after acute myocardial infarction to infarct size determined by technetium-99m sestamibi. Am J Cardiol 1991;68:21–26.

115. Christian TF, Behrenbeck T, Pellikka PA, Huber KC, Chesebro JH, Gibbons RJ: Mismatch of left ventricular function and infarct size demonstrated by technetium-99m isonitrile imaging after reperfusion therapy for acute myocardial infarction: Identification of myocardial stunning and hyperkinesia. J Am Coll Cardiol 1990;16:1632–1638.

116. Verani MS, Jeroudi MO, Mahmarian JJ, Boyce TM, Borges-Neto S, Patel B, Bolli R: Quantification of myocardial infarction during coronary occlusion and myocardial salvage after reperfusion using cardiac imaging with technetium-99m hexakis 2-methoxyisobutyl isonitrile. J Am Coll Cardiol 1988;12:1573–1581.

117. Sinusas AJ, Trautman KA, Bergin JD, Watson DD, Ruiz M, Smith WH, Beller GA: Quantification of area at risk during coronary occlusion and degree of myocardial salvage after reperfusion with technetium-99m methoxyisobutyl isonitrile. Circulation 1990;82:1424–1437.

118. Christian TF, Schwartz RS, Gibbons RJ: Determinants of infarct size in reperfusion therapy for acute myocardial infarction. Circulation 1992;86:81–90.

118a. McCallister BD, Christian TF, Gersh B, Gibbons RJ: Prognosis of myocardial infarctions involving more than 40% of the left ventricle after acute reperfusion therapy. Circulation 1993;88:1470–1475.

118b. Udelson JE, Coleman PS, Metherall J, Pandian NG, Gomez AR, Griffith JL, Shea NL, Oates E, Konstam MA: Predicting recovery of severe regional ventricular dysfunction: Comparison of resting scintigraphy with ^{201}Tl and ^{99m}Tc-sestamibi. Circulation 1994;89:2552–2561.

119. Schwaiger M, Brunken R, Grover-McKay M, Krivokapich J, Child J, Tillisch JH, Phelps ME, Schelbert HR: Regional myocardial metabolism in patients with acute myocardial infarction assessed by positron emission tomography. J Am Coll Cardiol 1986;8:800–808.

119a. Tamaki N, Kawamoto M, Takahashi N, et al.: Prognostic value of an increase in fluorine-18 deoxyglucose uptake in patients with myocardial infarction: Comparison with stress thallium imaging. J Am Coll Cardiol 1993;22:1621–1627.

120. Walsh MN, Geltman EM, Brown MA, Henes CG, Weinheimer CJ, Sobel BE, Bergmann SR: Noninvasive estimation of regional myocardial oxygen consumption by positron emission tomography with carbon-11 acetate in patients with myocardial infarction. J Nucl Med 1989;30:1798–1808.

121. Hanes C, Bergman S, Perez J, Sobel B, Geltman A: The time course of restoration of nutritive perfusion, myocardial oxygen consumption, and regional function after coronary thrombosis. Cor Artery Dis 1990;1:687–696.

122. Williams KA, Ryan JW, Resnekov L, Stark V, Peterson EL, Gustafson GC, Martin WB, Freier PA, Harper PV: Planar positron imaging of rubidium-82 for myocardial infarction: A comparison with thallium-201 and regional wall motion. Am Heart J 1989;118:601–610.

123. O'Rourke RA: Management of patients after myocardial infarction and thrombolytic therapy. Curr Prob Cardiol 1994;19:177–228.

124. Verani MS: Should all patients undergo cardiac catheterization after a myocardial infarction? J Nucl Cardiol 1994;7:S134–S146.

125. Grines CL: Should every patient undergo cardiac catheterization after myocardial infarction? J Nucl Cardiol 1994;7:S131–S133.

Chapter 7

Radionuclide Imaging in Unstable Angina Pectoris

Unstable angina is a syndrome that appears to be intermediate between acute myocardial infarction (MI) and stable angina. Angina that is of recent onset and occurs at rest or with minimal exertion is included under the rubric of unstable angina. The most common presentation of this entity is an abrupt change in anginal pattern in which episodes become more frequent or prolonged, are brought on by less effort or develop at rest, and/or are more refractory to usual pharmacologic measures for relief (e.g., nitroglycerin). Most commonly, acute ST-segment changes (depression or elevation) are recorded during attacks of acute chest pain. Some patients develop T-wave inversions on the electrocardiogram (ECG), which can then "pseudonormalize" during attacks of rest angina. The dominant mechanism for unstable angina is rupture or fracture of an atherosclerotic plaque with subsequent platelet activation and aggregation, frequently followed by intraluminal thrombus formation.[1] Silent ischemia is common in patients with unstable angina (see Chapter 5) and can be detected by continuous ECG monitoring. However, most patients respond favorably to aggressive medical management and can undergo a noninvasive strategy for further risk stratification.

Noninvasive techniques are useful in the evaluation of patients with unstable angina, particularly in the subacute phase, when medical management with antithrombotic therapy and antiischemic drugs have proven successful in stabilizing the patient and preventing recurrence of rest pain. In this chapter, the role of radionuclide imaging techniques in unstable angina is reviewed. Table 7–1 summarizes the clinical applications of nuclear cardiology techniques in patients who present with unstable angina.

REST THALLIUM-201 IMAGING IN PATIENTS KNOWN OR SUSPECTED TO HAVE UNSTABLE ANGINA PECTORIS

Serial myocardial thallium-201 (Tl-201) imaging at rest has been employed to evaluate myocardial perfusion and viability in patients with unstable angina pectoris. Several groups of investigators have demonstrated myocardial defects on resting Tl-201 scintigrams when the radionuclide is injected during the pain-free state, with no evidence of acute ST-segment changes or recent or old MI in patients with unstable angina.[2–4] Most patients with unstable angina who have defects at rest and demonstrate delayed rest redistribution on angiography have associated severe coronary artery stenoses. In such patients resting Tl-201–redistribution defects often revert to normal Tl-201 uptake when

Table 7–1. **Applications of Nuclear Cardiology Techniques for the Clinical Presentation of Unstable Angina**

1. Injection of radionuclide perfusion agent during spontaneous chest pain with subsequent imaging to detect ischemia
2. Perfusion imaging in pain-free state at rest for detection of hypoperfusion (rest Tl-201 redistribution)
3. Stress perfusion imaging after stabilization to identify high risk for CAD
4. Stress perfusion imaging to identify culprit lesion
5. Assessment of efficacy of revascularization after bypass surgery or angioplasty
6. Resting Tl-201 scintigraphy or positron-emission tomography to assess viability in patients with severe left ventricular dysfunction

repeat testing is performed after successful revascularization.[3] Berger et al.[3] showed that 13 of 18 preoperative persistent defects in a series of patients with severe stable or unstable angina also showed improved Tl-201 uptake after revascularization. Some patients with unstable angina who have resting Tl-201–redistribution defects have severe associated wall motion abnormalities. This asynergy could be due to either hibernation or myocardial stunning from repeated episodes of rest angina marked by cyclical transient decreases in coronary blood flow. This would most likely be the case when repeated episodes of coronary vasospasm result in sustained ischemic dysfunction. Figure 7–1 shows sequential planar Tl-201 images from a patient with unstable angina from the paper by Berger et al.[3] Note the marked initial defects in multiple myocardial regions, which show delayed rest redistribution. The postoperative images after bypass surgery shows marked improvement in Tl-201 uptake.

Smitherman et al.[4a] reported that rest Tl-201 scintigraphy could be used to distinguish between unstable angina and acute infarction in patients admitted with prolonged chest pain. Patients were given intravenous Tl-201 in the emergency room, and images were obtained shortly thereafter. In patients whose enzymatic and electrocardiographic findings subsequently fulfilled the criteria for MI, persistent defects were shown on serial imaging. Patients in whom MI was ruled out demonstrated resting defects that exhibited delayed redistribution. Freeman et al.[5] evaluated the role of resting Tl-201 scintigraphy in predicting coronary anatomy, left ventricular (LV) wall motion, and hospital outcome in unstable angina pectoris. In a group of 66 unstable-angina patients undergoing quantitative Tl-201 scintigraphy an average of 5.6 hours after rest pain, defects or washout abnormalities were present in 50% of those who had coronary stenoses smaller than 50%, in 82% of those with coronary stenoses of at least 50% who had no history of MI, and in all patients with a history of MI. Sensitivity of Tl-201 defects or a washout abnormality for detection of significant coronary stenoses was 67%, and specificity, 59%. As expected, patients with unstable angina and resting Tl-201 defects had a higher incidence of regional wall motion abnormalities than patients with normal perfusion or washout abnormalities only. In this study, 11 of 18 patients who experienced in-hospital cardiac events but had no history of MI had resting Tl-201 defects, whereas only eight of 25 patients without cardiac events had resting defects ($P = 0.056$). Figure 7–2 shows the distribution of Tl-201 perfusion abnormalities in patients with and without prior infarction in this study and in relation to the extent of angiographic coronary artery disease (CAD).

Hakki et al.[6] also evaluated the results of rest Tl-201 scintigraphy during angina-free periods in patients with unstable angina characterized by ischemic pain at rest but no acute MI. They found a high prevalence of perfusion abnormalities in these patients in the pain-free state. The more severe the coronary stenosis and the greater the collateral blood flow, the more prevalent were resting Tl-201 scan abnormalities. In a total of 40 patients, there were 26 persistent defects, 17 of which did not have corresponding Q waves on the ECG. As expected, these investigators found that occluded vessels had more corresponding perfusion defects (63%) than vessels with subtotal occlusion (30%). As shown in Figure 7–3, defect size at rest in patients with unstable angina was larger in those who had a low ejection fraction (EF) than in those whose EF was normal or high ($r = -0.47$). Thus, these studies indicate that many pa-

L. R. E0056

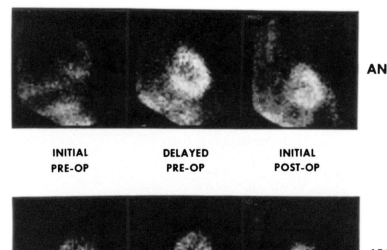

ANTERIOR

INITIAL   DELAYED   INITIAL
PRE-OP   PRE-OP   POST-OP

45° LAO

Figure 7–1. Resting planar Tl-201 images from a patient with unstable angina and three-vessel disease. The first two images represent preoperative (PRE-OP) initial and delayed images in the anterior and 45-degree left anterior oblique projections. Note extensive defects that show rest-redistribution. The third panel shows a repeat initial image obtained postoperatively of the bypass surgery. There is marked improvement in early Tl-201 uptake. (From Berger BC, et al.: Circulation 1979;60:1114–1125.)

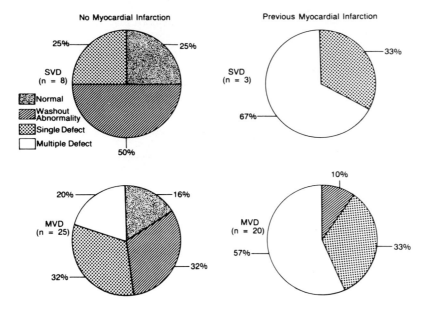

Figure 7–2. The distribution of resting Tl-201 perfusion abnormalities in unstable angina patients with and without previous MI according to the presence of single-vessel disease (SVD) or multivessel disease (MVD). The evaluation of Tl-201 washout enhanced the detection of CAD. (Freeman MR, et al.: Am Heart J 1989;117:306–314.)

tients with unstable angina have a severely reduced flow in the supply region of the coronary vessel that is considered the *culprit artery*—the one responsible for the abrupt change in symptoms or for new onset of angina. However, a normal Tl-201 scan does not rule out severe CAD as the cause of the chest pain syndrome. Some unstable angina patients have mild to moderate coronary artery stenosis, which becomes only severe enough to cause a decrement in resting blood flow during episodes of spasm or when a thrombus totally or subtotally occludes the vessel. When imaged, the stenosis may not be in spasm and the thrombus may have undergone lysis, spontaneously or in response to antithrombotic therapy.

REST THALLIUM-201 SCINTIGRAPHY IN PATIENTS WITH PRINZMETAL'S VARIANT ANGINA

When Tl-201 is injected during an acute episode of coronary vasospasm in patients with variant angina pectoris, significant defects can be observed in myocardial regions that correspond to the ECG leads that show acute ST-segment elevation. Maseri et al.[7] reported that such regional perfusion abnormalities most often show rest redistribution over a period of several hours. When imaging is repeated at rest in the pain-free period, no defects are apparent unless the stenosis in the involved vessel is 90% or greater. Tl

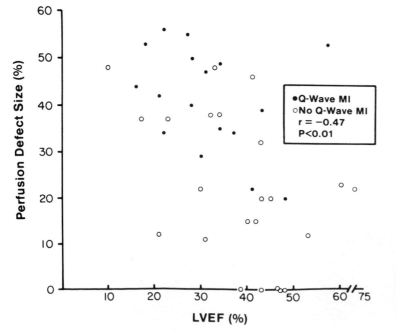

Figure 7–3. Correlation between the resting Tl-201 perfusion defect size (percentage of left ventricular perimeter) and LVEF in patients with unstable angina pectoris. Perfusion defect size was larger in patients with a lower LVEF. (Hakki AH, et al.: Am Heart J 1984;108:326–332.)

201 scintigraphy has been used in conjunction with ergonovine maleate infusion in patients with atypical chest pain suspected of having coronary vasospasm.[8] In such patients, incremental intravenous doses of ergonovine are administered and Tl-201 scintigraphy is performed at the peak dose and again during recovery. Patients who demonstrate both ECG and scintigraphic evidence of ischemia with ergovine tend to have less chest pain following therapy than patients who have chest pain induced by ergonovine but no associated ECG or scintigraphic markers of ischemia. Patients with spasm of the right coronary artery may have predominant right ventricular (RV) ischemia on the basis of a normal Tl-201 scan, a normal LVEF, and normal LV wall motion. Some of these patients have transiently abnormal RV function as assessed by first-pass angiography.[9] A regional perfusion abnormality is also observed if Tl-201 is injected into patients who show normalization of negative T waves during an episode of chest pain.[10]

If Tl-201 is administered during vasospastic angina induced during an exercise test, the severity of the myocardial defect is greater than it would be with exercise-induced ST depression and chest pain.[11] The explanation for this is most likely transmural compared with subendocardial flow diminution in the former situation. There has been one report of exercise-induced ST depression and an associated large Tl-201 perfusion defect in a patient with angiographically normal coronary arteries and exercise-induced coronary vasospasm. After treatment with nitrates and nifedipine, this patient had no further chest pain or ECG changes, and a repeat exercise Tl-201 perfusion scan revealed normal findings and enhanced exercise tolerance.[12] Figure 7–4 shows

the serial anterior and 45-degree left anterior oblique (LAO) planar images in this patient before drug therapy. Note marked ST depression and a severe septal defect on the stress images which show total delayed redistribution.

Single-photon emission computed tomography (SPECT) Tl-201 imaging was used by Kugiyama et al.[13] to assess drug therapy in patients with Prinzmetal's variant angina. They found that exercise-induced vasospasm occurred in 11 patients who took placebo, in 14 who took propranolol, and in none who took nifedipine. The size of the perfusion abnormality, as measured by Tl-201 tomography, was significantly larger in patients receiving propranolol compared with placebo, but significantly smaller in those who took nifedipine than in those who took placebo. Thus, these investigators showed that serial exercise Tl-201 scintigraphy could be used to assess the efficacy of pharmacologic therapy aimed at suppressing episodes of exercise-induced vasospastic angina.

TECHNETIUM-99m–SESTAMIBI IMAGING IN PATIENTS WITH UNSTABLE ANGINA

Many patients who present with chest pain at rest have no associated diagnostic ECG changes of ischemia. Such patients are often admitted to a monitored critical care unit to rule out an MI or exclude unstable angina as the cause of the chest pain syndrome. Technetium-99m–methoxyisobutyl isonitrile (Tc-99m–sestamibi) imaging at rest is particularly suitable for distinguishing patients with unstable angina pectoris from those with atypical rest pain who are

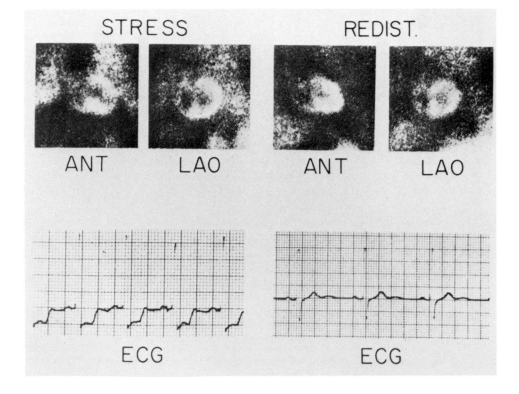

Figure 7–4. Stress and redistribution images in a patient with angiographically normal coronary arteries who had exercise-induced vasospasm of the LAD coronary artery. Note the apical and septal defects on the anterior (ANT) and 45-degree left anterior oblique (LAO) stress (STRESS) images, respectively. The redistribution (REDIST) images on the right show almost total resolution of these defects. The ECG showed resolution of marked stress-induced ischemic ST-segment depression. (Reprinted from American Journal of Cardiology: 48:1; July, 1981: 193–197.)

admitted to the hospital for evaluation. An intravenous dose of Tc-99m sestamibi can be injected at the bedside during episodes of chest pain. Because Tc-99m sestamibi shows negligible delayed redistribution, imaging can be performed as long as several hours after the episode of pain subsides. The perfusion pattern at the time of injection is assessed at the time of imaging. This permits immediate treatment of rest angina with nitrates or calcium blockers without affecting the perfusion defect that might be present at the time of tracer administration. Imaging can then be repeated with a second injection of Tc-99m sestamibi when the patient is pain free, to determine if there are any abnormalities in resting perfusion between episodes of resting ischemia. Figure 7–5 shows Tc-99m–sestamibi images in a patient receiving an intravenous dose of the tracer during pain and then a second injection during a pain-free period.[13]

Bilodeau et al.[14] determined the sensitivity and specificity of Tc-99m–sestamibi SPECT imaging for the diagnosis of CAD in 45 patients admitted to the hospital for clinical suspicion of unstable angina pectoris. SPECT studies obtained after injection of Tc-99m sestamibi during an episode of spontaneous chest pain showed a sensitivity of 96% for the detection of CAD; the ECG obtained at the time of Tc-99m–sestamibi injection during pain had a sensitivity of only 35%. Of interest, perfusion defects on Tc-99m–sestamibi imaging were also seen in 65% of patients during the pain-free state. Specificity of Tc-99m sestamibi for detection of CAD was 79% during pain and 84% in the pain-free state. Figure 7–6 depicts a summary of the results of this study. The location of the resting Tc-99m–sestamibi perfusion defect corresponded to the most severe coronary artery lesion in 88% of patients. The severity of the perfusion defect was shown directly to correlate well with the extent of underlying CAD. Thus, Tc-99m–sestamibi SPECT imaging at rest is associated with good accuracy for detection of CAD and identification of the involved coronary arteries in patients with spontaneous chest pain. Varetto et al.[14a] administered Tc-99m sestamibi in the emergency room to 64 patients with chest pain and a nondiagnostic ECG. Of the 30 patients who had an abnormal Tc-

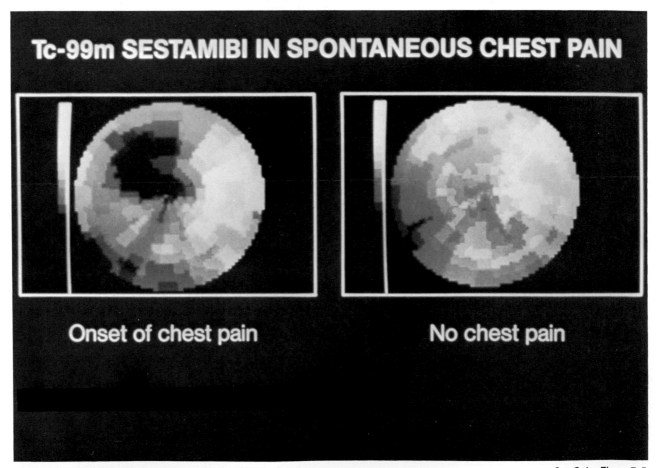

See Color Figure 7–5.

Figure 7–5. Two-dimensional polar map display of a Tc-99m–sestamibi study obtained in a 48-year-old man admitted for atypical chest pain at rest. The study obtained during an episode of chest pain *(left)* shows a large perfusion defect involving anterior and septal walls. The polar map image in the absence of chest pain *(right)* shows almost complete recovery of the perfusion defect. A 70% left anterior descending stenosis was found in angiography (see Color Figure 7–5). (Courtesy of Drs. J. Grégoire and P. Théroux.)

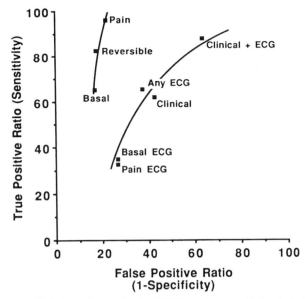

Figure 7–6. Tc-99m–sestamibi SPECT studies obtained during spontaneous chest pain (Pain) show higher sensitivity than any other combination of criteria. A reversible Tc-99m–sestamibi defect (Reversible) also is a very sensitive indicator. Similarly, specificity of SPECT studies is greater than with any of the clinical and ECG criteria. Note that SPECT studies obtained in the pain-free state (Basal) have a sensitivity in the range of 62% compared to basal ECG abnormalities in the range of 38%. (Reprinted with permission from the American College of Cardiology (Journal of the American College of Cardiology, 1991, Vol. 18, pp. 1684–1691).)

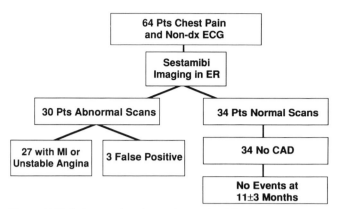

Figure 7–7. Outcome of patients who received Tc-99m–sestamibi in the emergency room during spontaneous chest pain to exclude ischemia in patients with a nondiagnostic ECG. Note that 27 of 30 patients with abnormal scans ultimately were shown to have an MI or unstable angina. None of the 34 patients with normal scans had evidence of CAD and none had cardiac events during follow-up. (Reprinted with permission of the American College of Cardiology (Journal of the American College of Cardiology, 1993, Vol. 22, pp. 1804–1808).)

99m–sestamibi scan, 27 were ultimately diagnosed as having an acute MI or unstable angina (Figure 7–7). In contrast, none of the 34 patients with a normal scan had evidence for CAD, and no events had occurred in that group

at 11 ± 3 months' follow-up. Hilton et al.[14b] gave Tl-99m sestamibi to 102 patients with chest pain and nondiagnostic ECGs in the emergency room. An abnormal scan was the only independent predictor of adverse cardiac events. Only 1 of 70 patients with a normal scan had an event, compared with a 71% event rate in patients with an abnormal scan. Figure 7–8 shows the ECG and corresponding Tc-99m sestamibi scan obtained during pain in a representative patient who had a left circumflex stenosis. The ECG shows nonspecific changes but the scan demonstrates a reversible posterolateral defect. Figure 7–9 shows that Tc-99m sestamibi

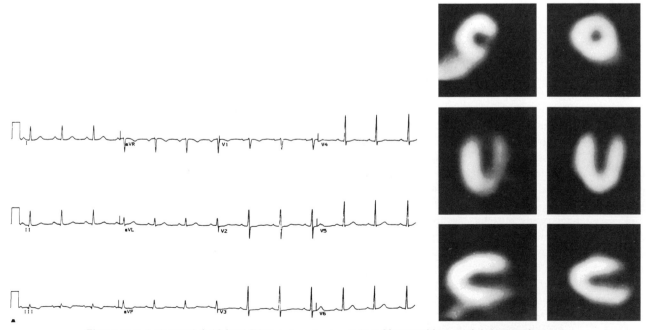

Figure 7–8. *Left panel:* A 12-lead ECG during chest pain in a 60-year-old man, showing no changes indicative of acute ischemia. *Right panel:* SPECT Tc-99m sestamibi images obtained in the emergency room *(left row)* and before discharge *(right row)*. The representative short-axis and horizontal long-axis tomograms show a reversible posterolateral defect.

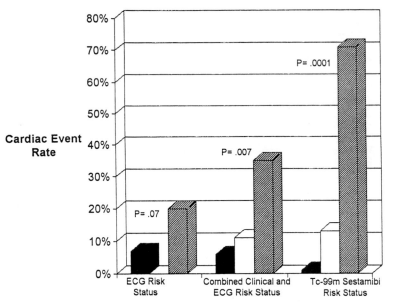

Figure 7–9. Risk status based on ECG results *(left bars)*, a combination of clinical and ECG variables *(middle bars)*, and results of Tc-99m sestamibi scans *(right bars)* in the 102 patients with chest pain who were injected with Tc-99m sestamibi in the emergency room during symptoms. *(Solid bars* = normal or low risk; *open bars* = equivocal or intermediate risk; *hatched bars* = abnormal or high risk.) (Reprinted with permission from the American College of Cardiology (Journal of the American College of Cardiology, 1994, Vol. 23, pp. 1016–1022).)

imaging identified both low- and high-risk groups and was superior to clinical and ECG variables alone for risk stratification.

EXERCISE OR PHARMACOLOGIC STRESS IMAGING IN PATIENTS WITH UNSTABLE ANGINA

As undertaken in patients with uncomplicated acute MI, exercise or pharmacologic stress perfusion imaging can be performed before hospital discharge of patients with unstable angina for purposes of risk stratification and identification of those at high risk for CAD who may benefit from coronary revascularization. A recently released practice guideline for diagnosis and management of unstable angina proposes noninvasive and invasive strategies for risk stratification in patients with unstable angina to supplement clinically based risk assessment.[14c] A substantial number of patients respond satisfactorily to medical management with antithrombotic therapy or antiischemic drug therapy. Such patients may not require routine coronary angiography to determine if revascularization is preferred to sustained medical therapy. Noninvasive testing can often be undertaken within 72 hours of presentation in low-risk nonhospitalized patients with unstable angina and at a minimum of 48 hours after angina has resolved in low- or intermediate-risk patients hospitalized with unstable angina.[14c] Figure 7–10 depicts the patient flow for cardiac catheterization and myocardial revascularization as recommended in the guideline.[14c] Findings on predischarge exercise or pharmacologic stress Tl-201 scintigraphy in patients with unstable angina that would suggest an indication for coronary angiography include (1) a large perfusion abnormality with delayed redistribution in the distribution of the coronary artery thought to be the culprit lesion in the unstable angina syn-

drome, (2) multiple defects in more than one coronary supply region, and (3) increased lung Tl-201 uptake with evidence of one or more redistribution defects. Exercise ST depression of at least 2.0 mm with a light workload with

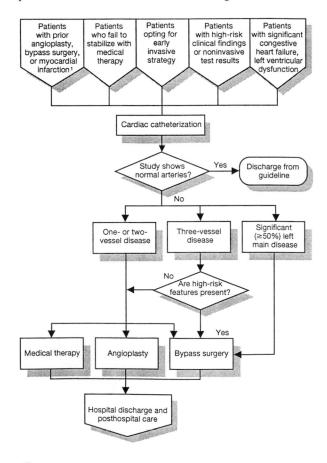

[1] Those patients who are candidates for revascularization.

Figure 7–10. Patient flow diagram for referral for cardiac catheterization in patients with unstable angina. (Clinical Practice Guideline Number 10, AHCPR Publication No. 94-0602, March 1994.)

Table 7–2. **Predictive Value of Exercise Testing for Patients Whose Unstable Angina Has Stabilized in Response to Medical Therapy**

Investigator	Pts (No.)	Sensitivity (%)	Specificity (%)	Positive Predictive Value (%)	Negative Predictive Value (%)
Nixon[15]	55	71	70	71	70
Butman[16]	125	76	85	88	71
Swahn[17]	275	92	70	40	98
Wilcox[18]	107	38	85	48	79
Brown[19]	52	86	32	32	86

(Adapted from Coplan NL, Wallach ID: Am Heart J 1992;124:252–256.)

only mild Tl-201 or Tc-99m–sestamibi perfusion defects is an indication for further invasive evaluation. The resting ECG may provide some useful prognostic information in patients with unstable angina.[14d] In that study, 54 patients with a normal resting ECG and a negative exercise test all survived at 1 year. Also, of the 86 patients with a normal resting ECG who had a positive exercise test, 97% were alive at 1 year.

Exercise Electrocardiographic Stress Testing

Standard exercise ECG stress testing in CAD patients whose condition has stabilized in response to medical therapy for unstable angina can provide important prognostic information. Table 7–2 summarizes the results of studies in the literature pertaining to the predictive value for adverse cardiac events of exercise testing in patients with unstable angina who respond to medical therapy.[15–19] Nixon et al.[15] reported a 71% positive predictive value and a 71% negative predictive value for the development of severe angina or recurrent unstable angina during follow-up in 55 patients with either new-onset or crescendo angina. Exercise was stopped because of the appearance of ischemic ECG changes, inducible chest pain, or reaching the target heart rate of 120 bpm. Butman[16] had 125 patients with unstable angina who had been free of pain for at least 3 days on medications perform submaximal exercise. After 1 year or more of follow-up, 87% of patients with inducible chest pain or at least 1.0 mm ST depression had an event as compared with 29% of patients whose exercise test was negative for ischemia. The positive predictive value of limiting chest pain, more than 1.0 mm of ST depression, or a rate-pressure product below 13,500 for events during follow-up in 400 patients with unstable angina or non-Q myocardial infarction studied by Swahn et al.[17] was only 40%. However, 98% of patients who had none of these findings had a favorable outcome. Wilcox et al.[18] reported that independent predictors of an adverse outcome by multivariate analysis in 107 patients with unstable angina included diabetes mellitus, evolutionary T-wave changes after admission, rest pain during hospitalization, ST depression during exercise, and low maximal rate-pressure product. The authors derived a predictive model using the regression equation and all independent predictors to stratify patients into high- and low-risk groups (41% and 5% risk of adverse outcome, respectively). Figure 7–11 shows a comparison of event-free survival using the logistic regression model in patients identified as being at low and high risk.

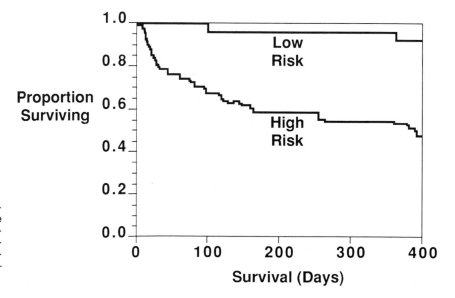

Figure 7–11. Survival rate in patients with low- or high-risk exercise test results after unstable angina utilizing a logistic regression model. (Reprinted with permission from the American College of Cardiology (Journal of the American College of Cardiology, 1991, Vol. 18, pp. 677–683).)

Table 7–3. **Multivariate Predictors of Cardiac Death or Nonfatal Myocardial Infarction in 52 Patients**

	Step 0: Before Variables Entered into Model		Step 1: After Tl-201 Redistribution Entered into Model	
	χ^2	*P Value*	χ^2	*P Value*
Tl-201 redistribution	5.98	0.014	(5.98)	(0.014)
History of MI	3.29	0.07	2.36	0.09
No. of Segments with Tl-201 redistribution	2.46	0.12	0.00	0.97
No. of fixed defects	1.32	0.25	1.83	0.22
Gender	0.73	0.39	0.43	0.51
Presence of fixed defect	0.73	0.39	1.49	0.22
Presenting syndrome	3.27	0.51	5.71	0.22
Exercise ECG	0.26	0.61	0.24	0.62
Presenting ECG	0.17	0.67	0.57	0.45
Age	0.06	0.80	0.44	0.51

(Reprinted with permission from the American College of Cardiology (Journal of the American College of Cardiology, 1991, Vol. 17, pp. 1053–1057).)

Thallium-201 Stress Scintigraphy

Several studies have shown that Tl-201 variables derived from stress perfusion imaging have superior predictive value for separating high- and low-risk subsets than variables derived solely from exercise ECG.[19–25]

Brown et al.[19] performed exercise Tl-201 scintigraphy within 1 week of discharge in 52 consecutive patients whose unstable angina responded to medical therapy. Patients were followed for up to 39 months. Tl-201 redistribution was the only significant predictor of subsequent cardiac death or nonfatal infarction (Table 7–3). The number of myocardial segments with Tl-201 redistribution and a history of infarction were the only significant predictors of all cardiac events. Of patients with Tl-201 redistribution 26% died or experienced a nonfatal infarction compared with a 3% rate of these events in those without redistribution. The exercise ECG had only 55% positive predictive value and 59% negative predictive value for future cardiac events, as compared with 70% and 76%, respectively, for Tl-201 redistribution. This study concluded that stress Tl-201 scintigraphy does have an important prognostic role in patients whose unstable angina responds to medical therapy. Both high- and low-risk subgroups for future cardiac events can be well separated by stress imaging variables.

Hillert et al.[20] also performed submaximal Tl-201 scintigraphy after initial successful treatment of unstable angina. They found that 15 of 19 patients who showed initial defects with delayed redistribution developed either infarction or severe angina by 12 weeks after discharge. This compared with only 2 of 18 patients without redistribution who experienced such an event. Marmur et al.[21] prospectively compared 24-hour ambulatory ST-segment monitoring soon after admission, predischarge quantitative exercise Tl-201 tomography, and cardiac catheterization 5 ±2 days after admission for their prognostic value in predicting cardiac events in unstable angina. When event-free patients were compared with those who had events, no difference was

found in the duration of ST-segment shifts of 1 mm or more on Holter monitoring. Similarly, there was no difference between event and nonevent groups with respect to exercise-induced ST depression and the resting EF. Figure 7–12 compares the 40 patients who had a favorable outcome and the 14 whose outcome was unfavorable in this study with respect to total reversible defect size expressed as a percentage of total myocardium. Patients with a favorable outcome were distinguished from those with an unfavorable outcome by a higher rate-pressure product during exercise and smaller Tl-201 redistribution defects as expressed as a percentage of the total myocardium (6% vs. 17%). As expected, patients who had a favorable outcome had a smaller number of significant coronary stenoses. In patients without MI, Tl-201 perfusion abnormality on exercise scintigraphy was the only predictor of a subsequent unfavorable outcome.

Freeman et al.[22] performed exercise Tl-201 imaging at 4.6 ± 1.6 days after admission in 67 patients with unstable angina who stabilized after medical therapy. By multiple regression analysis, Tl-201 defect size was the best predictor of extent of CAD, but exercise heart rate and chest pain during exercise were also predictive of extent of CAD. Exercise Tl-201 defect size was also the best noninvasive predictor of in-hospital cardiac events. There were no significant complications of early exercise stress testing in this patient population. In the study of Amanullah et al.,[24] the presence of Tl-201 redistribution was the only significant noninvasive predictor of a cardiac event ($P < 0.005$) in patients who underwent predischarge exercise testing and exercise Tl-201 scintigraphy. Table 7–4 depicts step 0 in the stepwise logistic regression model and lists the significant predictors of cardiac events. Among unstable angina patients who underwent both exercise echocardiography and exercise Tl-201 scintigraphy after responding to medical therapy, the number of segments with Tl-201 redistribution was the only significant predictor ($P < 0.0005$) of future cardiac events. This finding is comparable to what is

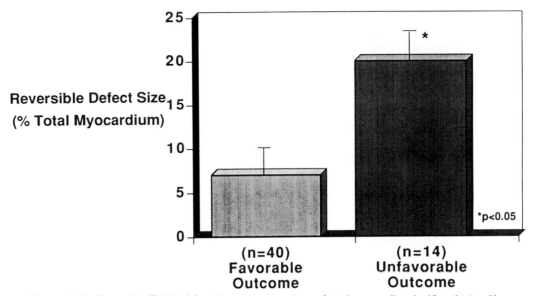

Figure 7–12. Reversible Tl-201 defect size as a percentage of total myocardium in 40 patients with a favorable outcome and 14 patients with an unfavorable outcome after unstable angina. (Marmur JD, et al.: Ann Intern Med 1991;113:575–579.)

observed in postinfarction patients undergoing predischarge risk stratification (see Chap. 6).

Pharmacologic Stress Imaging

Dipyridamole or adenosine Tl-201 imaging should not be performed during the acute phase of unstable angina since exacerbation of ischemia or even acute infarction can occur. There should be a minimum of 2 days between the last episode of rest pain and the performance of pharmacologic stress imaging in patients with unstable angina pectoris. Zhu et al.[23] evaluated the safety, accuracy, and potential clinical utility of dipyridamole Tl-201 imaging in 78 patients with suspected and 92 with known unstable angina. Interestingly, rates of noncardiac side effects (26%), chest pain (44%), and ST-segment alterations (12%) were similar in the two groups. Although no arrhythmias occurred, two patients developed prolonged chest pain associated with extensive redistribution defects and associated creatine kinase-MB release. Sensitivity and specificity for CAD detection were 91% and 79%, respectively. Per-vessel sensitivity

was 74% and per-vessel specificity, 78%, without differences between the two groups. Figure 7–13 shows the sensitivity and specificity for detecting left anterior descending, right coronary, and left circumflex (LCx) disease in this

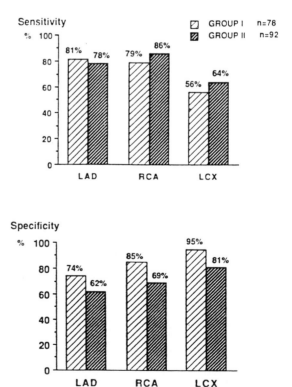

Figure 7–13. Individual vessel sensitivity and specificity for dipyridamole Tl-201 scintigraphy in patients with unstable angina. Note the reduced sensitivity for detection of left circumflex stenoses. Group I included patients with atypical or ambiguous chest pain. Group II comprised patients with a clear diagnosis of unstable angina. (Zhu YY, et al.: Am Heart J 1991;121:33–52.)

Table 7–4. **Stepwise Logistic Regression to Predict Events After Unstable Angina**

Variable	χ^2	P Value
Tl-201 redistribution	16.92	0.00004
No. Tl-201 redistribution segments	16.27	0.00006
Male sex	9.24	0.002
Abnormal exercise ECG	5.11	0.02
Maximum workload	0.85	0.36
Maximum heart rate	0.57	0.45

(From Amanullah AM: Int J Cardiol 1993;39:71.)

study. As expected, detection of LCx disease was lower than detection of stenosis in the other two major coronary vessels. The subsequent cardiac event rate was higher for patients with Tl-201 defects.

Thus, dipyridamole imaging is clinically useful for detecting significant CAD in patients with suspected or known unstable angina, though there are more side effects than in stable CAD patients who undergo this procedure. Adenosine Tl-201 imaging should yield similar results. A more detailed discussion of the use of pharmacologic stress imaging for risk stratification can be found in Chapter 8.

SUMMARY

Figure 7–14 is a focused decision-making algorithm that can be employed in patients with unstable angina who are stabilized on medical therapy. Most patients with unstable angina can be stabilized with antiplatelet and anticoagulant therapy as well as with nitrates and other antiischemic drugs (e.g., calcium antagonists, beta-blockers). Some patients are referred for urgent coronary angiography because of ongoing episodes of angina despite adequate medical therapy or because of extensive ECG changes in multiple

leads suggestive of a large area of myocardium in jeopardy. Patients with no recurrent ischemia who are hemodynamically stable and have no history of MI are candidates for exercise or pharmacologic stress Tl-201 or Tc-99m–sestamibi imaging for further risk stratification. Those who demonstrate significant ischemia or other high-risk findings are candidates for coronary angiography with an intent to revascularize myocardium at risk. As demonstrated for patients with stable angina and for post-MI patients, the number of reversible perfusion defects appears to be an important variable for predicting an adverse outcome. Also, increased lung Tl-201 uptake identifies high-risk patients whose risk of future ischemic events is increased. Certainly, angioplasty could be suitable for patients with one- or even two-vessel CAD, but bypass surgery is the approach of choice for left main or extensive multivessel disease. Presence of residual thrombus is associated with a higher risk of angioplasty.

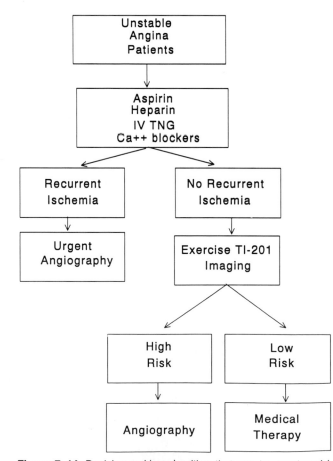

Figure 7–14. Decision-making algorithm that can be employed in patients with unstable angina who are stabilized in the hospital receiving medical therapy.

REFERENCES

1. Gorlin R, Fuster V, Ambrose JA: Anatomic-physiologic links between acute coronary syndromes. Circulation 1986;74:6–9.
2. Gewirtz H, Beller GA, Strauss HW, Dinsmore RE, Zir LM, McKusick KA, Pohost GM: Transient defects of resting thallium scans in patients with coronary artery disease. Circulation 1979;59:707–713.
3. Berger BC, Watson DD, Burwell LR, Crosby IK, Wellons HA, Teates CD, Beller GA: Redistribution of thallium at rest in patients with stable and unstable angina and the effect of coronary artery bypass surgery. Circulation 1979;60:1114–1125.
4. Wackers FJ, Lie KI, Liem KL, Sokole EB, Samson G, van der Schoot JB, Durrer D: Thallium-201 scintigraphy in unstable angina pectoris. Circulation 1978;57:738–742.
4a. Smitherman TC, Osborn RC Jr, Narahara KA: Serial myocardial scintigraphy after a single dose of thallium-201 in men after acute myocardial infarction. Am J Cardiol 1978;42:177–182.
5. Freeman MR, Williams AE, Chisholm RJ, Patt NL, Greyson ND, Armstrong PW: Role of resting thallium-201 perfusion in predicting coronary anatomy, left ventricular wall motion, and hospital outcome in unstable angina pectoris. Am Heart J 1989;117:306–314.
6. Hakki AH, Iskandrian AS, Kane SA, Amenta A: Thallium-201 myocardial scintigraphy and left ventricular function at rest in patients with rest angina pectoris. Am Heart J 1984;108:326–332.
7. Maseri A, Parodi O, Severi S, Pesola A: Transient transmural reduction of myocardial blood flow demonstrated by thallium-201 scintigraphy, as a cause of variant angina. Circulation 1976;54:280–288.
8. DiCarlo L, Botvinick E, Canhasi S, Schwartz A, Chatterjee K: Value of noninvasive assessment of patients with atypical chest pain and suspected coronary spasm using ergonovine infusion and thallium-201 scintigraphy. Am J Cardiol 1984;54:744–748.
9. Parodi O, Marzullo P, Neglia D, Galli M, Distante A, Rovai D, L'Abbate A: Transient predominant right ventricular ischemia caused by coronary vasospasm. Circulation 1984;70:170–177.
10. Parodi O, Uthurralt N, Severi S, Bencivelli W, Michelassi C, L'Abbete A, Maseri A: Transient reduction of regional myocardial perfusion during angina at rest with ST-segment depression or normalization of negative T waves. Circulation 1981;63:1238–1247.
11. Shimokawa H, Matsuguchi T, Koiwaya Y, Fukuyama T, Orita Y, Nakamura M: Variable exercise capacity in variant angina and greater exertional thallium-201 myocardial defect during vasospastic ischemic ST segment elevation than with ST depression. Am Heart J 1982;103:142–145.
12. Boden WE, Bough EW, Korr KS, Benham I, Gheorghiade M, Caputi A, Shulman RS: Exercise-induced coronary spasm with S-T segment depression and normal coronary arteriography. Am J Cardiol 1981;48:193–197.
13. Kugiyama K, Yasue H, Horio Y, Morikami Y, Fujii H, Koga Y,

Kojima A, Takahashi M: Effects of propranolol and nifedipine on exercise-induced attack in patients with variant angina: Assessment by exercise thallium-201 myocardial scintigraphy with quantitative rotational tomography. Circulation 1986;74:374–380.

13a. Gregoire J, Theroux P: Detection and assessment of unstable angina using myocardial perfusion imaging: Comparison between technetium 99m sestamibi SPECT and 12-lead electrocardiogram. Am J Cardiol 1990;66:42E–46E.

14. Bilodeau L, Theroux P, Gregoire J, Gagnon D, Arsenault A: Technetium-99m sestamibi tomography in patients with spontaneous chest pain: Correlations with clinical, electrocardiographic and angiographic findings. J Am Coll Cardiol 1991;18:1684–1691.

14a. Varetto T, Cantalupi D, Altieri A, Orlandi C: Emergency room technetium-99m sestamibi imaging to rule out acute myocardial ischemic events in patients with nondiagnostic electrocardiogram. J Am Coll Cardiol 1993;22:1804–1808.

14b. Hilton TC, Thompson RC, Williams HJ, Saylors R, Fulmer H, Stowers SA: Technetium-99m sestamibi myocardial perfusion imaging in the emergency room for evaluation of chest pain. J Am Coll Cardiol 1994;23:1016–1022.

14c. Clinical Practice Guideline Number 10: Unstable angina: Diagnosis and Management. AHCPR Publication No. 94-0602, U.S. Department of Health and Human Services, March 1994.

14d. Severi S, Orsini E, Marracini P, Michelassi C, L'Abbate A: The basal electrocardiogram and the exercise test in assessing prognosis in patients with unstable angina. Eur Heart J 1998;9:441–446.

15. Nixon JV, Hillert MC, Shapiro W, Smitherman TC: Submaximal exercise testing after unstable angina. Am Heart J 1980;99:772–778.

16. Butman SM, Olson HG, Gardin JM, Piters KM, Hullett M, Butman LK: Submaximal exercise testing after stabilization of unstable angina pectoris. J Am Coll Cardiol 1984;4:667–673.

17. Swahn E, Areskog M, Berglund U, Walfridsson H, Wallentin L: Predictive importance of clinical findings and a predischarge exercise test in patients with suspected unstable coronary artery disease. Am J Cardiol 1987;59:208–214.

18. Wilcox I, Freeman SB, Allman KC, Collins FL, Leitch JW, Kelly DT, Harris PJ: Prognostic significance of a predischarge exercise test in risk stratification after unstable angina pectoris. J Am Coll Cardiol 1991;18:677–683.

19. Brown KA: Prognostic value of thallium-201 myocardial perfusion imaging in patients with unstable angina who respond to medical treatment. J Am Coll Cardiol 1991;17:1053–1057.

20. Hillert MC Jr, Narahara KA, Smitherman TC, Burden LL, Wyatt JC: Thallium 201 perfusion imaging after the treatment of unstable angina pectoris—relationship to clinical outcome. Western J Med 1986; 145:335–340.

21. Marmur JD, Freeman MR, Langer A, Armstrong PW: Prognosis in medically stabilized unstable angina: Early Holter ST-segment monitoring compared with predischarge exercise thallium tomography. Ann Intern Med 1990;113:575–579.

22. Freeman MR, Chisholm RJ, Armstrong PW: Usefulness of exercise electrocardiography and thallium scintigraphy in unstable angina pectoris in predicting the extent and severity of coronary artery disease. Am J Cardiol 1988;62:1164–1170.

23. Zhu YY, Chung WS, Botvinick EH, Dae MW, Lim AD, Ports TA, Danforth JW, Wolfe CL, Goldschlager N, Chatterjee K: Dipyridamole perfusion scintigraphy: The experience with its application in one hundred seventy patients with known or suspected unstable angina. Am Heart J 1991;121:33–43.

24. Amanullah AM, Lindvoll K, Bevegård S: Prognostic significance of exercise thallium-201 myocardial perfusion imaging compared to stress echocardiography and clinical variables in patients with unstable angina who respond to medical treatment. Int J Cardiol 1993;39:71–78.

25. Coplan NL, Wallach ID: The role of exercise testing for evaluating patients with unstable angina. Am Heart J 1992;124:252–256.

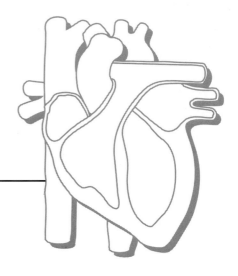

Chapter 8

Pharmacologic Stress Imaging

Pharmacologic stress imaging is increasingly being employed as an alternative to exercise perfusion or function imaging for detection of physiologically significant coronary artery disease (CAD) and for prognostication. Intravenous infusion of dipyridamole, adenosine, or dobutamine is an acceptable alternative to exercise stress for determining presence and extent of CAD, employing either planar or single-photon emission computed tomography (SPECT) perfusion imaging utilizing thallium-201 (Tl-201) or one of the new technetium-99m (Tc-99m)–radiolabeled imaging agents. Similarly, pharmacologic stress echocardiography is another noninvasive technique aimed at detecting ischemia-induced wall motion abnormalities in patients with CAD. Pharmacologic stress is of considerable clinical value in patients judged unable to adequately exercise for a variety of noncardiac conditions (Table 8–1). Some reasons for inability to perform an exercise test include disabling arthritis, amputation, limiting orthopedic abnormalities, stroke-related neurologic deficit, claudication, and lack of motivation or fear of the treadmill.

VASODILATOR STRESS IMAGING

Rationale for Use of Dipyridamole or Adenosine for Stress Imaging

Coronary Flow Reserve

The rationale for vasodilator stress imaging is based on the concept of coronary flow reserve. Under normal resting conditions, the epicardial coronary vessels are widely patent, but there is a significant degree of vascular tone at the arteriolar level. If this tone is reversed by dilating the pe-

ripheral coronary bed with a vasodilator such as papaverine, dipyridamole, or adenosine, coronary flow can increase as much as fivefold. Coronary flow reserve is defined as the ratio of flow during maximal vasodilatation to flow under control conditions at rest. Gould has proposed that coronary flow reserve is an accurate functional measure of stenosis severity and is experimentally related to the geometric dimensions of the stenosis.[1–5] Assessment of percentage of stenosis alone is inadequate for determination of true physiologic severity of a coronary stenotic lesion. Figure 8–1 represents the relation between coronary flow and pressure during maximal vasodilatation over a wide range of pressures.[5a] Changes in aortic pressure and heart rate influence cardiac workload, which, in turn, will affect baseline coronary flow, as well as alter maximal coronary flow during maximal vasodilatation. Therefore, absolute coronary flow reserve is independent of stenosis geometry, owing to the differential effects of heart rate and arterial blood pressure on both basal resting flow and maximal coronary flow. From one patient to another, absolute coronary flow reserve may not reliably reflect the severity of stenosis, since it can

Table 8–1. Limitations to Exercise Stress Testing

Peripheral arteriosclerotic vascular disease
Disabling arthritis
History of stroke
Orthopedic problems (e.g., low back pain)
Chronic pulmonary disease
Extremity amputation
Poor motivation to exercise
Poor exercise capacity due to noncardiac endpoints (e.g., fatigue)
Beta-blocking drugs limiting heart rate response
Left bundle branch block (false-positive exercise perfusion scans)
Early post–MI (<5 days)

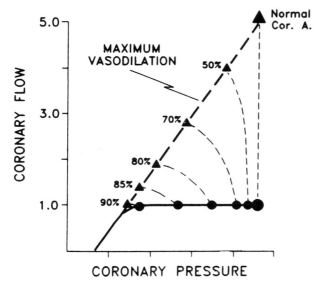

Figure 8–1. Coronary flows at rest and after vasodilation for individual stenotic lesions. Flows at rest and after vasodilation for individual stenotic lesions are connected by thin dashed lines, which are curvilinear. The flow increase that can be attained during maximal coronary vasodilation varies inversely with the degree of stenosis. (Key: Cor. A., coronary artery.) (Reprinted with permission from the American College of Cardiology (Journal of the American College of Cardiology, 1990, Vol. 16, pp. 763–769).)

be altered by physiologic variables and differences in resting flow (e.g., as with left ventricular hypertrophy).[6] Figure 8–2 depicts how hypertrophy shifts the pressure-flow relation during maximal vasodilatation.[5a] Vasodilator reserve is also reduced in reperfused patients with an acute myocardial infarction.[5b] Abnormal flow reserve can remain abnormal for up to 6 months following infarction in resistance vessels perfused by normal coronary arteries remote from the infarct zone as well as in resistance vessels of the infarct-related artery.

Relative maximal coronary flow or relative flow reserve is defined as maximal flow in a stenotic artery divided or normalized by the normal maximal flow in the absence of stenosis and is more independent of aortic pressure, heart rate, and varying baseline flow influenced by the change in cardiac work. Relative coronary flow reserve is what is evaluated on a stress myocardial perfusion scan. During maximal vasodilatation, normal and stenotic myocardial beds are equally affected by hemodynamic variables, and conditions like hypertrophy, which affect resting and maximal flow. Figure 8–3 illustrates the difference between absolute and relative flow reserve from experimental data reported by Gould et al. in dogs with calibrated stenoses of the left circumflex coronary artery.[5]

Autoregulation in the coronary microcirculation maintains normal resting coronary blood flow until the stenosis becomes severely narrowed, perhaps by more than 90%.[7] When blood flow is increased with a vasodilator, an impair-

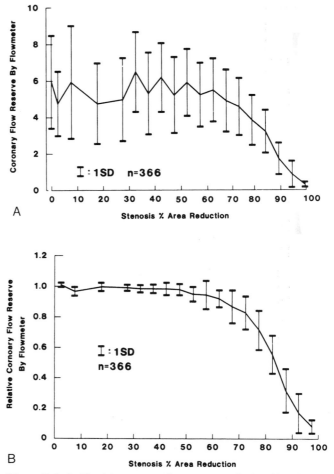

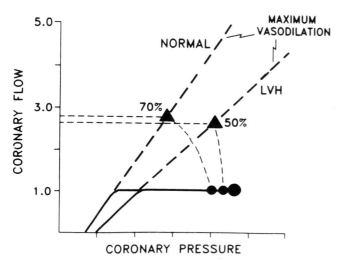

Figure 8–2. Hypertrophy-induced shift in the pressure-flow relation during maximal vasodilation. As noted, flow reserve is identical for 70% stenosis in a normal left ventricle and 50% stenosis in a ventricle with left ventricular hypertrophy (LVH). (Reprinted from the American College of Cardiology (Journal of the American College of Cardiology, 1990, Vol. 16, pp. 763–769).)

Figure 8–3. A. Absolute coronary flow reserve calculated by dividing the maximal flow by the resting flow for 366 experiments over the full range of changes in aortic pressure and stenosis severity (% area reduction). **B.** Relative maximal coronary flow or relative flow reserve calculated as the maximal flow in the stenotic artery divided by normal maximal flow in the absence of stenosis for the 366 experiments over the range of changes in aortic pressure with progressive coronary stenosis. (Reprinted with permission from the American College of Cardiology (Journal of the American College of Cardiology, 1990, Vol. 15, pp. 459–474).)

ment in flow reserve is seen before a stenosis is narrowed to a severe degree, owing to failure to augment flow comparably to that flow in the normal nonstenotic vascular bed. This results in "relative" inhomogeneity of regional myocardial perfusion with a gradient in flow between normal and stenotic myocardial beds.

Stenosis Severity and Flow Reserve

Impaired coronary flow reserve is a more accurate approach to determining severity of stenosis than merely measuring the percentage of anatomic stenosis in the large epicardial segment of a diseased coronary vessel. The amount of flow that can be achieved during maximal vasodilatation varies inversely with the degree of stenosis. This inverse relationship has been confirmed in humans utilizing Doppler velocity probe data. Flow reserve varies not only with changes in arterial pressure but also with changes in other hemodynamic variables, such as heart rate and ventricular preload. Ventricular hypertrophy affects coronary flow reserve because the growth of the microcirculatory vessels does not keep up with growth of the ventricular myocytes. Nevertheless, *relative* flow reserve should not be as influenced by these variables when comparing flow reserve in normally perfused myocardium with the reserve in myocardium perfused by stenotic coronary arteries.

The principle of vasodilator stress myocardial perfusion imaging was first introduced by Strauss and Pitt, who used dimethyladenosine in dogs with experimental coronary artery stenosis.[8] They showed that dimethyladenosine increased coronary blood flow and Tl-201 uptake to normal areas of myocardium, whereas regions of myocardium perfused by a coronary vessel with a hemodynamically significant coronary stenosis had reduced flow reserve and, thus, less Tl-201 uptake. Thus, during coronary hyperemia, normal myocardium accumulates a greater amount of a flow-dependent imaging agent than myocardium supplied by a vessel containing a hemodynamically significant stenosis.

Coronary Steal

In a normally perfused nonstenotic coronary bed, infusion of a vasodilator such as dipyridamole or adenosine results in a greater increase in subepicardial than in endocardial flow. When these agents are infused intravenously in the presence of a critical stenotic coronary artery, blood flow is redistributed away from the endocardium to epicardial layers; this redistribution has been referred to as intramural or transmural coronary steal.[9–11] This steal results in an absolute decrease in endocardial flow coupled with an attenuated increase in epicardial flow consequent to vasodilation. Figure 8–4 depicts the alterations in regional transmural blood flow consequent to coronary steal produced by intravenous dipyridamole in an experimental canine stenosis model.[9] The endocardial underperfusion has clinical rel-

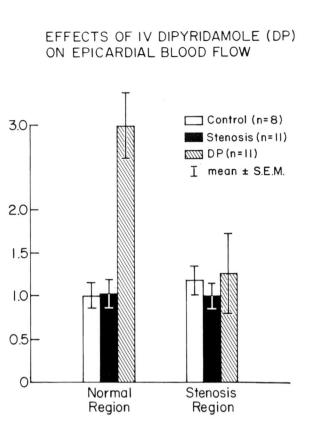

EFFECTS OF IV DIPYRIDAMOLE (DP) ON EPICARDIAL BLOOD FLOW

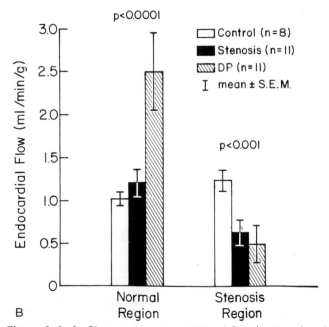

EFFECTS OF IV DIPYRIDAMOLE (DP) ON ENDOCARDIAL BLOOD FLOW

Figure 8–4. A. Changes in epicardial blood flow in normal and stenotic regions after intravenous dipyridamole (DP) in dogs with a partial left anterior descending coronary stenosis. **B.** Changes in endocardial blood flow in normal and stenotic regions after intravenous DP in the same group of dogs showing a decrease in flow after DP in the stenotic region consistent with transmural coronary steal. As in **A**, epicardial flow increased slightly in the same zone. (Beller GA, et al.: Circulation 1983;68:1328–1338.)

evance as it may be the principal mechanism producing ST-segment depression or angina consequent to vasodilator stress in patients undergoing pharmacologic imaging. Coronary narrowings as mild as 45% may diminish vasodilatory reserve in a coronary vascular bed.

Mechanism of Action of Dipyridamole and Adenosine

Dipyridamole most likely induces coronary vasodilatation by elevating interstitial adenosine concentration through blockade of cellular uptake of adenosine.[12, 13] Dipyridamole inhibits adenosine uptake in vascular endothelium and in red blood cell membranes. Dipyridamole is a complex pyrimidine derivative with a molecular weight of 504. It is lipophilic, and the presence of hydroxyl groups on the diethanolamino portion of the molecule promotes metabolism by hepatic biotransformation with subsequent primary biliary and fecal excretion. Only small amounts of dipyridamole are excreted in the urine, and caution should be utilized when administering this drug to patients with hepatic failure.

In the heart, adenosine causes coronary vascular smooth muscle relaxation, inhibits norepinephrine released from sympathetic nerve endings, reduces atrioventricular (AV) node conduction velocity, and has negative inotropic and chronotropic effects.[12] Endogenous adenosine is released from myocardial cells during hypoxia and ischemia. The source of adenosine is degradation of adenine nucleotides in the hypoperfused or hypoxic cardiac myocyte. Adenosine moves between plasma and interstitial fluid by simple diffusion, and vascular endothelial cells act as a source of sink for plasma adenosine. At physiologic levels, 75% to 90% of exogenously administered adenosine does not reach vascular smooth muscle cells and myocardium because of endothelial cell uptake. After intravenous administration, adenosine has rapid onset and offset of action with respect to coronary vasodilatation. Intravenous adenosine at a dose of 140 mg/kg/minute for a minimum of 2 minutes causes coronary vasodilatation similar to that caused by intracoronary papaverine. The metabolism of adenosine occurs through active cellular uptake and enzymatic degradation (adenosine deaminase), and the half-life of exogenously infused adenosine is approximately 10 seconds.[14]

Hemodynamic Effects of Dipyridamole and Adenosine

In humans, intravenous dipyridamole infusion results in a mild decrease in systemic blood pressure, a slight reflex increase in heart rate, a slight increase in cardiac output, but no change in myocardial oxygen consumption.[15] Coronary vascular resistance significantly decreases and coronary sinus flow increases, with a small increase in pulmonary artery pressure. In one published study, a group of 1008 patients had vital sign data measured in a nonstanding position at baseline and at least one subsequent time after the infusion of dipyridamole.[16] In this group, there was an average 4.7% decrease in systolic pressure, a 7.8% decrease in diastolic pressure, and a 22.1% increase in pulse rate. In patients who performed mild exercise (e.g., standing or walking, handgrip, or bicycle exercise) after infusion of dipyridamole, the mean maximum percentage changes in vital signs from baseline consisted of a 6.6% increase in systolic blood pressure, a 3.0% increase in diastolic blood pressure, and a 27.0% increase in pulse rate. Brown et al.[17] reported a mean increase of 2.8 and 3.8 times the control value in coronary sinus flow by thermodilution during dipyridamole and dipyridamole plus handgrip, respectively, in subjects with angiographically normal coronary arteries. The infusion of 20 mg of dipyridamole intravenously over 10 seconds in patients undergoing cardiac catheterization was associated with a fall in coronary vascular resistance from a control value of 1.00 ± 0.07 mm Hg/ml/minute to 0.63 ± 0.05 mm Hg/ml/minute 1 minute after dipyridamole administration.[18] Total resistance remained decreased for 15 minutes. Coronary sinus flow rose by 75% and also remained elevated for 15 minutes. Figure 8–5 shows the serial measurements of total and regional coronary venous flow after intravenous dipyridamole in the patients included in this study.[18] Note that flow increased more in normal regions than in abnormal ones.

Adenosine infusion of 140 µg/kg/minute over 6 minutes resulted in a heart rate increase from 74.5 to 91.8 bpm in a group of 607 patients reported by Abreu et al.[19] In that study, the baseline systolic blood pressure fell from 138 to 121 mm Hg and the diastolic blood pressure fell from 78 to 67 mm Hg. Kern et al.[20] showed that constant infusion of adenosine resulted in a $198 \pm 59\%$ increase in coronary flow velocity. In that study, the coronary vasodilator reserve ratio (calculated as the ratio of hyperemic to basal mean flow velocity) was 2.94 for adenosine, which was identical to that measured with intracoronary papaverine. Adenosine infusion causes prolongation of the PR interval of the electrocardiogram (ECG). Coyne et al.[21] reported that 72.3% of subjects with CAD versus 43.4% of normal subjects experienced prolongation of the PR interval above baseline measurements. O'Keefe et al.[22] reported that 28 of 340 consecutive patients who received intravenous adenosine for Tl-201 imaging developed either second-degree AV block ($N = 24$) or third-degree AV block ($N = 4$). A more detailed discussion of side effects of dipyridamole is presented later in this chapter.

Comparison of Dipyridamole and Adenosine

Although both dipyridamole and adenosine exhibit similar physiologic effects on the coronary and systemic circu-

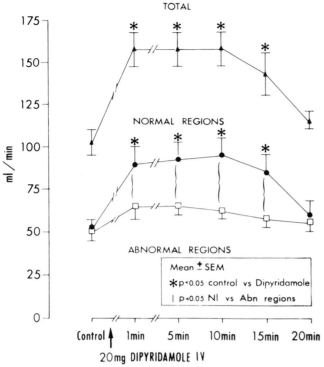

Figure 8–5. Total and regional coronary venous flow during a control period and serially 1, 5, 10, 15, and 20 minutes after dipyridamole in normal (Nl) and abnormal (Abn) regions. One minute after dipyridamole, flow increased in normal regions *(solid circles)* and remained elevated for 15 minutes, whereas flow to abnormal regions *(open squares)* was not significantly increased at any point after administration of the vasodilator. (Feldman RL, et al.: Circulation 1981;64:333–344.)

lation, the vasodilator effect of dipyridamole is more prolonged (up to 20 to 40 min) than that of adenosine.[23] Rossen et al.[24] directly compared the vasodilator potency of adenosine and dipyridamole. They found that the increase in heart rate at peak coronary vasodilator effect was comparable with adenosine (11 ± 9 bpm) and dipyridamole (11 ± 7 bpm). The decrease in mean arterial pressure, however, was larger with adenosine (− 16 ± 5 mm Hg) than with dipyridamole (− 10 ± 3 mm Hg). There was no difference between adenosine and dipyridamole with respect to the ratio of peak to rest coronary blood flow velocity (3.4 ± 1.2 vs. 3.1 ± 1.2). Figure 8–6 shows the individual values for myocardial flow during adenosine infusion and after dipyridamole infusion for patients in this study. Neither adenosine nor dipyridamole produced changes in the diameter of the proximal nonstenotic coronary artery segments. The authors measured what they referred to as the ''coronary vasodilator potency,'' which was assessed by a coronary vascular resistance index which incorporates the change in arterial pressure. Using this index, they concluded that the coronary vasodilator effect of adenosine was greater than that of dipyridamole and equal to that of intracoronary papaverine. Nevertheless, this greater vasodilatory response induced by adenosine compared to dipyridamole may not translate to enhanced detection of coronary steno-

ses. This is because of the decreased myocardial extraction of Tl-201 as flow rises above the physiologic range. More hyperemia at greater than 2.5 times normal flow does not translate into greater Tl-201 uptake in nonischemic myocardium and, therefore, no enhancement of defect contrast.

Chan et al.[25] quantitated the magnitude of hyperemia and the hyperemia–baseline blood flow ratios during intravenous adenosine and dipyridamole infusion using positron-emission tomography (PET) and nitrogen-13 (N-13)–ammonia imaging. In 20 normal volunteers, myocardial blood flow averaged 1.1 ± 0.2 ml/minute/g and increased significantly to 4.4 ± 0.9 ml/minute/g during adenosine and 4.3 ± 1.3 ml/minute/g after dipyridamole infusion. Hyperemia–baseline flow ratios averaged 4.3 ± 1.6 for adenosine and 4.0 ± 1.3 for dipyridamole (P = NS). These authors concluded that both agents were equally effective in producing myocardial hyperemia. Thus, based on these physiologic studies, no difference in stenosis detection should be observed between dipyridamole and adenosine imaging protocols with currently employed tracers like Tl-201.

PHARMACOLOGIC STRESS IMAGING WITH THALLIUM-201

Dipyridamole-Induced Vasodilatation and Thallium-201 Kinetics

The initial myocardial distribution of intravenously administered Tl-201 is proportional to blood flow when the tracer is administered following dipyridamole or adenosine infusion.[9] Figure 8–7 shows a good relationship between Tl-201 activity and myocardial blood flow in five individual intact conscious dogs with a total occlusion of the left circumflex coronary artery (LCx) receiving intravenous di-

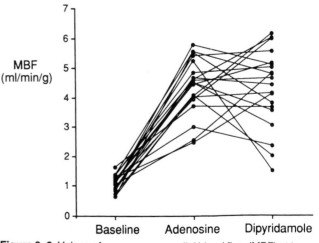

Figure 8–6. Values of average myocardial blood flow (MBF) at baseline, during adenosine infusion, and after dipyridamole administration. Although there is a wide variation in individual responses, mean flows were comparable for dipyridamole and adenosine. (Reprinted with permission from the American College of Cardiology (Journal of the American College of Cardiology, 1992, Vol. 20, pp. 979–985).)

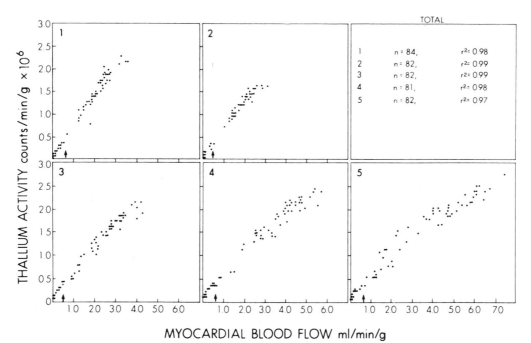

Figure 8–7. Relationship between Tl-201 activity and myocardial blood flow in five dogs during dipyridamole infusion and total occlusion of the left circumflex coronary artery. The arrows designate the value for resting myocardial blood flow. (Reproduced from *The Journal of Clinical Investigation*, 1984, Vol. 78, pp. 1359–1366 by copyright permission of The Society for Clinical Investigation.)

pyridamole.[26] There appears to be a higher myocardial than total body extraction fraction for Tl-201. That is, under normal basal conditions, myocardial Tl-201 activity, expressed as a percentage of injected dose, overestimates LV blood flow when expressed as a percentage of cardiac output.[27] We and others have demonstrated that, under conditions of an experimental coronary stenosis in canine models of ischemia or in humans, dipyridamole- or adenosine-induced vasodilatation results not only in diminished Tl-201 uptake but also in delayed redistribution similar to that observed with exercise scintigraphy.[9, 10, 28] Redistribution defects are seen with comparable frequency on serial myocardial scintigrams acquired with vasodilator stress or exercise stress in patients with CAD who underwent both tests at different times.

Mechanism of Redistribution with Dipyridamole Infusion

The mechanism and significance of Tl-201 redistribution after dipyridamole imaging have been elucidated. In a study using serial myocardial needle biopsy specimens from anesthetized dogs with a critical left anterior descending coronary artery (LAD) stenosis, when Tl-201 was injected intravenously after infusion of dipyridamole, net clearance of Tl-201 from the region of the stenosis was slower than from normal myocardium (Fig. 8–8).[9] The difference in net clearance rates resulted in normalization of the initial defect (redistribution). In a subsequent study, the intrinsic Tl-201 washout rate after intracoronary Tl-201 injection under normal conditions and after dipyridamole-induced hyperemia

was measured.[10] (See Chap. 2 for description of Tl-201 kinetic parameters.) In normal dogs, dipyridamole-induced coronary vasodilatation resulted in a more rapid intrinsic myocardial washout rate of Tl-201 coincident with increases in both epicardial and endocardial blood flow. In a group of dogs with an experimental LAD stenosis, the half-time ($T_{1/2}$) for the intrinsic Tl-201 washout rate was 70 ± 5 minutes at control conditions and slowed significantly to 108 ± 6 minutes after production of the stenosis. After intravenous dipyridamole infusion, the intrinsic Tl-201 washout rate slowed further to 169 ± 21 minutes. Figure 8–9 shows the changes in the $T_{1/2}$ of intrinsic Tl-201 washout rate in one of the dogs with a critical stenosis receiving dipyridamole after intracoronary Tl-201 administration. The $T_{1/2}$ for Tl-201 washout was slow during occlusion (102 minutes) compared with the preocclusion state (51 minutes) and was slowed even further after dipyridamole. These changes in intrinsic Tl-201 washout rate from the stenotic region correlated with the severity of endocardial hypoperfusion consequent to dipyridamole infusion. As blood flow becomes subnormal and progressively decreases, the intrinsic Tl-201 washout rate becomes progressively more prolonged (Fig. 8–10).

This observation of reduced Tl-201 efflux in regions of decreased perfusion is an important mechanism in understanding Tl-201 redistribution. The disparate Tl-201 efflux rates in normal and underperfused myocardium can explain delayed redistribution observed after dipyridamole infusion in the presence of a coronary stenosis. After the initial uptake phase, the defect zone distal to a coronary stenosis would tend to lose Tl-201 more slowly than the normally

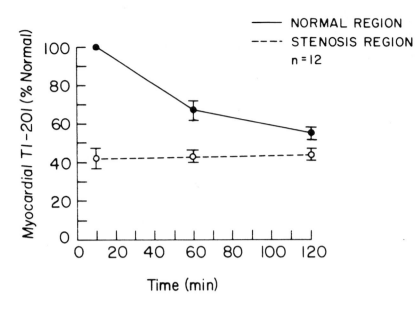

Figure 8–8. Serial changes in myocardial Tl-201 activity in normal *(solid line)* and stenotic *(dotted line)* regions in 12 dogs receiving intravenous dipyridamole before Tl-201 administration. Values are expressed as a percentage of initial normal myocardial Tl-201 activity, designated as 100%. Note that initial Tl-201 uptake is reduced to 40% of normal, but by 120 minutes shows significant normalization secondary to redistribution. (Beller GA, et al.: Circulation 1983;68:1328–1338.)

perfused area. Eventually, the defect tends to normalize. This is because the net loss rate of Tl-201 from myocardium is a balance between the influx from systemic recirculation and the intrinsic efflux rate. Intravenous aminophylline, or adenosine antagonist, reverses the dipyridamole-induced abnormal Tl-201 washout rate as well as the systemic hypotension and transmural coronary steal.[23] Pretreatment with aminophylline prevents the dipyridamole-induced vasodilatation and prolongation of Tl-201

efflux rate. Aminophylline alone had no significant hemodynamic or coronary flow effects in this study.[23]

Clinical Imaging Protocols

Dipyridamole Imaging Protocol

Figure 8–11 summarizes the Tl-201 imaging protocols for use with either dipyridamole infusion. Dipyridamole Tl-

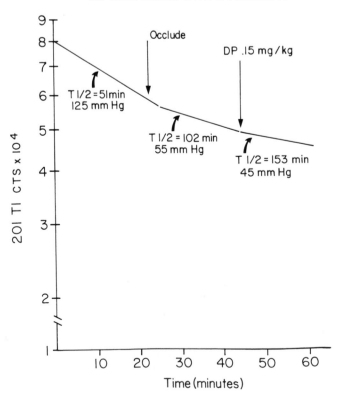

Figure 8–9. Changes in the $T_{1/2}$ of intrinsic Tl-201 washout in a dog with a critical stenosis receiving intravenous dipyridamole (DP) after intracoronary administration of Tl-201. The $T_{1/2}$ for Tl-201 washout is slow during occlusion as compared with the control state and is slowed even further after dipyridamole. (Beller GA, et al.: Circulation 1985;71:378–386.)

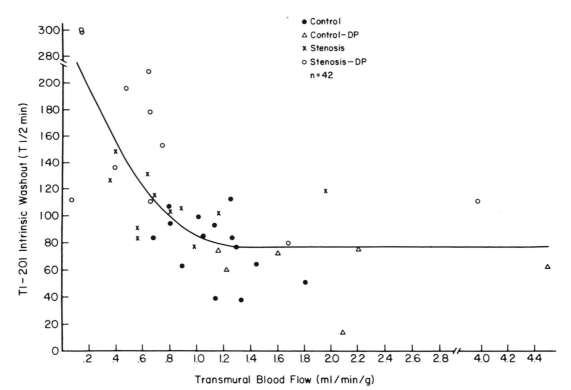

Figure 8–10. Relationship between blood flow and the $T_{1/2}$ of the intrinsic washout rate of Tl-201. Points on this graph were derived from Tl-201 washout and microsphere flow values under control conditions *(solid circles)* after creation of the stenosis (x) and after dipyridamole (DP) under control (△) and during the stenosis (○). (Beller GA, et al.: Circulation 1985;71:378–386.)

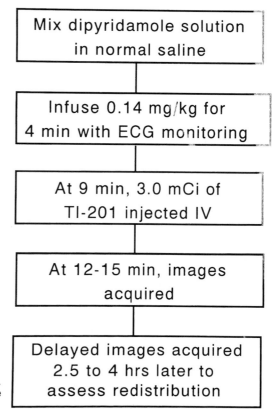

Figure 8–11. Outline of dipyridamole Tl-201 pharmacologic stress imaging protocol. Some investigators have advocated low-level treadmill exercise after dipyridamole infusion and prior to tracer administration.

201 stress scintigraphy is performed in the following manner: first, no caffeinated beverages and tea are permitted for 12 hours prior to imaging. Patients receiving theophylline-type drugs (e.g., for bronchospasm) cannot be considered for testing unless these drugs are discontinued. Interestingly, Heller et al.[28a] showed that theophylline alone can significantly delay the onset of exercise-induced ischemia and cause ischemia to occur at a higher rate-pressure product and oxygen uptake. This occurs without greater ischemia as determined by ST segment depression, angina pectoris, or size of Tl-201 scan abnormalities. The authors hypothesize that the increased ischemic threshold with theophylline may occur through the inhibition of adenosine, thereby preventing coronary steal with exercise stress. After baseline hemodynamics are measured, 0.56 mg/kg of dipyridamole is infused over a period of 4 minutes. A dose of 2.0 to 3.0 mCi of Tl-201 is injected at 9 minutes, and initial images are obtained 3 to 5 minutes later. As with exercise scintigraphy, delayed images are obtained 2½ to 4 hours later, to evaluate for presence or absence of redistribution. Handgrip exercise[29] or low-level treadmill exercise[30] can be combined with dipyridamole imaging to attenuate systemic hypotension and to further increase coronary blood flow. The adjunctive measures would also increase myocardial oxygen demand and therefore increase the frequency of symptomatic ischemia. Vital signs and serial 12-lead ECG are obtained before and every minute during dipyridamole infusion and for at least 5 minutes after the infusion is completed.

Aminophylline, 50 to 100 mg, can be administered intravenously to reverse dipyridamole-associated side effects such as systemic hypotension, chest pain, and nausea.

Adenosine Imaging Protocol

Adenosine imaging is performed following the infusion of adenosine in a peripheral vein with incremental doses every minute. An infusion rate of 140 μg/kg/minute is maintained for 6 minutes. After 3 minutes at this dose of adenosine, 3 mCi of Tl-201 is injected in a contralateral vein and flushed with normal saline. The adenosine infusion is maintained for 3 minutes more after Tl-201 administration. As with dipyridamole, vital signs are obtained and ECG monitoring performed during and for 5 minutes after adenosine infusion. Early and delayed images are acquired in a manner similar to what is undertaken after exercise or for dipyridamole imaging. Aminophylline is rarely administered to counteract side effects of adenosine infusion, since mere cessation of the infusion results in rapid disappearance of unwanted side effects because of the extremely short half-life of the drug.

Detection of Coronary Artery Disease

Dipyridamole Imaging

The principal clinical application of dipyridamole Tl-201 imaging is for detection of CAD in patients judged unable to exercise adequately. The sensitivity and specificity of dipyridamole Tl-201 imaging for detection of CAD is comparable to that observed with Tl-201 exercise scintigraphy.[15, 31–34] In a pooled analysis of data from multiple published series, the sensitivity and specificity of dipyridamole Tl-201 scintigraphy for CAD detection averaged 85.4% and 86.8%,[35–47] respectively (Table 8–2). Both exercise and dipyridamole infusion induce heterogeneity of blood flow at the time of tracer administration, so it is not surprising that the pattern of Tl-201 uptake on initial images after either dipyridamole or exercise stress is similar. In a review of five series in the literature compiled by Leppo,[31] comprising 215 patients who underwent both exercise and dipyridamole–Tl-201 scintigraphy for the detection of CAD, the sensitivity was 79% for both tests, and the specificity 95% for dipyridamole imaging and 92% for exercise imaging. Absolute myocardial Tl-201 activity in

Table 8–2. Sensitivity and Specificity of Dipyridamole Stress Tl-201 Scintigraphy for Detection of Coronary Artery Disease

Investigator	(No.) Patients With CAD	(No.) Patients Without CAD		Sensitivity (%)	Specificity (%)
Albro[35]	51	11		67	91
Leppo[36]	40	20		93	80
Schmoliner[37]	60	—		95	—
Francisco[38]	51	35		90	96
Timmis[39]	20	—		85	—
Narita[40]	35	15		69	100
Machencourt[41]	58	10		90	90
Okada[42]	23	7		91	100
Sochor[43]	149	45		92	81
Ruddy[44]	53	27		85	93
Taillefer[45]	19	6		79	86
Lam[47]	101	31		85	71
Laarman[46]	18	12		89	67
Total	678	219	Mean	85.4	86.8

normal myocardium is greater with dipyridamole than with exercise stress (491 counts/pixel versus 409 counts/pixel).[34a] In this study, myocardial Tl-201 clearance was lower with dipyridamole than with exercise (9.9% per hour vs. 13% per hour).

Varma et al.[34] compared segmental Tl-201 uptake and washout after exercise scintigraphy and dipyridamole scintigraphy performed 2 weeks apart in 21 patients with chest pain. Agreement between the two tests was observed in 92% (61 of 63) of coronary supply regions determined to be normal (41 of 41) or abnormal (20 of 22). In this group of patients, exercise and dipyridamole Tl-201 scintigraphy each detected 61% of stenotic vessels. As shown in Figure 8–12, the number of segments with normal Tl-201 uptake and the number of numerically significant defects by quantitative criteria were similar with exercise and dipyridamole (76% vs. 73%; 24% vs. 27%, respectively). Redistribution was slightly but significantly more prevalent in the dipyridamole scintigrams (17% vs. 10%). Agreement between 87% (165 of 189) of segment pairs was found when each was classified as either normal or abnormal. These data further indicate that exercise and dipyridamole–Tl-201 imaging when performed in the same patients are comparable for detecting and localizing regions of abnormal myocardial perfusion.

Quantitative image analysis can be applied to dipyridamole–Tl-201 scintigraphy similar to the analysis employed for exercise scintigraphy. Figure 8–13A and B are examples of postdipyridamole and delayed planar Tl-201 images with quantitative count profiles shown below the images obtained prior to and after coronary angioplasty of a stenotic left anterior descending coronary artery. Note a septal defect on the preprocedure imaging study, which shows almost total delayed redistribution. A repeat exercise scintigraphic study after angioplasty shows improved early Tl-201 uptake in the images acquired immediately post-exer-

cise. Isolated washout abnormalities in the absence of defects in other segments on dipyridamole–Tl-201 scans should not be interpreted as abnormal. Tl-201 clearance between initial and delayed images in normal myocardium is slower after dipyridamole-induced vasodilation than after exercise testing, and isolated regional washout abnormality may be within the limits of normal.[34]

Figure 8–14 shows normal uptake of Tl-201 in a patient with left ventricular hypertrophy and normal coronary arteries. Note the excellent clarity of the myocardial walls in these images obtained with dipyridamole stress.

Ruddy et al.[44] showed by stepwise logistic regression analysis that the best quantitative Tl-201 correlate of the presence of CAD on dipyridamole scintigrams was a combination variable of "either abnormal uptake or abnormal linear clearance, or both." This yielded sensitivity of 85% and specificity of 93% for detection of CAD stenoses. Borges-Neto et al.,[48] employing quantitative SPECT dipyridamole–Tl-201 scintigraphy, reported overall sensitivity of 92% and corresponding specificity of 84%. In that study, patients with significant multivessel disease (greater than 70% stenosis) were identified with sensitivity of 79% and specificity of 87%. Using a dose of 0.84 mg/kg of dipyridamole, Lalonde et al.[48a] showed that defect extent and detection of reversibility with Tl-201 were greater than using the 0.56 mg/kg dose when both protocols were undertaken in the same patient population. Interestingly, the side-effect rate was only 20% higher using the larger dose.

More recent studies utilizing the SPECT technique demonstrate sensitivity and specificity values in the range of 90% and per-vessel sensitivity in the range of 70% to 80% as compared with coronary angiography.[49, 50] In a study of 79 patients who underwent both dipyridamole–Tl-201 imaging and coronary angiography, the overall detection rate of CAD was 89% for SPECT and 67% for planar imaging.[50] Receiver operating characteristic (ROC) curves generated

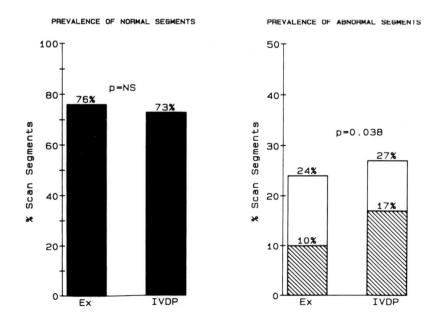

Figure 8–12. Prevalence of normal and abnormal Tl-201 scan segments after intravenous dipyridamole (IVDP) infusion and exercise (Ex). The frequency of defects observed after exercise and dipyridamole imaging is similar (24% vs. 27%). The frequency of redistribution defects was significantly greater after dipyridamole. (From Varma SK, et al.: Am J Cardiol 1989;64:871–877.)

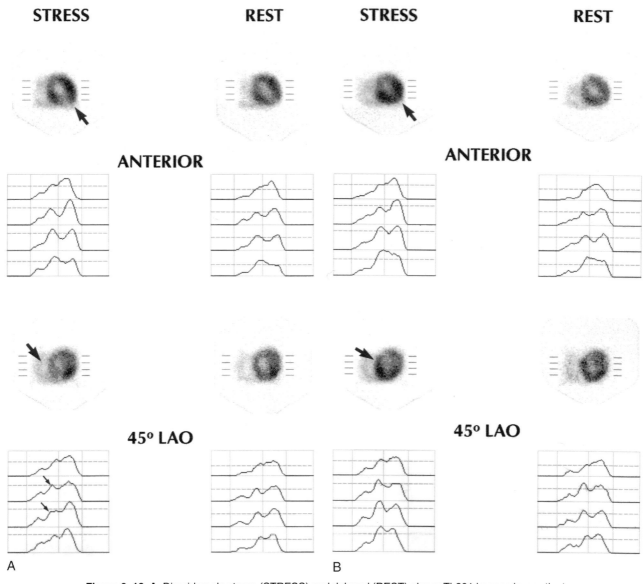

Figure 8–13. A. Dipyridamole stress (STRESS) and delayed (REST) planar Tl-201 images in a patient with a small defect on the anterior projection stress image and a mild interventricular septal defect *(arrow)* on the 45° left anterior oblique (LAO) image. The count profiles below the images verify the significance of these defects *(arrows)*. The REST images demonstrate redistribution. **B**. Dipyridamole Tl-201 images obtained after angioplasty in the same patient, showing improved post-dipyridamole Tl-201 uptake in the apex and interventricular septum *(arrow)*.

for SPECT and planar studies in this study demonstrated improved diagnostic performance by SPECT in the anterior vascular territory, but showed similar performance in the posterior territory because of lower SPECT specificity despite higher sensitivity (Fig. 8–15). Using ROC analysis and cutoff points of greater than 0% (any defect), and at least 4%, 8% and 12%, respectively, for definitions of an abnormal quantitative SPECT scan, Popma et al.[49] found that the optimal balance between sensitivity and specificity occurred at a defect size of at least 8% for the LAD, at least 4% for the LCx, and greater than 0% for the right coronary artery (RCA). This yielded sensitivities and specificities of 82% and 76% for the LAD, 71% and 71% for the LCx, and 76% and 82% for the RCA. No difference was found in accuracy of dipyridamole–Tl-201 imaging for detecting CAD in women and in men.[51] However, adverse effects were more common in women (62% vs. 38%). Figure 8–16 shows a SPECT dipyridamole myocardial perfusion scan obtained with Tc-99m sestamibi that demonstrates defects in the posterolateral and inferior regions.

Adenosine Imaging

The sensitivity and specificity of adenosine SPECT Tl-201 scintigraphy for detection of CAD is similar to values reported for both dipyridamole scintigraphy and exercise

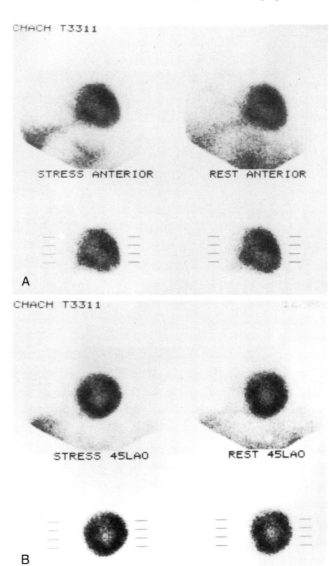

Figure 8–14. A. Unprocessed and background-subtracted anterior planar dipyridamole Tl-201 images showing uniform uptake after exercise and at rest. **B**. Unprocessed and background-subtracted 45° left anterior oblique (LAO) images from the same patient, showing uniform Tl-201 uptake in all segments.

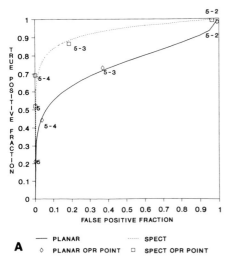

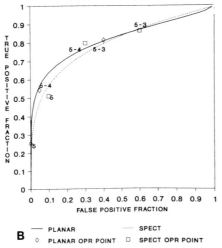

Figure 8–15. A. Receiver-operating characteristic curve for diagnosis of CAD in the anterior circulation perfusion zone. **B**. ROC curve for diagnosis of CAD in the posterior circulation perfusion zone. The solid line represents planar imaging, and the dotted line, SPECT imaging. (Mendelson MA, et al.: Am J Cardiol 1992;69:1150–1155.)

STRESS   REST

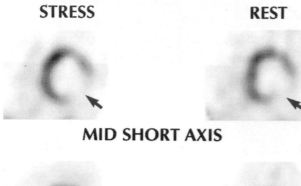

MID SHORT AXIS

DISTAL SHORT AXIS

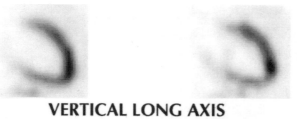

VERTICAL LONG AXIS

HORIZONTAL LONG AXIS

Figure 8–16. Dipyridamole (STRESS) and rest (REST) Tc-99m sestamibi SPECT images, showing defects in the posterolateral wall *(arrows)* that appear nonreversible.

SPECT scintigraphy.[51a] Miller reviewed a total of seven adenosine SPECT Tl-201 imaging studies published between 1989 and 1991, in which 500 patients comprised the pooled study analysis.[52] He found a cumulative average sensitivity of 88% ± 6%, a specificity of 91% ± 6%, and diagnostic accuracy of 88% ± 5% in those studies. Nishimura et al.[53] reported that individual stenoses were identified in 68% of patients with two-vessel disease and in 65 patients with three-vessel disease, employing adenosine SPECT Tl-201 scintigraphy. Table 8–3 summarizes the sensitivity of adenosine Tl-201 tomography related to extent of CAD in 70 patients in this study classified as having or not having a history of myocardial infarction (MI). A large multicenter trial was undertaken to compare adenosine to exercise Tl-201 SPECT imaging in a prospective, crossover fashion, in the same patients.[54] As expected, a high degree of concordance (89%) for defect versus no defect was observed between the adenosine and exercise images. The sensitivity, specificity, and predictive accuracy for detection of CAD with use of quantitative analysis in

Table 8–3. Sensitivity* of Adenosine Tl-201 Tomography Related to the Extent of Coronary Artery Disease in 70 Patients

Extent of CAD	Visual Tomography (%)	(No.)	Quantitative Tomography (%)	(No.)
Single-vessel disease				
All patients	72	(23/32)	81	(26/32)
No MI	62	(13/21)	76	(16/21)
MI	91	(10/11)	91	(10/11)
Double-vessel disease				
All patients	95	(21/22)†	91	(20/22)
No MI	93	(13/14)†	86	(12/14)
MI	100	(8/8)	100	(8/8)
Triple-vessel disease				
All patients	94	(15/16)	94	(15/16)
No MI	90	(9/10)†	90	(9/10)
MI	100	(6/6)	100	(6/6)

*Sensitivity refers to detection of significant stenosis in at least one coronary artery.

†*P* < 0.05 versus single-vessel disease.

(Reprinted with permission from the American College of Cardiology (Journal of the American College of Cardiology, 1991, Vol. 18, pp. 736–745).)

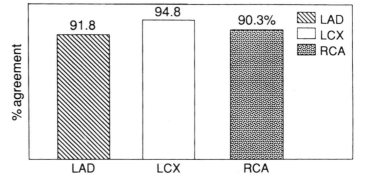

Figure 8–17. Comparative efficacy of adenosine SPECT in exercise treadmill SPECT imaging studies for detection of CAD in a multicenter trial comprising 51 healthy subjects and 93 patients with suspected CAD. Percent agreement between the two studies for identifying disease in the CAD, LCx, and RCA are shown. (Reprinted with permission from the American College of Cardiology (Journal of the American College of Cardiology, 1992, Vol. 19, pp. 248–257).)

this trial were, respectively, 83%, 87% and 84% for adenosine SPECT and 82%, 80%, and 81% for exercise SPECT studies (Fig. 8–17). Most false-negative studies in both adenosine and exercise SPECT groups were seen in patients with single-vessel disease. Sensitivity of both adenosine and exercise SPECT studies was 94% for detection of multivessel CAD. Figure 8–17 depicts a dipyridamole SPECT Tl-201 image in a patient with CAD.

Nishimura et al.[55] compared adenosine Tl-201 scintigraphy and exercise stress imaging using the SPECT technique in 175 subjects in a multicenter prospective crossover trial. Agreement on the presence of normal or abnormal tomograms by adenosine and exercise SPECT imaging was 82.8% by visual analysis and 86% by computer quantification. A good correlation was observed between quantified perfusion defect size by adenosine and exercise ($r = 0.80$; $P < 0.0001$), but values for defect size were greater with adenosine SPECT. Figure 8–18 shows the correlation of perfusion defect size by adenosine and exercise Tl-201 SPECT using quantitation. O'Keefe et al.[55a] found that adenosine SPECT imaging was superior to exercise Tl-201 imaging for detection of CAD in patients with left bundle branch block. The overall predictive accuracy was 93% in

the adenosine Tl-201 group, as compared with 68% in the exercise group ($P = 0.01$). Specificity of septal perfusion abnormalities was only 42% for exercise, as compared with 82% for adenosine ($P < 0.0002$).

Differentiation Between Ischemia and Scar

As with exercise Tl-201 scintigraphy, dipyridamole imaging can be employed to differentiate between transient ischemia and scar on perfusion scans. Okada et al.[56] compared various dipyridamole Tl-201 scan patterns with global and regional LV function changes on exercise radionuclide angiography in patients undergoing both perfusion and functional testing. Redistribution defects on dipyridamole scans were associated with normal regional wall motion and a normal exercise left ventricular ejection fraction (LVEF). Mild persistent defects were associated with normal regional wall motion at rest but with deterioration during exercise. Severe persistent Tl-201 defects on dipyridamole scans were associated with a subnormal resting EF and abnormal regional wall motion in the resting state, but no further deterioration with exercise. Reinjection of a second dose of Tl-201 following the acquisition of redistri-

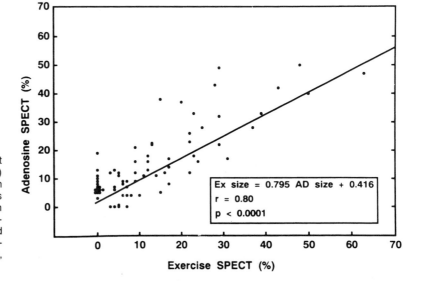

Figure 8–18. Correlation of SPECT perfusion defect size by quantitative adenosine (AD) and exercise (Ex) Tl-201 imaging. The correlation coefficient between adenosine and exercise tomographic defect size was 0.80 ($P < 0.0001$) by linear regression analysis. Mean ± SD of the difference in the extent of abnormal myocardium by the two tests was 2.7 ± 8.3%. (Reprinted with permission from the American College of Cardiology (Journal of the American College of Cardiology, 1992, Vol. 20, pp. 265–275).)

Ex size = 0.795 AD size + 0.416
r = 0.80
p < 0.0001

bution images during adenosine–Tl-201 scintigraphy was shown to enhance the detection rate of viable myocardium.[57] This is comparable to the enhanced detection of defect reversibility with reinjection of a second dose of Tl-201 at rest with exercise imaging protocols (see Chap. 9).

Dipyridamole perfusion scintigraphy has been used to distinguish between ischemic and nonischemic cardiomyopathy. Eichorn et al.[58] correctly classified 20 of 22 patients (91%) using dipyridamole scanning when a perfusion defect of at least 15% was used as an indication of nonischemic LV dysfunction. Patients with nonischemic cardiomyopathy demonstrated more homogeneous myocardial perfusion than those with ischemic cardiomyopathy. In that study, the mean perfusion defect was 25% ± 11% with nonischemic cardiomyopathy and 6% ± 6% with idiopathic cardiomyopathy.

Leppo et al.[36] found that the segmental Tl-201 defect patterns on dipyridamole images predicted abnormal wall motion by angiography better than ECG Q waves. Seventy-four per cent of myocardial scan segments that demonstrated complete redistribution of an initial dipyridamole-induced perfusion abnormality had normal wall motion on ventriculography. Conversely, 71% of scan segments that demonstrated a persistent reduction in Tl-201 activity over time had akinetic or dyskinetic wall motion. Figure 8–19 shows the relationship between asynergic or normal regional wall motion and the type of delayed Tl-201 scan pattern (redistribution or no redistribution) for the 537 segments in the 60 patients who comprised this study.

Thus, distinguishing between stress-induced ischemia and myocardial scar can be accomplished with dipyridamole–Tl-201 scintigraphy in a manner comparable to what has been undertaken using exercise stress. Again, it should be pointed out that as many as 20% to 25% of mild persistent defects may represent viable myocardium rather than scar on either dipyridamole or exercise scintigraphy. Care-

ful serial quantitation of redistribution, or reinjection of a second dose of Tl-201 after redistribution images have been acquired, should enhance the ability to detect defect reversibility and identify viable but ischemic myocardium. A detailed discussion concerning radionuclide detection of myocardial viability can be found in Chapter 9.

Markers of High-Risk Coronary Artery Disease

Left Ventricular Cavity Dilatation

As observed after exercise, some patients may develop increased lung Tl-201 uptake and LV cavity dilatation after either dipyridamole or adenosine infusion.[59–66] Transient LV cavity dilation during dipyridamole–Tl-201 imaging was reported in 9% of consecutive patients referred for dipyridamole–Tl-201 imaging.[59] Patients with transient LV cavity dilatation during dipyridamole–Tl-201 imaging had a high prevalence of either left main, three-vessel or "high-risk" two-vessel CAD. Sixty-four per cent of patients with transient cavity dilatation who were not referred for coronary vascularization suffered a cardiac event during a mean follow-up of 1 year. Most events were cardiac deaths (75%), most of which occurred within 4 months of the test. Thus, this study demonstrated that transient LV dilatation during dipyridamole–Tl-201 imaging is a marker of severe underlying CAD and denotes a poor prognosis. Iskandrian et al.[60] also reported that dipyridamole-induced increase in LV cavity size correlated with the extent and severity of underlying CAD. Transient dilatation occurred in patients with extensive perfusion abnormalities that were severe in nature. The dilatation observed was primarily due to an increase in cavity dimension, and to a lesser extent due to increased LV size. Therefore, it was postulated that this abnormality is due to diffuse subendocardial ischemia with resultant diminished Tl-201 uptake in the endocardial layers of the left ventricle.

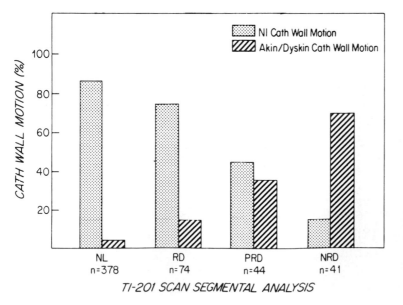

Figure 8–19. Percentage of normal (nl) and akinetic or dyskinetic (akin/dyskin) wall motion observed at catheterization (cath) versus the type of segmental Tl-201 findings interpreted as normal (nl), showing complete redistribution (RB), partial redistribution (PRB), or no redistribution (NRD). Note that the majority of akinetic or dyskinetic segments had either partial or no delayed Tl-201 redistribution. (Leppo JA, et al.: Circulation 1982;66:649–656.)

Chouraqui et al.[63] reported that transient dilatation of the left ventricle associated with dipyridamole–Tl-201 scintigraphy was related to a significantly higher frequency of three critical (at least 90%) coronary stenoses, higher prevalence of collaterals, more extensive myocardial Tl-201 redistribution defects, and a higher incidence of vasodilator-induced anginal chest pain than are seen in patients without transient LV dilatation. In that study, an abnormal transient dilatation ratio of at least 1.12 was a specific marker for multivessel (87%) or three-vessel (85%) critical CAD.

Increased Lung Thallium-201 Uptake

An increased lung-heart Tl-201 ratio is observed in approximately 20% of patients who undergo dipyridamole–Tl-201 imaging. In a study reported by Villanueva et al.[62] the lung-heart ratios for patients with normal and abnormal dipyridamole stress images (0.41 ± 0.05 and 0.48 ± 0.08, respectively) were similar to those for normal and abnormal exercise images (0.39 ± 0.06 and 0.46 ± 0.09). Patients with an increased lung-heart ratio on dipyridamole–Tl-201 scintigrams were more likely to have had a higher incidence of previous infarction and had a slightly higher rate-pressure product than patients with a normal lung-heart Tl-201 ratio. Significantly more patients with an increased lung-heart Tl-201 ratio had myocardial segments that showed initial defects, redistribution, and fixed defects compared to those with a normal ratio. LV cavity dilatation on the initial anterior planar image was also more prevalent in patients with an increased (compared to a normal) lung-heart Tl-201 ratio. As shown in Figure 8–20, patients with an increased lung-heart ratio had more segments that exhibited initial defects, redistribution defects, and persistent defects than did those with a normal ratio. Multiple stepwise linear regression analysis showed that the presence of Tl-201 redistribution was the strongest correlate of the lung-heart Tl-201 ratio.

Iskandrian et al.[60] also found that the lung-heart Tl-201 ratio on initial dipyridamole scintigrams was significantly higher in patients with coronary disease than in normal subjects. Patients with multivessel disease had a significantly higher lung-heart ratio (0.48) than those who had single-vessel disease (0.43). In that study, normal subjects had a lung-heart ratio of 0.36. There was a significant correlation between the severity and extent of the perfusion abnormality (determined from the polar SPECT maps) and the lung-heart Tl-201 ratio. Nishimura et al.[66] found that the lung-heart Tl-201 ratio on adenosine Tl-201 images was significantly higher in patients with multivessel CAD than in those with single-vessel disease. Patients with elevated lung Tl-201 activity during adenosine infusion had more segments with redistribution ($P = 0.04$), more hypoperfused segments ($P = 0.007$), and a larger Tl-201 defect than those with normal lung activity.

Okada et al.[65] did not find a significant difference in the prevalence of increased lung-heart ratio between patients with one-vessel and patients with multivessel CAD; however, only 40 patients with CAD were included in this study. The resting LV end-diastolic pressure was higher in patients with abnormal dipyridamole lung Tl-201 uptake

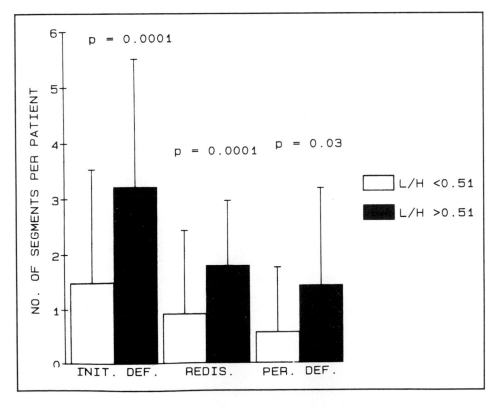

Figure 8–20. Number (no.) of segments showing initial (INIT) Tl-201 defects (DEF), redistribution (REDIS), and persistent (PER) defects (Def) in patients with normal *(open bars)* and abnormal *(solid bars)* lung-heart (L/H) ratios on planar dipyridamole Tl-201 scans. (Villanueva FS, et al.: Am J Cardiol 1990;66:1324–1328.)

than in those with normal lung uptake in this study. The LVEF in patients with CAD and abnormal dipyridamole lung Tl-201 uptake tended to be lower than those for patients with CAD and normal lung Tl-201 uptake.

Taken together, these studies suggest that abnormal transient LV dilatation and an increased lung-heart Tl-201 ratio are variables that indicate functionally more severe CAD. The mechanism for increased lung Tl-201 uptake with dipyridamole infusion may be an increase in LV filling pressure consequent to subendocardial ischemia caused by the transmural coronary steal. This would cause pulmonary interstitial edema similar to what has been observed with exercise-induced increased lung Tl-201 uptake. Evidence against this mechanism is a preliminary report from McLaughlin et al.,[67] who showed that patients with an increased lung-heart Tl-201 ratio on dipyridamole scans did not have a higher LV diastolic pressure during drug infusion as assessed by pulmonary capillary wedge pressure and coronary sinus lactate and adenosine levels. Also, coronary sinus lactate levels were comparable in patients with CAD and patients with normal coronary arteries who received intravenous dipyridamole.

The hemodynamic and radionuclide ventriculographic responses to intravenous dipyridamole were assessed by Klein et al.[68] In normal subjects, LV function was shown to improve with dipyridamole administration secondary to peripheral vasodilatation and the "unloading" effect of the drug. Eighty-seven per cent of the CAD patients in their study showed an abnormal response of the EF, decreasing from 49% ± 11% to 43% ± 13% ($P < 0.0001$). Wall motion worsened in 66% of patients, and the pressure-volume ratio deteriorated in 72%. These authors concluded that dipyridamole may induce true ischemia in CAD. The degree of LV dysfunction was related to the angiographic severity of CAD. Ogilby et al.[69] reported a 77% ± 38% increase in pulmonary capillary wedge pressure in normal subjects and a 125% ± 83% increase in patients with CAD during adenosine infusion. Interestingly, LVEF did not change significantly after adenosine infusion, and few (8%) regional wall motion abnormalities appeared. Thus, despite an elevation of wedge pressure consequent to drug infusion, no evidence of regional or global ischemia was observed by functional criteria. McLaughlin et al.[68a] did not find a difference in the pulmonary capillary wedge pressure between CAD and non-CAD patients receiving intravenous dipyridamole. Coronary sinus lactate and adenosine levels during dipyridamole infusion were also similar in CAD and non-CAD patients, suggesting that "true ischemia" was not induced in CAD patients receiving intravenous dipyridamole. It should be pointed out that no significant fall in systemic arterial pressure was observed in the CAD patients during dipyridamole infusion in this study.

Risk Stratification and Prognostication

Dipyridamole– or adenosine–Tl-201 scintigraphy can provide useful prognostic information in patients with oc-

cult or known CAD, particularly those who are unable to exercise and require risk assessment before major peripheral vascular or aortic surgery.[68b] High-risk scintigraphic variables on dipyridamole or adenosine scans are similar to those variables identified on exercise scans. They include multiple scan segments demonstrating hypoperfusion, an increased lung-heart ratio of Tl-201 uptake, and transient LV cavity dilatation.

Iskandrian et al.[69a] reported that adenosine Tl-201 SPECT imaging could help differentiate patients with left main or three-vessel CAD from patients with no CAD or one- or two-vessel disease. High-risk patients had more abnormal Tl-201 images (95% vs. 74%; $P < 0.0001$), a higher prevalence of a multivessel scan abnormality (76% vs. 39%; $P < 0.0001$), greater extent of perfusion defects (24% vs. 19%; $P < 0.0001$), and more increased lung Tl-201 uptake (39% vs. 15%; $P < 0.01$), findings similar to those reported for exercise imaging in comparable patient populations (see Chap. 4). Table 8–4 summarizes the results of stepwise discriminant analysis of the independent predictors of three-vessel and left main CAD in this study. A multivessel Tl-201 scan abnormality was the best predictor of high-risk disease.

Younis et al.[70] reported on their evaluation of the prognostic utility of dipyridamole–Tl-201 imaging in 107 asymptomatic patients, including 33 with a history of MI and 47 who had undergone bypass surgery or angioplasty. In nearly half of the patients, the indications for the dipyridamole–Tl-201 stress test were symptomatic peripheral vascular disease and preoperative clearance for major noncardiac surgery. Fifty-one patients had poor exercise tolerance. Despite the heterogeneity of this patient cohort, the authors found that, by stepwise logistic regression analysis, presence of Tl-201 redistribution defects was the only significant predictor of subsequent cardiac events during the 14 months of follow-up. Of the 13 asymptomatic patients who subsequently died or had a nonfatal infarction, 12 had a reversible dipyridamole–Tl-201 defect at the index imaging study. As shown in Figure 8–21, the event rate was comparable in patients with a reversible Tl-201 defect and patients with combined reversible and persistent Tl-201 defects. None of the 36 patients with a normal dipyridamole–Tl-201 scan died or had a nonfatal infarction. The majority of patients who died or who had a subsequent nonfatal infarction had underlying multivessel CAD. These findings are remarkably similar to the findings of reported prognostic studies utilizing exercise Tl-201 scintigraphy (see Chap.

Table 8–4. Stepwise Discriminant Analysis of Independent Predictors of Three-Vessel and Left Main Disease

Variable	χ^2
Multivessel thallium abnormality	27
Increased lung thallium uptake	10
ST-segment depression	5

(Iskandrian AS, et al.: Am Heart J 1993;125:1130–1135.)

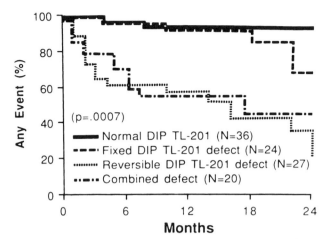

Figure 8–21. Incidence of cardiac events in 107 asymptomatic patients with CAD who were stratified by intravenous dipyridamole (DIP) Tl-201 scintigraphic results. A cardiac event was defined as cardiac death, nonfatal myocardial infarction, unstable angina, functional class III or IV angina, or the need for a revascularization procedure. (Reprinted with permission from the American College of Cardiology (Journal of the American College of Cardiology, 1989, Vol. 14, pp. 1635–1641).)

4). These observations are also similar to those made in an earlier study by Younis et al.[71] assessing the prognostic value of dipyridamole–Tl-201 scintigraphy after either unstable angina or acute MI. In that study, logistic regression analysis revealed that a reversible Tl-201 defect and the extent of angiographic CAD were the only independent predictors of a subsequent cardiac event. When only death or recurrent infarction was considered as an *event*, the extent of CAD and LVEF proved to be the only variables that were predictive. Figure 8–22 is an example of a high-risk dipyridamole Tl-201 scan showing redistribution defects in both inferior and anteroseptal segments and increased lung Tl-201 uptake in a patient with multivessel CAD.

In yet another study from the St. Louis University group, the utility of dipyridamole–Tl-201 imaging for assessing risk of subsequent events was evaluated in 373 patients with stable chest pain.[72] A history of MI, congestive heart failure, or coronary bypass surgery before the study, or an abnormal scan or one with a fixed perfusion defect was associated with a significantly increased frequency of subsequent cardiac events ($P < 0.05$). Interestingly, the presence of a reversible perfusion defect was not associated with increased risk. Stepwise logistic regression analysis showed that a history of coronary artery bypass surgery before the study and the presence of a fixed perfusion defect were the only variables that had independent predictive value for occurrence of a subsequent cardiac event. Although redistribution defects were predictive of perioperative cardiac events, Hendel et al.[73] reported a persistent defect increased the relative risk for late cardiac events more than redistribution in patients followed up after dipyridamole–Tl-201 imaging. Patients with a persistent defect had a 24% late event rate, as compared with 4.9% for those with a normal scan. Cox regression analysis showed that a persistent Tl-201 defect was the strongest predictor of a late

event and increased the relative risk nearly fivefold. This finding may be due to the fact that persistent Tl-201 defects reflect the degree of irreversible myocardial damage and should correlate with depressed LVEF and, thus, increased mortality on long-term follow-up. Of course, some persistent defects represent severe ischemia, which may also contribute to an adverse late outcome.

In an earlier study, Hendel et al.[74] examined the prognostic utility of dipyridamole–Tl-201 imaging in 516 consecutive patients undergoing the test for a variety of clinical indications. Of these, 23 died and 43 experienced a nonfatal infarction during a mean follow-up of 21 months. By logistic regression analysis, an abnormal dipyridamole scan was

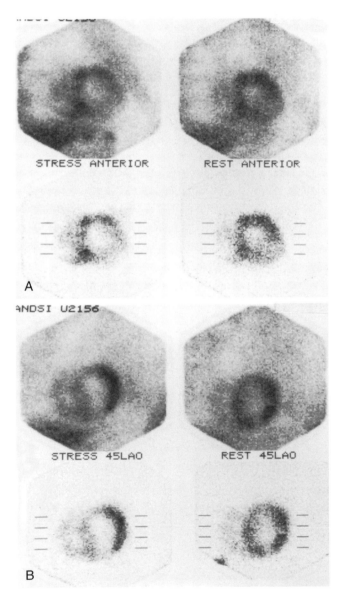

Figure 8–22. A. Anterior dipyridamole Tl-201 planar images obtained at stress and 2½ hours later (REST), which shows anterolateral, apical, and inferoapical defects with partial delayed redistribution. Increased lung Tl-201 uptake can be seen in the stress image. **B.** Stress and 2½ hour delayed (REST) 45° left anterior oblique (LAO) images in the same patient, showing an extensive anteroseptal defect that fills in almost totally.

an independent and significant predictor of subsequent infarction or death and increased the relative risk of an event more than threefold (Table 8–5). The presence of redistribution on the dipyridamole–Tl-201 perfusion scan further increased the risk of a cardiac event. Figure 8–23 shows the event-free survival for patients with a normal and patients with an abnormal dipyridamole–Tl-201 scan in this study. In patients with an abnormal scan, the presence of more than one segment demonstrating redistribution, as well as persistent abnormalities, was found more often in the group that experienced cardiac events. The combination of diabetes mellitus, congestive heart failure, and an abnormal dipyridamole–Tl-201 scintigram was associated with the highest predicted probability of experiencing subsequent infarction or death, and raised the relative risk of a cardiac event more than 26-fold. One limitation of this study is the absence of a measure of LV function. Depressed global function may have provided similar or additional information.

Zhu[75] evaluated the potential clinical utility of intravenous dipyridamole perfusion imaging with Tl-201 in a group of 170 patients, 78 with suspected angina and 92 with unstable angina. All underwent coronary angiography, which revealed 28 patients with normal coronary arteries and 35 with single-vessel disease. Dipyridamole scintigraphy yielded a per-vessel sensitivity of 74% and specificity of 78%. Patients with complicated courses and those who subsequently required revascularization had more extensive dipyridamole-induced defects.

Rose et al.[76] evaluated 236 patients with peripheral vascular disease who underwent dipyridamole–Tl-201 scintigraphy. Follow-up ranged from 9 to 30 months. Dipyridamole–Tl-201 lung-heart ratio and LVEF added significant prognostic information to clinical variables. Figure 8–24 shows the survival curves generated from the Cox model

Table 8–5. Predictive Value of Various Clinical Variables

Variable	All Cardiac Events	
	P Value*	Relative Risk†
Abnormal scan	0.0004	3.1
Congestive heart failure	0.0137	3.0
Diabetes mellitus	0.0002	2.8
Gender	0.0834	—
Prior MI	0.0254	—
Peripheral vascular disease	0.3204	—

*P values reflect values from step 0 of regression analysis.
†Relative risk refers to odds ratio after completion of regression model.
(Adapted from Hendel RC, et al.: J Am Coll Cardiol 1990;15:109–116.)

for patients with a heart-lung Tl-201 ratio of above or below 1.8.

Adenosine Tl-201 imaging provides comparable prognostic information as dipyridamole imaging in CAD patients. Kamal et al.[76a] found that the size of the SPECT perfusion abnormality was the strongest predictor of cardiac death or nonfatal infarction in 177 patients with follow-up for a mean of 22 months after adenosine Tl-201 imaging. Life table analysis showed that patients with perfusion defects of 15% or greater had a worse prognosis than had patients with normal scans or smaller defects ($P < 0.0001$).

Risk Stratification in the Elderly

Advanced age is a major variable that influences prognosis in symptomatic patients with CAD. Approximately 55% of all patients who experience an MI are older than 65 years; of those who die, approximately four of five are older than 65 years. Also, among the elderly, women are twice

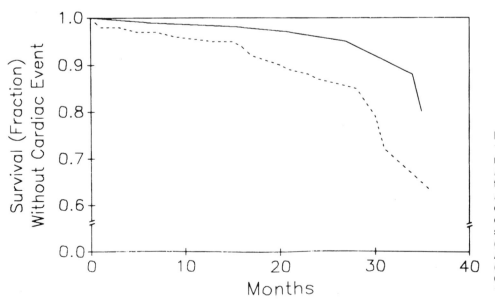

Figure 8–23. Event-free survival in 172 patients with a normal dipyridamole Tl-201 perfusion scan *(solid line)* compared to survival of 332 patients with an abnormal scan *(dashed line).* Events were defined as death or myocardial infarction. The difference in these survival curves was statistically significant ($P < 0.005$). (Reprinted with permission from the American College of Cardiology (Journal of the American College of Cardiology, 1990, Vol. 15, pp. 109–116).)

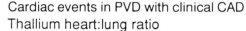

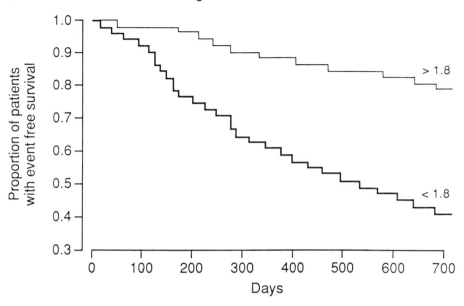

Figure 8–24. Event-free survival curves by Cox analysis in patients with peripheral vascular disease (PVD) and clinical CAD based on a heart-lung Tl-201 ratio >1.8 or <1.8. (Rose EL, et al.: Am J Cardiol 1993;71:40–44.)

as likely as men to die within several weeks of their infarction.[77] Left main or three-vessel CAD is more prevalent in elderly patients who present with angina symptoms and no history of infarction than in their younger counterparts.[78] The data from the CASS registry show that coronary artery bypass graft surgery has a beneficial effect on survival in patients with angina who were older than 65 years.[79] The survival rate at 6 years was 80% for the surgical cohort and 63% for the medical group.

A substantial number of elderly patients have occult high-risk CAD but are asymptomatic or have minimal angina symptoms. Many present with manifestations of carotid, peripheral, or aortic vascular disease. Hertzer's review of previously published studies revealed a greater than 50% prevalence of associated CAD in patients who present with either abdominal aortic aneurysms, carotid artery disease, or peripheral vascular disease.[80] Many elderly patients are unable to adequately perform an exercise test, for any of a variety of reasons. Pharmacologic stress myocardial perfusion imaging with intravenous dipyridamole or adenosine can be utilized in such patients to detect physiologically significant CAD and for prognostication. Shaw et al.[81] determined the predictive value of intravenous dipyridamole–Tl-201 imaging for subsequent cardiac death or nonfatal infarction in patients at least 70 years of age who were known or suspected to have CAD. They evaluated 348 patients, of whom 207 were symptomatic and 141 asymptomatic. The 2-year hard event rate was high and included 52 cardiac deaths and 24 nonfatal infarctions. The overall cardiac event rate (cardiac death or nonfatal infarction) was 5% for patients with a normal scan, as compared with 35% for patients with an abnormal scan, and it increased with the number of Tl-201 defects. By multivariate stepwise

logistic regression analysis of clinical and scintigraphic variables, an abnormal Tl-201 scan was the single best predictor of cardiac events. Patients with an abnormal scan were 7.2 times more likely to experience a subsequent cardiac event than were patients with a normal scan. As expected, symptoms of congestive heart failure (odds ratio, 2.1) and previous infarction (odds ratio, 2.2) were additional independent predictors of events. Figure 8–25 shows the actuarial event-free survival rate in the 149 patients who had a normal dipyridamole–Tl-201 scan in this study and the 199 patients with who had an abnormal one. Thus, elderly patients with functionally high-risk CAD can be identified by noninvasive pharmacologic stress imaging. This group of patients with limited exercise capacity and potential for advanced CAD are at high risk for future cardiac events.

Risk Stratification Before Vascular Surgery

Dipyridamole Imaging

Dipyridamole–Tl-201 imaging has proven useful for risk stratification before surgery in patients with peripheral vascular or aortic disease.[81a] Such patients often have underlying risk factors that promote the development of both peripheral atherosclerotic disease and CAD.[81b] Patients with peripheral vascular disease may be limited by claudication and therefore may not manifest exercise-induced angina. In these patients, CAD may be occult but pose a significant perioperative risk for infarction and cardiac death to the patient. Table 8–6 summarizes operative and 5-year mortality rates in patients undergoing operation for vascular disease as a function of preoperative cardiac status.[82, 83] Patients suspected to have CAD had a 6.8% operative

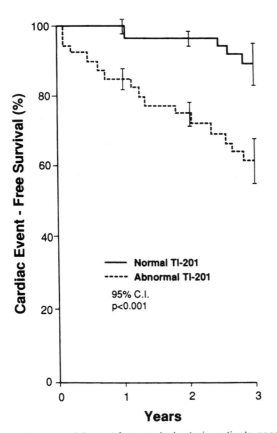

Figure 8–25. Actuarial event-free survival rate in patients aged 70 years or older who have a normal *(solid line)* or abnormal *(dotted line)* dipyridamole Tl-201 scan result. Stepwise logistic regression analysis of clinical and radionuclide variables revealed that an abnormal scan was the single best predictor of cardiac events (relative risk, 7.2; *P*<0.001). (Key: C.I., confidence interval.) (Reprinted with permission from the American College of Cardiology (Journal of the American College of Cardiology, 1992, Vol. 19, pp. 1390–1398).)

mortality and 41% 5-year late mortality rate, as compared to 1.3% and 20% mortality rates, respectively, for patients with no "overt" CAD. Figure 8–26 depicts the prevalence of associated CAD in patients with peripheral vascular disease summarized by Gersh et al.[83] from multiple series representing approximately 10,000 patients analyzed by Hertzer.[82] As shown, approximately 50% of patients with abdominal aortic aneurysm, carotid artery disease, or lower extremity ischemia had associated CAD. Criqui et al.[84] reported a 15-fold increase in rates of mortality due to cardio-

vascular disease and CAD among subjects with large-vessel peripheral arterial disease that was both severe and symptomatic.

Pharmacologic stress imaging offers an approach for detection of physiologically important coronary lesions which may be associated with an increased risk of a cardiac event during or following surgery and after hospital discharge. Table 8–7 summarizes the positive and negative predictive values for dipyridamole Tl-201 scintigraphy for predicting perioperative cardiac events in patients undergoing noncardiac surgery. Note that the negative predictive value of a normal scan for a good outcome is better than the positive predictive value of an abnormal scan for perioperative ischemic events.

Boucher et al.[85] first reported that in patients with a history of angina or MI, the presence of Tl-201 redistribution on dipyridamole scintigrams preoperatively was superior to any other clinical variable in predicting perioperative death, infarction, unstable angina, or pulmonary edema. There were no cardiac events in patients whose scan was normal or demonstrated only persistent defects.

In another study from the Massachusetts General Hospital group published by Eagle et al.,[86] all patients who underwent dipyridamole–Tl-201 imaging before major vascular surgery were stratified into clinically low-risk and high-risk groups on the basis of a history of angina, MI, congestive heart failure, diabetes mellitus, or ECG Q waves. Based on clinical variables, 52 (47%) patients were assigned to the low-risk group. Dipyridamole-induced Tl-201 redistribution occurred in 17% of these low-risk patients, and one patient had subsequent angina. Redistribution occurred in 56% of the clinically high-risk patients, with 45% of them experiencing postoperative ischemic events. In this study, Tl-201 redistribution was observed in 89% of patients with ischemic events. Figure 8–27 shows the outcome of patients stratified first on the basis of clinical risk factors and then on the basis of the dipyridamole Tl-201 scan results. No events were seen in patients with no clinical risk factors, even though 6 of the 23 had reversible defects on the dipyridamole scan. In contrast 10 of the 27 clinically high-risk patients had a postoperative ischemic event and eight had redistribution defects. This study points out that clinically low-risk patients may not benefit from dipyridamole–

Table 8–6. **Mortality in Patients Undergoing Operation for Vascular Disease**

	Operative Mortality*		5-Year Mortality†	
Cardiac Status	*(No.)*	*(%)*	*(No.)*	*(%)*
Overall	14,180	3.3	7,805	31
No "overt" CAD	1,782	1.3	1,185	20
Suspected CAD	1,337	6.8	1,092	41
History of coronary artery bypass graft	1,237	1.5	1,172	21

*Based on 29 reported series, representing 14,180 patients.
†Based on 23 reported series, representing 7,805 patients (53% of deaths were cardiac related).
Data from Hertzer.[80] Data collected by Gersh et al.[83]
(Reprinted with permission from the American College of Cardiology (Journal of the American College of Cardiology, 1991, Vol. 16, pp. 203–214).)

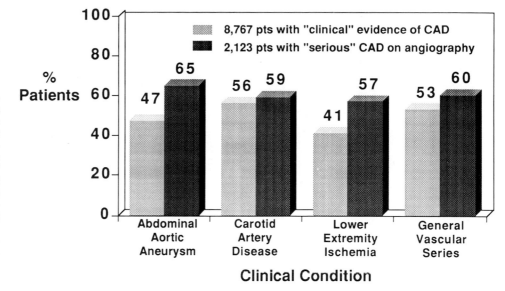

Figure 8–26. Prevalence of associated CAD (vertical axis) in patients (pts) with peripheral vascular disease. Data are from a review by Hertzer[82] from multiple series comprising approximately 10,000 patients. Stippled bars indicate 8767 patients with "clinical" evidence of CAD. Hatched bars represent 2123 subjects with "serious" CAD on angiography. (Key: AAA, abdominal aortic aneurysm.) (Reprinted with permission from the American College of Cardiology (Journal of the American College of Cardiology, 1991, Vol. 18, pp. 203–214).)

Tl-201 imaging for preoperative risk stratification because of a low prevalence of redistribution defects and a low perioperative event rate.

In a subsequent study published several years later by Eagle et al.,[87] 254 patients referred for dipyridamole–Tl-201 imaging before major vascular surgery were evaluated. Of these, 44 patients had surgery canceled or postponed for clinical or scintigraphic reasons. In another 10 patients, surgery was not confirmed. Thirty of the remaining 200 patients who underwent surgery (15%) experienced one or more postoperative ischemic events (3% cardiac death rate, 4.5% nonfatal infarction rate, 9.5% rate of unstable angina, 4.5% rate of pulmonary edema). Logistic regression identified five clinical predictors (Q waves, history of ventricular ectopic activity, diabetes, advanced age, angina) and two dipyridamole–Tl-201 predictors of postoperative events. Of the 64 patients with none of the clinical risk variables, only two had ischemic events with no deaths. In contrast, 50% of the patients with three or more clinical markers had events. In the group who had either one or two clinical predictors, only 2 of 62 patients without Tl-201 redistribution had events, all compared with a 30% event rate in the 54 patients with Tl-201 redistribution. This study confirmed the earlier one cited previously, as patients classified as low risk by clinical criteria had very few cardiac events. The

multivariate model using both clinical and Tl-201 variables showed significantly higher specificity at equivalent sensitivity levels in models using either clinical or Tl-201 variables alone. The authors of this study concluded that preoperative dipyridamole Tl-201 imaging appears most useful for stratifying vascular disease patients determined by clinical evaluation to be at intermediate risk. However, for nearly half of the patients, dipyridamole imaging may have been unnecessary because of very high or low cardiac risk predicted by clinical variables alone.

Hendel et al.,[73] using stepwise logistic regression analysis, also found that Tl-201 redistribution was the most predictive of 32 clinical and scan variables for occurrence of perioperative nonfatal infarction, yielding almost a ninefold increase in relative risk. The predicted probability of death or infarction was 1.3% in the absence of any predictors selected from the regression model, which included Tl-201 redistribution, ST-segment depression during vasodilator stress, diabetes mellitus, and advanced age. The greater the magnitude of the Tl-201 redistribution defect, the greater the probability of a perioperative event.

Leppo et al.[88] evaluated 100 consecutive patients admitted for vascular surgery. All underwent dipyridamole–Tl-201 imaging. Using multivariate analysis of clinical variables and imaging data, the risk of experiencing a post-

Table 8–7. Predictive Value of Dipyridamole Tl-201 Scintigraphy for Perioperative Cardiac Events

| Investigator | Patients (No.) | Predictive Value (%) | | Risk Ratio |
		Positive	Negative	
Boucher[85]	48	50	100	16.0
Cutler[89]	101	23	100	14.3
Leppo[88]	89	33	98	15.7
Eagle[86]	200	30	96	7.2
Mangano[93]	60	27	82	1.5

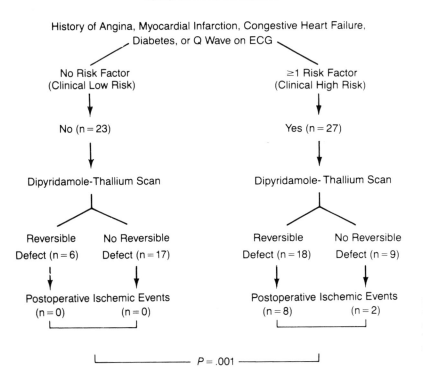

Validation Set of 50 Patients

History of Angina, Myocardial Infarction, Congestive Heart Failure, Diabetes, or Q Wave on ECG

No Risk Factor (Clinical Low Risk) — No (n = 23) — Dipyridamole-Thallium Scan — Reversible Defect (n = 6) / No Reversible Defect (n = 17) — Postoperative Ischemic Events (n = 0) (n = 0)

≥1 Risk Factor (Clinical High Risk) — Yes (n = 27) — Dipyridamole-Thallium Scan — Reversible Defect (n = 18) / No Reversible Defect (n = 9) — Postoperative Ischemic Events (n = 8) (n = 2)

P = .001

Figure 8–27. Risk stratification algorithm applied to 50 patients undergoing peripheral vascular surgery. Groups are separated on the basis of presence or absence of clinical risk factors and then stratified on the basis of the dipyridamole Tl-201 scan results. (Eagle KA, et al.: JAMA 1987;257:2185–2189. Copyright 1987, American Medical Association.)

operative cardiac event was 23 times greater for patients with perfusion abnormalities than for those without evidence of redistribution defects. In addition, diabetes patients or patients who demonstrated ST-segment depression after dipyridamole infusion in combination with Tl-201 redistribution were at even higher risk. These latter findings are comparable to those reported by Hendel et al.[73]

Cutler and Leppo[89] found that Tl-201 redistribution showed the best statistical correlation with postoperative myocardial infarction in 116 consecutive patients referred for aortic reconstructive surgery. For a patient with Tl-201 scintigraphic abnormalities on dipyridamole imaging the odds of having a postoperative infarction in this group of patients was 12 times greater than for those with a normal scan. Of interest, the incidence of postoperative infarction was similar regardless of whether these patients had symptomatic or asymptomatic CAD. Lette et al.,[90] employing a scintigraphic scoring system that took into account dipyridamole-induced reversible LV cavity dilatation on serial dipyridamole scans with indices of severity and extent of redistribution, found that patients could be successfully classified into low-, intermediate-, and high-risk subgroups. Patients classified as low risk underwent noncardiac surgery uneventfully. In contrast, eight of ten patients with high-risk scintigraphic abnormalities had a postoperative event (seven deaths and one nonfatal myocardial infarction).

Levinson[91] determined the usefulness of semiquantitative analysis of dipyridamole–Tl-201 redistribution for improving risk stratification before vascular surgery. They determined which patients with Tl-201 redistribution were at

greatest risk of an event after surgery. Scans were analyzed to determine the number of myocardial segments out of 15 which showed redistribution. Seventeen of 64 patients with redistribution (27%) had postoperative ischemic events. Tl-201 predictors of ischemic operative complications included Tl-201 redistribution in at least four myocardial segments ($P = 0.03$), at least two of the three planar views showing a segment with redistribution ($P = 0.005$), and at least two coronary vascular territories showing redistribution ($P = 0.007$). No patient with redistribution in only one view had an ischemic event. Thus, these authors concluded that determining the extent of redistribution on dipyridamole–Tl-201 scans improves risk stratification for vascular surgery. Patients with the greater numbers of myocardial segments and greater numbers of coronary territories showing Tl-201 redistribution are at higher risk for ischemic cardiac events in the postoperative period.

Lette et al.[92] also reported data relative to the prognostic utility of preoperative dipyridamole–Tl-201 imaging using quantitative image analysis in 360 patients. Of interest was that clinical descriptors were not useful in predicting outcome. In patients with normal scans or solely persistent defects, postoperative and long-term cardiac event rates (myocardial infarction on death) were 1% and 3.5%, respectively. These rates were 17.5% and 22% for patients with redistribution defects. The greater the amount of hypoperfusion on Tl-201 scintigrams, the higher was the risk of a subsequent event. A subsequent study by Lette et al.[92a] presented a three-step, three-segment model to improve accuracy of dipyridamole–Tl-201 imaging for preoperative cardiac risk assessment before noncardiac vascular surgery or major general surgery. In step 1, the postoperative cardiac event rate was 1.3% in 225 patients with normal anterior, inferior, and posterolateral region perfusion and no transient LV cavity dilatation. Step 2 consists of identifying those with a high probability of left main, three-vessel or high risk two-vessel CAD, or a significant risk area of jeopardy in the supply zone of a critically stenotic artery. Of 29 patients with redistribution defects of all three segments, transient LV dilatation or at least one severe reversible defect, 52% sustained a cardiac event. The remaining group of 101 patients was stratified according to age older than 70 years, diabetes, and number of redistribution segments. The event rate ranged from 5% to 36%.

Mangano et al.[93] also examined the value of dipyridamole Tl-201 scintigraphy as a preoperative screening test for perioperative myocardial ischemia and infarction. Myocardial ischemia was assessed during the intraoperative period using continuous 12-lead ECG and transesophageal echocardiography, and during the postoperative period using continuous ambulatory monitoring. Twenty-two patients (37%) had defects that showed reversibility on delayed scintigrams, eighteen (30%) had persistent defects and twenty (33%) had normal scans. There was no association between redistribution defects and adverse cardiac outcome: 54% of adverse outcomes occurred in patients without redistribution defects, and the risk of an adverse outcome was not significantly increased in patients with redistribution defects (relative risk 1.5, 95% confidence interval 0.6 to 3.9, $P = 0.43$). In addition, these authors found no association between redistribution defects and perioperative ischemia. More than half of the ischemic episodes detected by ECG or transesophageal echocardiography occurred in patients who had no redistribution defects. Baron et al.[92b] also found that dipyridamole Tl-201 SPECT imaging did not accurately predict cardiac events in patients undergoing cardiac risk assessment prior to abdominal surgery. The best correlates of perioperative cardiac complications were definite clinical evidence of CAD (odds ratio:

2.6) and age greater than 65 years (odds ratio: 2.3). Quantitative scan analysis was not undertaken in this study. Also, 75% of the events were nonfatal, and "prolonged myocardial ischemia" was the most frequently observed event. Finally, 11 patients with severe but correctable CAD were subsequently excluded from outcome analysis. Thus, these results differ from those of previous studies with respect to the usefulness of dipyridamole imaging for risk stratification.

The extent of reversible ischemia by dipyridamole Tl-201 scintigraphy, and not just its presence, is also an important factor for risk stratification before noncardiac surgery. Brown and Rowen[93a] found that the number of myocardial segments with transient Tl-201 defects ($P < 0.0005$) and a history of diabetes mellitus ($P < 0.05$) were the only multivariate predictors of perioperative cardiac death or nonfatal infarction in a cohort of 231 consecutive patients who underwent noncardiac surgery. Figure 8–28 shows that the probability of perioperative death or nonfatal infarction is a function of the number of myocardial segments with redistribution Tl-201 defects and presence or absence of diabetes.

Urbanati et al.[93b] demonstrated the long-term prognostic value of exercise Tl-201 scintigraphy in patients with symptomatic carotid vascular disease but no symptoms of CAD. Event-free survival after carotid endarterectomy in patients with silent ischemia by Tl-201 scintigraphy was only 51% at 5.4 years follow-up, as compared with 98% in patients without scintigraphic ischemia. This study points out that patients with carotid vascular disease who can exercise are successfully risk stratified by exercise perfusion imaging. Pharmacologic stress imaging should be reserved for those patients with coexisting peripheral vascular disease that precludes achieving adequate levels of exercise stress.

Rose et al.[93c] found that the dipyridamole Tl-201 lung-heart ratio and the LV ejection fraction at rest added significantly and incrementally to prediction of cardiac events once the clinical history, physical findings, and rest ECG findings were known in 236 patients with peripheral vas-

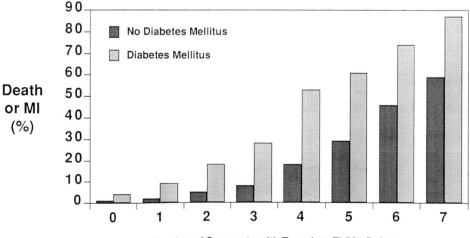

Figure 8–28. Probability of perioperative cardiac death (CD) or nonfatal MI (NFMI) relative to the number of scan segments with transient Tl-201 defects and further stratified by presence or absence of diabetes mellitus. Note that patients with diabetes have a significantly higher event rate than nondiabetic patients at all values depicting number of abnormal reversible segments. (Reprinted with permission from the American College of Cardiology (Journal of the American College of Cardiology, 1993, Vol. 21, pp. 2325–2330).)

Death or MI (%)

Number of Segments with Transient Tl-201 Defects

cular disease undergoing vascular surgery. Results of ambulatory ECG monitoring did not add significant prognostic information.

Nonvascular Surgery

There are few data concerning the value of preoperative dipyridamole Tl-201 imaging for evaluation of risk for nonvascular surgery.[94–94b] Coley et al.[94] determined the ability of clinical and dipyridamole–Tl-201 scan variables for risk stratification in 100 consecutive patients who proceeded to nonvascular surgery. Of these, only 9% experienced an ischemic cardiac event. Logistic regression identified age over 70 years, a history of heart failure, and Tl-201 redistribution as predictors of events. Of the 45 patients who had neither clinical variable, none (0%) had events. In the remaining 55 patients with a clinical marker, the event rate was 3.2% for those without redistribution (1 of 31) and 33.3% for those with redistribution (8 of 24). Younis et al.[94a] studied 161 patients referred for dipyridamole Tl-201 imaging prior to intraabdominal surgery (n = 39), orthopaedic surgery (n = 45), thoracic surgery (n = 12), renal transplantation (n = 26), or miscellaneous procedures (n = 39). Sixty patients had evidence for CAD and 101 did not. However, 50% of the latter group had two or more CAD risk factors. Forty-five percent of the entire cohort had an abnormal scan. Presence of two or more abnormal Tl-201 scan segments was the only independent predictor of cardiac death or nonfatal infarction. Thus, dipyridamole Tl-201 is useful for risk stratification in patients with clinical markers of cardiac disease who are referred for nonvascular surgery.

Adenosine Imaging

Scant data are available on the prognostic utility of adenosine–Tl-201 scintigraphy for risk stratification before vascular surgery. Shaw et al.[95] found by stepwise logistic regression that presence of a combined persistent and reversible adenosine Tl-201 defect, three-vessel CAD, and left bundle branch block was predictive of subsequent cardiac events with relative risk ratios of 4.9, 2.9, and 2.2, respectively (Table 8–8). Since adenosine–Tl-201 imaging has comparable sensitivity and specificity for CAD detection to dipyridamole imaging, the prognostic value of this pharmacologic stress technique should also be similar to what is achieved with dipyridamole vasodilator stress.

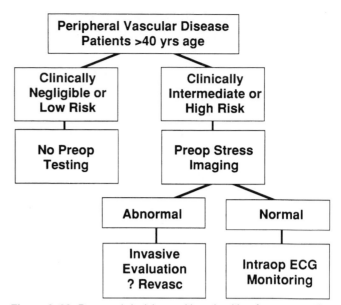

Figure 8–29. Proposed decision-making algorithm for preoperative risk stratification in patients with peripheral vascular disease referred for noncardiac surgery. (See text for explanation.)

Which Patients Should Undergo Preoperative Stress Perfusion Imaging?

The data presented in the previous paragraphs clearly show that many patients with peripheral vascular or aortic disease have asymptomatic CAD. Figure 8–29 depicts a decision-making algorithm for selection of patients to undergo preoperative pharmacologic perfusion imaging for risk stratification. Patients with physiologically important CAD manifested by abnormal perfusion scans are at higher risk for both in-hospital perioperative complications and a long-term increase in fatal and nonfatal ischemic events. Patients under 60 years of age with no clinical markers of CAD and a normal resting ECG do not usually require pharmacologic stress imaging before peripheral vascular surgery, since the prevalence of events is low. In contrast, older patients who have at least one clinical marker of CAD should benefit from pharmacologic stress imaging before elective surgery. A normal scan has excellent predictive value for a good prognosis. Conversely, the greater the number of defects detected, particularly of the redistribution type, the greater the early and late risk for cardiac events. Presently, there are no convincing data on the cost-effectiveness of pharmacologic stress imaging in asymptomatic patients who are being evaluated before nonvascular surgery. The prevalence of CAD would be low in the absence of clinical evidence of CAD or peripheral vascular disease, or risk factors such as smoking and hypertension, known to be associated with a higher incidence of atherosclerosis. Certainly, if such patients have a history of CAD or if arterial bruits are detected on physical examination, pharmacologic or exercise stress scintigraphy may be useful for identifying functionally significant CAD.

Table 8–8. Stepwise Logistic Regression Analysis for Prediction of Perioperative Events

Variable	P Value	Risk Ratio
1. Combined fixed and reversible adenosine Tl-201 defect	0.0007	4.9
2. Three-vessel coronary artery disease	0.001	2.9
3. Left bundle branch block	0.02	2.2

(Shaw L, et al.: Am Heart J 1992;124:861–869.)

Risk Stratification in Diabetic Patients

The incidence of dipyridamole-induced Tl-201 scan abnormalities is extremely high in diabetic patients scheduled for vascular surgery. Lane et al.[96] found an 80% prevalence of Tl-201 scan abnormalities in 101 diabetic patients undergoing dipyridamole scintigraphy before vascular surgery. Cardiac complications occurred in 10 of the 71 patients (14%) who showed at least one reversible defect, as compared to 1 of 30 (3.3%) who demonstrated no redistribution defects. In that study for more optimal predictive accuracy for identifying high-risk patients, quantitation of the total number of redistribution defects, as well as assessment of ischemia in the distribution of the LAD coronary artery were required. Brown et al.[97] determined the ability of dipyridamole–Tl-201 imaging and resting radionuclide angiography to predict perioperative and long-term cardiac events in 36 uremic diabetic and 20 nondiabetic patients before renal transplant surgery. By logistic regression analysis of multiple clinical and radionuclide variables, presence of Tl-201 redistribution and LVEF were the only significant predictors of future cardiac events. No other patient variables, including diabetes or receiving a renal allograft, had either univariate or multivariate predictive value. Overall, five of six patients with cardiac events had either Tl-201–redistribution defects or a depressed EF.

Nesto et al.[98] investigated the incidence of silent myocardial ischemia and infarction as assessed by dipyridamole–Tl-201 scintigraphy in 30 diabetes patients with peripheral vascular disease but no clinical evidence of CAD. Fifty-seven per cent had Tl-201 perfusion abnormalities. Tl-201 scan defects were most frequent in patients who had hypertension and smoked cigarettes. The authors concluded that unsuspected CAD is common in this particular group of patients with diabetes.

Risk Stratification in Patients with Chronic Renal Disease

Pharmacologic stress imaging is helpful for identifying underlying CAD in patients with chronic renal disease and is often performed in working up such patients when renal transplantation is being contemplated. Marcen et al.[99] found perfusion defects on dipyridamole scans in 50% of patients receiving long-term hemodialysis who had no clinical manifestations of CAD. Perfusion abnormalities were associated with age over 50 years and aortic calcification. Camp et al.[100] reported that cardiac events occurred only in patients with reversible defect on Tl-201 scan who had diabetes and chronic renal disease. Of the six patients who experienced events, three had them before renal transplantation and three in the early postoperative phase.

Risk Stratification After Myocardial Infarction

Dipyridamole Imaging

Dipyridamole–Tl-201 imaging has proven useful and safe for risk assessment before hospital discharge for patients with an uncomplicated MI.[101, 102] The clinical applications of predischarge stress Tl-201 imaging after myocardial infarction are reviewed in Chapter 6. Leppo et al.[103] were first to show that dipyridamole–Tl-201 scintigraphy was safe in asymptomatic stable patients when performed 1 to 2 weeks after infarction. Fifty-one patients undergoing predischarge pharmacologic stress imaging were followed for an average of 19 months after discharge. Eleven of 12 patients who died during follow-up or sustained a recurrent infarction showed redistribution perfusion defects on their predischarge scans, as did 22 of 24 patients who required readmission for management of angina. Among all clinical and scintigraphic variables tested, the presence of redistribution on the dipyridamole Tl-201 scan was the only significant predictor of these subsequent cardiac events (Table 8–9). Exercise stress ECG was a less sensitive predictor of events than was dipyridamole imaging.

Pirelli et al.[104] performed predischarge Tl-201 scintigraphy in 35 patients with uncomplicated myocardial infarction and found that 11 had vasodilator-induced redistribution. They reported 93% sensitivity and 100% specificity for detecting inferior infarction, 87% sensitivity and 100% specificity for detecting anterior infarction, and 70% sensitivity and 100% specificity for detecting remote noninfarct stenotic vessels in inferior infarction, and 67% sensitivity and 100% specificity for detecting anterior infarction. Of the 11 patients with redistribution, 7 developed recurrent angina, as compared with 2 of 24 patients without redistribution.

Dipyridamole Tl-201 scintigraphy can safely be performed very soon (62 ± 21 hours) after hospitalization for acute MI.[105] No serious adverse reactions were experienced with the dipyridamole infusion protocol in this patient population. By stepwise multivariate logistic regression analysis, the best and only statistically significant predictor of in-hospital ischemic cardiac events was the presence of dipyridamole-induced Tl-201 redistribution within the infarct zone ($P = 0.0001$). Forty-five per cent of patients who demonstrated infarct zone redistribution developed in-hospital cardiac events. No patients without infarct zone redistribution had an event.

In postinfarction patients, Gimple et al.[106] reported that dipyridamole-induced Tl-201 redistribution defects outside of the infarct zone had a 63% sensitivity and 75% specificity for subsequent cardiac events. Redistribution outside the infarct zone was seen in 40% of patients who underwent testing. This implies that, like exercise scintigraphy, pharmacologic stress imaging is useful for identifying functionally significant multivessel CAD in postinfarction patients.

Miller et al.[107] assessed the acute hemodynamic effects of intravenous dipyridamole imaging on an average of 7 days following acute infarction in 10 stable patients. They showed that 30% of the patients developed ischemic ST-segment depression, and one third of those developed angina consequent to dipyridamole administration. There was a significant rise in the pulmonary capillary wedge pressure (from 13 to 17 mm Hg), and three patients developed new V waves in the pulmonary capillary wedge tracing. All

Table 8–9. Stepwise Logistic Regression Model to Predict Cardiac Events by Myocardial Infarction Patients After Dipyridamole Tl-201 Imaging

Predictor Term*	Step 0 No Predictor in Model		Step 1 After Redistribution in Model	
	χ^2	P Value	χ^2	P Value
Presence of redistribution (^{201}Tl)	5.92	0.02	5.92	0.02
Inferior MI	2.20	0.14	1.75	0.19
Propranolol use	2.14	0.14	1.79	0.18
Ejection fraction <35 (GBPS)	1.79	0.18	2.66	0.10
Mean no. of defects (^{201}Tl)	1.62	0.20	1.14	0.29
Anterior MI	1.44	0.23	1.99	0.16
Ejection fraction (GBPS)	0.89	0.35	1.89	0.17
Readmission for angina	0.80	0.37	0.11	0.74
No. of transient defects (^{201}Tl)	0.59	0.44	0.73	0.39
Nontransmural MI	0.11	0.74	0.01	0.93
Sex	0.11	0.74	0.01	0.93
Age	0.04	0.84	0.10	0.75
No. of persistent defects (^{201}Tl)	0.00	0.96	1.51	0.22

Key: ^{201}Tl, thallium-201 myocardial scan; GBPS, gated blood-pool scan.
(Reprinted by permission of *The New England Journal of Medicine* from Leppo JA, et al.: N Engl J Med 1984;310:1014–1018, copyright 1984, Massachusetts Medical Society.)

three patients had associated Tl-201 redistribution in segments appropriate to the LAD. Those patients who developed an abnormal elevated wedge pressure but who had a normal baseline wedge pressure had underlying multivessel disease with Tl-201 redistribution on dipyridamole scintigrams. Nienaber et al.[108] showed that redistribution within or remote from an infarct zone on dipyridamole scans yielded sensitivity of 85% and specificity of 78% for the detection of significant collateral circulation in a group of 80 consecutive postinfarction patients. In the presence of collaterals, remote reversible defects were larger than in their absence. Similarly, the extent of combined periinfarctional and remote redistribution was greater in collateralized patients, whereas the size of persistent defects was similar in collateralized and noncollateralized groups.

Hendel et al.[109] examined the utility of dipyridamole–Tl-201 scintigraphy in the prediction of late cardiac death and recurrent MI in 71 postinfarction patients who received thrombolytic therapy. They found that no scintigraphic variable was predictive of MI or death in this patient population; however, it should be pointed out that coronary angioplasty was performed in 29 patients before hospital discharge. There were only two deaths in this study, and most events were recurrent infarction in the 10 patients who experienced a subsequent event.

Adenosine Imaging

Adenosine–Tl-201 SPECT imaging was utilized to risk stratify patients early after MI in a series of 125 patients.[110] The test proved to be safe in this patient subgroup and revealed areas of residual myocardial ischemia. The group from Baylor University related adenosine SPECT infarct size on adenosine–Tl-201 imaging to future cardiac events in patients who were imaged after an uncomplicated MI.[111] The perfusion defect size was larger ($P = 0.0001$) in pa-

tients who had in-hospital cardiac events (45% ± 18%) than in those who did not (22% ± 15%). Ninety per cent of patients with events had at least a 20% perfusion defect, as compared with only 38% of those without events ($P = 0.0001$). Perfusion defect size was 51% ± 14% in patients who developed congestive heart failure, died, or developed ventricular tachycardia. Also in that study, the overall sensitivity for detecting individual coronary stenosis was 87%. Sixty-three per cent of patients with two-vessel CAD and 91% of patients with three-vessel CAD had a multivessel scan pattern. Table 8–10 relates the total adenosine perfusion defect size to subsequent cardiac events in patients enrolled in this study.

Thus, both dipyridamole and adenosine pharmacologic stress perfusion imaging are useful for separating high- and low-risk subsets of postinfarction patients who have experienced an uncomplicated hospital course. Either technique can be safely employed as a substitute for exercise stress scintigraphy and can be performed as early as three days after onset of symptoms of infarction. The advantage of pharmacologic stress over exercise stress is that it can be used early in the course of an uncomplicated infarction when patients are not yet ready to exercise on a treadmill or bicycle. This permits identifying low-risk patients early who might be candidates for early discharge at 4 to 5 days. Such low-risk patients would not require coronary arteriography.

Side Effects: Dipyridamole

Considerable data are available on the safety and side effects of intravenous dipyridamole infusion using the 0.56-mg/kg dose that is often employed in the United States for scintigraphy. Ranhosky and Kempthorne-Rowson reported on dipyridamole safety data from 3911 patients collected

Table 8–10. **Adenosine SPECT Perfusion Defect Size: Cardiac Events**

	No Complications (N = 52)	Chest Pain (N = 14)	CHF/Death/VT (N = 25/1/2)	Total Complications (N = 41)
PDS (total)	22% ± 15%	33% ± 19%*	51% ± 14%‡	45% ± 18%‡
PDS (ischemia)	10% ± 10%	21% ± 16%†	18% ± 14%§	19% ± 14%‖
PDS (scar)	12% ± 10%	12% ± 8%	33% ± 10%‡	26% ± 16%‡

Key: CHF, congestive heart failure; PDS, perfusion defect size; VT, ventricular tachycardia.
*P = 0.047 vs. no complications.
†P = 0.01 vs. no complications.
‡P = 0.0001 vs. no complications.
§P = 0.004 vs. no complications.
‖P = 0.001 vs. no complications.
(Mahmarian JJ, et al.: Circulation 1993;87:1197–1210.)

from 64 investigators, which comprised the Boehringer Ingelheim Pharmaceuticals registry.[16] All adverse events that occurred within 24 hours after administration of dipyridamole were recorded. Ten patients (0.26%) had major adverse events, and 1820 (46.5%) had minor side effects. Two patients (0.05%) died as a consequence of myocardial infarction within 24 hours of testing, and two (0.05%) had nonfatal infarctions. One of the two patients who died and both patients with a nonfatal infarction had unstable angina just before dipyridamole imaging. It is not stated whether these three patients had "stabilized" with resolution of ischemic chest pain before the dipyridamole study was conducted. Six patients (0.15%) developed acute bronchospasm, which was reversed in all instances with intravenous aminophylline. Table 8–11 lists the frequency of lesser side effects recorded in patients who underwent dipyridamole Tl-201 imaging. Lesser side effects included chest pain (19.7%), headache (12.2%), dizziness (11.8%), nausea (4.6%), and hypotension (4.6%). ST-segment depression was seen in 7.5%, and chest pain developed in 19.7%. Ninety-seven per cent of patients receiving aminophylline to treat side effects experienced complete relief of symptoms.

Reports published since 1985 have suggested that, with appropriate patient selection and adequate monitoring during the dipyridamole infusion, the incidence of serious adverse reactions is negligible. Homma et al.[112] reported no deaths or infarctions in 293 consecutive patients who underwent dipyridamole–Tl-201 imaging. Hendel et al.[74] reported no life-threatening reactions from more than 500 procedures. In that study, chest pain occurred in 18% of patients during dipyridamole infusion, and ST-segment depression was reported in only 7%. Interestingly, aminophylline was required for only 17% of that patient population for management of side effects. Lewen et al.[113] reported a single patient who developed severe myocardial ischemia which persisted for 90 minutes and required emergency coronary angioplasty after dipyridamole imaging.

Dipyridamole–Tl-201 scintigraphy appears to be safe for elderly patients undergoing testing. Lam et al.[114] found comparable side-effect profiles for 101 patients who were at least 70 years of age and for 236 younger patients. No deaths or infarctions were observed in this total group of 337 patients undergoing testing. Similarly, Gerson et al.[115] found comparable incidences of side effects among patients less than 65 years of age and older than 65 years.

More and more patients who have recovered from an uncomplicated MI are undergoing dipyridamole–Tl-201 imaging for purposes of risk stratification. In five such studies comprising 247 patients who underwent intravenous dipyridamole–Tl-201 imaging within a few weeks after the onset of infarction, no major adverse cardiac events were reported.[116]

Most reports in the literature indicate that the incidence of chest pain is significantly higher than the incidence of ischemic ST-segment depression after dipyridamole infusion.[15] Some instances of chest pain after dipyridamole infusion are not secondary to myocardial ischemia from underlying CAD. Angina-like chest pain can be provoked by intravenous adenosine administration and subsequently reversed by aminophylline in normal healthy volunteers.[117] Pearlman and Boucher[118] reported that 9% of patients with angiographically normal coronary arteries developed chest pain during dipyridamole administration.

Table 8–11. **Adverse Events in Patients Who Underwent Intravenous Dipyridamole Thallium Imaging**

Adverse Event	Patients (N)	(%)
Chest pain	770	(19.7)
Headache	476	(12.2)
Dizziness	460	(11.8)
ST-T changes on ECG	292	(7.5)
Ventricular extrasystoles	204	(5.2)
Nausea	180	(4.6)
Hypotension	179	(4.6)
Flushing	132	(3.4)
Tachycardia	127	(3.2)
Pain (unspecified)	102	(2.6)
Dyspnea	100	(2.6)
Blood pressure lability	61	(1.6)
Hypertension	59	(1.5)
Paresthesia	49	(1.3)
Fatigue	45	(1.2)
Dyspepsia	38	(1.0)

Values are for adverse events reported by at least 1.0% of total (100.0%) number of patients (3911) studied.
(Ranhosky A, et al.: Circulation 1990;81:1205–1209.)

ST Depression and Vasodilator Stress

Ischemic ST-segment depression appears likely to be secondary to "coronary steal," which results in subendocardial underperfusion in the distribution of a stenotic coronary artery. Chambers and Brown[119] found that the presence of coronary collaterals and an increased rate-pressure product after dipyridamole infusion were significant predictors of ST-segment depression. They speculated that coronary collaterals facilitate steal when hyperemia occurs in the feeder vessel. Blood is directed away from the ischemic zone to the normally perfused myocardial zone, resulting in diminished collateral flow and, then, subendocardial ischemia. Villanueva et al.[120] showed that patients with more extensive perfusion abnormalities after dipyridamole infusion were more likely to develop ST depression than patients with lesser degrees of hypoperfusion. Tl-201 redistribution was seen in 64% of patients who exhibited ST depression during dipyridamole infusion, as compared with 38% of patients who had no associated ST depression. Those with ST depression had 2.3 ± 0.04 redistribution segments per patient; those without ST depression had 0.9 ± 0.1 redistribution segments ($P < 0.001$). Patients with ST depression, compared to those without, were older (64 ± 1 vs. 60 ± 1 years, $P < 0.03$) and had a higher frequency of chest pain ($57\% \pm 23\%$, $P < 0.001$) and a higher heart rate–pressure product (12.7 ± 0.6 vs. $11.2 \pm 0.2 \times 10^3$, $P < 0.008$) after dipyridamole.

Nishimura et al.[120a] examined the angiographic, hemodynamic, and Tl-201 scintigraphic determinants of adenosine-induced ECG ST-segment depression in patients with CAD. The presence of coronary collateral vessels ($P = 0.001$), systolic blood pressure at baseline ($P = 0.006$), and adenosine-induced ischemic chest pain ($P = 0.011$) were the only independent predictors of ischemic ST depression by logistic regression analysis. Perfusion defect size, number of diseased vessels, and age did not correlate with ST-segment depression. The latter finding is different from that reported by Villanueva et al.,[120] who found more ischemia by Tl-201 scintigraphy in patients who manifested ST segment depression with dipyridamole imaging.

Thus, the ECG reflection of ischemia during vasodilatation may be related to presence of collaterals, hemodynamic factors, the severity of hypoperfusion, evidenced by a larger number of redistribution-type defects and an increase in myocardial oxygen demand reflected by a higher double product.[120b]

Caution should be exercised in performing dipyridamole Tl-201 imaging in patients with pulmonary disease and a history of recent bronchospasm. If a patient with pulmonary disease and evidence for bronchospasm requires stress scintigraphy, then dobutamine is an adequate alternative agent to dipyridamole or adenosine. This is assuming that an exercise test cannot be performed.

Thus, with respect to side effects, it appears that dipyridamole scintigraphy is relatively safe for patients without active unstable angina or recent manifestations of bronchospasm. Aminophylline and nitroglycerin are both effective in rapidly reversing both minor and major side effects. All patients receiving intravenous dipyridamole for myocardial perfusion imaging should be monitored continuously. If chest pain, ST-segment depression, or hemodynamic instability occurs, aminophylline should be promptly administered intravenously.

Side Effects: Adenosine

According to Verani,[121] of 5552 patients who underwent adenosine Tl-201 imaging, only one instance of MI occurred. One case of pulmonary edema and one episode of syncope were observed in this cohort. A side effect unique to adenosine and rarely seen with dipyridamole is high-grade AV conduction block. It is seen in approximately 6% of patients. The degree and duration of AV block appear to be related to preexisting sick sinus syndrome, AV conduction system disease, the concomitant use of beta-adrenergic and calcium-blocking drugs, and the rate and concentration of adenosine infusion. Third-degree block is reported in fewer than 1% of patients receiving the drug. AV block is not responsive to atropine[14] but promptly resolves with cessation of adenosine infusion. Aminophylline also rapidly reverses AV block secondary to adenosine administration. Minor side effects with adenosine are quite prevalent: flushing, nausea, headache, lightheadedness, and dizziness are common complaints. In one reported study by Coyne et al.,[21] shortness of breath was a complaint in 62% of patients receiving adenosine infusion. This sensation of dyspnea is due to adenosine-induced hyperventilation.

The safety profile of adenosine infusion was analyzed in 607 patients enrolled in a multicenter study.[19] In this patient population, flushing occurred in 35%, chest pain in 34%, headache in 21%, and dyspnea in 19%. As with dipyridamole, many patients may develop chest pain during adenosine infusion without associated redistribution defects. In this multicenter trial, concomitance of chest pain and ischemic ST depression was seen in only 6% of patients, but, when present it predicted perfusion abnormalities in 73% of patients. Despite the high incidence of side effects, for only six patients (1%) was it necessary to discontinue the infusion. No cases of cardiac death or infarction were reported. In another multicenter trial reported by Gupta et al.,[54] adenosine infusion caused side effects in 82% of patients. The most common side effects were flushing (41%), chest pain (24%), dyspnea (23%), throat or neck tightness (20%), and dizziness (20%). No subject experienced a life-threatening or serious adverse reaction such as MI, hypotension (systolic pressure below 90 mm Hg), or complete heart block. Table 8–12 summarizes the incidence of cardiac and noncardiac side effects from adenosine infusion in the 144 patients who comprised this study cohort. Finally, Cerqueira et al.[121a] reported the safety profile of adenosine

Table 8–12. **Incidence of Cardiac and Noncardiac Side Effects from Adenosine Infusion in 144 Patients**

Side Effects	(No.)	(%)
Cardiac		
Chest pain	35	(24)
Dyspnea	33	(23)
ST depression >1 mm	12	(8)
AV block		
First-degree	3	(2)
Second degree	1	(1)
Third degree	0	
Noncardiac		
Flushing	59	(41)
Temporomandibular joint discomfort	29	(20)
Lightheadedness	29	(20)
Nausea	15	(10)
Headache	17	(12)
Paresthesia	6	(4)
Miscellaneous	10	(7)
Total number of patients reporting side effects	118	(82)

(Reprinted with permission from the American College of Cardiology (Journal of the American College of Cardiology, 1992, Vol. 19, pp. 248–257).)

stress perfusion imaging from a registry comprising 9256 consecutive patients receiving 140 µg/kg/minute infusion of adenosine. The protocol was terminated early in 7% of patients with 81.1% reporting minor and well-tolerated side effects. There were no deaths, one MI, and seven episodes of bronchospasm. Seventy-two patients experienced transient third-degree AV block. Interpretable nuclear studies were obtained in 98.7% of patients.

Limitations of Vasodilator Thallium-201 Scintigraphy

In some patients, significant hepatic and splanchnic Tl-201 uptake with dipyridamole infusion can be seen which only occasionally interferes with cardiac Tl-201 analysis. This uptake occurs because the vascular bed of the liver and other splanchnic organs dilates in response to dipyridamole or adenosine, thus enhancing Tl-201 uptake in these organs. With exercise stress there is splanchnic constriction, and less Tl-201 uptake adjacent to the diaphragmatic border of the heart is observed. With dipyridamole scintigraphy, regional clearance abnormalities are not as reliable a reflection of abnormal Tl-201 kinetics as with exercise scintigraphy. The clearance of Tl-201 is significantly slower after intravenous dipyridamole than after exercise.[34, 34a] In the study by Varma et al.,[34] where exercise scintigraphy and dipyridamole scintigraphy were compared in the same patient population, there was a 21% decrease in Tl-201 activity between initial and delayed images after exercise, but only a 12% reduction in Tl-201 activity after dipyridamole ($P < 0.001$). In that study, 34% of myocardial segments demonstrated flat Tl-201 washout after dipyridamole, as compared to only 15% of segments showing flat Tl-201 washout after exercise. Thus, if abnormal segmental clear-

ance were employed as a criterion for a perfusion abnormality, more false-positive interpretations would result with dipyridamole than with exercise scintigraphy.

As with exercise scintigraphy, attenuation artifacts causing false-positive interpretation are seen with dipyridamole scintigraphy. The most common attenuation artifacts are due to an overlying breast shadow or a high diaphragm causing diminishing Tl-201 activity measured from the posterior wall.

PHARMACOLOGIC STRESS IMAGING WITH TECHNETIUM-99m–LABELED AGENTS

Technetium-99m Sestamibi

The basic myocardial kinetics of Tc-99m–sestamibi uptake are reviewed in Chapter 2. Pharmacologic stress myocardial perfusion imaging can be performed in conjunction with intravenous administration of Tc-99m sestamibi. Glover and Okada[122] showed that the initial myocardial uptake of Tc-99m sestamibi was linearly related ($r = 0.97$) to regional myocardial blood flow at rates up to 2.0 ml/min/g in dogs with an experimental stenosis receiving intravenous dipyridamole infusion. Gamma camera images showed initial defects without delayed redistribution over 4 hours. Patients with or without CAD have been shown to have comparable Tc-99m sestamibi uptake by SPECT imaging using exercise, dipyridamole, or adenosine as the form of stress.[122a] Similarly, no differences were observed between dipyridamole and adenosine images performed in the same patients with respect to defect size, ischemia extent, and defect severity. Figure 8–30 summarizes the results of this study.

Results of several clinical studies have been reported in patients known or suspected to have CAD who underwent dipyridamole Tc-99m–sestamibi perfusion imaging.[123–126a] Figure 8–31 shows dipyridamole and rest Tc-99m–sestamibi images in a patient who recently had an acute MI. Note that defects in the infarct zone of the inferior wall show residual stress-induced ischemia characterized by increasing Tc-99m sestamibi uptake after the resting injection. Tartagni[123] reported comparable sensitivity and specificity values for CAD detection for Tc-99m sestamibi and Tl-201. Sensitivity for identification of stenotic vessels by Tl-201 was 68% for the LAD, 89% for the RCA, and 80% for the Cx vessel, as compared with 75%, 89%, and 80%, respectively, for Tc-99m sestamibi. Specificity values were also comparable with respect to individual stenosis detection. Kettunen et al.[124] combined high-dose dipyridamole infusion (0.7 mg/kg) and handgrip stress in conjunction with Tc-99m–sestamibi tomographic imaging. The sensitivity for detection of CAD was 95% with this technique: 82% of stenotic lesions (more than 50% diameter narrowing) were correctly identified. Overall, the individual vessel de-

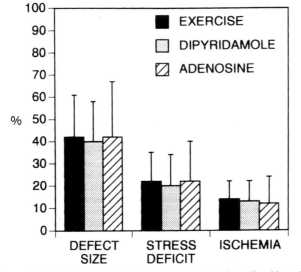

Figure 8–30. Percentage defect sizes after exercise, dipyridamole, and adenosine are similar, as shown in the first three bars. The stress deficit (middle bars), reflecting both extent and severity of perfusion defects, and percentage ischemia (right three bars) were also similar for the three stress modalities. (Santos-Ocampo CD, Herman SD, Travin MI, et al.: J Nucl Cardiol 1994;1:57–64.)

tection rate was 78%. The percent diameter reduction in the diameter of the stenoses were more severe in the vessels detected with Tc-99m sestamibi than in those not detected (87 vs. 76%; $P < 0.01$). A subgroup of these patients also underwent dipyridamole SPECT Tl-201 scintigraphy with an overall stenotic vessel detection rate comparable to that for Tc-99m sestamibi in the same patients (76% for Tl-201 and 83% for Tc-99m sestamibi).

In a multicenter trial comprising 101 patients with exertional chest pain and no history of MI reported by Parodi et al.,[125] high-dose dipyridamole stress imaging yielded an overall sensitivity, specificity, and predictive accuracy for Tc-99m–sestamibi SPECT imaging of 81%, 90%, and 83%, respectively. The criterion for significant CAD in this study was at least 50% reduction in luminal diameter. Sensitivity for detection of single-vessel disease (68%) was less than that for two-vessel (100%) or three-vessel (87%) disease. Side effects occurred in 57% of patients receiving large doses of dipyridamole. Thus, despite a lower first-pass extraction fraction for Tc-99m sestamibi than for Tl-201 (see Chap. 2), the ability to detect significant coronary stenoses is comparable for both radionuclides.

Cuocolo et al.[125a] reported a 90% concordance rate between exercise and adenosine Tc-99m SPECT sestamibi studies with respect to identification of the perfusion status in 22 patients with CAD. Adenosine Tc-99m sestamibi imaging should yield comparable diagnostic accuracy as dipyridamole Tc-99m sestamibi imaging for CAD detection and risk stratification.

Tc-99m sestamibi imaging with dipyridamole stress is reported to also provide useful prognostic information.

Miller et al.[76b] followed up 137 consecutive patients with either unstable angina (n = 106) or recent uncomplicated infarction (n = 31) who underwent predischarge risk stratification with intravenous dipyridamole stress Tc-99m myocardial SPECT imaging. At 10 ± 5 months, cardiac events occurred more frequently in patients with abnormal scintigraphic results (Fig. 8–32A). Multivariate stepwise logistic regression models identified an abnormal Tc-99m sestamibi study and either fixed or reversible perfusion defects as being predictive of death or nonfatal myocardial infarction.

STRESS   **REST**

MID SHORT AXIS

DISTAL SHORT AXIS

VERTICAL LONG AXIS

HORIZONTAL LONG AXIS

Figure 8–31. Post-dipyridamole (STRESS) and rest (REST) Tc-99m sestamibi SPECT images in a patient with a recent inferior wall infarction. Note inferoapical and inferior defects on stress images, which show partial reversibility on the rest images. This pattern is consistent with residual viable myocardium at jeopardy in the infarct zone.

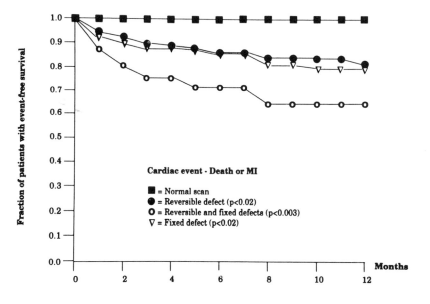

Figure 8–32. Event-free survival related to type of perfusion abnormalities on dipyridamole Tc-99m sestamibi SPECT images. (Miller DD: J Nucl Cardiol 1994;1:172–174.)

Technetium-99m Teboroxime

The basic physiologic properties of Tc-99m teboroxime are reviewed in Chapter 2. Tc-99m teboroxime can be used in conjunction with dipyridamole or adenosine infusion for detection of CAD.[126–127] Labonte et al.,[126] employing a planar imaging technique, found good correlation between dipyridamole Tl-201 and Tc-99m–teboroxime imaging for detecting significant coronary artery stenosis. Seventy-three per cent of significantly stenotic coronary arteries were detected by Tl-201 dipyridamole imaging and 64% by dipyridamole Tc-99m–teboroxime imaging. Tc-99m–teboroxime imaging has also been undertaken with adenosine infusion.[127] In this study, 4 minutes into the adenosine infusion, 20 to 25 mCi of Tc-99m teboroxime was injected, and imaging started 2 minutes later. SPECT imaging was characterized by the use of a 180-degree anterior arc and 32 stops at 10 seconds per stop. This yielded a total imaging time of 7.8 minutes. Rest images were obtained 60 and 90 minutes later. In the 20 patients enrolled, Tc-99m–teboroxime images were abnormal in 15 of 16 (94%) patients with CAD and in two of four (50%) normal subjects. There was agreement between Tc-99m–teboroxime and exercise SPECT Tl-201 imaging, performed in the same patients within 2 weeks of the teboroxime studies, in 80% of patients and 80% of segments. Of interest, the two normal subjects with abnormal adenosine Tc-99m teboroxime images had apparent fixed inferior wall defects. The SPECT Tl-201 scans were normal in these patients. These two normal patients exhibited intense Tc-99m–teboroxime uptake in the left lobe of the liver. The authors point out that uptake of teboroxime in the liver is considerable since adenosine does not result in a redistribution of regional cardiac output as exercise stress does. Figure 8–33 shows

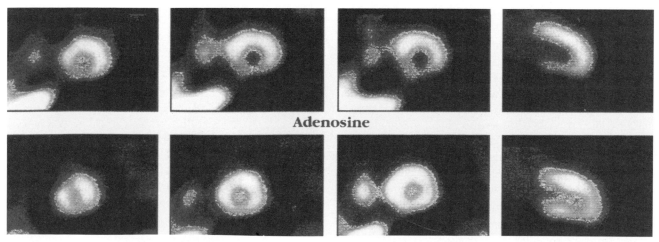

See Color Figure 8–33.

Figure 8–33. Teboroxime SPECT images obtained after adenosine and after rest demonstrating a reversible inferior defect. (See Color Figure 8–33.) (Reprinted with permission from the American College of Cardiology (Journal of the American College of Cardiology, 1992, Vol. 19, pp. 307–312).)

Tc-99m–teboroxime images in a patient included in this study. Chua et al.,[127a] employing rapid back-to-back adenosine stress and rest Tc-99m–teboroxime imaging protocol using a triple-detector camera, found that image quality was only fair to good for three-quarters of the patients studied. The frequency of severe liver interference increased with duration of imaging time and was 30% with the 2- to 8-minute images (compared to 3% for the 1- to 2-minute images).

The technical limitations of acquiring SPECT images with Tc-99m teboroxime may be significant. Because of the rapid washout of Tc-99m teboroxime after initial uptake (Chap. 2), a rapid imaging protocol must be utilized (Chap. 3). Marked hepatic uptake of the tracer with pharmacologic stress imaging may interfere with optimal image analysis.

VASODILATOR STRESS ECHOCARDIOGRAPHY

Echocardiography performed in conjunction with pharmacologic stress for detection of ischemia-induced regional wall motion abnormalities is an alternative to radionuclide imaging for detection of CAD and for assessing prognosis. The quality of the test results is very operator dependent, and adequate images for interpretation are obtained from approximately 90% of subjects. True ischemia with regional systolic dysfunction is required to render a test result abnormal. Theoretically, the sensitivity of stress echocardiography for CAD detection should be lower than the sensitivity of stress perfusion imaging, since the latter requires only abnormal flow reserve for a positive or abnormal test response. Abnormal flow reserve–producing heterogeneity of tracer uptake can occur without ischemic myocardial dysfunction.

Detection of Myocardial Ischemia

Continuous two-dimensional (2-D) echocardiographic recording during dipyridamole infusion can be employed for detection of CAD. An abnormal test is usually defined as one demonstrating transient asynergy of contraction that was absent or of lesser degree in the baseline examination. The dipyridamole dose employed to obtain maximum sensitivity is often larger (0.75 to 0.84 mg/kg) than that utilized for myocardial Tl-201–dipyridamole imaging (0.56 mg/kg). In a study by Picano et al.,[128] of 93 patients with exertional chest pain, 38 had a positive low-dose dipyridamole echocardiography test (0.56 mg/kg), and 15 additional patients had a positive test only with the large dose (0.84 mg/kg). The overall sensitivity for CAD detection was 74%, and specificity 100%. In 83 patients with exertional chest pain and either a negative or a nondiagnostic exercise ECG stress test, large-dose dipyridamole echocardiography was positive in 54% of the patients with CAD who had electro-

cardiographically "silent" myocardial ischemia.[129] Dipyridamole echocardiography was shown to be associated with significantly greater specificity than exercise electrocardiography (93% vs. 52%, $P < 0.001$) in 83 consecutive women evaluated for a chest pain syndrome.[130] The sensitivity and predictive value for a negative test were similar for dipyridamole echocardiography and exercise electrocardiography (79% vs. 72% and 84% vs. 68%; respectively) in this study.

Dipyridamole 2-D echocardiography was compared to Tl-201 perfusion imaging in the same patients in a study by Ferrara et al.[131] There was excellent correlation between the wall-by-wall comparison of the distribution of dipyridamole-induced echocardiographic asynergy with reversible Tl-201 perfusion defects. Dipyridamole-induced wall motion abnormalities and myocardial perfusion defects were detected, respectively, in 63% and 70% of patients with significant CAD.

Assessing Functional Severity of Coronary Artery Disease

Picano et al.[132] utilized dipyridamole 2-D echocardiography to assess the functional significance of a coronary artery stenosis. Patients with CAD who demonstrated increased coronary blood flow, as measured by the coronary sinus thermodilution technique, showed no regional asynergy in response to dipyridamole. In contrast, impairment in regional contractility was associated with a lesser increase in coronary sinus blood flow. Thus, coronary artery stenoses of similar angiographic severity can produce different reductions in coronary reserve capacity. Only patients with significantly abnormal flow reserve demonstrated an impairment in regional systolic function by echocardiography after dipyridamole infusion. Severity of an anatomic stenosis and impairment of flow reserve are greater when dipyridamole-induced wall motion abnormalities appear early during the test.[132a] In this study, regional flow by PET measurements was lower in zones becoming akinetic with dipyridamole infusion compared with zones demonstrating hypokinesia.

Margonato et al.[133] showed that in patients with severe angina and multivessel CAD, dipyridamole 2-D echocardiography appeared to identify the "culprit" vessel in which flow reserve was most limited. Nine of eleven patients with multivessel disease and a positive echocardiographic response exhibited angina and ST-segment depression.

As with dipyridamole Tl-201 scintigraphy, dipyridamole echocardiography can yield important prognostic information. Picano et al.[134] determined the value of dipyridamole echocardiography in comparison with clinical and ECG variables in predicting cardiac events in 539 consecutive patients referred for the dipyridamole echocardiography tests. A Cox survival analysis identified "echocardiographic positivity" after dipyridamole administration as the best predictor of cardiac events (relative risk ratio, 2:7).

The next most powerful predictor was angina after dipyridamole administration.

Bolognese et al.[135] showed that large-dose dipyridamole echocardiography could identify high-risk multivessel disease patients after uncomplicated MI. Transient remote asynergy on echocardiography was present in 27 of 40 patients with multivessel disease and in none of 33 patients without multivessel disease. The sensitivity of dipyridamole-induced transient remote asynergy for multivessel disease detection was 68%, compared with 52% for treadmill testing. The overall accuracy of dipyridamole echocardiography (81%) was better than that of dipyridamole stress ECG (63%), or exercise ECG (60%) ($P < 0.02$).

Dipyridamole echocardiography has been useful in detecting patients with restenosis after coronary angioplasty.[136, 137] Picano et al.[137] reported that at an average follow-up of 10.8 months after angioplasty, angina recurred in 8 of 47 patients (17%) whose high-dose dipyridamole echocardiogram was negative, as compared with 11 of 16 (69%) whose echocardiogram was positive.

Cates et al.[138] employed radionuclide ventriculography to assess changes in regional function with dipyridamole infusion rather than 2-D echocardiography. In normal patients, the EF increased 5.6% ± 2% during exercise and 7.9 ± 1 units after dipyridamole. However, in patients with CAD, the EF failed to increase during exercise or after dipyridamole. ROC analysis demonstrated general comparability between the sensitivity and specificity of exercise and dipyridamole ventriculography. In patients with more than 70% coronary stenosis, the sensitivity of dipyridamole ventriculography was 67%, and specificity 92%. This compared with 89% sensitivity and 67% specificity for exercise ventriculography. Thus, dipyridamole radionuclide ventriculography does not provide adequate sensitivity for detection of CAD. This technique is rarely used in clinical practice.

Whitfield et al.[139] sought to determine if isometric handgrip performed in conjunction with dipyridamole echocardiography would enhance detection of regional wall motion abnormalities induced by the drug in patients with CAD. In this study, only five of 24 patients with Tl-201 redistribution had new wall motion abnormalities after dipyridamole infusion. The addition of isometric handgrip to the imaging protocol did not distinguish between patients with and without new wall motion abnormalities on Tl-201 redistribution. Interestingly, the extent of Tl-201 redistribution was greater in the five patients who demonstrated new asynergy on echocardiography as compared with the 19 who did not.

The incremental diagnostic information of Tl-201 scintigraphic data was greater than that of data from dipyridamole echocardiography in 102 patients with a clinical suspicion of CAD studied by DiBello et al.[139a] Clinical data were 73% accurate in the prediction of CAD. The addition of dipyridamole echocardiographic data to the clinical model yielded a diagnostic accuracy of 88%, whereas the addition of Tl-201 scintigraphic variables to the clinical model improved diagnostic accuracy to 94%.

Risk Stratification Prior to Vascular Surgery

Dipyridamole echocardiography can be employed to identify high-risk patients undergoing peripheral vascular surgery. Tischler evaluated the role of dipyridamole echocardiography in predicting major cardiac events in 109 unselected patients undergoing elective peripheral vascular surgery.[140] Of the 109 patients, nine (8%) had positive studies, defined as development of new regional wall motion abnormalities or worsening of a preexisting wall motion abnormality. Of these nine patients, seven had postoperative events—three cardiac deaths, one nonfatal MI, and two cases of unstable angina. Only one cardiac event occurred among the 100 patients with negative studies. The sensitivity and specificity of dipyridamole echocardiography for predicting cardiac events after vascular surgery were 88% and 98%, respectively. The relative risk of a cardiac event if the dipyridamole echocardiogram was abnormal was 78.

Dipyridamole Echocardiography After Myocardial Infarction

Bolognese et al.[141] performed dipyridamole echocardiography 8 to 10 days after acute MI in 76 consecutive patients treated with urokinase. Large-dose dipyridamole infusion, 0.84 mg/kg over 10 minutes, was employed. A patent infarct-related vessel with a critical residual stenosis was significantly more prevalent in patients with dipyridamole-induced wall motion abnormalities in the infarct zone than in those without such wall motion abnormalities. Among 23 patients with occluded infarct-related vessels, nine had collateral flow to the distal vessel; six of these had a positive dipyridamole echocardiogram. Thus, the sensitivity and specificity for identifying a critically stenotic but patent infarct-related vessel or the presence of a collateral-dependent zone were 66% and 93%, respectively. Camerieri et al.[141a] evaluated the prognostic utility of dipyridamole echocardiography in patients older than 65 years who survived an uncomplicated MI. Figure 8–34 shows that the mortality rate at a mean follow-up of 14 ± 9.8 months was 13% for patients with a positive test and 3% for those with a negative test result ($P < 0.01$).

Dipyridamole Magnetic Resonance Imaging

Large-dose (0.75 mg/kg over 10 minutes) dipyridamole infusion in conjunction with magnetic resonance imaging (MRI) has also been undertaken for detection of CAD. Baer et al.[142] reported abnormal dipyridamole MRI images (deterioration of wall motion) in 78% of patients with CAD; sensitivity was 69% and 90%, respectively, for detection of one- and two-vessel disease. Sensitivities for detection of LAD, LCx, and RCA lesions were 78%, 73%, and 88%, respectively, and specificities of 100%, 100%, and 87%. Pennell et al.[143] reported 96% sensitivity for CAD detection

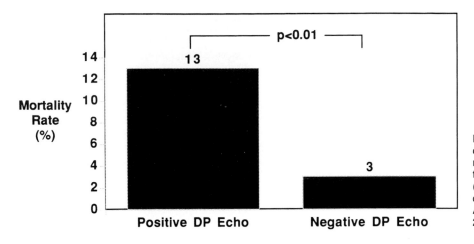

Figure 8–34. Mortality rate after uncomplicated MI in patients with a positive dipyridamole (DP) echocardiogram (echo) and patients with a negative DP echocardiogram. (Reprinted with permission from the American College of Cardiology (Journal of the American College of Cardiology, 1993, Vol. 22, pp. 1809–1815).)

in 25 patients with exertional chest pain using dobutamine Tl-201 tomography. Ninety-one percent had reversible wall motion abnormalities as shown by dobutamine cine-MRI. Comparison of abnormal segments of perfusion and wall motion showed 96% agreement at rest, 90% agreement during stress, and 91% agreement of functional reversibility. van Rugge et al.[143a] studied 39 CAD patients and 10 normal volunteers with gradient echo MRI imaging at rest and during peak dobutamine stress. Using a modification of the centerline methods for quantitative wall motion analysis, the overall sensitivity of dobutamine MRI for the detection of significant CAD (≥50% stenosis) was 91% with a specificity of 80%. All patients with three-vessel CAD were detected. Thus, it appears that dobutamine MRI could yield greater sensitivity for detection of CAD than small-dose dipyridamole imaging with myocardial perfusion tracers or large-dose dipyridamole echocardiography or MRI, though the expense of this technique is substantial.

Adenosine Stress Echocardiography

Adenosine infusion at a dose of 140 μg/kg/minute has been used in combination with 2-D echocardiography for detection of CAD similar to the approach utilized for dipyridamole echocardiography.[144–145a] Zoghbi et al.[144] assessed the diagnostic accuracy of adenosine echocardiography in 73 patients with known or suspected CAD. Sensitivity for CAD detection (more than 75% stenosis) was 85%, with a specificity of 92% in patients with normal coronary arteries. In patients with a normal baseline ECG, sensitivity was reduced to 60%. Detection of all coronary arteries was observed in 69% of the 87 diseased vessels. Figure 8–35 summarizes the results of this study. Heinle et al.[145a] found 92% concordance between adenosine echocardiography and adenosine Tl-201 imaging in patients being evaluated for suspected CAD.

DOBUTAMINE STRESS IMAGING

Dobutamine Thallium-201 Imaging

Intravenous dobutamine infusion has been utilized in combination with Tl-201 scintigraphy and 2-D echocardiography for detection of CAD and for assessing cardiac risk before vascular surgery.[146–148d] The rationale for using this pharmacologic approach is that, in the presence of a significant coronary stenosis, dobutamine infusion produces systolic wall motion abnormalities because it increases myocardial oxygen demand by increasing heart rate, blood pressure, and myocardial contractility. This results in a mismatch between oxygen supply and demand in the presence of a functionally significant coronary stenosis. In an experimental study reported by Fung et al.,[146] dobutamine was more effective than dipyridamole in inducing regional myo-

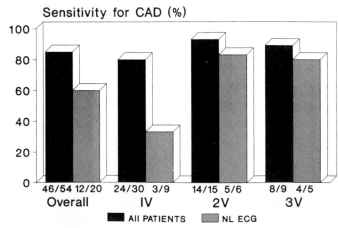

Figure 8–35. Overall sensitivity of adenosine echocardiography for detection of CAD in patients with a normal baseline ECG as well as all patients enrolled in the study. Data are also shown for sensitivity of detecting one-vessel (1V), two-vessel (2V), and three-vessel (3V) disease. Note the low sensitivity of adenosine echocardiography for detecting single-vessel disease in patients with a normal resting ECG. (Reprinted with permission from the American College of Cardiology (Journal of the American College of Cardiology, 1991, Vol. 18, pp. 1271–1279).)

Table 8–13. **Overall Sensitivity and Specificity of Dobutamine Tl-201 Tomography for Detection of Coronary Artery Disease**

Coronary Artery Disease	Dobutamine Tl-201 Myocardial Perfusion Tomography			
	Abnormal	Normal	Sensitivity	Specificity
Present (N = 40)	39	1	97%	——
Absent (N = 10)	2	8	——	80%

Tl-201 tomography was significantly superior to exercise ECG in the detection of CAD (P < 0.01).
(Reprinted with permission from the American College of Cardiology (Journal of the American College of Cardiology, 1991, Vol. 18, pp. 1471–1479).)

cardial dysfunction for similar coronary lesions. These authors concluded that, for imaging modalities that rely on functional assessment, such as echocardiography, dobutamine may be superior to a vasodilator stress agent. In contrast, dipyridamole induces greater blood flow heterogeneity than dobutamine, which prompted the authors to conclude that, for myocardial perfusion scintigraphy, dipyridamole (or adenosine) may be superior to dobutamine as the pharmacologic stressor of choice. With this technique dobutamine is first diluted to a concentration of 1 mg/ml and then infused at incremental doses of 5, 10, 20, 30, and 40 μg/kg/minute at 3-minute intervals.[148b] After 1 minute of the maximally tolerated dose, 3.0 mCi of Tl-201 is injected through a peripheral intravenous line (not the same line used for drug infusion). The dobutamine infusion is continued for another 2 minutes after Tl-201 administration. Blood pressure, heart rate, and the 12-lead ECG are recorded every minute during the test. Hays et al.[148b] terminated the infusion for systolic blood pressure over 230 mm Hg or diastolic pressure over 130 mm Hg, a decrease in blood pressure below 80 mm Hg, more than 2.0 mm of ST-segment depression, severe angina, or the appearance of cardiac arrhythmia.

Pennell et al.[147] determined the value of dobutamine SPECT Tl-201 imaging in 50 patients with exertional chest pain undergoing coronary arteriography. Of the forty patients with CAD, 39 (97%) had a reversible perfusion defect on dobutamine tomograms, whereas 8 of 10 patients with normal coronary arteries had normal dobutamine scintigrams. In this study, dobutamine was infused in 5-minute stages at incremental rates from 5 to 20 μg/kg/minute or until symptoms appeared. Table 8–13 summarizes the findings of this study. Note that, as with exercise Tl-201 scintigraphy, the detection rate for LCx disease is less (40%) than for LAD and RCA lesions. Seventy-eight per cent of patients developed chest pain as the limiting symptom. Thirty-eight per cent developed some arrhythmia, most being ventricular or atrial premature beats. Noncardiac side effects were chiefly skin tingling and flushing. Systolic blood pressure rose from 135 to 162 mm Hg, and heart rate from 72 to 120 bpm from baseline to the maximum dose of 20 μg/kg/minute. Hays et al.[148] reported a large series of 144 patients who underwent SPECT dobutamine Tl-201 imaging. Overall sensitivity for CAD detection was 86% (90% specificity), values comparable to those achieved with

exercise or vasodilator stress imaging. Sensitivity was 84%, 82%, and 100%, respectively, in patients with single-, double-, and triple-vessel CAD. Table 8–14 shows the individual stenosis detection rate for dobutamine SPECT Tl-201 imaging in this study, a significant stenosis was defined as more than 50% narrowing. Sixty-eight per cent of all lesions were identified. Heart rate with dobutamine increased from 75 to 120 bpm and systolic blood pressure rose from 136 to 148 mm Hg. Approximately 75% of patients had some side effect, and 97% tolerated a dose of 30 μg/kg/minute.

Elliott et al.[148a] reported the feasibility of using dobutamine Tl-201 imaging for assessing cardiac risk before vascular surgery. Of 126 patients who underwent preoperative dobutamine Tl-201 imaging, 33% had reversible defects. Of those who underwent vascular surgery and had not previously had bypass surgery or angioplasty, 50% experienced a postoperative myocardial ischemic event. In this study, dobutamine Tl-201 scintigraphy was associated with sensitivity of 69%, specificity of 99%, and a predictive value of 82% for postoperative myocardial ischemic events. These results compare favorably with the data summarized previously regarding the prognostic utility of dipyridamole Tl-201 imaging for preoperative risk stratification. Dobutamine perfusion imaging can also be employed for risk stratification after uncomplicated myocardial infarction. Figure 8–36 shows post-dobutamine anterior and 45-degree left anterior oblique images with quantitative count profiles obtained six days after an acute anterior infarction treated within 1.5 hours with accelerated tissue plasminogen acti-

Table 8–14. **Individual Vessel Detection with Dobutamine SPECT**

Vessel	Overall Sensitivity	
	(No.)	(%)
Left anterior descending	14/25	56*†
Right coronary artery	34/39	87
Left circumflex	15/28	54
Total	63/92	68

*P = 0.005 versus right coronary artery.
†P = NS versus the left circumflex and the right coronary artery.
(Reprinted with permission from the American College of Cardiology (Journal of the American College of Cardiology, 1993, Vol. 21, pp. 1583–1590).)

vator infusion. Note that only very mild post-dobutamine apical and anteroseptal defects are observed.

Pennell et al.[148b] infused dobutamine into 30 asthmatic patients for SPECT Tl-201 imaging and found no episodes of bronchospasm, although limiting dyspnea appeared in association with reversible ischemia in eight patients. Tl-201 images were abnormal in ten of eleven with CAD and normal in seven of nine patients with normal coronary arteries. Chest pain occurred in 67% of patients.

Dobutamine Tc-99m Sestamibi Imaging

Dobutamine stress can be employed with Tc-99m sestamibi SPECT imaging for detection of CAD and for risk assessment. Herman et al.[148b] compared dobutamine Tc-99m sestamibi imaging with exercise stress imaging in 24 patients with a high likelihood of CAD. Global first-order agreement (normal vs. abnormal) between exercise and dobutamine studies was 96% (kappa value = 0.65; P = 0.02). Exercise and dobutamine stress scores were similar, as were defect size and number of abnormal segments.

Dobutamine Echocardiography

Dobutamine echocardiography has gained increasing popularity for stress imaging for detection of CAD and for identifying viability in regions of myocardial asynergy (see Chap. 9).[149–153o] The conventional protocol for dobutamine echocardiography is to record images in standard parasternal long-axis and short-axis, four-chamber and two-chamber views, digitized and displayed for comparison in a quad screen format. A 16-segment model is used for scoring wall motion abnormalities. Ischemia is considered to be present when a new wall motion abnormality is observed in a region with normal or only hypokinetic resting wall motion. A normal response to dobutamine is hyperdynamic wall motion, inward endocardial excursion of 5 mm, wall thickening, and a reduction in end-systolic cavity size. Sawada et al.[149] recorded echocardiograms during stepwise infusion of dobutamine to a maximum dose of 30 μg/kg/minute in 103 patients who also underwent quantitative coronary angiography. An abnormal test was defined as the development of a new regional wall motion abnormality. The sensitivity and specificity of dobutamine-induced wall motion abnormalities for CAD were 89% and 85%, respectively. Sensitivity was 81% for single-vessel disease and 100% for multivessel or left main disease. In that study, five patients experienced side effects deemed severe enough to terminate the dobutamine infusion. Overall, 18% experienced side effects during dobutamine infusion, which included nausea in five patients, apprehension or anxiety in five, headache and lightheadedness in three, tremors in three, palpitations in two, and chills in one. Cohen et al.[150] also reported high

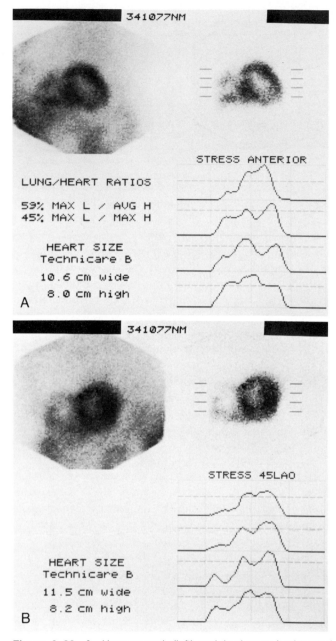

Figure 8–36. A. Unprocessed *(left)* and background-subtracted *(right)* anterior view Tl-201 image obtained with dobutamine stress in a patient with an uncomplicated anterior infarction treated with intravenous tissue plasminogen activator. The quantitative count profiles below the background-subtracted image show a mild reduction in apical Tl-201 activity *(bottom profile)*. **B.** A 45° left anterior oblique (LAO) post-dobutamine image in the same patient, showing a mild upper septal defect that just achieves numerical significance (second profile from the top) by quantitative criteria. Delayed images (not shown) demonstrated no redistribution.

rates of sensitivity (86%) and specificity (95%) for dobutamine echocardiography for detecting CAD. Heart rate was the most important physiologic determinant of ischemia induced by dobutamine.

Segar et al.[151] compared the results of dobutamine stress echocardiography with quantitative coronary angiography in 85 patients. The overall sensitivity of dobutamine echocardiography for detecting CAD (at least 50% stenosis) was 95%, with 82% specificity and 92% accuracy. Sensitivity for detecting individual stenoses in the three major coronary arteries was comparable. Stenosis detection improved when the lesion's minimal diameter was reduced to less than 1.0 mm. Dobutamine echocardiography is more sensitive than dobutamine ECG for CAD detection. Mazeika et al.[152] reported 78% sensitivity and 93% specificity for dobutamine echocardiography, as compared with sensitivity of 47% and specificity of 71% for the dobutamine ECG. These values for the exercise ECG were 72% and 71%, respectively. The peak rate-pressure product during dobutamine infusion was significantly less than that with exercise stress (18,845 vs. 23,740 mm Hg/minute; $P < 0.01$). Atropine can be added to dobutamine when no ischemia is induced by dobutamine alone and the peak heart rate is less than 85% of the age-predicted maximum heart rate. About one-third of these patients will develop new wall motion abnormalities.[152a] In this study an increased risk of ventricular arrhythmias with the combination of dobutamine and atropine was noted.

Side Effects

Cardiac side effects of dobutamine infusion are different from those encountered with pharmacologic stress and are similar to those seen with exercise testing. In 202 patients receiving dobutamine infusion in the University of Indiana experience, arrhythmias occurred in 15%.[149] No patient, however, had ventricular tachycardia or hypotension. Among a large number of patients (1118) collected by Mertes et al.[153a] dobutamine echocardiographic testing was terminated in 3% because of noncardiac side effects such as nausea, anxiety, headache, tremor, and urgency; 19.3% developed angina that required cessation of drug infusion, sublingual nitroglycerin, or a short-acting beta blocker. Frequent ventricular premature beats (at least 6/minute) was observed in 15% and frequent atrial premature beats was seen in 8%. Forty of the 1118 patients had nonsustained ventricular tachycardia; only one required pharmacologic therapy to terminate it.

Martin et al.[153] compared the results of adenosine, dipyridamole, and dobutamine echocardiography performed in the same patients. The sensitivity of dobutamine echocardiography (76%) was significantly greater than that of adenosine (40%) and of dipyridamole (56%) echocardiography, but it had lower specificity (60%). Specificity for adenosine and dipyridamole echocardiography was 93% and 67%, respectively. Adenosine caused second-degree heart block in 10% of patients. Interestingly, treatment for persistent symptoms after cessation of drug infusion was required by more patients after dipyridamole (40%) than after dobutamine (12%; $P < 0.001$) or adenosine (0%; $P < 0.001$) echocardiography. On the other hand, more patients

preferred dobutamine (48%) or dipyridamole (40%) over adenosine (12%).

Comparison with Other Techniques

Hoffman et al.[153c] reported no significant differences in sensitivity between exercise echocardiography (80%), dobutamine stress echocardiography (79%), and exercise sestamibi SPECT perfusion imaging (89%) for detection of CAD in 66 patients who underwent all three tests. All had higher sensitivity than the exercise ECG (52%). Specificity of SPECT sestamibi (71%) was lower than that of exercise echocardiography (87%) and dobutamine echocardiography (81%). These differences were not statistically significant. Günlap et al.[153e] compared dobutamine echocardiography with dobutamine Tc-99m–sestamibi SPECT imaging in 27 patients who also underwent coronary arteriography. Sensitivity and specificity of dobutamine sestamibi imaging were 94% and 88%, respectively, as compared with 84% and 88% for dobutamine echocardiography. Marwick et al.[153h] found that the sensitivity of adenosine sestamibi (86%), dobutamine sestamibi (80%), and dobutamine echocardiography (85%) was significantly better than that of adenosine echocardiography (58%) for detection of CAD. In this study the accuracy was comparable for adenosine sestamibi, dobutamine sestamibi, and dobutamine echocardiography. All were superior to the accuracy of adenosine echocardiography. In another study by Marwick et al.[153m] in 217 patients without previous infarction, sensitivity for detection of CAD was 72% for dobutamine echocardiography and 76% for dobutamine Tc-99m sestamibi imaging (Fig. 8–37). Specificity was higher for echocardiography (83% vs. 67%; $P = 0.05$). Of 31 patients with a negative submaximal dobutamine echocardiogram, 80% had a positive Tc-99m sestamibi perfusion scan. Simek et al.[153l] from the University of Virginia reported greater detection of ischemic zones by dipyridamole Tl-201 scintigraphy compared to dobutamine echocardiography. Verani[153n] presents a comprehensive critical discussion of the strengths and weaknesses of stress echocardiography and stress perfusion imaging. He suggests that perhaps the major weakness of 2-D echocardiography is the highly subjective assessment of wall motion abnormalities.

PHARMACOLOGIC STRESS IMAGING WITH POSITRON EMISSION TOMOGRAPHY

PET is clinically applicable for detection of CAD using intravenous dipyridamole or adenosine in conjunction with N-13 ammonia or rubidium-82 (Rb-82) as tracers of blood flow.[6, 154–161] The basis for using PET clinically for evaluation of blood flow is discussed in depth in Chapter 2. Utilizing this technique, baseline myocardial perfusion is first assessed, followed by evaluation of regional perfusion

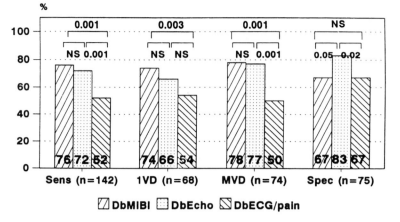

Figure 8–37. Results of dobutamine (Db) Tc-99m–sestamibi perfusion scintigraphy (MIBI), echocardiography (Echo), and ECG changes or anginal pain for the diagnosis of CAD. As shown, sensitivity for Db echo and Db MIBI for detection of one-vessel disease (1VD) and multivessel disease (MVD) was comparable. Specificity (spec) was better for Db echo than for Db MIBI. (Reprinted with permission from the American College of Cardiology (Journal of the American College of Cardiology, 1993, Vol. 22, pp. 159–167).)

after pharmacologic stress. A transmission image is initially acquired for correction for photon attenuation. An automated quantitative analysis program may enhance accuracy and reproducibility of cardiac PET flow studies.[161] Demer et al.[4] reported 94% sensitivity and 95% specificity for CAD detection in 193 patients with PET Rb-82 imaging. Several studies have compared PET imaging with Rb-82 with SPECT Tl-201 imaging. In a study by Go et al.,[158] sensitivity for CAD detection following the same pharmacologic stress was 93% for PET and 76% for Tl-201 SPECT. Overall specificities were comparable: 78% and 80%, respectively. The authors stated, ''The improved contrast resolution of PET resulted in markedly superior images and a more confident identification of defects.'' In another study by Stewart et al.[159] comprising 81 patients, the sensitivity, specificity, and overall accuracy were 84%, 88%, and 85%, respectively, with Rb-82 dipyridamole PET, as compared with 84%, 53%, and 79% for SPECT Tl-201 imaging. This study had an extraordinarily low specificity value for SPECT imaging and may reflect the study design where patients were referred to angiography principally because of an abnormal Tl-201 perfusion scan. The issue of ''referral bias'' was previously reviewed in Chapter 3. In contrast, Tamaki et al.[160] reported comparable sensitivity and specificity values for PET and SPECT imaging.

In summary, pharmacologic stress imaging using PET methods probably yields sensitivity and specificity values for CAD detection comparable to those for single-photon imaging techniques. To date, no large-scale studies have been undertaken comparing PET and SPECT using the most recent advances for both imaging technologies as well as comparing results to those obtained with the new Tc-99m perfusion agents. A cost-benefit analysis of the competing imaging approaches also appears warranted. The use of oxygen-15 water and other newer PET radiopharmaceuticals for regional flow determination by PET is discussed in Chapter 2.

SUMMARY

In summary, pharmacologic stress is an attractive alternative to exercise stress imaging for detecting myocardial

ischemia and determining its extent in patients suspected or known to have CAD or those who have recovered from a recent MI. Dipyridamole and adenosine are the most commonly employed pharmacologic stress imaging agents and are utilized in conjunction with myocardial perfusion imaging, whereas dobutamine is the pharmacologic agent most commonly used for stress echocardiography. Sensitivity, specificity, and diagnostic accuracy for CAD detection for dipyridamole or adenosine Tl-201 scintigraphy are comparable to values achieved with exercise stress. Similarly, the prognostic value of the pharmacologic stress technique for the detection of high-risk CAD patients has clearly been demonstrated and appears to be comparable to the prognostic worth of exercise scintigraphy. High-risk patients have multiple defects in more than one coronary vascular territory, increased lung-heart Tl-201 ratio, and transient LV cavity dilatation. High-risk patients by dipyridamole or adenosine scan criteria who also have clinical risk factors for CAD are prone to an increased incidence of perioperative complications with vascular surgery as well as an increased risk of events during long-term follow-up. The use of pharmacologic stress imaging is, perhaps, most valuable in patients with aortic or peripheral vascular disease who cannot exercise and have a high prevalence of symptomatic or occult CAD. Preoperative vasodilator or dobutamine stress perfusion imaging should be seriously considered for all such patients over age 60 years who manifest at least one risk factor for CAD (e.g., smoking, hypertension, hyperlipidemia, Q waves on the rest ECG). Coronary arteriography is considered for any patient who exhibits redistribution defects on Tl-201 imaging or reversible Tc-99m–sestamibi or teboroxime defects, particularly when they involve the territory of the LAD. Revascularization is then undertaken, depending upon anatomic findings on angiography. Both dipyridamole and adenosine scintigraphy are relatively safe, and most side effects are minor and transitory. Dobutamine perfusion imaging can be substituted for vasodilator stress imaging in patients with bronchospasm or those who are receiving theophylline compounds.

Dipyridamole or dobutamine echocardiography, although less sensitive for CAD detection than vasodilator stress perfusion imaging (particularly for single-vessel disease or

50% stenosis), may also provide important prognostic information. To maximize the application of dipyridamole echocardiography, larger intravenous doses of dipyridamole must be utilized, which are associated with more side effects. Dobutamine echocardiography as a pharmacologic stress is an intriguing approach that might prove useful in detecting residual myocardial viability in asynergic segments in patients who have undergone reperfusion therapy for MI (see Chap. 9). Large-scale studies have not yet been undertaken to compare dobutamine echocardiography with dipyridamole, adenosine, or dobutamine radionuclide perfusion imaging to determine which is more accurate for detection of CAD.

REFERENCES

1. Gould KL, Goldstein RA, Mullani NA, Kirkeeide RL, Wong WH, Tewson TJ, Berridge MS, Bolomey LA, Hartz RK, Smalling RW, et al.: Noninvasive assessment of coronary stenoses by myocardial perfusion imaging during pharmacologic coronary vasodilation. VIII. Clinical feasibility of positron cardiac imaging without a cyclotron using generator-produced rubidium-82. J Am Coll Cardiol 1986;7:775–789.
2. Kirkeeide RL, Gould KL, Parsel L: Assessment of coronary stenoses by myocardial perfusion imaging during pharmacologic coronary vasodilation. VII. Validation of coronary flow reserve as a single integrated functional measure of stenosis severity reflecting all its geometric dimensions. J Am Coll Cardiol 1986;7:103–113.
3. Gould KL: Identifying and measuring severity of coronary artery stenosis. Quantitative coronary arteriography and positron emission tomography. Circulation 1988;78:237–245.
4. Demer LL, Gould KL, Goldstein RA, Kirkeeide RL, Mullani NA, Smalling RW, Nishikawa A, Merhige ME: Assessment of coronary artery disease severity by positron emission tomography. Comparison with quantitative arteriography in 193 patients. Circulation 1989;79:825–835.
5. Gould KL, Kirkeeide RL, Buchi M: Coronary flow reserve as a physiologic measure of stenosis severity. J Am Coll Cardiol 1990;15:459–474.
5a. Klocke FJ: Cognition in the era of technology: "Seeing the shades of gray." J Am Coll Cardiol 1990;16:763–769.
5b. Uren NG, Crake T, Lefroy DC, DeSilva R, Davies GJ, Maseri A: Reduced coronary vasodilator function in infarcted and normal myocardium after myocardial infarction. N Engl J Med 1994;331:222–227.
6. Gould KL: PET perfusion imaging and nuclear cardiology. J Nucl Med 1991;32:579–606.
7. Gould KL, Lipscomb K, Hamilton GW: Physiologic basis for assessing critical coronary stenosis. Instantaneous flow response and regional distribution during coronary hyperemia as measures of coronary flow reserve. Am J Cardiol 1974;33:87–94.
8. Strauss HW, Pitt B: Noninvasive detection of subcritical coronary arterial narrowings with a coronary vasodilator and myocardial perfusion imaging. Am J Cardiol 1977;39:403–406.
9. Beller GA, Holzgrefe HH, Watson DD: Effects of dipyridamole-induced vasodilation on myocardial uptake and clearance kinetics of thallium-201. Circulation 1983;68:1328–1338.
10. Beller GA, Holzgrefe HH, Watson DD: Intrinsic washout rates of thallium-201 in normal and ischemic myocardium after dipyridamole-induced vasodilation. Circulation 1985;71:378–386.
11. Becker LC: Conditions for vasodilator-induced coronary steal in experimental myocardial ischemia. Circulation 1978;57:1103–1110.
12. Sparks HV Jr, Bardenheuer H: Regulation of adenosine formation by the heart. Circulation Res 1986;58:193–201.
13. Knabb RM, Gidday JM, Ely SW, Rubio R, Berne RM: Effects of dipyridamole on myocardial adenosine and active hyperemia. Am J Physiol 1984;247:H804–H810.
14. Belardinelli L, Linden J, Berne R: Cardiac effects of adenosine. Progr Cardiovasc Dis 1989;32:73–91.
15. Beller GA: Pharmacologic stress imaging. JAMA 1991;265:633–638.
16. Ranhosky A, Kempthorne-Rawson J: The safety of intravenous dipyridamole thallium myocardial perfusion imaging. Intravenous dipyridamole thallium imaging study group. Circulation 1990;81:1205–1209.
17. Brown BG, Josephson MA, Petersen RB, Pierce CD, Wong M, Hecht HS, Bolson E, Dodge HT: Intravenous dipyridamole combined with isometric handgrip for near maximal acute increase in coronary flow in patients with coronary artery disease. Am J Cardiol 1981;48:1077–1085.
18. Feldman RL, Nichols WW, Pepine CJ, Conti CR: Acute effect of intravenous dipyridamole on regional coronary hemodynamics and metabolism. Circulation 1981;64:333–344.
19. Abreu A, Mahmarian JJ, Nishimura S, Boyce TM, Verani MS: Tolerance and safety of pharmacologic coronary vasodilation with adenosine in association with thallium-201 scintigraphy in patients with suspected coronary artery disease. J Am Coll Cardiol 1991;18:730–735.
20. Kern MJ, Deligonul U, Tatineni S, Serota H, Aguirre F, Hilton TC: Intravenous adenosine: Continuous infusion and low dose bolus administration for determination of coronary vasodilator reserve in patients with and without coronary artery disease. J Am Coll Cardiol 1991;18:718–729.
21. Coyne EP, Belvedere DA, Vande Streek PR, Weiland FL, Evans RB, Spaccavento LJ: Thallium-201 scintigraphy after intravenous infusion of adenosine compared with exercise thallium testing in the diagnosis of coronary artery disease. J Am Coll Cardiol 1991;17:1289–1294.
22. O'Keefe JH Jr, Bateman TM, Silvestri R, Barnhart C: Safety and diagnostic accuracy of adenosine thallium-201 scintigraphy in patients unable to exercise and those with left bundle branch block. Am Heart J 1992;124:614–621.
23. Granato JE, Watson DD, Belardinelli L, Cannon JM, Beller GA: Effects of dipyridamole and aminophylline on hemodynamics, regional myocardial blood flow and thallium-201 washout in the setting of a critical coronary stenosis. J Am Coll Cardiol 1990;16:1760–1770.
24. Rossen JD, Quillen JE, Lopez AG, Stenberg RG, Talman CL, Winniford MD: Comparison of coronary vasodilation with intravenous dipyridamole and adenosine. J Am Coll Cardiol 1991;18:485–491.
25. Chan SY, Brunken RC, Czernin J, Porenta G, Kuhle W, Krivokapich J, Phelps ME, Schelbert HR: Comparison of maximal myocardial blood flow during adenosine infusion with that of intravenous dipyridamole in normal men. J Am Coll Cardiol 1992;20:979–985.
26. Mays AE Jr, Cobb FR: Relationship between regional myocardial blood flow and thallium-201 distribution in the presence of coronary artery stenosis and dipyridamole-induced vasodilation. J Clin Invest 1984;73:1359–1366.
27. Melin JA, Becker LC: Quantitative relationship between global left ventricular thallium uptake and blood flow: Effects of propranolol, ouabain, dipyridamole, and coronary artery occlusion. J Nucl Med 1986;27:641–652.
28. Okada RD, Leppo JA, Boucher CA, Pohost GM: Myocardial kinetics of thallium-201 after dipyridamole infusion in normal canine myocardium and in myocardium distal to a stenosis. J Clin Invest 1982;69:199–209.
28a. Heller GV, Barbour MM, Dweik RB, Corning JJ, McClellan JR, Garber CE: Effects of intravenous theophylline on exercise-induced myocardial ischemia. Impact on the ischemic threshold. J Am Coll Cardiol 1993;21:1075–1079.
29. Rossen JD, Simonetti I, Marcus ML, Winniford MD: Coronary dilation with standard dose dipyridamole and dipyridamole combined with handgrip. Circulation 1989;79:566–572.
30. Casale PN, Guiney TE, Strauss HW, Boucher CA: Simultaneous low level treadmill exercise and intravenous dipyridamole stress thallium imaging. Am J Cardiol 1988;62:799–802.
31. Leppo JA: Dipyridamole-thallium imaging: The lazy man's stress test. J Nucl Med 1989;30:281–287.
32. Botvinick E, Dae M: Dipyridamole-perfusion imaging (Abstract). Am J Cardiac Imaging 1991;5:7–15.
33. Beer SG, Heo J, Iskandrian AS: Dipyridamole thallium imaging. Am J Cardiol 1991;67:18D–26D.
34. Varma SK, Watson DD, Beller GA: Quantitative comparison of thallium-201 scintigraphy after exercise and dipyridamole in coronary artery disease. Am J Cardiol 1989;64:871–877.
34a. Lee J, Chae SC, Lee K, Heo J, Iskandrian AS: Biokinetics of thallium-201 in normal subjects: Comparison between adenosine,

dipyridamole, dobutamine, and exercise. J Nucl Med 1994;35:535–541.

35. Albro PC, Gould KL, Westcott RJ, Hamilton GW, Ritchie JL, Williams DL: Noninvasive assessment of coronary stenoses by myocardial imaging during pharmacologic coronary vasodilatation. III. Clinical trial. Am J Cardiol 1978;42:751–760.

36. Leppo J, Boucher CA, Okada RD, Newell JB, Strauss HW, Pohost GM: Serial thallium-201 myocardial imaging after dipyridamole infusion: diagnostic utility in detecting coronary stenoses and relationship to regional wall motion. Circulation 1982;66:649–657.

37. Schmoliner R, Dudczak R, Kronik G, Hutterer B, Kletter K, Mosslacher H, Frischauf H: Thallium-201 imaging after dipyridamole in patients with coronary multivessel disease. Cardiology 1983;70:145–151.

38. Francisco DA, Collins SM, Go RT, Ehrhardt JC, Van Kirk OC, Marcus ML: Tomographic thallium-201 myocardial perfusion scintigrams after maximal coronary artery vasodilation with intravenous dipyridamole. Comparison of qualitative and quantitative approaches. Circulation 1982;66:370–379.

39. Timmis AD, Lutkin JE, Fenney LJ, Strak SK, Burwood RJ, Gishen P, Chamberlain DA: Comparison of dipyridamole and treadmill exercise for enhancing thallium-201 perfusion defects in patients with coronary artery disease. Eur Heart J 1980;1:275–280.

40. Narita M, Kurihara T, Usami M: Noninvasive detection of coronary artery disease by myocardial imaging with thallium-201—the significance of pharmacologic interventions. Jpn Circulation J 1981; 45:127–140.

41. Machecourt J, Denis B, Wolf JE, Comet M, Pellet J, Martin-Noel P: Respective sensitivity and specificity of 201 Tl myocardial scintigraphy during effort, after injection of dipyridamole and at rest. Comparison in 70 patients who had undergone coronary radiography. [French] Arch Malad Coeur Vaisseaux 1981;74:147–156.

42. Okada RD, Lim YL, Rothendler J, Boucher CA, Block PC, Pohost GM: Split dose thallium-201 dipyridamole imaging: A new technique for obtaining thallium images before and immediately after an intervention. J Am Coll Cardiol 1983;1:1302–1310.

43. Sochor H, Pachinger O, Ogris E, Probst P, Kaindl F: Radionuclide imaging after coronary vasodilation: Myocardial scintigraphy with thallium-201 and radionuclide angiography after administration of dipyridamole. Eur Heart J 1984;5:500–509.

44. Ruddy TD, Dighero HR, Newell JB, Pohost GM, Strauss HW, Okada RD, Boucher CA: Quantitative analysis of dipyridamole-thallium images for the detection of coronary artery disease. J Am Coll Cardiol 1987;10:142–149.

45. Taillefer R, Lette J, Phaneuf DC, Leveille J, Lemire F, Essiambre R: Thallium-201 myocardial imaging during pharmacologic coronary vasodilation: Comparison of oral and intravenous administration of dipyridamole. J Am Coll Cardiol 1986;8:76–83.

46. Laarman GJ, Verzijlbergen JF, Ascoop CA: Ischemic ST-segment changes after dipyridamole infusion. Int J Cardiol 1987;14:383–386.

47. Lam JY, Chaitman BR, Glaenzer M, Byers S, Fite J, Shah Y, Goodgold H, Samuels L: Safety and diagnostic accuracy of dipyridamole-thallium imaging in the elderly. J Am Coll Cardiol 1988;11:585–589.

48. Borges-Neto S, Mahmarian JJ, Jain A, Roberts R, Verani MS: Quantitative thallium-201 single photon emission computed tomography after oral dipyridamole for assessing the presence, anatomic location and severity of coronary artery disease. J Am Coll Cardiol 1988;11:962–969.

48a. Lalonde D, Taillefer R, Bisson G, Basile F, Prieto I, Benjamin C: Thallium-201–dipyridamole imaging: Comparison between a standard dose and a high dose of dipyridamole in the detection of coronary artery disease. J Nucl Med 1994;35:1245–1253.

49. Popma JJ, Dehmer GJ, Walker BS, Simon TR, Smitherman TC: Analysis of thallium-201 single-photon emission computed tomography after intravenous dipyridamole using different quantitative measures of coronary stenosis severity and receiver operator characteristic curves. Am Heart J 1992;124:65–74.

50. Mendelson MA, Spies SM, Spies WG, Abi-Mansour P, Fintel DJ: Usefulness of single-photon emission computed tomography of thallium-201 uptake after dipyridamole infusion for detection of coronary artery disease. Am J Cardiol 1992;69:1150–1155.

51. Kong BA, Shaw L, Miller DD, Chaitman BR: Comparison of accuracy for detecting coronary artery disease and side-effect profile of dipyridamole thallium-201 myocardial perfusion imaging in women versus men. Am J Cardiol 1992;70:168–173.

51a. Iskandrian AS, Verani MS, Heo J: Pharmacologic stress testing: Mechanism of action, hemodynamic responses, and results in detection of coronary artery disease. J Nucl Cardiol 1994;1:94–111.

52. Miller D: Pharmacologic vasodilator stress alternatives for cardiac perfusion imaging. Am Coll Cardiol, Learning Center Highlights 1991;7:7–11.

53. Nishimura S, Mahmarian JJ, Boyce TM, Verani MS: Quantitative thallium-201 single-photon emission computed tomography during maximal pharmacologic coronary vasodilation with adenosine for assessing coronary artery disease. J Am Coll Cardiol 1991;18:736–745.

54. Gupta NC, Esterbrooks DJ, Hilleman DE, Mohiuddin SM: Comparison of adenosine and exercise thallium-201 single-photon emission computed tomography (SPECT) myocardial perfusion imaging. The GE SPECT Multicenter Adenosine Study Group. J Am Coll Cardiol 1992;19:248–257.

55. Nishimura S, Mahmarian JJ, Boyce TM, Verani MS: Equivalence between adenosine and exercise thallium-201 myocardial tomography: A multicenter, prospective, crossover trial. J Am Coll Cardiol 1992;20:265–275.

55a. O'Keefe JH, Bateman TM, Barnhart CS: Adenosine Tl-201 is superior to exercise Tl-201 for detecting coronary artery disease in patients with left bundle branch block. J Am Coll Cardiol 1993;21:1332–1338.

56. Okada RD, Dai YH, Boucher CA, Pohost GM: Serial thallium-201 imaging after dipyridamole for coronary disease detection: Quantitative analysis using myocardial clearance. Am Heart J 1984;107:475–481.

57. Iskandrian AS, Heo J, Nguyen T, Beer SG, Cave V, Ogilby JD, Untereker W, Segal BL: Assessment of coronary artery disease using single-photon emission computed tomography with thallium-201 during adenosine-induced coronary hyperemia. Am J Cardiol 1991;67:1190–1194.

58. Eichhorn EJ, Kosinski EJ, Lewis SM, Hill TC, Emond LH, Leland OS: Usefulness of dipyridamole-thallium-201 perfusion scanning for distinguishing ischemic from nonischemic cardiomyopathy. Am J Cardiol 1988;62:945–951.

59. Lette J, Lapointe J, Waters D, Cerino M, Picard M, Gagnon A: Transient left ventricular cavitary dilation during dipyridamole-thallium imaging as an indicator of severe coronary artery disease. Am J Cardiol 1990;66:1163–1170.

60. Iskandrian AS, Heo J, Nguyen T, Lyons E, Paugh E: Left ventricular dilatation and pulmonary thallium uptake after single-photon emission computer tomography using thallium-201 during adenosine-induced coronary hyperemia. Am J Cardiol 1990;66:807–811.

61. Hurwitz GA, O'Donoghue JP, Powe JE, Gravelle DR, MacDonald AC, Finnie KJ: Pulmonary thallium-201 uptake following dipyridamole-exercise combination compared with single modality stress testing. Am J Cardiol 1992;69:320–326.

62. Villanueva FS, Kaul S, Smith WH, Watson DD, Varma SK, Beller GA: Prevalence and correlates of increased lung/heart ratio of thallium-201 during dipyridamole stress imaging for suspected coronary artery disease. Am J Cardiol 1990;66:1324–1328.

63. Chouraqui P, Rodrigues EA, Berman DS, Maddahi J: Significance of dipyridamole-induced transient dilation of the left ventricle during thallium-201 scintigraphy in suspected coronary artery disease. Am J Cardiol 1990;66:689–694.

64. Takeishi Y, Tono-oka I, Ikeda K, Komatani A, Tsuiki K, Yasui S: Dilatation of the left ventricular cavity on dipyridamole thallium-201 imaging: A new marker of triple-vessel disease. Am Heart J 1991;121:466–475.

65. Okada RD, Dai YH, Boucher CA, Pohost GM: Significance of increased lung thallium-201 activity on serial cardiac images after dipyridamole treatment in coronary heart disease. Am J Cardiol 1984;53:470–475.

66. Nishimura S, Mahmarian JJ, Verani MS: Significance of increased lung thallium uptake during adenosine thallium-201 scintigraphy. J Nucl Med 1992;33:1600–1607.

67. McLaughlin D, Beller G, Ayers C, Ripley M, Taylor H, Linden J, Feldman M: Increased lung/heart ratio on dipyridamole thallium-201 imaging does not imply severe myocardial ischemia. Circulation 1992;86:I44.

68. Klein HO, Ninio R, Eliyahu S, Bakst A, Levi A, Dean H, Oren V, Beker B, Kaplinsky E, Gilboa S, et al.: Effects of the dipyridamole test on left ventricular function in coronary artery disease. Am J Cardiol 1992;69:482–488.

68a. McLaughlin DP, Beller GA, Linden J, Ayers CR, Ripley ML, Taylor H, Watson DD, Feldman MD: Hemodynamic and metabolic correlates of dipyridamole-induced myocardial thallium-201 perfusion abnormalities in multivessel coronary artery disease. Am J Cardiol 1994;74:1159–1164.

68b. Brown KA: The role of stress redistribution thallium-201 myocardial perfusion imaging in evaluating coronary artery disease and perioperative risk. J Nucl Med 1994; 35:703–706.

69. Ogilby JD, Iskandrian AS, Untereker WJ, Heo J, Nguyen TN, Mercuro J: Effect of intravenous adenosine infusion on myocardial perfusion and function. Hemodynamic/angiographic and scintigraphic study. Circulation 1992;86:887–895.

69a. Iskandrian AS, Heo J, Lemlek J, Ogilby JD, Untereker WJ, Iskandrian B, Cave V: Identification of high-risk patients with left main and three-vessel coronary artery disease by adenosine-single photon emission computed tomographic thallium imaging. Am Heart J 1993;125:1130–1135.

70. Younis LT, Byers S, Shaw L, Barth G, Goodgold H, Chaitman BR: Prognostic importance of silent myocardial ischemia detected by intravenous dipyridamole thallium myocardial imaging in asymptomatic patients with coronary artery disease. J Coll Cardiol 1989;14:1635–1641.

71. Younis LT, Byers S, Shaw L, Barth G, Goodgold H, Chaitman BR: Prognostic value of intravenous dipyridamole thallium scintigraphy after an acute myocardial ischemic event. Am J Cardiol 1989;64:161–166.

72. Stratmann HG, Younis LT, Kong B: Prognostic value of dipyridamole thallium-201 scintigraphy in patients with stable chest pain. Am Heart J 1992;123:317–323.

73. Hendel RC, Whitfield SS, Villegas BJ, Cutler BS, Leppo JA: Prediction of late cardiac events by dipyridamole thallium imaging in patients undergoing elective vascular surgery. Am J Cardiol 1992;70:1243–1249.

74. Hendel RC, Layden JJ, Leppo JA: Prognostic value of dipyridamole thallium scintigraphy for evaluation of ischemic heart disease. J Am Coll Cardiol 1990;15:109–116.

75. Zhu YY, Chung WS, Botvinick EH, Dae MW, Lim AD, Ports TA, Danforth JW, Wolfe CL, Goldschlager N, Chatterjee K: Dipyridamole perfusion scintigraphy: The experience with its application in one hundred seventy patients with known or suspected unstable angina. Am Heart J 1991;121:33–43.

76. Rose EL, Liu XJ, Henley M, Lewis JD, Raftery EB, Lahiri A: Prognostic value of noninvasive cardiac tests in the assessment of patients with peripheral vascular disease. Am J Cardiol 1993;71:40–44.

76a. Kamal AM, Fattah AA, Pancholy S, Aksut S, Cave V, Heo J, Iskandrian AS: Prognostic value of adenosine single-photon emission computed tomographic thallium imaging in medically treated patients with angiographic evidence of coronary artery disease. J Nucl Cardiol 1994;1:254–261.

76b. Miller DD, Strattman HG, Shaw L, et al.: Dipyridamole technetium-99m sestamibi myocardial tomography as an independent predictor of cardiac events—free survival after acute ischemic events. J Nucl Cardiol 1994;1:172–182.

77. Heart and Stroke Facts. Dallas, American Heart Association 1991.

78. Chaitman BR, Ryan TJ, Kronmal RA, Foster ED, Frommer PL, Killip T: Coronary Artery Surgery Study (CASS): Comparability of 10 year survival in randomized and randomizable patients. J Am Coll Cardiol 1990;16:1071–1078.

79. Gersh BJ, Kronmal RA, Schaff HV, Frye RL, Ryan TJ, Mock MB, Myers WO, Athearn MW, Gosselin AJ, Kaiser GC, et al.: Comparison of coronary artery bypass surgery and medical therapy in patients 65 years of age or older. A nonrandomized study from the Coronary Artery Surgery Study (CASS) registry. N Engl J Med 1985;313:217–224.

80. Hertzer NR, Beven EG, Young JR, O'Hara PJ, Ruschhaupt WF, Graor RA, Dewolfe VG, Maljovec LC: Coronary artery disease in peripheral vascular patients. A classification of 1000 coronary angiograms and results of surgical management. Ann Surg 1984;199:223–233.

81. Shaw L, Chaitman BR, Hilton TC, Stocke K, Younis LT, Caralis DG, Kong BA, Miller DD: Prognostic value of dipyridamole thallium-201 imaging in elderly patients. J Am Coll Cardiol 1992;19:1390–1398.

81a. Abraham SA, Eagle KA: Preoperative cardiac risk assessment for noncardiac surgery. J Nucl Cardiol 1994;1:389–398.

81b. Eagle KA, Rihal CS, Foster ED, Mickel MC, Gersh BJ, for the Coronary Artery Surgery Study (CASS) investigators: Long-term survival in patients with coronary artery disease: Importance of peripheral vascular disease. J Am Coll Cardiol 1994;23:1091–1095.

82. Hertzer NR: Basic data concerning associated coronary disease in peripheral vascular patients. Ann Vasc Surg 1987;1:616–620.

83. Gersh BJ, Rihal CS, Rooke TW, Ballard DJ: Evaluation and management of patients with both peripheral vascular and coronary artery disease. J Am Coll Cardiol 1991;18:203–214.

84. Criqui MH, Langer RD, Fronek A, Feigelson HS, Klauber MR, McCann TJ, Browner D: Mortality over a period of 10 years in patients with peripheral arterial disease. N Engl J Med 1992;326:381–386.

85. Boucher CA, Brewster DC, Darling RC, Okada RD, Strauss HW, Pohost GM: Determination of cardiac risk by dipyridamole-thallium imaging before peripheral vascular surgery. N Engl J Med 1985;312:389–394.

86. Eagle KA, Singer DE, Brewster DC, Darling RC, Mulley AG, Boucher CA: Dipyridamole-thallium scanning in patients undergoing vascular surgery. Optimizing preoperative evaluation of cardiac risk. JAMA 1987;257:2185–2189.

87. Eagle KA, Coley CM, Newell JB, Brewster DC, Darling RC, Strauss HW, Guiney TE, Boucher CA: Combining clinical and thallium data optimizes preoperative assessment of cardiac risk before major vascular surgery. Ann Intern Med 1989;110:859–866.

88. Leppo J, Plaja J, Gionet M, Tumolo J, Paraskos JA, Cutler BS: Noninvasive evaluation of cardiac risk before elective vascular surgery. J Am Coll Cardiol 1987;9:269–276.

89. Cutler BS, Leppo JA: Dipyridamole thallium 201 scintigraphy to detect coronary artery disease before abdominal aortic surgery. J Vasc Surg 1987;5:91–100.

90. Lette J, Waters D, Lapointe J, Gagnon A, Picard M, Cerino M, Kerouac M: Usefulness of the severity and extent of reversible perfusion defects during thallium-dipyridamole imaging for cardiac risk assessment before noncardiac surgery. Am J Cardiol 1989;64:276–281.

91. Levinson JR, Boucher CA, Coley CM, Guiney TE, Strauss HW, Eagle KA: Usefulness of semiquantitative analysis of dipyridamole-thallium-201 redistribution for improving risk stratification before vascular surgery. Am J Cardiol 1990;66:406–410.

92. Lette J, Waters D, Bernier H, Champagne P, Lassonde J, Picard M, Cerino M, Nattel S, Boucher Y, Heyen F, et al.: Preoperative and long-term cardiac risk assessment. Predictive value of 23 clinical descriptors, 7 multivariate scoring systems, and quantitative dipyridamole imaging in 360 patients. Ann Surg 1992;216:192–204.

92a. Lette J, Waters D, Cerino M, Picard M, Champagne P, Lapointe J: Preoperative coronary artery disease risk stratification based on dipyridamole imaging and a simple three-step, three-segment model for patients undergoing noncardiac vascular surgery or major general surgery. Am J Cardiol 1992;69:1553–1558.

92b. Baron J-F, Mundler O, Bertrand M, et al.: Dipyridamole-thallium scintigraphy and gated radionuclide angiography to assess cardiac risk before abdominal aortic surgery. N Engl J Med 1994;330:663–669.

93. Mangano DT, London MJ, Tubau JF, Browner WS, Hollenberg M, Krupski W, Layug EL, Massie B: Dipyridamole thallium-201 scintigraphy as a preoperative screening test. A reexamination of its predictive potential. Study of Perioperative Ischemia Research Group. Circulation 1991;84:493–502.

93a. Brown KA, Rowen M: Extent of jeopardized viable myocardium determined by myocardial perfusion imaging best predicts perioperative cardiac events in patients undergoing noncardiac surgery. J Am Coll Cardiol 1993;21:325–330.

93b. Urbinati S, Di Pasquale G, Andreoli A, Lusa AM, Ruffini M, Lanzino G, Pinelli G: Frequency and prognostic significance of silent coronary artery disease in patients with cerebral ischemia undergoing carotid endarterectomy. Am J Cardiol 1992;69:1166–1170.

93c. Rose EL, Liu XJ, Henley M, Lewis JD, Raftery EB, Lahiri A: Prognostic value of noninvasive cardiac tests in the assessment of patients with peripheral vascular disease. Am J Cardiol 1993;71:40–44.

94. Coley CM, Field TS, Abraham SA, Boucher CA, Eagle KA: Usefulness of dipyridamole-thallium scanning for preoperative evaluation of cardiac risk for nonvascular surgery. Am J Cardiol 1992;69:1280–1285.

94a. Younis L, Stratmann H, Takase B, Byers S, Chartman B, Miller DD: Preoperative clinical assessment and dipyridamole thallium-201 scintigraphy for prediction and prevention of cardiac events in patients having major nonvascular surgery and known or suspected coronary artery disease. Am J Cardiol 1994;74:311–317.

94b. Takase B, Younis LT, Byers SL, Shaw LJ, Labovitz AJ, Chaitman BR, Miller DD: Comparative prognostic value of clinical risk indexes, resting two-dimensional echocardiography, and dipyridamole stress thallium-201 myocardial imaging for perioperative cardiac events in major nonvascular surgery patients. Am Heart J 1993;126:1099–1106.

95. Shaw L, Miller DD, Kong BA, Hilton T, Stelken A, Stocke K, Chaitman BR: Determination of perioperative cardiac risk by adenosine thallium-201 myocardial imaging. Am Heart J 1992;124:861–869.

96. Lane SE, Lewis SM, Pippin JJ, Kosinski EJ, Campbell D, Nesto RW, Hill T: Predictive value of quantitative dipyridamole-thallium scintigraphy in assessing cardiovascular risk after vascular surgery in diabetes mellitus. Am J Cardiol 1989;64:1275–1279.

97. Brown KA, Rimmer J, Haisch C: Noninvasive cardiac risk stratification of diabetic and nondiabetic uremic renal allograft candidates using dipyridamole-thallium-201 imaging and radionuclide ventriculography. Am J Cardiol 1989;64:1017–1021.

98. Nesto RW, Watson FS, Kowalchuk GJ, Zarich SW, Hill T, Lewis SM, Lane SE: Silent myocardial ischemia and infarction in diabetics with peripheral vascular disease: Assessment by dipyridamole thallium-201 scintigraphy. Am Heart J 1990;120:1073–1077.

99. Marcen R, Lamas S, Orofino L, Quereda C, Barcia F, Castro JM, Alonso de Caso P, Ortuno J: Dipyridamole thallium-201 perfusion imaging for the study of ischemic heart disease in hemodialysis patients. Int J Artificial Organs 1989;12:773–777.

100. Camp AD, Garvin PJ, Hoff J, Marsh J, Byers SL, Chaitman BR: Prognostic value of intravenous dipyridamole thallium imaging in patients with diabetes mellitus considered for renal transplantation. Am J Cardiol 1990;65:1459–1463.

101. Verani M: Pharmacologic stress myocardial perfusion imaging. Curr Prob Cardiol 1993;18:481–528.

102. Okada RD, Glover DK, Leppo JA: Dipyridamole 201Tl scintigraphy in the evaluation of prognosis after myocardial infarction. Circulation 1991;84:I132–I139.

103. Leppo JA, O'Brien J, Rothendler JA, Getchell JD, Lee VW: Dipyridamole-thallium-201 scintigraphy in the prediction of future cardiac events after acute myocardial infarction. N Engl J Med 1984;310:1014–1018.

104. Pirelli S, Inglese E, Suppa M, Corrada E, Campolo L: Dipyridamole-thallium 201 scintigraphy in the early post-infarction period. (Safety and accuracy in predicting the extent of coronary disease and future recurrence of angina in patients suffering from their first myocardial infarction). Eur Heart J 1988;9:1324–1331.

105. Brown KA, O'Meara J, Chambers CE, Plante DA: Ability of dipyridamole-thallium-201 imaging one to four days after acute myocardial infarction to predict in-hospital and late recurrent myocardial ischemic events. Am J Cardiol 1990;65:160–167.

106. Gimple LW, Hutter AM Jr, Guiney TE, Boucher CA: Prognostic utility of predischarge dipyridamole-thallium imaging compared to predischarge submaximal exercise electrocardiography and maximal exercise thallium imaging after uncomplicated acute myocardial infarction. Am J Cardiol 1989;64:1243–1248.

107. Miller DD, Scott RA, Riesmeyer JS, Chaudhuri TK, Blumhardt R, Boucher CA, O'Rourke RA: Acute hemodynamic changes during intravenous dipyridamole thallium imaging early after infarction. Am Heart J 1989;118:686–694.

108. Nienaber CA, Salge D, Spielmann RP, Montz R, Bleifeld W: Detection of human collateral circulation by vasodilation-thallium-201 tomography. Am J Cardiol 1990;65:991–998.

109. Hendel RC, Gore JM, Alpert JS, Leppo JA: Prognosis following interventional therapy for acute myocardial infarction: Utility of dipyridamole thallium scintigraphy. Cardiology 1991;79:73–80.

110. Abreu A, Nishimura S, Mahmarian J, Verani M: Safety of adenosine thallium-201 scintigraphy. Circulation 1990;82:730.

111. Mahmarian JJ, Pratt CM, Nishimura S, Abreu A, Verani MS: Quantitative adenosine 201Tl single-photon emission computed tomography for the early assessment of patients surviving acute myocardial infarction. Circulation 1993;87:1197–1210.

112. Homma S, Gilliland Y, Guiney TE, Strauss HW, Boucher CA: Safety of intravenous dipyridamole for stress testing with thallium imaging. Am J Cardiol 1987;59:152–154.

113. Lewen MK, Labovitz AJ, Kern MJ, Chaitman BR: Prolonged myocardial ischemia after intravenous dipyridamole thallium imaging. Chest 1987;92:1102–1104.

114. Lam JY, Chaitman BR, Glaenzer M, Byers S, Fite J, Shah Y, Goodgold H, Samuels L: Safety and diagnostic accuracy of dypyridamole-thallium imaging. J Am Coll Cardiol 1988;11:585–589.

115. Gerson MC, Moore EN, Ellis K: Systemic effects and safety of intravenous dipyridamole in elderly patients with suspected coronary artery disease. Am J Cardiol 1987;60:1399–1401.

116. Beller GA: Dipyridamole thallium 201 imaging. How safe is it? (comment). Circulation 1990;81:1425–1427.

117. Sylven C, Beermann B, Jonzon B, Brandt R: Angina pectoris-like pain provoked by intravenous adenosine in healthy volunteers. Br Med J Clin Res 1986;293:227–230.

118. Pearlman JD, Boucher CA: Diagnostic value for coronary artery disease of chest pain during dipyridamole-thallium stress testing. Am J Cardiol 1988;61:43–45.

119. Chambers CE, Brown KA: Dipyridamole-induced ST segment depression during thallium-201 imaging in patients with coronary artery disease: Angiographic and hemodynamic determinants. J Am Coll Cardiol 1988;12:37–41.

120. Villanueva FS, Smith WH, Watson DD, Beller GA: ST-segment depression during dipyridamole infusion, and its clinical, scintigraphic and hemodynamic correlates. Am J Cardiol 1992;69:445–448.

120a. Nishimura S, Kimball KT, Mahmarian JJ, Verani MS: Angiographic and hemodynamic determinants of myocardial ischemia during adenosine thallium-201 scintigraphy in coronary artery disease. Circulation 1993;87:1211–1219.

120b. Marshall ES, Raichlen JS, Tighe DA, Paul JS, Breuninger KM, Chung EK: ST-segment depression during adenosine infusion as a predictor of myocardial ischemia. Am Heart J 1994;127:305–311.

121. Verani M: Adenosine stress imaging. Coronary Artery Dis 1992;3:1145.

121a. Cerqueira MD, Verani M, Schwaiger M, Heo J, Iskandrian A: Safety profile of adenosine stress perfusion imaging: Results from the adenoscan multicenter trial registry. J Am Coll Cardiol 1994;23·384–389.

122. Glover D, Okada R: Myocardial kinetics of Tc-MIBI in canine myocardium after dipyrimidole. Circulation 1990;81:628–636.

122a. Santos-Ocampo CD, Herman SD, Travin MI, et al.: Comparison of exercise dipyridamole and adenosine by use of technetium-99m sestamibi tomographic imaging. J Nucl Cardiol 1994;1:57–64.

123. Tartagni F, Dondi M, Limonetti P, Franchi R, Maiello L, Monetti N, Magnani B: Dipyridamole technetium-99m-2-methoxy isobutyl isonitrile tomoscintigraphic imaging for identifying diseased coronary vessels: Comparison with thallium-201 stress-rest study. J Nucl Med 1991;32:369–376.

124. Kettunen R, Huikuri HV, Heikkila J, Takkunen JT: Usefulness of technetium-99m-MIBI and thallium-201 in tomographic imaging combined with high-dose dipyridamole and handgrip exercise for detecting coronary artery disease. Am J Cardiol 1991;68:575–579.

125. Parodi O, Marcassa C, Casucci R, Sambuceti G, Verna E, Galli M, Inglese E, Marzullo P, Pirelli S, Bisi G, et al.: Accuracy and safety of technetium-99m hexakis 2-methoxy-2-isobutyl isonitrile (sestamibi) myocardial scintigraphy with high dose dipyridamole test in patients with effort angina pectoris: A multicenter study. Italian Group of Nuclear Cardiology. J Am Coll Cardiol 1991;18:1439–1444.

125a. Cuocolo A, Soricelli A, Pace L, et al.: Adenosine technetium-99m—methoxyisobutyl isonitrile myocardial tomography in patients wtih coronary artery disease: Comparison with exercise. J Nucl Med 1994;35:1110–1115.

126. Labonte C, Taillefer R, Lambert R, Basile F, TonThat T, Jarry M, Leveille J: Comparison between technetium-99m-teboroxime and thallium-201 dipyridamole planar myocardial perfusion imaging in detection of coronary artery disease. Am J Cardiol 1992;69:90–96.

126a. Sciagrà R, Bisi G, Santoro GM, Briganti V, Leoncini M, Fazzini PF: Evaluation of coronary artery disease using technetium-99m—

sestamibi first-pass perfusion imaging with dipyridamole infusion. J Nucl Med 1994;35:1254–1264.

127. Iskandrian AS, Heo J, Nguyen T, Beer S, Cave V, Cassel D, Iskandrian BB: Tomographic myocardial perfusion imaging with technetium-99m teboroxime during adenosine-induced coronary hyperemia: Correlation with thallium-201 imaging. J Am Coll Cardiol 1992;19:307–312.

127a. Chua T, Kiat H, Germano G, Takemoto K, Fernandez G, Biasio Y, Friedman J: Rapid back to back adenosine stress/rest technetium-99m teboroxime myocardial perfusion SPECT using a triple-detection camera (Abstract). J Nucl Med 1993;34:1485–1493.

128. Picano E, Lattanzi F, Masini M, Distante A, L'Abbate A: High dose dipyridamole echocardiography test in effort angina pectoris. J Am Coll Cardiol 1986;8:848–854.

129. Picano E, Masini M, Lattanzi F, Distante A, L'Abbate A: Role of dipyridamole-echocardiography test in electrocardiographically silent effort myocardial ischemia. Am J Cardiol 1986;58:235–237.

130. Masini M, Picano E, Lattanzi F, Distante A, L'Abbate A: High dose dipyridamole-echocardiography test in women: Correlation with exercise-electrocardiography test and coronary arteriography. J Am Coll Cardiol 1988;12:682–685.

131. Ferrara N, Bonaduce D, Leosco D, Longobardi G, Abete P, Morgano G, Salvatore M, Rengo F: Two-dimensional echocardiographic evaluation of ventricular asynergy induced by dipyridamole: Correlation with thallium scanning. Clin Cardiol 1986;9:437–442.

132. Picano E, Simonetti I, Masini M, Marzilli M, Lattanzi F, Distante A, De Nes M, L'Abbate A: Transient myocardial dysfunction during pharmacologic vasodilation as an index of reduced coronary reserve: A coronary hemodynamic and echocardiographic study. J Am Coll Cardiol 1986;8:84–90.

132a. Picano E, Parodi O, Lattanzi F, et al.: Assessment of anatomic and physiological severity of single-vessel coronary artery lesions by dipyridamole echocardiography: Comparison with positron emission tomography and quantitative arteriography. Circulation 1994; 89:753–761.

133. Margonato A, Chierchia S, Cianflone D, Smith G, Crea F, Davies G, Maseri A, Foale R: Limitations of dipyridamole-echocardiography in effort angina pectoris. Am J Cardiol 1987;59:225–230.

134. Picano E, Severi S, Michelassi C, Lattanzi F, Masini M, Orsini E, Distante A, L'Abbate A: Prognostic importance of dipyridamole-echocardiography test in coronary artery disease. Circulation 1989;80:450–457.

135. Bolognese L, Sarasso G, Aralda D, Bongo AS, Rossi L, Rossi P: High dose dipyridamole echocardiography early after uncomplicated acute myocardial infarction: Correlation with exercise testing and coronary angiography. J Am Coll Cardiol 1989;14:357–363.

136. Pirelli S, Danzi GB, Alberti A, Massa D, Piccalo G, Faletra F, Picano E, Campolo L, De Vita C: Comparison of usefulness of high-dose dipyridamole echocardiography and exercise electrocardiography for detection of asymptomatic restenosis after coronary angioplasty. Am J Cardiol 1991;67:1335–1338.

137. Picano E, Pirelli S, Marzilli M, Faletra F, Lattanzi F, Campolo L, Massa D, Alberti A, Gara E, Distante A, et al.: Usefulness of high-dose dipyridamole echocardiography test in coronary angioplasty. Circulation 1989;80:807–815.

138. Cates CU, Kronenberg MW, Collins HW, Sandler MP: Dipyridamole radionuclide ventriculography: A test with high specificity for severe coronary artery disease. J Am Coll Cardiol 1989;13:841–851.

139. Whitfield S, Aurigemma G, Pape L, Leppo J: Two-dimensional Doppler echocardiographic correlation of dipyridamole-thallium stress testing with isometric handgrip. Am Heart J 1991;121:1367–1373.

139a. DiBello V, Gori E, Bellina CR, et al.: Incremental diagnostic value of dipyridamole echocardiography and exercise Tl-201 scintigraphy in the assessment of presence and extent of coronary artery disease. J Nucl Cardiol 1994;1:372–381.

140. Tischler MD, Lee TH, Hirsch AT, Lord CP, Goldman L, Creager MA, Lee RT: Prediction of major cardiac events after peripheral vascular surgery using dipyridamole echocardiography. Am J Cardiol 1991;68:593.

141. Bolognese L, Sarasso G, Bongo AS, Rossi L, Aralda D, Piccinino C, Rossi P: Dipyridamole echocardiography test. A new tool for detecting jeopardized myocardium after thrombolytic therapy. Circulation 1991;84:1100–1106.

141a. Camerieri A, Picano E, Landi P, et al.: Prognostic value of dipyr-

idamole echocardiography early after myocardial infarction in elderly patients. J Am Coll Cardiol 1993;22:1809–1815.

142. Baer FM, Smolarz K, Jungehulsing M, Theissen P, Sechtem U, Schicha H, Hilger HH: Feasibility of high-dose dipyridamole-magnetic resonance imaging for detection of coronary artery disease and comparison with coronary angiography. Am J Cardiol 1992;69:51–56.

143. Pennell DJ, Underwood SR, Manzara CC, Swanton RH, Walker JM, Ell PJ, Longmore DB: Magnetic resonance imaging during dobutamine stress in coronary artery disease. Am J Cardiol 1992;70:34–40.

143a. van Rugge PF, van der Wall EE, Spanjersberg SS, et al.: Magnetic resonance imaging during dobutamine stress for detection and localization of coronary artery disease. Quantitative wall motion analysis using a modification of the centerline method. Circulation 1994;90:127–138.

144. Zoghbi WA, Cheirif J, Kleiman NS, Verani MS, Trakhtenbroit A: Diagnosis of ischemic heart disease with adenosine echocardiography. J Am Coll Cardiol 1991;18:1271–1279.

145. Zoghbi WA: Use of adenosine echocardiography for diagnosis of coronary artery disease. Am Heart J 1991;122:285–292.

145a. Heinle S, Hanson M, Gracey L, Coleman E, Kisslo J: Correlation of adenosine echocardiography and thallium scintigraphy. Am Heart J 1993;125:1606–1613.

146. Fung AY, Gallagher KP, Buda AJ: The physiologic basis of dobutamine as compared with dipyridamole stress interventions in the assessment of critical coronary stenosis. Circulation 1987;76:943–951.

147. Pennell DJ, Underwood SR, Swanton RH, Walker JM, Ell PJ: Dobutamine thallium myocardial perfusion tomography. J Am Coll Cardiol 1991;18:1471–1479.

148. Hays JT, Mahmarian JJ, Cochran AJ, Verani MS: Dobutamine thallium-201 tomography for evaluating patients with suspected coronary artery disease unable to undergo exercise or vasodilator pharmacologic stress testing. J Am Coll Cardiol 1993;21:1583–1590.

148a. Elliott BM, Robison JG, Zellner JL, Hendrix GH: Dobutamine-201Tl imaging. Assessing cardiac risks associated with vascular surgery. Circulation 1991;84:III54–III60.

148b. Pennell D, Underwood S, Ell P: Safety of dobutamine stress for thallium-201 myocardial perfusion tomography in patients with asthma (Abstract). Am J Cardiol 1993;71:1346–1350.

148c. Coma-Canella I, Martinez M, Rodrigo F, Bieras J: The dobutamine stress test with thallium-201 single-photon emission computed tomography and radionuclide angiography: Postinfarction study (Abstract). J Am Coll Cardiol 1993;22:399–406.

148d. Herman SD, LaBresh KA, Santos-Ocampo CD, et al.: Comparison of dobutamine and exercise using technetium-99m–sestamibi imaging for the evaluation of coronary artery disease. Am J Cardiol 1994;73:164–169.

149. Sawada SG, Segar DS, Ryan T, Brown SE, Dohan AM, Williams R, Fineberg NS, Armstrong WF, Feigenbaum H: Echocardiographic detection of coronary artery disease during dobutamine infusion. Circulation 1991;83:1605–1614.

150. Cohen JL, Greene TO, Ottenweller J, Binenbaum SZ, Wilchfort SD, Kim CS: Dobutamine digital echocardiography for detecting coronary artery disease. Am J Cardiol 1991;67:1311–1318.

151. Segar DS, Brown SE, Sawada SG, Ryan T, Feigenbaum H: Dobutamine stress echocardiography: Correlation with coronary lesion severity as determined by quantitative angiography. J Am Coll Cardiol 1992;19:1197–1202.

152. Mazeika PK, Nadazdin A, Oakley CM: Dobutamine stress echocardiography for detection and assessment of coronary artery disease. J Am Coll Cardiol 1992;19:1203–1211.

152a. Poldermans D, Fioretti PM, Boersma E, Forster T, van Urk H, Cornel JH, Arnese M, Roelandt JRTC: Safety of dobutamine-atropine stress echocardiography in patients with suspected or proven coronary artery disease. Am J Cardiol 1994;73:456–459.

153. Martin TW, Seaworth JF, Johns JP, Pupa LE, Condos WR: Comparison of adenosine, dipyridamole, and dobutamine in stress echocardiography. Ann Intern Med 1992;116:190–196.

153a. Mertes H, Sawada S, Ryan T, Segar D, Kovacs R, Foltz J, Feigenbaum H: Symptoms, adverse effects, and complications associated with dobutamine stress echocardiography (Abstract). Circulation 1993;88:15–19.

153b. Bach DS, Hepner A, Marcovitz PA, Armstrong WF: Dobutamine stress echocardiography: Prevalence of a nonischemic response in a low-risk population. Am Heart J 1993;125:1257–1261.

153c. Hoffman R, Lethan H, Kleinhans E, Weiss M, Flaschkempf F, Hanrath P: Comparitive evaluation of bicycle and dobutamine stress echocardiography with perfusion scintigraphy and bicycle electrocardiogram for identification of coronary artery disease (Abstract). Am J Cardiol 1993;72:555–559.

153d. Eichelberger J: Predictive value of dobutamine echo just before noncardiac vascular surgery (Abstract). Am J Cardiol 1993;72:602–607.

153e. Günlap B, Dokumaci B, Uyan C, Vardareli E, Isik E, Bayhan H, Özgüven M, Öztürk E: Value of dobutamine technetium-99m-sestamibi SPECT and echocardiography in the detection of coronary artery disease compared with coronary angiography. J Nucl Med 1993;34:889–894.

153f. Smart S, Sawada S, Ryan T, Segar D, Atherton L, Berkovitz K, Bourdillion P, Feigenbaum H: Low dose dobutamine echocardiography detects reversible dysfunction after thrombolytic therapy of acute myocardial infarction. Circulation 1993;88:405–415.

153g. Cigarroa C, deFlippi C, Bricker M, Alverez L, Wait M, Graybin P: Dobutamine stress echocardiography identifies hibernating myocardium and predicts recovery of left ventricular function after coronary revascularization (Abstract). Circulation 1993;88:430–436.

153h. Marwick T, Willemart B, D'Hondt AM, Baudhuin T, Wijns W, Detry JM, Melin J: Selection of the optimal nonexercise stress for the evaluation of ischemic regional myocardial dysfunction and malperfusion. Comparison of dobutamine and adenosine using echocardiography and 99mTc-MIBI single photon emission computed tomography. Circulation 1993;87:345–354.

153i. Marwick T, Willemart B, D'Hondt AM, Baudhuin T, Wijns W, Detry JM, Melin J: Selection of the optimal nonexercise stress for the evaluation of ischemic regional myocardial dysfunction and malperfusion. Comparison of dobutamine and adenosine using echocardiography and 99mTc-MIBI single photon emission computed tomography. Circulation 1993;87:345–354.

153j. Poldermans D, Fioretti PM, Forster T, Thomson IR, Boersma E, el-Said EM, du Bois NA, Roelandt JR, van Urk H: Dobutamine stress echocardiography for assessment of perioperative cardiac risk in patients undergoing major vascular surgery. Circulation 1993; 87:1506–1512.

153k. Marcovitz PA, Bach DS, Mathias W, Shayna V, Armstrong WF: Paradoxic hypotension during dobutamine stress echocardiography: Clinical and diagnostic implications. J Am Coll Cardiol 1993;21:1080–1086.

153l. Simek CL, Watson DD, Smith WII, Vinson E, Kaul S: Dipyrida-

mole thallium-201 imaging versus dobutamine echocardiography for the evaluation of coronary artery disease in patients unable to exercise. Am J Cardiol 1993;72:1257–1262.

153m. Marwick T, D'Hondt AM, Baudhuin T, Willemart B, Wijns W, Detry JM, Melin J: Optimal use of dobutamine stress for the detection and evaluation of coronary artery disease combination with echocardiography or scintigraphy, or both? J Am Coll Cardiol 1993;22:158–167.

153n. Verani MS: Myocardial perfusion imaging versus two-dimensional echocardiography: Comparative value in the diagnosis of coronary artery disease. J Nucl Cardiol 1994;1:399–414.

153o. Bach DS, Muller DWM, Gros BJ, Armstrong WF: False positive dobutamine stress echocardiograms: characterization of clinical, echocardiographic and angiographic findings. J Am Coll Cardiol 1994;24:928–933.

154. Schelbert HR: Current status and prospects of new radionuclides and radiopharmaceuticals for cardiovascular nuclear medicine. Semin Nucl Med 1987;17:145–181.

155. Gould KL: Clinical cardiac positron emission tomography: State of the art. Circulation 1991;84:I22–I36.

156. Schwaiger M, Hutchins G: Qualitative and quantitative assessment of perfusion imaging: Evaluation of coronary flow by PET (Abstract). Am J Card Imag 1991;5:25–31.

157. Schwaiger M, Muzik O: Assessment of myocardial perfusion by positron emission tomography. Am J Cardiol 1991;67:35D–43D.

158. Go RT, Marwick TH, MacIntyre WJ, Saha GB, Neumann DR, Underwood DA, Simpfendorfer CC: A prospective comparison of rubidium-82 PET and thallium-201 SPECT myocardial perfusion imaging utilizing a single dipyridamole stress in the diagnosis of coronary artery disease. J Nucl Med 1990;31:1899–1905.

159. Stewart RE, Schwaiger M, Molina E, Popma J, Gacioch GM, Kalus M, Squicciarini S, al-Aouar ZR, Schork A, Kuhl DE: Comparison of rubidium-82 positron emission tomography and thallium-201 SPECT imaging for detection of coronary artery disease. Am J Cardiol 1991;67:1303–1310.

160. Tamaki N, Yonekura Y, Senda M, Kureshi SA, Saji H, Kodama S, Konishi Y, Ban T, Kambara H, Kawai C, et al.: Myocardial positron computed tomography with 13N-ammonia at rest and during exercise. Eur J Nucl Med 1985;11:246–251.

161. Laubenbacher C, Rothley J, Sitomer J, Beanlands R, Sawada S, Sutor R, Muller D, Schwaiger M: An automated analysis program for the evaluation of cardiac PET studies: Initial results in the detection and localization of coronary artery disease using nitrogen-13-ammonia. J Nucl Med 1993;34:968–978.

Chapter 9

Assessment of Myocardial Viability

An accurate noninvasive determination of myocardial viability is vitally important for clinical decision making, since it permits the identification of those patients with coronary artery disease (CAD) and left ventricular (LV) dysfunction who will most benefit from revascularization. Prior results of clinical trials evaluating the efficacy of coronary bypass surgery have shown that patients with multivessel CAD and a depressed left ventricular ejection fraction (LVEF) benefit most from revascularization, even if symptoms of angina are minimal or absent.[1–3] In recent years, there has been a greater appreciation among clinicians of the phenomena of "stunned" and of "hibernating" myocardium.[4, 5] Both these pathophysiologic states may result in profound regional LV dysfunction in the absence of necrosis. Thus, mere assessment of regional systolic function, by echocardiography, radionuclide angiography, or contrast ventriculography, is insufficient to distinguish between irreversibly injured and viable but dysfunctional myocardium.

Both experimental and clinical data indicate that imaging of myocardial perfusion and/or metabolism provides clinically relevant information about the status of myocardial viability in the presence of regional and global myocardial systolic dysfunction.[6–10a] This ability to differentiate irreversibly damaged from viable but asynergic myocardium can help clinicians in identifying those patients with CAD and depressed LV function who might benefit most from coronary bypass surgery or coronary angioplasty. This is because many surgeons are reluctant to perform bypass surgery in CAD patients who have a marked diminution in LV function unless angina symptoms are severe. Many of these patients have poor distal coronary vessels for grafting, are elderly, have concomitant renal disease, or are diabetic.

All these variables have been associated with a less than satisfactory outcome after bypass surgery. Table 9–1 lists some of the clinical and noninvasive test variables that indicate preserved myocardial viability.

STUNNED AND HIBERNATING MYOCARDIUM

Stunned Myocardium

Evidence has accumulated that, under various experimental conditions and in certain clinical syndromes, postischemic myocardial dysfunction (stunning) can be observed.[4, 11] Myocardial stunning implies a reversible form of contractile dysfunction that can occur after restoration of coronary blood flow following a relative brief period of coronary occlusion (e.g., 15 minutes).[12] Stunning can also be observed after multiple serial transient decreases in coronary blood flow, where cessation of flow with any one episode rarely exceeds 5 minutes.[13, 14] This myocardial dysfunction may be prolonged, despite full restoration of blood flow after the transient obstruction(s) of a coronary vessel. The precise pathophysiology of the stunning phenomenon is not entirely understood. Some mechanisms proposed have included impairment of myocardial energy production,[15] disruption or inefficient transfer of energy into myocyte contraction,[16, 17] impairment of sympathetic nerve activity due to ischemic damage,[18] altered calcium sensitivity at the myofilament level,[19] calcium overload,[20, 21] microvascular capillary obstruction by neutrophils,[22] ischemic damage to the extracellular collagen matrix,[23] and detrimental effects of oxygen-free radicals liberated during reperfusion, which cause membrane lipid peroxidation.[24]

Table 9–1. Clinical and Noninvasive Variables Suggestive of Preserved Myocardial Viability

Clinical, ECG, and resting echocardiographic parameters
  Presence of angina
  Preserved systolic thickening on echocardiography
  Asynergy out of proportion to extent of Q waves
  Asynergy after infarction out of proportion to creatine kinase levels
  Microcirculatory integrity by contrast echocardiography
  Enhanced systolic thickening after dobutamine infusion
  Worsening of wall motion with larger dose of dobutamine
Myocardial perfusion imaging parameters
  Normal initial TI-201 uptake after stress
  Delayed TI-201 redistribution at 2.5 to 4 hours
  Enhanced TI-201 uptake after "reinjection"
  18- to 24-hour late TI-201 redistribution
  TI-201 uptake ($\geq$50% of normal) on rest redistribution
Tc-99m–sestamibi or –tetrofosmin imaging parameters
  Normal uptake after stress or rest
  Mild decreased uptake (>50% of normal) at rest
  Reversible defects from stress to rest
  Preserved systolic thickening on gated perfusion imaging
MRI parameters
  Preserved thickness on end-diastolic images
  Enhanced thickening after dobutamine on gated images
PET parameters
  Mismatch between perfusion and FDG uptake
  Preserved C-11 acetate kinetics
  Normal extraction and washout of Rb-82

The myocardial stunning phenomenon has been extensively studied in animal models of experimental coronary occlusion followed by reperfusion.[4] In chronically instrumented intact dogs, Buxton et al.[25] examined the time course of blood flow and metabolic and regional systolic functional changes after 3 hours of left anterior descending coronary artery (LAD) occlusion followed by reperfusion. Regional myocardial function assessed by two-dimensional (2-D) echocardiography was markedly depressed during occlusion and did not improve significantly until 1 week after reperfusion. Despite rapid normalization of blood flow in reversibly injured regions, myocardial oxygen consumption (MVo_2) remained depressed and did not improve from occlusion levels until 1 week after flow restoration, indicating that oxygen extraction in the stunned myocardium was depressed for a prolonged period. Early (3 hours) after reperfusion, there was a decrease in fatty acid oxidation but also no increase in glucose metabolism. At 24 hours postreperfusion, there was increased glucose extraction and increased glucose metabolism relative to the normal myocardial tissue remote from the infarct. Thus, oxidative metabolism and regional function showed parallel recovery with time in postischemic myocardial tissue.

Clinical Correlates of Stunned Myocardium

In the clinical setting, myocardial stunning probably occurs after thrombolytic therapy in acute myocardial infarction (MI) since regional and global LV function demonstrate delayed improvement during days or weeks after coronary reperfusion.[26, 27] Stunning may also be observed in some patients with unstable angina who experience repeated episodes of coronary flow diminution caused by coronary vasospasm or cyclical obstruction by intraluminal thrombi.[28, 29] Also, stunning could occur after exercise-induced regional myocardial ischemia, which can be detected in the postexercise period using 2-D echocardiographic techniques.

Anderson et al.[27] serially assessed regional wall motion by 2-D echocardiography in patients who were treated with intracoronary streptokinase for acute MI. Gradual improvement in regional wall motion, as compared with prethrombolysis assessment, was seen between 1 and 10 days after thrombolytic therapy. Similarly, Stack et al.[30] employing serial LV angiography in patients undergoing thrombolytic therapy, found that the percentage of radial shortening of segments in the infarct zone showed no significant change on day 1, but that significant improvement was demonstrated 2 weeks following reperfusion. Touchstone et al.[31] evaluated regional systolic function by 2-D echocardiography in a group of MI patients receiving intravenous streptokinase. All patients were treated within 4 hours of the onset of symptoms. Improvement in wall motion was observed in approximately half of the patients, but this functional recovery was not evident during the first 3 days after infarction. By day 10, improvement was noted in patients with a patent infarct-related vessel, with continued enhancement of systolic function by 6 weeks after discharge.

Thus, studies conducted in patients with acute MI treated early with thrombolytic therapy show that, soon after flow restoration, myocardial systolic function in the infarct zone remains depressed. Such patients may manifest hemodynamic instability or even cardiogenic shock in the early postreperfusion period as a consequence of postischemic cardiac dysfunction. It may be important to determine at that time whether the dysfunction in the infarct zone indeed represents stunning or is a manifestation of irreversible cellular injury. Urgent revascularization with the former state would most likely be beneficial, whereas with the latter situation of extensive necrosis, revascularization may not prove beneficial. If one had a sensitive and cost-effective noninvasive approach to distinguishing stunned from necrotic myocardium in postthrombolytic patients with hemodynamic compromise, selection of patients for revascularization could be made on a more rational basis.

Hibernating Myocardium

Hibernating myocardium describes a state of persistently impaired LV dysfunction in the resting basal state attributed to a chronic reduction in coronary blood flow. This term, first used by Rahimtoola,[5] represents a state of reduced blood flow where neither ischemic pain nor myocardial necrosis is identified but myocardial function is substantially "down-regulated." Hibernating myocardium implies that if regional flow is enhanced or the oxygen supply-demand relation improved, then cardiac function will improve. Transmural myocardial dysfunction, the hallmark of hibernation, can be observed in the presence of subendocardial hypoperfusion with preservation of subepicardial blood flow. Using a single-crystal pulsed Doppler system in open-chest dogs, Edwards et al.[32] from the University of Virginia showed that under conditions of low coronary flow produced by a stenosis of the LAD, dysfunction was observed in endocardial, midwall, and epicardial layers, although ischemia was confined to the subendocardium. In fact, in this canine model, systolic thinning of the epicardial layers occurred despite nearly normal subepicardial blood flow (Fig. 9–1). Data from this study showed that marked depression of transmural function occurred with a chronic diminution in subendocardial flow. This severe subendocardial hypoperfusion may be a mechanism for severe transmural asynergy in the absence of infarction. Hibernation and stunning could occur simultaneously when brief periods of transient total or subtotal coronary occlusion are superimposed on a prolonged low-flow state (i.e., episodes of coronary vasospasm in the setting of a chronic severe stenosis causing a decrease in resting flow). Patients with chronic ischemic dysfunction may present with clinical symptoms and signs of ischemic cardiomyopathy characterized by a depressed LVEF and multiple regional wall motion abnormalities, which often correspond to severe and extensive underlying multivessel CAD.

Clinical Correlates of Hibernating Myocardium

Lewis et al.[33] determined the frequency and significance of LV wall motion abnormalities in patients without clinical evidence of MI. They reviewed the 2-D echocardiograms of 252 patients with no clinical or electrocardiographic (ECG) evidence of MI who subsequently underwent coronary angiography. There were 77 separate echocardiographic regions showing resting wall motion abnormalities in the 66 patients with CAD, of which 49 were hypokinetic, 22 akinetic, and 6 dyskinetic. After revascularization in a subset of 19 patients examined by serial preoperative and postoperative echocardiography, 85% of the segments with preoperative wall motion abnormalities improved, and 75% normalized. Only two of seven akinetic dyskinetic segments failed to show improvement. Thus, most of these asynergic segments were of the "hibernating" type.

Other studies have also shown improvement in regional and global LV function after revascularization. Brundage et al.[34] showed a high frequency of improvement and normalization of wall motion late after revascularization if bypass grafts were patent and improved perfusion was demonstrated. Topol et al.[35] reported that improvement in segmental function after bypass surgery was greatest in segments that preoperatively exhibited the most severe dysfunction. A similar improvement in wall motion after coronary angioplasty with some akinetic segments reverting to normal wall motion after successful dilatation has been reported by Nienaber et al.[36] Interestingly, these investigators found that wall motion did not improve early after angioplasty (4 days) but did improve significantly by 5 months after the procedure. Perfusion improved immediately after angioplasty, with no further improvement at late follow-up. Improvement in segmental function after angioplasty has been seen in zones of prior infarction, suggesting some hibernation in myocardium within the risk area of the infarct-related vessel.[37]

Linderer et al.[38] reported an improvement in LVEF from 60% ± 13% to 64% ± 13% (P < 0.001) and improvement in 40% of resting regional wall motion abnormalities in 145 patients who had successful coronary angioplasty of the

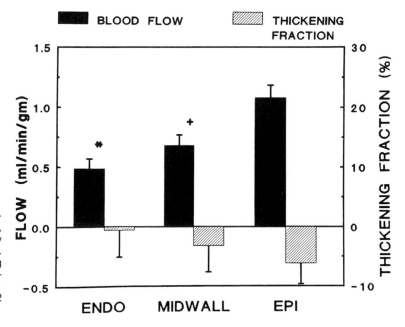

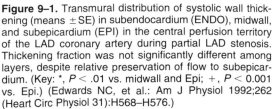

Figure 9–1. Transmural distribution of systolic wall thickening (means ± SE) in subendocardium (ENDO), midwall, and subepicardium (EPI) in the central perfusion territory of the LAD coronary artery during partial LAD stenosis. Thickening fraction was not significantly different among layers, despite relative preservation of flow to subepicardium. (Key: *, P < .01 vs. midwall and Epi; +, P < 0.001 vs. Epi.) (Edwards NC, et al.: Am J Physiol 1992;262 (Heart Circ Physiol 31):H568–H576.)

infarct-related artery at an average of 5 months after infarction. Montalescot et al.[39] also showed that patients randomized to coronary angioplasty after Q-wave MI had a significant improvement in segmental wall motion (11.5% ± 2.2%, $P < 0.001$ from baseline) 2 months after the procedure. The change was greater than that for patients randomized to conservative treatment (4.1% ± 1.4%; Fig. 9–2). None of these patients manifested symptomatic ischemia, and none had redistribution thallium-201 (Tl-201) defects on stress imaging. Myocardial hibernation can also be observed in myocardial regions remote from the infarct zone in the setting of multivessel CAD. Smucker et al.[40] reported two patients whose LV dysfunction after MI was far in excess of infarct size as evidenced by ECG changes and the magnitude of creatine kinase release. Both patients demonstrated Tl-201 redistribution in the myocardial beds remote from the infarct zone on rest Tl-201 images, and both had multivessel CAD on coronary angiography. Improvement in regional and global LV function was seen after revascularization surgery.

As with the ''stunned'' myocardial state, the demonstration of viability in asynergic ''hibernating'' myocardial segments by noninvasive means in patients with chronic CAD or after MI[40a] might suggest that coronary revascularization would be of benefit in enhancing cardiac dynamics and improving indices of systolic ventricular performance. Revascularization for chronic underperfusion, rather than extensive scar, should result in enhancement in exercise tolerance with concomitant improvement in heart failure functional class.

EXPERIMENTAL BASIS FOR THALLIUM-201 IMAGING FOR DETECTION OF MYOCARDIAL VIABILITY

Thallium-201 Uptake in Stunned or Hibernating Myocardium

As described in Chapter 2, after intravenous injection, the early myocardial uptake of Tl-201 is proportional to regional blood flow and the extraction fraction of Tl-201 by the myocardium. The extraction fraction under normal basal flow conditions is in the range of 85%. Acidosis and hypoxemia have little effect on myocardial extraction of Tl-201 as long as sarcolemmal membrane injury is avoided. Transient ischemia, characterized by a fall in coronary perfusion pressure, does not alter the myocardial extraction fraction for Tl-201.

Tl-201 uptake and washout kinetics were shown to be unaltered in an experimental canine model of stunned myocardium characterized by severe postischemic dysfunction observed after repetitive brief periods of flow reduction.[13] To produce myocardial stunning, open-chested dogs with a critical LAD stenosis were subjected to ten 5-minute periods of total LAD coronary artery occlusion, each interspersed by 10 minutes of reperfusion by reflow through the critical stenosis. The stenosis, itself, did not significantly reduce resting blood flow. Systolic thickening was serially measured by echocardiography. The myocardial stunning protocol resulted in a reduction of systolic thickening in the LAD zone to 0.4% ± 2.4% as compared with 32% ± 2% thickening in control dogs (Fig. 9–3A). Despite virtual akinesis in the LAD zone, the first-pass ejection fraction of Tl-201 was 0.78, a value identical to that measured in control animals (Fig. 9–3B). The half-time ($T_{1/2}$) for the intracellular Tl-201 washout was also not significantly different for stunned (60 ± 13 minutes) and control (53 ± 14 minutes) dogs. In another experimental study by Sinusas et al.,[41] Tl-201 uptake was not affected by postischemic dysfunction produced by stunning the myocardium with 15 minutes of total LAD occlusion followed by reperfusion. These experimental data are consistent with normal myocardial Tl-201 extraction and washout kinetics in canine models of myocardial stunning.

Sinusas et al.[41] examined Tl-201 uptake in a low-flow canine model of ''short-term'' hibernating myocardium characterized by a sustained reduction in systolic function without necrosis. Myocardial Tl-201 uptake was not impaired out of proportion to the flow diminution when resting flow was reduced by approximately 40% in these experiments (Fig. 9–4).

Thallium-201 Uptake and Irreversibly-Injured Myocardium

Irreversibly-damaged myocardial tissue cannot concentrate Tl-201 intracellularly (see Chap. 2). If necrotic myocardial cells were able to bind Tl-201, then the radionuclide could not be utilized as a viability agent for myocardial scintigraphy. Goldhaber et al.,[42] in a cultured fetal mouse heart preparation, found that accumulation of Tl-201 in hearts subjected to ischemia-like myocardial injury was related in a decreasing fashion to the loss of lactic dehydrogenase. Loss of this enzyme has characteristically been associated with cell death. In a study performed in open-chest anesthetized dogs by Granato et al.,[43] necrotic myocardium did not concentrate Tl-201 intracellularly when administered after reperfusion preceded by 3 hours of LAD occlusion. Tl-201 was administered after 40 minutes of coronary occlusion, and Tl-201 activity was serially measured in nonischemic and ischemic zones utilizing transmural myocardial biopsy. In these dogs, the occlusive snare around the vessel was quickly released, allowing rapid reflow. Figure 9–5 shows the Tl-201 time-activity curves from ischemic and normal myocardium for this group of animals. At the end of the 3-hour occlusion period, Tl-201 activity in the central ischemic zone was reduced to 24% ± 6% of initial normal activity. After 2 hours of reperfu-

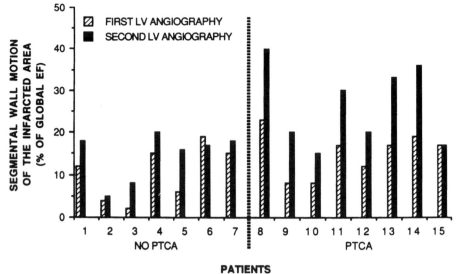

Figure 9–2. Bar graph shows individual changes of segmental area ejection fraction indexes (expressed as a percentage of global area ejection fraction) in postinfarction patients treated conservatively with no coronary angioplasty (NO PTCA; patients 1 to 7) and by revascularization with PTCA (patients 8 to 15). Mean change was +11.5 ± 2.2% in PTCA patients, as compared to +4.1 ± 1.4% in the no PTCA group. (Key: EF, ejection fraction; LV, left ventricle.) (Montalescot G, et al.: Circulation 1992;86:47–55.)

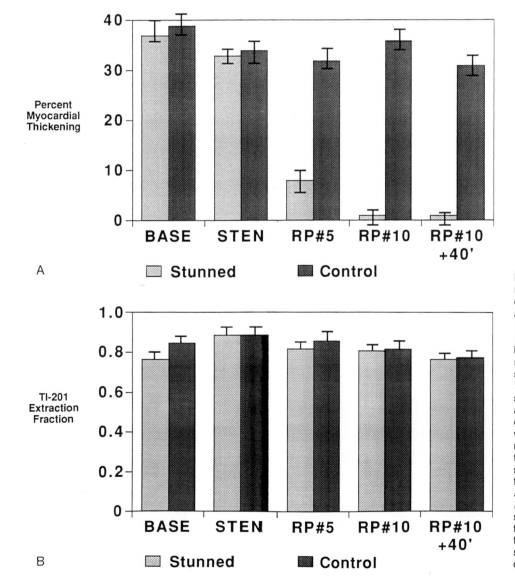

A

Figure 9–3. A. Bar graph shows serial changes in percentage of myocardial thickening in the LAD coronary artery perfusion zone in stunned dogs *(lightly shaded bars)* and controls *(darkly shaded bars).* (Key: Base, baseline; Sten, stenosis; RP#5, after reperfusion 5; RP#10, after reperfusion 10; R-10E +40, 40 minutes after 10th reflow.) Note that, in dogs in the stunning protocol there was virtual absence of myocardial systolic thickening after the 10th reflow period, whereas control dogs with LAD stenosis alone exhibited no change in thickening at that point. **B.** Bar graph shows first-pass Tl-201 extraction fractions in stunned dogs *(lightly shaded bars)* and control dogs *(darkly shaded bars).* Note that despite severe abnormalities in systolic thickening, the first-pass Tl-201 extraction fraction is unaltered in the stunned group. (Moore CA, et al.: Circulation 1990;81:1622–1632.)

B

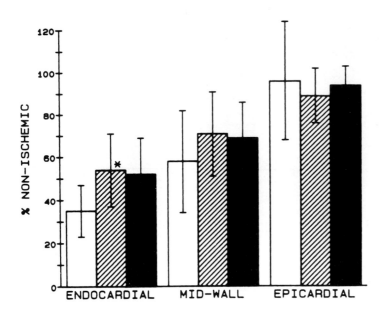

Figure 9–4. Regional blood flow *(open bars)*, Tl-201 activity *(crosshatched bars)*, and Tc-99m–sestamibi activity *(solid bars)*, expressed as a percentage of the nonischemic values, in dogs subjected to a sustained reduction in LAD coronary artery flow. Note that Tl-201 and Tc-99m–sestamibi activities were comparable and increased proportionally with flow. (Key: *, $P = 0.05$ vs. flow.) (Reprinted with permission from the American College of Cardiology (Journal of the American College of Cardiology, 1989, Vol. 14, pp. 1785–1793).)

sion, ischemic zone Tl-201 activity rose only slightly but not significantly to 28% ± 5%. Regional transmural blood flow, however, was restored to 89% ± 10% of normal flow. The Tl-201 defect magnitude decreased from 78% ± 6% during occlusion to 51% ± 9% after 2 hours of reflow. This diminution in defect magnitude was chiefly due to washout of Tl-201 from normal myocardium perfused by the left circumflex coronary artery. Infarct size averaged 29% ± 4% of the left ventricle by weight. Thus, in these experiments the extent of Tl-201 uptake in reperfused myocardium reflected the extent of myocardial salvage. Although transmural flow was restored to near nonischemic levels, Tl-201 uptake remained depressed, since myocardial Tl-201 activity reflected viability rather than just mere flow restoration.

Taken together, this experimental work suggests that the intracellular extraction of Tl-201 is not altered unless there is ischemia-induced irreversible sarcolemmal membrane injury. Chronic low-flow states alone and myocardial stunning after brief periods of transient coronary occlusion do not adversely affect Tl-201 extraction or intracellular washout as along as some residual blood flow is preserved to ensure adequate delivery of the radionuclide to the myocardial cells. Even akinetic myocardial segments can exhibit normal or nearly normal Tl-201 uptake as long as some residual flow is present and necrosis has been avoided.

Thallium-201 Redistribution and Viability

Following the initial myocardial uptake phase after intravenous injection, there is a continuous exchange of myocar-

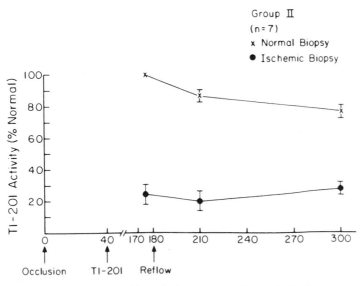

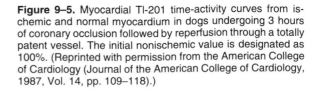

Figure 9–5. Myocardial Tl-201 time-activity curves from ischemic and normal myocardium in dogs undergoing 3 hours of coronary occlusion followed by reperfusion through a totally patent vessel. The initial nonischemic value is designated as 100%. (Reprinted with permission from the American College of Cardiology (Journal of the American College of Cardiology, 1987, Vol. 14, pp. 109–118).)

dial Tl-201 and Tl-201 in the blood pool (see Chap. 2). Tl-201 is continually clearing from normally perfused myocardium and replaced by recirculating Tl-201 from the residual activity in the vascular compartment.[44, 45] Normal myocardial zone washout of Tl-201 parallels washout of the tracer from the blood pool. This process of continuous exchange forms the basis of Tl-201 ''redistribution.'' Redistribution implies delayed defect resolution and is observed when Tl-201 is administered during transient underperfusion of the myocardium or with a chronic reduction in myocardial blood flow (''rest redistribution'').[46] With respect to myocardial Tl-201 scintigraphy, *redistribution* refers to the total or partial resolution of initial defects when assessed by repeat imaging at 2.5 to 4 hours after Tl-201 administration.[47] That is, the magnitude of the ischemic zone–normal zone ratio of Tl-201 activity, as measured quantitatively using computer-assisted techniques during image analysis, tends to normalize over time. The degree of resolution of an ischemic defect over the serial imaging period reflects the amount of redistribution.

When Tl-201 is injected during peak exercise or vasodilator stress, the disparity of flow between normal myocardium and myocardium that was relatively underperfused is substantial in the presence of a hemodynamically significant coronary stenosis.[48] With cessation of exercise stress or reversal of dipyridamole-induced vasodilation, there is restoration of relatively homogeneous flow to normal myocardium and previously underperfused myocardial regions. If Tl-201 is injected intravenously at the time of peak stress, delayed Tl-201 redistribution is subsequently observed as Tl-201 washes out of the normal region and exhibits late accumulation or flat washout in the previously ischemic segment. However, redistribution can only occur if myocardial cells supplied by the stenotic artery are metabolically viable and have functioning cell membranes, and if adenosine triphosphate (ATP) is available for active transport processes.

When myocardial necrosis is present, no delayed Tl-201 redistribution is seen in the zone of irreversibly injured myocardial tissue.[44] That is, the infarct-normal ratio of Tl-201 activity remains constant over time. Thus, a persistent Tl-201 defect is recognized in the supply region of the vessel perfusing the irreversibly damaged area. As will be subsequently discussed, some persistent Tl-201 defects in which no redistribution is visually observed on images obtained 4 hours after tracer injection, show improved Tl-201 uptake following revascularization.[49] Thus, in the clinical setting, not all persistent defects represent myocardial scar or acute myocardial damage. Partial redistribution is seen when there is a mixture of necrosis and reversibly ischemic myocardium or under conditions of severe ischemia in which redistribution is not ''complete'' at 2.5 to 4 hours after Tl-201 administration.

Figure 9–6 is a schematic diagram that summarizes the principles of Tl-201 kinetics as applied to the determination of myocardial viability by assessment of initial tracer uptake and delayed redistribution during the equilibrium phase.

Rest Thallium-201 Redistribution

Tl-201 redistribution over time when the tracer is injected in the resting state (rest redistribution) can be observed in patients with chronic asymptomatic CAD, unstable angina, severe stable angina, or after acute MI.[50–52] Many patients who demonstrate rest redistribution may have hibernating myocardial segments with persistent systolic dysfunction.[51, 52] These patients have ''resting'' hypoperfusion or resting ischemia with initial perfusion defects at rest that show subsequent total or delayed redistribution. The mechanism for ''rest redistribution'' with a chronic reduction in blood flow is discussed in Chapter 2. There is substantially slower washout of Tl-201 over time from chronically underperfused regions, as compared with more rapid Tl-201 washout from nonischemic regions. These disparate washout rates from hypoperfused and normal myocardium result in near normalization of Tl-201 activity between nonischemic and stenotic regions by 4 hours.[45]

EXERCISE THALLIUM-201 SCINTIGRAPHY AND MYOCARDIAL VIABILITY

Table 9–2 summarizes the various approaches utilized to assess myocardial viability with exercise or rest perfusion scintigraphy employing Tl-201.

Initial and 2.5- to 4-Hour Redistribution Imaging

Myocardial Tl-201 scintigraphy is most often performed in conjunction with exercise stress in patients suspected or known to have CAD (see Chap. 3). In addition to detection of stress-induced ischemia with exercise, the radionuclide test permits simultaneous assessment of regional myocardial viability. Perfusion defects observed on the Tl-201 images obtained 5 to 10 minutes after exercise indicate transient ischemia or a scar, or a combination of the two. To differentiate between viable and nonviable myocardium in defect regions, delayed images are obtained 2.5 to 4 hours later to determine whether or not redistribution is

Table 9–2. Approaches to Assessment of Myocardial Viability by Tl-201 Imaging

1. Stress and 2.5- to 4-hour redistribution
2. Stress, 2.5- to 4-hour redistribution, and 24-hour delayed images
3. Stress, 2.5- to 4-hour redistribution, and reinjection images
4. Stress, immediate reinjection, and delayed images
5. Early and 4-hour delayed resting images

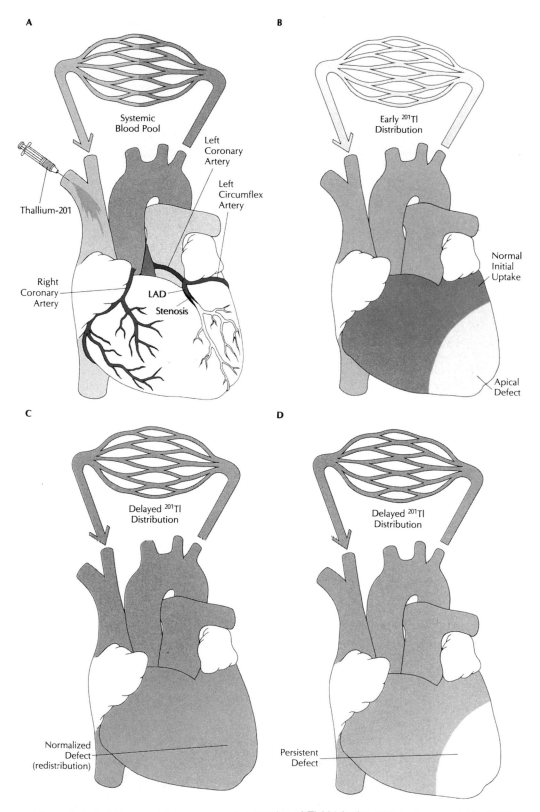

Figure 9–6. A. Diagram of intravenous administration of Tl-201 in the setting of severe LAD artery stenosis. **B.** After the initial myocardial uptake phase of early Tl-201 distribution, an apical defect is observed in the supply zone of the narrowed LAD. **C.** After initial uptake, continuous tissue-blood exchange results in delayed redistribution, which results in normalization of the defect depicted in **B**. **D.** In the presence of myocardial scar, the apical defect noted in **B** would remain persistent. (Reprinted with permission. Beller GA: Hospital Practice Volume 23, issue 9, pages 96–97. Illustration by Seward Hung.)

evident. As described in the preceding paragraphs, an initial postexercise perfusion defect demonstrating delayed redistribution implies ischemia and viability. Detection of redistribution is enhanced by utilizing quantitative planar image analysis where relative regional Tl-201 uptake and washout are measured after appropriate interpolative background subtraction[53] (see Chap. 2). Figure 9–7 is an example of significant delayed Tl-201 redistribution in a zone of infarction, indicating substantial residual viability despite presence of Q waves on the resting ECG on serial planar images. Single-photon emission computed tomography (SPECT) Tl-201 imaging with quantitation of regional activity can also be undertaken for viability determination with exercise stress.

Some persistent Tl-201 defects represent ischemia rather than scar. Gibson et al.[49] evaluated 47 patients with CAD who underwent quantitative planar Tl-201 exercise scintigraphy before and 4.3 ± 3.1 weeks after coronary bypass surgery. Figure 9–8 illustrates the frequency with which the various types of perfusion Tl-201 abnormalities normalized after surgery. Ninety-three percent of defects showing total redistribution preoperatively showed normal uptake and washout of Tl-201 postoperatively. Seventy-three percent of partial redistributing defects showed improved Tl-201 uptake and washout after revascularization. Forty-five percent of persistent defects thought preoperatively to represent scar showed significant improvement in Tl-201 uptake postoperatively. The persistent defects that normalized

postoperatively were usually mild, showing no more than 25% to 50% reduction in Tl-201 activity relative to normal zone activity preoperatively. Fifty-seven percent of these mild defects normalized postoperatively. In contrast, only 3 of 14 severe persistent defects that exhibited more than 50% reduction in regional Tl-201 activity showed improvement after revascularization. Figure 9–9 shows that the percentage of reduction in regional Tl-201 uptake for persistent defects that normalized or improved after surgery was significantly smaller than that of those that did not improve.

More recently, Yamamoto et al.[53a] reported that improvement in regional wall motion in infarct zones after angioplasty was more likely to occur when mean Tl-201 uptake on delayed images was more than 50% of nonischemic uptake. The data from this study are summarized in Table 9–3. In zones of more than 50% uptake mean regional EF in the infarct zone increased from 39% ± 18% before angioplasty to 47% ± 14% after angioplasty. In contrast, preangioplasty regional EF was 23% ± 9% and remained at 24% ± 12% postangioplasty in zones of not more than 50% Tl-201 uptake on delayed images.

In a patient cohort undergoing coronary angioplasty, Liu et al.[54] reported that 75% of persistent Tl-201 defects on 3-hour delayed images normalized after angioplasty. Ohtani et al.[55] reported that 47% of segments showing persistent Tl-201 defects on 4-hour delayed images showed improvement in perfusion and function postoperatively. Cloninger

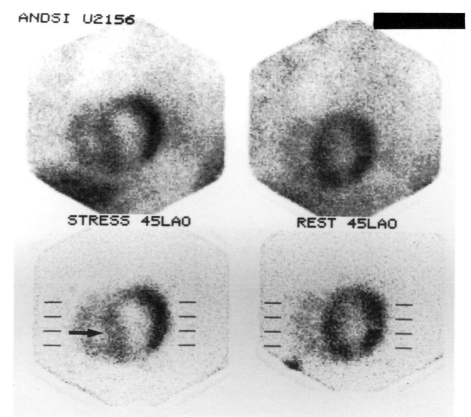

Figure 9–7. Postexercise and delayed 45-degree left anterior oblique images in a patient who experienced an anterior myocardial infarction with Q waves on the resting ECG. Note significantly delayed Tl-201 redistribution in the septum, which is the supply zone of the LAD coronary artery on this view.

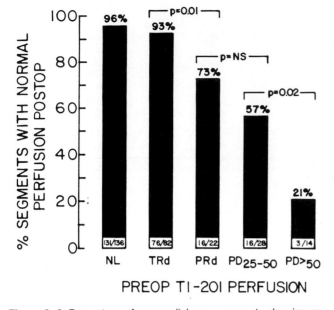

Figure 9–8. Percentage of myocardial scan segments showing normalization of Tl-201 perfusion abnormalities postoperatively (POSTOP) related to the preoperative (PREOP) Tl-201 perfusion patterns. (Key: Nl, normal; TRd, total redistribution; PRd, partial redistribution; PD$_{25-50}$, mild persistent defect showing 25% to 50% reduction in Tl-201 counts; PD$_{>50}$, severe persistent defects with greater than 50% reduction in Tl-201 counts.) (Reprinted with permission from the American College of Cardiology (Journal of the American College of Cardiology, 1983, Vol. 1, pp. 804–815).)

Table 9–3. **Delayed Tl-201 Uptake and Improvement in Wall Motion After PTCA in Infarct Zones**

	Mean Tl-201 Uptake	
	REF ≤50%	*REF* >50%
Pre-PTCA	23 ± 9%	39 ± 18%
Post-PTCA	24 ± 12%	47 ± 14%*

*P < 0.05, c/w Post-PTCA REF ≤50%
REF = regional ejection fraction; PTCA = percutaneous transluminal coronary angioplasty.
(Adapted from Yamamoto K: Am Heart J 1993;125:33.)

et al.[56] evaluated extent of delayed Tl-201 redistribution before and after angioplasty in 141 patients undergoing 160 successful dilation procedures. Sixty-seven percent of the imaging studies in patients without a history of infarction showed partial redistribution at 4 hours prior to coronary angioplasty. After angioplasty, 76% showed improvement on the 4-hour delayed image; 34% showed complete defect normalization. All patients with non–Q-wave infarction had redistribution on 4-hour delayed images prior to angioplasty. After angioplasty, 80% showed improved final Tl-201 uptake 4 hours after tracer administration, and a third showed complete defect normalization. In contrast, only half of Q-wave patients showed more Tl-201 uptake after angioplasty, and 6% demonstrated total normalization of the scan.

Other evidence that some persistent Tl-201 defects on exercise scintigraphy represent ischemic but viable myocardium rather than scar comes from studies correlating Tl-201 images with positron emission tomography (PET) images of fluorine-18 2,deoxyglucose (FDG) uptake in the same patients.[57]

Late Redistribution Imaging

Late redistribution imaging at 18 to 24 hours after Tl-201 administration, following acquisition of 2.5- to 4-hour redistribution images, has been undertaken to enhance the detection of viability in defects that at 2.5 to 4 hours appear

to be persistent.[56, 58, 59] The rationale for this approach is that redistribution is an ongoing kinetic process that depends on continued reuptake of Tl-201 in areas perfused by stenotic lesions and differential Tl-201 washout rates between stenotic and normal myocardial zones. Redistribution also requires an adequate residual blood pool concentration of Tl-201 that recirculates in the myocardium during the period between initial uptake and the equilibrium phase. Gutman et al.[60] found late redistribution at 18 to 24 hours in 21% of postexercise defects in 59 patients with CAD. Cloninger et al.[56] obtained 8- to 24-hour delayed images of 40 patients who demonstrated "incomplete" redistribution at 4 hours with exercise SPECT scintigraphy. The late imaging studies showed further redistribution in approximately 45% of patients who had a history of MI and 92%

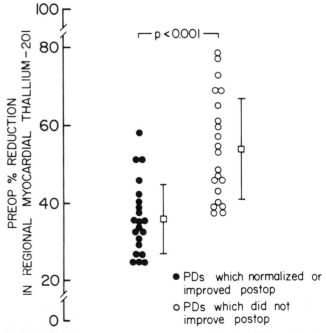

Figure 9–9. Percentage of reduction in regional Tl-201 uptake for persistent defects (PDs) that normalized after surgery *(solid circles)* as compared with persistent defects that did not improve after surgery *(open circles)*. Note that the persistent defects that normalized or improved postoperatively (postop) had a significantly smaller reduction in regional myocardial Tl-201 activity preoperatively (preop). (Reprinted with permission from the American College of Cardiology (Journal of the American College of Cardiology, 1983, Vol. 1, pp. 804–815).)

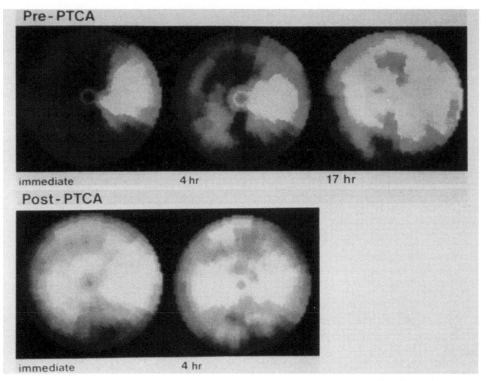

See Color Figure 9–10.

Figure 9–10. Bull's-eye maps from SPECT Tl-201 images obtained in a patient with angina pectoris before angioplasty (pre-PTCA) and 2 days after angioplasty (post-PTCA). Pre-PTCA, images were obtained immediately (immediate) after stress and 4 and 17 hours later and the post-PTCA scintigrams immediately and 4 hours after Tl-201 injection. Note the additional delayed redistribution at 17 hours compared to 4 hours in the pre-PTCA series of bull's-eye maps. After PTCA, Tl-201 activity is normal in both the stress and the 4-hour delayed images. (See Color Figure 9–10.) (Reprinted with permission from the American College of Cardiology (Journal of the American College of Cardiology, 1988, Vol. 12, pp. 955–963.).)

of patients without such a history. No patient who had had an MI demonstrated complete redistribution on 18- to 24-hour delayed images. Figure 9–10 shows the SPECT bull's-eye images from a patient in this study. Although some redistribution is perceived at 4 hours after Tl-201 injection, further filling in of the defect is apparent at 17 hours. After angioplasty, perfusion markedly improves after exercise stress.

Kiat et al.[58] reported that the presence or absence of late

Tl-201 redistribution at 18 to 24 hours predicted the post–coronary bypass or postangioplasty regional Tl-201 uptake pattern (Fig. 9–11). Ninety-five percent of segments showing late redistribution at 18 to 24 hours improved after revascularization, whereas only 37% of the segments that remained persistent at 18 to 24 hours showed improvement after revascularization. In that study comprising 21 patients, there were 220 perfusion defects on initial postexercise or dipyridamole SPECT Tl-201 images preintervention. Of

Figure 9–11. Relation between the percentage of Tl-201 scan segments that improve after intervention (angioplasty or bypass surgery) and the preintervention late (18- to 72-hour) imaging pattern. Significantly more segments showed postintervention improvement *(left bar)* that demonstrated late reversibility on 18- to 72-hour images as compared to segments showing nonreversibility on late imaging *(right bar)*. (Reprinted with permission from the American College of Cardiology (Journal of the American College of Cardiology, 1988, Vol. 12, pp. 1456–1463).)

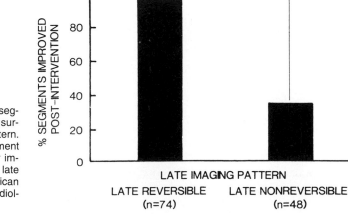

these, 40% showed redistribution and 60% were persistent at 4 hours as assessed by a visual scoring system. Sixty-four percent of the persistent defects showed late redistribution at 18 to 72 hours. After either bypass surgery or angioplasty, 85% of the segments that before the procedure showed redistribution at 4 hours after Tl-201 administration, improved after bypass surgery or angioplasty. Similarly, 82% of segments with partial redistribution at 4 hours showed improvement; however, 72% of persistent defects at 4 hours also improved after the intervention. Thus, in this study the Tl-201 scintigraphic patterns analyzed on 18- to 72-hour late imaging were more predictive of the postintervention scintigraphic response than the 4-hour image patterns. Nevertheless, 37% of late persistent defects still showed improvement after surgery or angioplasty, indicating that more than a third of segments judged to be nonviable on 18- to 72-hour late imaging were indeed viable (see Fig. 9–11).

In another study from the Cedars-Sinai group,[59] the frequency of late redistribution was assessed prospectively in a larger cohort of 118 patients who underwent SPECT exercise Tl-201 scintigraphy. Fifty-three percent of patients in this study showed late redistribution in regions that appeared as persistent defects on the 4-hour delayed images (Fig. 9–12). Thirty-five percent of patients had late redistribution in two or more segments that appeared persistent on 4-hour redistribution images. A total of 22% of 762 segments analyzed in these 118 patients showed late redistribution at 24 hours (Fig. 9–12). Of the total 1047 stress defects, 27% showed redistribution at 4 hours, and on late imaging an additional 16% showed redistribution. Thus, a total of 43% of segments showed redistribution on either 4-hour images or late imaging.

There are potential limitations of 24-hour imaging for detecting late redistribution not seen on 4-hour redistribution images. One problem is suboptimal count statistics, which can result in reduced image quality because of excess "noise." If one is undertaking this approach to differentiate between ischemia and scar, an initial dose of 3 to 4 mCi of Tl-201 should be administered at peak exercise and at least a 50% longer imaging time should be employed when acquiring the 24-hour redistribution images. Other limitations of 24-hour delayed imaging include patient inconvenience because of the necessity of returning the following day for repeat imaging and difficulty in prospectively identifying which patients will need to return for 24-hour imaging, since quantitative image analysis and interpretation of the scans may only be performed at the end of the first day. In one experience using quantitative early and 2.5- to 4-hour redistribution Tl-201 scintigraphy, few defects showed redistribution only on the 24-hour images and not on 4-hour images. Most defects that exhibit late redistribution at 24 hours demonstrate evidence of some redistribution on 4-hour images. In a study performed by Watson et al.,[61] mean defect magnitude after exercise in a group of CAD patients being evaluated for presence of ischemia was 43.8% ± 5.6%. Mean defect magnitude in segments showing redistribution was 31.0% ± 5.6% at 2.5 hours and 30.6% ± 7.6% at 24 hours (P = NS). Figure 9–13 summarizes the results of this study. No segments showed redistribution at 24 hours but not at 2.5 or 4.0 hours. Thus, quantitative planar imaging is a sensitive technique for detecting defect reversibility on early imaging and no benefit derives from 24-hour imaging to enhance appreciation of redistribution.

Reinjection Thallium-201 Imaging

An alternative to 24-hour delayed redistribution imaging for detection of viable myocardium is injection of a second dose of Tl-201 at rest following acquisition of the 2.5- to 4-hour redistribution images.[62–74b] Most often, 50% of the original dose that was administered during exercise is reinjected. Dilsizian et al.[62] studied 100 CAD patients using SPECT Tl-201 scintigraphy. Each patient received 2 mCi of Tl-201 intravenously during exercise, and immediate postexercise and 3- to 4-hour delayed images were made. Then, after obtaining the redistribution images, a second dose of 1 mCi of Tl-201 was injected while the patient was at rest. As shown in Figure 9–14, 33% of the abnormal segments in the patients reported by Dilsizian et al.[62] showed persistent defects on the 3- to 4-hour redistribution

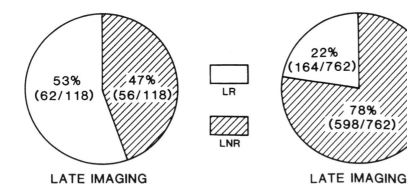

PATIENTS (n = 118)

53% (62/118)   47% (56/118)

LR

LNR

LATE IMAGING

SEGMENTS (n = 762)

22% (164/762)

78% (598/762)

LATE IMAGING

Figure 9–12. Frequency of late reversibility (LR) and late nonreversibility (LNR) in patients who underwent 18- to 72-hour Tl-201 redistribution imaging in relation to the number of patients *(left)* and number of segments *(right)*. (Reprinted with permission from the American College of Cardiology (Journal of the American College of Cardiology, 1990, Vol. 15, pp. 334–340).)

MAGNITUDE OF PERFUSION DEFECTS VS TIME POST INJECTION

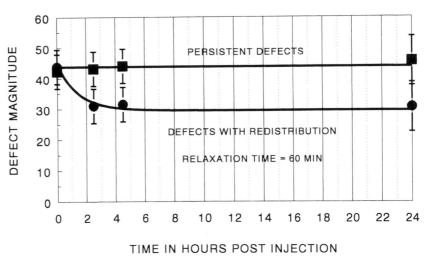

Figure 9–13. Defect magnitude by quantitative planar Tl-201 imaging at 2.5, 4, and 24 hours postinjection. Values are averages of 22 persistent defects and 20 defects graded as showing redistribution. Note that the redistribution process appears to follow an exponential relaxation curve with a half-time constant of approximately 60 minutes as predicted from kinetic models. (Watson DD: In: Zaret BL, Beller GA (eds): Nuclear Cardiology: State of the Art and Future Direction. St. Louis, CV Mosby, 1993, pp 65–76.)

images. Approximately half of these persistent Tl-201 defects demonstrated improved or normal Tl-201 uptake after reinjection of the second Tl-201 dose. Figure 9–15 shows stress, redistribution and reinjection tomographic images from a CAD patient in this study. Tl-201 uptake is enhanced in the anterior wall and septum after reinjection, as compared with uptake on the 4-hour images. In a subset of 20 patients, 87% of regions that exhibit enhanced Tl-201 uptake on preprocedure reinjection images showed normal Tl-201 uptake and improved regional wall motion after coronary angioplasty. In contrast, all regions with persistent Tl-201 defects on reinjection imaging before balloon dilatation had both abnormal Tl-201 uptake and persistently abnormal regional wall motion after the procedure. The authors concluded that reinjection of Tl-201 at rest after acquisition of redistribution images significantly enhanced the detection of viable myocardium.

Ohtani et al.[55] performed stress, 3-hour redistribution, and reinjection Tl-201 SPECT imaging in 24 patients before coronary bypass surgery. Tl-201 scan findings were compared with improvement in perfusion and function 1 to 2 months postoperatively. Reinjection imaging identified enhanced Tl-201 uptake in 47% of persistent defects on 3-hour delayed images. As expected, 79% of segments that exhibited redistribution before revascularization showed improved perfusion postoperatively. Forty-seven percent of

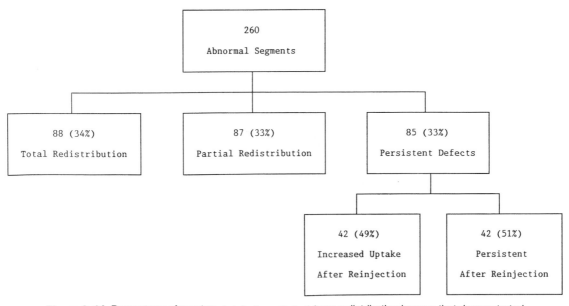

Figure 9–14. Percentage of persistent defects on 3- to 4-hour redistribution images that demonstrated improved or normal Tl-201 uptake after reinjection of a second dose of Tl-201. (Adapted from Dilsizian V, et al.: N Engl J Med 1990;323:141–146. Copyright 1990, Massachusetts Medical Society.)

Stress

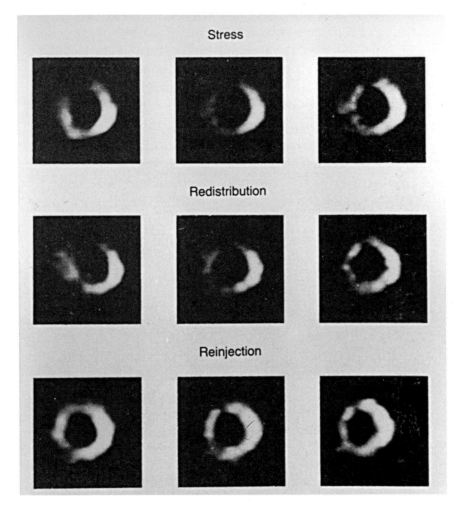

Redistribution

Reinjection

Figure 9–15. Short-axis Tl-201 tomograms during stress, redistribution, and reinjection in a patient with CAD. Note the extensive perfusion abnormalities in anterior and septal segments during stress imaging that showed only partial redistribution in the septum on the redistribution image but improved markedly on the reinjection image. (Reprinted by permission of *The New England Journal of Medicine* from Dilsizian V, et al.: N Engl J Med 1990;323:141–146. Copyright 1990, Massachusetts Medical Society.)

persistent defects on 3-hour delayed images also showed improved perfusion after surgery. Twelve of these fifteen persistent defects that showed improved perfusion after surgery had "new redistribution" on the preoperative reinjection images. Improved wall motion after surgery was similarly well predicted by preoperative scintigraphy. Seventy-four percent of segments with preoperative redistribution exhibited improved function and 71% of persistent defects at 3 hours that exhibited "new redistribution" after reinjection showed enhanced wall motion postoperatively. The predictive values for improvement in perfusion and wall motion by reinjection imaging were significantly higher (92% and 98%) than by 3-hour delayed imaging (69% and 62%, respectively; $P < 0.05$ for each).

Rocco et al.[63] performed reinjection imaging in 41 patients with persistent Tl-201 defects on 3- to 4-hour delayed images. Of 360 segments analyzed, concordance between the delayed and reinjected images occurred in 85%. Of 141 segments that demonstrated a persistent reduction in Tl-201 uptake on 3- to 4-hour delayed images, 44 (31%) exhibited enhanced Tl-201 uptake after reinjection. In nine patients in this study, data from the reinjection images provided the only evidence of ischemia. Most of the defects that demonstrated enhanced Tl-201 uptake after reinjection had evidence for sustained antegrade perfusion through a stenotic coronary artery or perfusion via collaterals.

Tamaki et al.[64] reported a series of 60 patients with CAD who showed improved tracer uptake following Tl-201 reinjection in 32% of segments with fixed defects on SPECT redistribution images. In this study, 29% of patients with persistent defects who had no evidence of redistribution in any segment on 3- to 4-hour delayed images showed enhanced Tl-201 uptake after reinjection. Thus, in this subgroup, the Tl-201 reinjection protocol was the only way to demonstrate myocardial viability.

There are some defects that remain irreversible after Tl-201 injection but are viable by the PET criteria of increased FDG uptake relative to flow (mismatch pattern). Despite remaining irreversible after reinjection, such defects can show a substantial increase in "absolute" Tl-201 counts in the defect zone as compared with the 4-hour delayed redistribution images.[65] Dilsizian et al.[65] showed that the mild to moderate (51% to 85% of normal activity) persistent defects were more likely to show this increase in absolute Tl-201 activity after reinjection than the severe (not more than 50% of normal activity) persistent defects. These data are consistent with the finding of Gibson et al.,[49] who reported that mild persistent defects showing no more than a 50%

reduction in Tl-201 counts, relative to normal zone activity, had the greatest likelihood of exhibiting improved perfusion and function after revascularization. Defects characterized by a severe persistent reduction in Tl-201 activity on 4-hour redistribution images are less likely to show enhanced uptake after reinjection.

Kiat et al.[66] explored the option of dispensing with the redistribution images altogether and reinjecting the second dose of Tl-201 immediately after the stress tomographic acquisition. Repeat SPECT images are acquired 4 hours after reinjection. This protocol was considered to be superior to the conventional poststress, redistribution, and reinjection sequence protocol. Time is provided for "rest redistribution," since the interval between reinjection and imaging is spread out to 4 hours. Despite the potential superiority of this approach, 58% of patients had further redistribution at 18 to 72 hours after reinjection than on their 4-hour images. The frequency of the need for 24-hour imaging to enhance detection of reversibility was not reduced by this early reinjection of a second dose of Tl-201 immediately after stress images were obtained, as compared to the conventional single-dose Tl-201 stress and redistribution imaging.

Eliminating the acquisition of the 2.5- to 4-hour redistribution images and just reinjecting Tl-201 at 4 hours may convert some myocardial segments that would have showed redistribution at 4 hours into irreversible defects on reinjection images.[67] This phenomenon is most likely due to a resting decrease in regional blood flow so that the defect seen when Tl-201 is reinjected, represents the flow diminution at the time of Tl-201 administration. Thus, the "redistribution" images should not be eliminated in favor of just acquiring "reinjection" images. Figure 9–16 shows peak Tl-201 activity in 14 regions exhibiting this phenomenon of reinjection making defects that showed reversibility on 3- to 4-hour redistribution images revert to persistent defects after reinjection.

Reinjection Thallium-201 Imaging Versus Positron Emission Tomography

Tl-201 scintigraphy employing the reinjection technique may be as sensitive as PET imaging with FDG for assessing myocardial viability. Theoretically, Tl-201 uptake at the redistribution phase or after reinjection of a Tl-201 dose at rest, should correlate well with metabolic integrity of the myocardial region in question. In one study, Tl-201 and FDG were compared in an open-chest canine model in which 2 hours of coronary occlusion was followed by 4 hours of reflow.[68] Tl-201 was injected before reperfusion and FDG was administered 3 hours after reflow. Both normal FDG uptake and delayed Tl-201 redistribution reflected myocardial viability after reperfusion. Lack of redistribution and depressed FDG uptake were observed in irreversibly injured myocardial zones. Bonow et al.[69] compared

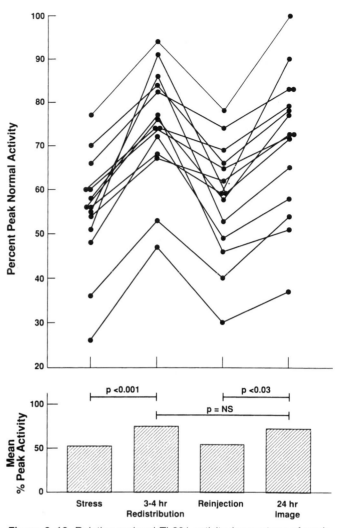

Figure 9–16. Relative regional Tl-201 activity (percentage of peak normal activity) in myocardial regions showing a reduction in Tl-201 activity in the defect region after reinjection compared to the 3- to 4-hour redistribution image. On images acquired 24 hours after reinjection, redistribution is again apparent. If 3- to 4-hour redistribution images were eliminated, and only reinjection images were acquired, perfusion in these regions would be determined (incorrectly) to have irreversible defects. The bottom panel depicts mean activity at all designated points in time. (Dilsizian V, et al.: Circulation 1992; 85:1032–1038.)

reinjection Tl-201 scintigraphy to PET imaging with FDG in the same patients. FDG uptake was observed in 94% of defects on conventional postexercise imaging that corresponded to complete or partial Tl-201 redistribution. Thirty-eight percent of 432 myocardial segments in 16 patients with chronic CAD demonstrated persistent Tl-201 defects on redistribution images before reinjection. FDG uptake suggesting preserved metabolic integrity was present in 51% of these segments with severe persistent defects. An identical number of persistent defects (51%) had enhanced Tl-201 uptake after reinjection. Detection of myocardial viability in these persistent defects by the two techniques was concordant in 88% of segments. The authors concluded that the Tl-201 reinjection protocol was as predictive as

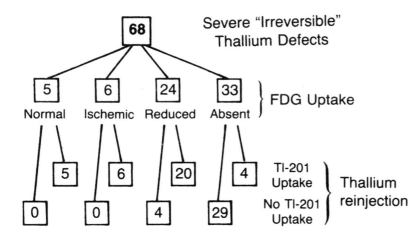

Figure 9–17. Nomogram of FDG uptake in 68 regions with severe irreversible Tl-201 defects on redistribution imaging. FDG uptake was observed in the majority of myocardial segments that showed Tl-201 uptake after Tl-201 reinjection. Only four segments that showed no FDG uptake on PET showed Tl-201 uptake after reinjection. (Bonow RO, et al.: Circulation 1991;83:26–37.)

FDG imaging for detecting viable myocardium in patients with chronic CAD and LV dysfunction.

Tamaki et al.[64] compared changes seen on exercise SPECT Tl-201 reinjection imaging with FDG uptake on PET imaging in 18 patients with CAD. Of 48 segments showing no redistribution on 3-hour delayed images, reinjection images identified further Tl-201 uptake in 20 segments (42%), all of which exhibited FDG uptake. In contrast, only seven of 28 segments (25%) that showed no enhanced Tl-201 uptake after reinjection were viable by FDG criteria. The majority of segments that showed defect reversibility on redistribution images (87%), or further defect reversibility after reinjection (65%), showed improved wall motion after bypass surgery. Only 25% of persistent defects after reinjection showed improved wall motion after surgery.

Bonow et al.[69] also showed that most mild persistent defects on 4-hour redistribution images showed evidence of myocardial viability by FDG criteria. Mild defects on SPECT images were defined as 60% to 84% of peak activity, moderate defects as 50% to 59% of peak activity, and severe defects less than 50% of peak activity. Of 166 regions corresponding to persistent Tl-201 defects on early and 4-hour delayed imaging, 53 (32%) had a "mild" reduction in Tl-201 uptake (74% of normal), 45 (27%) had a "moderate" reduction in activity (56% of normal), and 68 (41%) had a "severe" reduction (33% of normal) in Tl-201 activity. FDG uptake was identified in 73% of the 166 persistent defects. FDG uptake was seen in 91% of mild persistent defects, 84% of moderate persistent defects, and 51% of severe persistent defects. Again, the "absolute" level of Tl-201 activity in persistent defects can be used as an index to predict presence of viable myocardium. Figure 9–17 shows that severe irreversible defects on redistribution imaging that demonstrated Tl-201 uptake on reinjection almost always had preserved FDG uptake. Perrone-Filardi et al.[70] found in a subsequent study that systolic wall thickening as demonstrated by gated magnetic resonance imaging (MRI) was comparable in regions corresponding to mild or moderate persistent defects and in regions with

reversible Tl-201 defects (Fig. 9–18). Only regions with severe irreversible defects showed absence of thickening. Figure 9–19A depicts the percentage of regions showing viability by PET FDG criteria and the type of Tl-201 defect on redistribution images. The percentage of regions showing FDG uptake was similar among regions with normal Tl-201 uptake, reversible Tl-201 defects, and mild or moderate irreversible defects. In contrast, 64% of severe irreversible Tl-201 defects showed an absence of FDG uptake. After Tl-201 reinjection, 26% of regions with severe irreversible defects (less than 50% of maximal activity) showed enhanced Tl-201 uptake. All showed FDG uptake. Interestingly, impairment in regional thickening by MRI was not significantly different between Tl-201 defects with and without enhanced Tl-201 uptake after reinjection. The au-

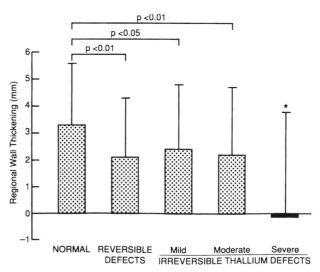

Figure 9–18. Bar graphs show regional wall thickening in myocardial segments that exhibit normal Tl-201 uptake, reversible defects, mild irreversible defects, moderate irreversible defects, and severe irreversible defects on SPECT 3- to 4-hour redistribution imaging. Regional systolic wall thickening was absent in regions with severe irreversible defects at redistribution, whereas mild and moderate irreversible defects associated with comparable regional thickening to defects showing reversibility. (Perrone-Filardi P, et al.: Circulation 1992;86:1125–1137.)

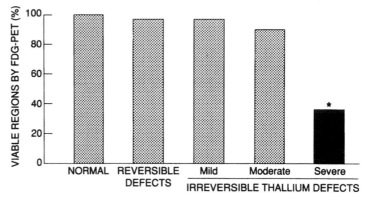

Figure 9–19. Bar graphs showing percentage of regions that by PET show evidence of metabolic activity in groups of defects classified as reversible or mild, moderate, or severe irreversible Tl-201 defects. The percentage of regions that on redistribution imaging show the presence of FDG uptake was similar among segments with normal Tl-201 uptake, reversible Tl-201 defects, and mild or moderate irreversible defects. (*P* < 0.01 compared with all other groups of regions.) (Perrone-Filardi P, et al.: Circulation 1992;86:1125–1137.)

thors concluded that the findings of increased Tl-201 uptake after reinjection and preserved FDG uptake, but lack of thickening, reflects presence of hibernating myocardium.

A conclusion that can be derived from these stress imaging studies is that a mild reduction in Tl-201 uptake on serial images (mild persistent defect) indicates preserved viability even if reversibility is not evident with reinjection. Mere demonstration of preserved Tl-201 uptake, albeit reduced, identifies myocardium that is viable in zones of hypoperfusion. Reinjection of a second dose of Tl-201 adds confirming evidence of viability if reversibility is detected or if the absolute Tl-201 counts in the defect are greater on the reinjection images than on the redistribution images.

Reinjection Versus 24-Hour Late Imaging

The "reinjection" protocol is preferred by many to 18- to 24-hour late redistribution imaging to detect viable myocardium in defects that remain persistent on 2.5- to 4-hour images. Late 24-hour imaging after reinjection did not ap-

pear to detect further improvement in Tl-201 uptake, as compared with images acquired 10 minutes after reinjection.[71] In this study, 92% of regions that showed improved Tl-201 uptake on early reinjection images showed no further improvement on the 24-hour late redistribution study. The mean normalized Tl-201 activity in regions with enhanced Tl-201 activity after reinjection increased from 57% ± 13% of normal on 4-hour redistribution images to 70% ± 14% after reinjection and to 71% ± 14% at 24 hours. In defects that remained persistent after reinjection, no enhanced activity was seen at 24 hours (57% ± 17% at reinjection versus 58% ± 17% at 24 hours). In fact, only three of 50 patients showed enhanced Tl-201 uptake at 24 hours in defects judged to be persistent after reinjection. Figure 9–20 shows that, of 30 defects that remained irreversible after reinjection, 29 were still irreversible 24 hours later when imaging was repeated.

Kayden et al.[72] addressed the issue of whether or not the reinjection protocol was superior to the stress-redistribution–24-hour delayed protocol for maximizing detection of viability. In their study, reinjection was performed imme-

Myocardial Regions

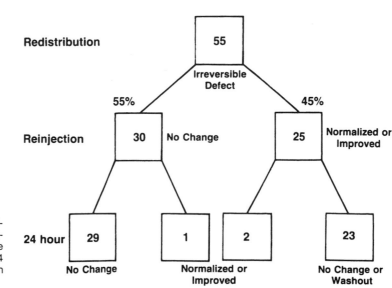

Figure 9–20. Diagram depicts the fate of irreversible Tl-201 defects on standard 3- to 4-hour redistribution imaging after reinjection and 24 hours after reinjection. There was little difference between the defect patterns at 24 hours and at reinjection. (Dilsizian V, et al.: Circulation 1991;83:1247–1255.)

diately after the acquisition of 24-hour redistribution images. They found that 38% of Tl-201 defects that remained irreversible on 24-hour redistribution images showed enhanced Tl-201 uptake after reinjection. Thus, the reinjection technique was superior to late 24-hour imaging for detecting defect reversibility after a single dose of Tl-201 administered during stress.

Reinjection Versus Quantitative Redistribution Imaging

In many instances, the amount of redistribution evident on 4-hour poststress images is slight and may not be adequately detected by qualitative visual scintigraphic analysis. If too much contrast enhancement or background suppression is performed during display of images, subtle degrees of redistribution in severe initial defects may be missed. The value of the addition of reinjection of a second dose of Tl-201 to standard postexercise and 2.5-hour quantitative planar redistribution imaging was evaluated in 50 consecutive patients with at least one defect on postexercise images.[73] Reinjection did not yield an appreciable increase in defect reversibility over that determined solely from quantitative analysis of the redistribution images. Figure 9–21 shows no significant difference in defect magnitude between redistribution and reinjection images in all defects that were determined to be persistent at 2.5 hours. Similarly, there was no significant increase in defect reversibility after reinjection in scan segments that showed evidence of redistribution at 2.5 hours. Although, by quantitative criteria, defect reversibility was not significantly enhanced by reinjection on these serial planar images, visual appreciation of increased Tl-201 uptake after reinjection was enhanced because of the increased Tl-201 counts in the reinjection images. Tl-201 counts increased proportionally the same in normal and defect regions, yielding the same relative defect magnitude but more "absolute" counts in the defect zone, thus improving image contrast. Figure 9–22 is an illustrative example of this phenomenon. Visually, the

reinjection images in this patient appear to show greater defect reversibility than that seen in the 2.5-hour redistribution images; however, defect magnitude is comparable on both redistribution and reinjection images.

Experimental studies in a canine model of coronary stenosis with ischemic dysfunction confirmed these clinical observations.[74] In dogs with a previous infarction and a residual critical stenosis undergoing poststress, redistribution, and reinjection imaging, the improvement in defect magnitude was slight between redistribution and reinjection images (Fig. 9–23).

DIPYRIDAMOLE THALLIUM-201 SCINTIGRAPHY AND MYOCARDIAL VIABILITY

Ischemia can be distinguished from scar with pharmacologic stress Tl-201 perfusion imaging employing dipyridamole or adenosine infusion in a manner similar to what was described for exercise scintigraphy in the previous section (see Chap. 8).

Dipyridamole Thallium-201 Defects and Regional Wall Motion

Myocardial regions showing defects with pharmacologic stress that exhibit delayed redistribution suggest preservation of some viability. Leppo et al.[75] reported that 74% of myocardial scan segments that demonstrated complete redistribution of an initial dipyridamole perfusion defect had normal wall motion on ventriculography. Conversely, 71% of scan segments that demonstrated persistent Tl-201 defects were associated with akinetic or dyskinetic wall motion. Thus, segmental Tl-201 defect patterns on dipyridamole imaging predicted normal or abnormal wall motion by ventriculography with predictive values comparable to those reported for exercise scintigraphy. Okada et al.[76] also compared various dipyridamole Tl-201 scan patterns with

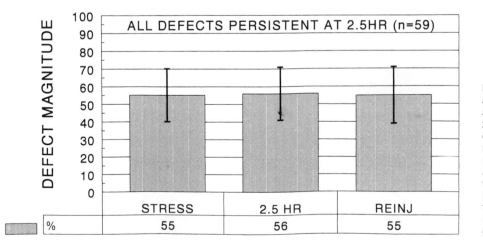

Figure 9–21. Mean defect magnitude at 2.5 hours after exercise stress and after reinjection of a second dose of Tl-201 in defects that were persistent by quantitative criteria at 2½ hours. The mean defect magnitude (percentage of reduction in Tl-201 counts) is depicted at the bottom of each of the bars. There was no significant difference in defect magnitude between values at reinjection and 2½ hours of redistribution. (Submitted to J Nucl Cardiol for publication.)

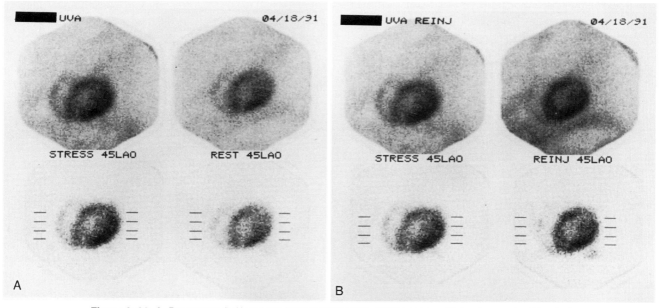

Figure 9–22. A. Poststress *(left)* and 2½-hour redistribution *(right)* images with background-subtracted images shown at the bottom. **B.** Poststress *(left)* and reinjection *(right)* Tl-201 images for the same patient. Although Tl-201 activity appears to be greater in the anteroseptal region on the reinjection image, as compared to the redistribution image, the quantitative count profiles showed comparable ratios of septum-posterolateral wall Tl-201 activity on the reinjection and 2½-hour redistribution images.

global and regional LV function changes on exercise radionuclide angiography. Redistribution defects on dipyridamole scans were associated with normal rest and exercise LVEF and preserved regional wall motion. Mild persistent Tl-201 defects were associated with a normal EF and normal regional wall motion at rest but with a deterioration during exercise. As would be expected, severe persistent Tl-201 defects on dipyridamole scans were associated with

reduced EF and normal wall motion at rest but without further deterioration during exercise.

Like exercise imaging, dipyridamole perfusion scintigraphy can help distinguish between ischemic and nonischemic cardiomyopathy. Eichorn et al.[77] were able to correctly classify 91% of patients with dipyridamole imaging when a perfusion defect of at least 15% was used as a cutoff for nonischemic cardiomyopathy. The mean perfu-

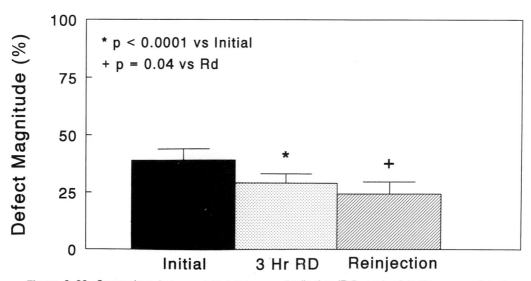

Figure 9–23. Comparison between initial, 3-hour redistribution (Rd), and reinjection mean defect magnitudes in dogs that had a small anterior infarction and a residual coronary stenosis and that received Tl-201 during intravenous dobutamine and adenosine infusion. Note that the defect magnitude diminishes only slightly after reinjection, as compared to the 3-hour redistribution images. In no instance was reversibility identified only on the reinjection image in this group of dogs.

sion defect magnitude was 25% ± 11% in patients with ischemic cardiomyopathy and 6% ± 6% in those with idiopathic dilated cardiomyopathy.

RESTING THALLIUM-201 IMAGING AND MYOCARDIAL VIABILITY

Tl-201 imaging can be performed solely in the resting state for evaluation of resting regional blood flow and myocardial cellular viability (see Chap. 2). This approach is most useful for assessing viability in patients who exhibit a severe reduction in global LV function, to determine if coronary revascularization would improve regional systolic dysfunction and symptoms of congestive heart failure.[77a, 77b] Figure 9–24 shows rest and delayed horizontal long-axis Tl-201 SPECT tomograms of a patient with severe asynergy of the anterior wall, apex, and septum. Note rest redistribution in the septum consistent with preserved viability.

Rest Imaging in Stable and Unstable Angina

Resting Tl-201 scintigraphy has proven useful in patients with severe chronic stable angina or unstable angina to assess myocardial viability before and after revascularization. Berger et al.[51] reported that 76% of scan segments in 29 patients with either severe stable angina (N = 15) or unstable angina (N = 14) showed defects at rest that showed delayed rest redistribution at 3 hours. Seventy-seven percent of these segments showed reversion to normal initial Tl-201 uptake at rest after bypass surgery. As was observed with exercise scintigraphy, 72% of persistent defects on the preoperative imaging study showed improved Tl-201 uptake after bypass surgery. Twelve of the thirteen persistent defects that improved did not have associated Q waves on the ECG. Improved wall motion on postoperative ventriculograms corresponded to scan segments showing improved perfusion. In this study, 80% of patients who showed initial resting defects with delayed rest redistribution preoperatively demonstrated at least a 5% increase in LVEF postoperatively. In contrast, only 22% of patients with persistent defects preoperatively on rest imaging showed comparable improvement. Gewirtz et al.[50] also reported that most defects at rest which showed delayed redistribution are associated with normal or hypokinetic wall motion. In that study, 50% of akinetic segments had normal Tl-201 uptake or rest redistribution. No quantitative scan analysis was undertaken, and no postoperative evaluation was conducted. Also, correlation of differing magnitudes of resting persistent Tl-201 defects (e.g., mild versus severe) and resting wall motion was not undertaken. Hakki et al.[78] found that 50% of 12 unstable angina patients with an LVEF of less than 30% had either normal Tl-201 uptake at rest or evidence of rest redistribution. Again, no postoperative assessment of LV function or perfusion was performed in this study.

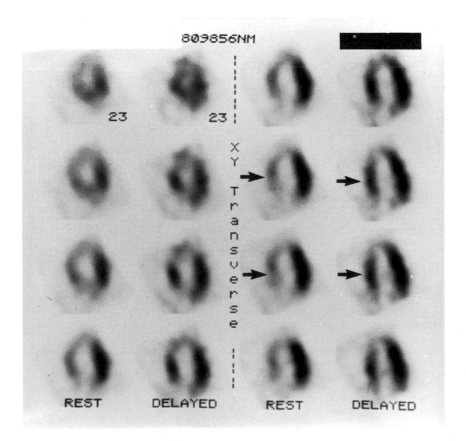

Figure 9–24. Early and 3-hour delayed rest, Tl-201 horizontal long-axis tomograms of a patient with a prior anteroseptal infarction who demonstrates "rest redistribution" in the interventricular septum *(arrow)* and apex indicative of preserved viability.

Mori et al.[79] evaluated the utility of initial and delayed rest Tl-201 scintigraphy for determining regional viability in severely asynergic regions. All had a history of infarction, and all underwent preoperative and postoperative radionuclide ventriculography. The percentage of Tl-201 uptake was calculated as the ratio of counts in asynergic segments to the maximum counts in normal segments. Eleven of fourteen regions with resting Tl-201 redistribution had improved wall motion after revascularization. Regions without redistribution that showed improved function had more mild persistent defects than those that did not improve, consistent with the concept discussed previously that mild persistent Tl-201 defects suggest preserved viability.

Rest Tl-201 scintigraphy can assist in identifying which patients with CAD and ischemic cardiomyopathy benefit most from coronary bypass surgery. Ragosta et al.[52] performed preoperative and postoperative rest Tl-201 scintigraphy in 21 patients whose mean LVEF was 27% ± 5%. Among akinetic or dyskinetic segments, 73% had evidence of viability, as defined as normal Tl-201 uptake, an initial rest defect with delayed redistribution at 3 hours, or a mild persistent defect that showed no more than a 25% to 50% reduction in Tl-201 activity (Fig. 9–25). Significantly more asynergic segments with preserved rest Tl-201 uptake showed postoperative wall motion improvement compared to scan segments corresponding to severe persistent defects exhibiting more than 50% reduction in Tl-201 activity. Figure 9–26 shows an example of a patient with a preoperative LVEF of 22%, which increased to 45% after revascularization. Note the substantial Tl-201 uptake in anterior and septal regions, which showed severe asynergy on radionuclide ventriculography preoperatively. A greater number of viable but asynergic segments correlated positively with improved global LV function after surgery. As shown in Figure 9–27 in 10 patients with more than 7 viable, asynergic segments (using a 15-segment model from anterior, 45-degree left anterior oblique [LAO], and 70-degree LAO projections), mean LVEF increased significantly (29% ± 7% to 41% ± 11%, P = 0.002) after surgery, whereas in 11 patients with no more than 7 viable asynergic segments, mean LVEF remained unchanged after revascularization (27% ± 5% vs. 30% ± 8%, P = NS).

Dilsizian et al.[79a] reported a concordance rate of 94% between Tl-201 stress-redistribution-reinjection imaging and rest-redistribution imaging regarding myocardial viability as defined by PET criteria in 41 patients with chronic stable CAD. Criteria for viability by rest Tl-201 imaging was demonstration of defect reversibility or 51% or greater uptake of Tl-201 relative to a normal region in a persistent resting defect.

Thus, the results of the studies cited above indicate that rest Tl-201 scintigraphy can be used to identify viability in asynergic myocardial segments in patients with stable or unstable CAD and in patients with ischemic cardiomyopathy where congestive heart failure may be a more prominent clinical presentation than angina. Patients with numerous asynergic but viable myocardial segments are likely to

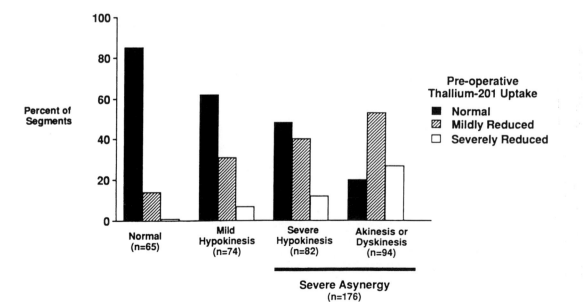

Figure 9–25. Bar graph shows relationship between preoperative regional wall motion and preoperative viability as determined by rest and redistribution Tl-201 scintigraphic criteria. The solid bars represent normal initial uptake or total rest redistribution. The crosshatched bars represent mildly reduced Tl-201 uptake, reflected by partial delayed redistribution or a persistent defect with no more than 25% to 50% reduction in counts. The open bars represent severely reduced Tl-201 uptake, reflected by a >50% persistent defect. Note that, in zones of severe asynergy, many myocardial segments show normal or only mildly reduced viability. (Ragosta M, et al.: Circulation 1993;87:1630–1641.)

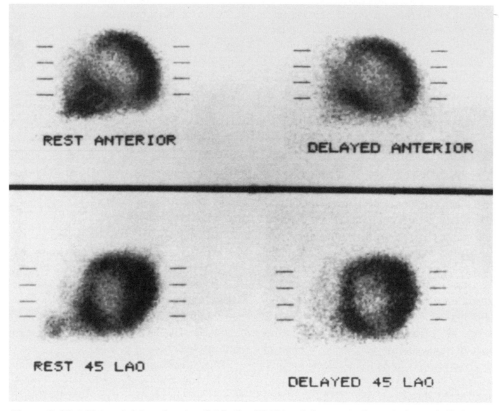

Figure 9–26. Initial and delayed rest-redistribution Tl-201 scintigrams in the anterior and 45-degree left anterior oblique (LAO) projection from a patient with a preoperative ejection fraction of 22% and multiple lesions of severe asynergy. Normal Tl-201 uptake was observed in the anterolateral and posterolateral walls, whereas mildly reduced viability was judged to exist in the inferior wall, apex, and septum. After revascularization, the postoperative ejection fraction increased to 45%. (Ragosta M, et al.: Circulation 1993;87:1630–1641.)

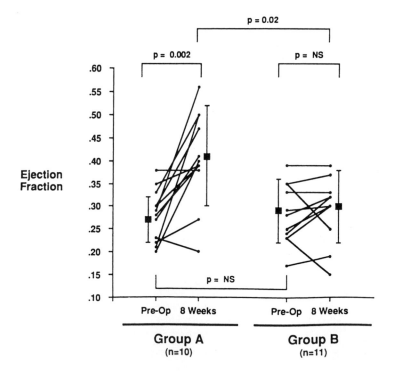

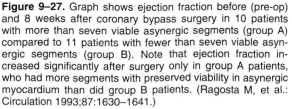

Figure 9–27. Graph shows ejection fraction before (pre-op) and 8 weeks after coronary bypass surgery in 10 patients with more than seven viable asynergic segments (group A) compared to 11 patients with fewer than seven viable asynergic segments (group B). Note that ejection fraction increased significantly after surgery only in group A patients, who had more segments with preserved viability in asynergic myocardium than did group B patients. (Ragosta M, et al.: Circulation 1993;87:1630–1641.)

experience significant improvement in global LV function after bypass surgery. Patients with extensive asynergy with residual Tl-201 activity on rest scintigraphy are unlikely to show an increase in LVEF after revascularization.

Rest Imaging After Thrombolytic Therapy in Acute Infarction

The application of Tl-201 scintigraphy for determination of efficacy of reflow and myocardial salvage after coronary reperfusion in patients with acute MI is described in detail in Chapter 6. To summarize, resting Tl-201 scintigraphy can be employed to assess the extent of reflow and myocardial salvage after coronary reperfusion. Several investigators have administered Tl-201 intravenously before infusing a thrombolytic agent and obtained postthrombolysis images several hours later. These studies demonstrated that patients who exhibit successful thrombolysis had more Tl-201 redistribution and smaller final Tl-201 defects than patients with persistently occluded infarct-related vessels.[80, 81] Patients who demonstrated redistribution 4 hours after institution of thrombolytic therapy may show even further improvement in Tl-201 uptake when imaging is repeated several weeks later.[81]

Resting Tl-201 scintigraphy is perhaps most useful when performed 24 hours or longer after thrombolytic therapy to determine success of reflow and to estimate the degree of salvage.[82] By delaying this injection of Tl-201 for 24 hours after thrombolytic therapy, the trapping of Tl-201 in the infarct region during the hyperemic flow phase that immediately follows reperfusion might be avoided[83] (see Chap. 6). In the Western Washington Intravenous Thrombolytic Trial, patients who received streptokinase had significantly more Tl-201 uptake in the infarct zone than controls.[84] The degree of regional Tl-201 uptake in the infarct zone is proportional to the mass of viable myocytes. Enhanced regional systolic function in the infarct zone after thrombolytic therapy can be predicted by rest Tl-201 scintigraphy. Improvement in LV function after angioplasty of the infarct vessel can also be predicted if there is preserved Tl-201 uptake before dilation. Figure 9–28 depicts short-axis and horizontal long-axis rest and delayed rest SPECT Tl-201 images in a patient who received thrombolytic therapy for an acute anterior myocardial infarction. Predominantly persistent apical and anterior wall defects are observed, but substantial uptake of Tl-201 is seen in the septum.

TECHNETIUM-99m MYOCARDIAL PERFUSION AGENTS AND MYOCARDIAL VIABILITY

In recent years, new technetium-99m (Tc-99m)–labeled perfusion agents have undergone clinical testing for their efficacy in detecting myocardial ischemia and distinguishing viable from irreversible myocardium (see Chaps. 2 and 3). The Tc-99m isonitriles and Tc-99m tetrofosmin appear to be the most promising of this new group of agents for determining myocardial viability. Tc-99m methoxyisobutyl isonitrile (sestamibi) is probably the most clinically applicable of the Tc-99m isonitrile agents for human myocardial imaging. Tc-99m teboroxime is not very suitable for imaging of myocardial viability and is predominantly a perfusion agent.

Technetium-99m Isonitrile Imaging for Viability Determination

The basic uptake and clearance kinetics of Tc-99m sestamibi in experimental laboratory models are discussed in Chapter 2. Like that of Tl-201, myocardial uptake of Tc-99m sestamibi after intravenous injection is proportional to myocardial blood flow.[85] The intracellular transport processes for Tc-99m sestamibi is less dependent than Tl-201 on active transport mechanisms.[86]

Myocardial stunning in anesthetized dogs produced by 15 minutes of transient coronary occlusion followed by total reperfusion did not affect Tc-99m–sestamibi uptake.[41] Myocardial uptake of Tc-99m sestamibi was also examined under conditions of a chronic low-flow state in anesthetized dogs intended to simulate short-term myocardial hibernation.[41] As reported for Tl-201 in this canine model, Tc-99m–sestamibi uptake was preserved and was proportional to blood flow. Even though significant myocardial asynergy was produced by the reduction in regional blood flow, Tc-99m–sestamibi uptake reflected the degree of viability. Other experimental studies (see Chap. 2) have clearly shown that Tc-99m sestamibi is a valid viability agent as long as there is flow preservation to deliver the tracer to myocardial tissue.[87, 88, 88a]

Recent experiments in intact anesthetized dogs receiving both Tl-201 and Tc-99m sestamibi in the setting of a critical stenosis and a small subendocardial infarction revealed almost comparable uptake of the two tracers as judged by serial imaging and by gamma well counting techniques (Fig. 9–29A).[89] However, during sustained low flow producing severe regional dysfunction in dogs with a stenosis of the LAD, Tl-201 uptake exceeded Tc-99m–sestamibi uptake (see Fig. 9–29B). Leon et al.[90] compared Tl-201 and Tc-99m–sestamibi uptake by SPECT imaging in the same dogs undergoing partial coronary occlusion during intravenous adenosine infusion. Counts in the defects were 39% higher for Tc-99m sestamibi than for Tl-201 (0.86 ± 0.08 of normal vs. 0.64 ± 0.09). Thus, tomographic imaging with Tc-99m sestamibi underestimated the degree of underperfusion. In contrast, with nearly total coronary occlusion, defect magnitude was comparable with the two agents. In normally perfused myocardium, there is greater retention of

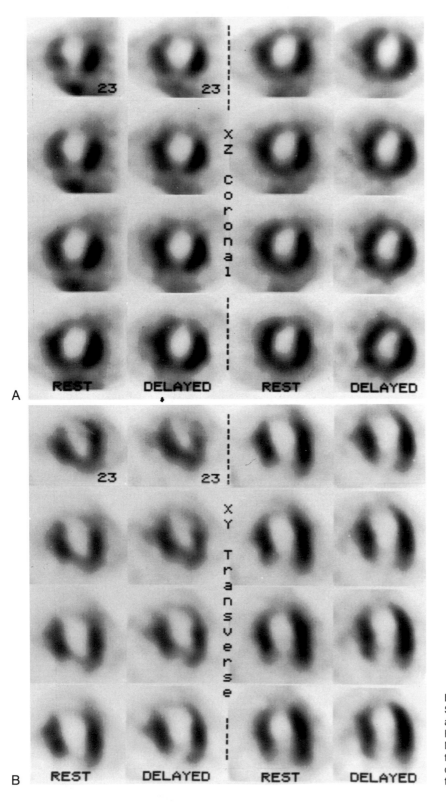

A

B

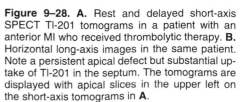

Figure 9–28. A. Rest and delayed short-axis SPECT Tl-201 tomograms in a patient with an anterior MI who received thrombolytic therapy. **B.** Horizontal long-axis images in the same patient. Note a persistent apical defect but substantial uptake of Tl-201 in the septum. The tomograms are displayed with apical slices in the upper left on the short-axis tomograms in **A**.

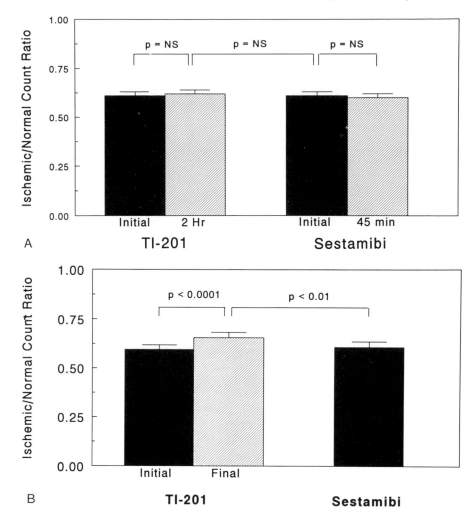

Figure 9–29. A. Ischemic-normal count ratios on initial and 2-hour resting Tl-201 images and initial and 45-minute Tc-99m–sestamibi images in 14 dogs with a sustained 50% reduction in LAD coronary artery flow and interspersed 1 hour of total LAD occlusion. Note the negligible rest Tl-201 redistribution and comparability of 2-hour Tl-201 and Tc-99m–sestamibi defect ratios. **B.** Tl-201 and Tc-99m–sestamibi ischemic-normal image defect ratios in dogs with a sustained reduction in flow. The final Tl-201–defect magnitude at 2 hours of redistribution *(crosshatched bar)* was significantly less than the Tc-99m–sestamibi defect magnitude. (Glover D, et al.: Circulation 1995; 91:813–820.)

Tl-201 than of Tc-99m sestamibi, particularly at high flow states.[91] Greater retention of Tl-201 in nonischemic myocardium may be the explanation for better defect contrast than that afforded by Tc-99m sestamibi. Another isonitrile compound, Tc-99m-[2(1-methoxybutyl) isonitrile] (MBI) shows better myocardial uptake relative to flow than sestamibi because it is avidly retained in the myocardium.[91a] Clinical studies to assess flow and viability have not been undertaken with this agent.

One reason that Tl-201 imaging may be preferable to Tc-99m–sestamibi imaging is the lack of substantial redistribution with the latter. Quan-Sheng Li et al.[91b] revealed slight filling in of Tc-99m sestamibi in transient perfusion defects on serial tomographic images in dogs. Animals received Tc-99m sestamibi at 6 minutes of coronary occlusion, which was followed by reperfusion.[91b] Glover et al.[91c] detected a small amount of redistribution of Tc-99m sestamibi by gamma well counting of myocardial specimens in dogs that received the agent after 15 minutes of left circumflex coronary artery occlusion followed by 2 hours' reflow. However, Tc-99m sestamibi was not observed to redistribute by serial gamma camera imaging in these animals. Posterior wall defects appeared persistent during the 2 hours of reperfusion. Sansoy et al.[89] showed some resting sestamibi redistribution in dogs with a chronic 50% reduction in coronary flow although significantly less redistribution than that seen with simultaneously administered Tl-201 in the same animals (Fig. 9–30).

Taillefer et al.[91d] showed ischemic-normal defect ratios to diminish from 1 to 3 hours after injection of Tc-99m sestamibi during exercise stress, indicating some redistribution (0.73 to 0.83). Myocardial Tc-99m–sestamibi washout was 26% for normally perfused zones and 15% for ischemic zones ($P < 0.001$). These authors concluded that faster washout from normal regions of myocardium was the explanation for redistribution of the tracer seen from 1 to 3 hours after intravenous administration. In contrast, Villanueva-Meyer et al.[91e] performed SPECT imaging 1 and 4 hours after Tc-99m sestamibi was injected during peak exercise or dipyridamole effect. The left ventricular defect size 1 hour after exercise or dipyridamole infusion was similar to that observed after 4 hours. Defect sizes were larger than the defect size seen after injection of the radionuclide at rest. This finding suggested that Tc-99m sestamibi did not redistribute over 4 hours in underperfused myocardium. Dilsizian et al.[92e] found that 38% of irreversi-

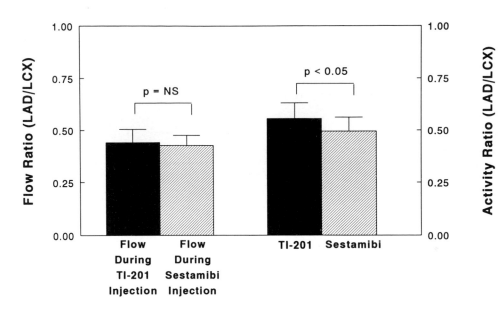

Figure 9–30. Comparison of Tl-201 and Tc-99m–sestamibi uptake in dogs with a 50% reduction in flow. The two bars on the left represent the LAD-LCx flow ratios by microspheres at the time of tracer injections. The two bars on the right represent LAD-LCx Tl-201 and Tc-99m sestamibi count ratios by gamma well counting 2 hours after tracer injections and demonstrate greater redistribution of Tl-201 than of Tc-99m sestamibi. (Glover D, et al.: Circulation 1995; 91:813–820.)

ble defects on rest-stress Tc-99m sestamibi SPECT imaging showed delayed redistribution when an additional 4-hour redistribution image was acquired. Although Tc-99m sestamibi does not redistribute significantly over time after injection, substantial uptake of the radionuclide in viable but asynergic myocardium occurs soon after injection, indicating that this agent may still provide clinically relevant information pertaining to viability in the clinical setting.

Several clinical studies have been undertaken investigating the utility of Tc-99m–sestamibi imaging for detection of viability.[92–94d] Cuocolo et al.[92] found that Tl-201 imaging with reinjection was superior to rest and stress Tc-99m–sestamibi imaging for detection of defect reversibility. Of 122 regions with irreversible defects on standard stress-redistribution Tl-201 imaging in 20 patients with CAD and LV dysfunction, 47% showed enhanced Tl-201 uptake after reinjection. Of the same 122 fixed Tl-201 defects on redistribution imaging, 18% were reversible on Tc-99m–sestamibi scans. Marzullo et al.[92a] performed resting Tc-99m sestamibi and before and after revascularization echocardiography in 14 patients with CAD and regional wall motion abnormalities. Sensitivity and specificity of Tc-99m–sestamibi uptake for prediction of postrevascularization recovery of function were 83% and 71%, respectively. Tc-99m sestamibi imaging underestimated the extent of viability in 25% of myocardial regions supplied by stenotic vessels that exhibited normal wall motion. Presence of a severe perfusion defect identified most segments that did not show improvement in wall motion after revascularization. In a subsequent study by the same group,[92b] asynergic segments showing improved wall motion after dobutamine administration had more early and redistribution Tl-201 uptake and a higher percentage of sestamibi uptake than unresponsive segments. Using improved function on postrevascularization echocardiography as the criterion for viability, delayed Tl-201 scans and dobutamine echocardiography had good

sensitivity and specificity for detecting viable myocardium. Tc-99m–sestamibi activity was significantly less than early and delayed Tl-201 activity in segments perfused by stenotic coronary arteries but showing normal systolic function. Tc-99m–sestamibi activity averaged 60% ± 15% of peak activity in dyssynergic segments, comparable to the delayed Tl-201 activity of 59% ± 13% of peak. Maurea et al.[92c] found that resting Tl-201 uptake was higher than Tc-99m–sestamibi uptake in segments supplied by a totally occluded coronary artery; however, uptake of the two tracers was comparable in segments supplied by vessels with 50% to 99% stenoses. The authors concluded that resting Tl-201 redistribution imaging may be more accurate that Tc-99m–sestamibi imaging for identifying the presence of viable myocardium in patients with chronic CAD, particularly when myocardial perfusion is severely impaired owing to a totally obstructed artery.

Rocco et al.[92d] injected Tc-99m sestamibi at rest into patients with CAD before and after coronary bypass surgery. Tc-99m–sestamibi uptake correlated well with preoperative wall motion but seemed to underestimate the extent of viable myocardium. Sixty-one percent of segments with severely reduced uptake preoperatively showed improved tracer uptake after revascularization. Dilsizian et al.[92e] studied 54 patients who underwent both stress-redistribution-reinjection Tl-201 SPECT imaging and same-day rest-stress sestamibi imaging within a mean of 5 days. They found that sestamibi imaging incorrectly identified 36% of myocardial regions as being irreversible and nonviable compared to both Tl-201 redistribution-reinjection and PET imaging. Sawada et al.[92f] also reported an underestimation of myocardial viability by resting SPECT Tc-99m sestamibi imaging compared to FDG uptake criteria by PET imaging. FDG evidence of viability was present in 50% of segments with Tc-99m sestamibi activity of less than 40% of normal Tc-99m sestamibi activity. It appeared that most of the

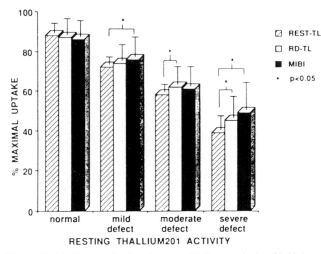

Figure 9–31. Bar graph showing quantitative analysis of initial rest Tl-201 activity (REST-TL), delayed rest redistribution Tl-201 activity (RD-TL), and 1-hour post-rest injection of Tc-99m sestamibi (MIBI). Segments are grouped according to mean normalized resting Tl-201 activity. (Udelson JE, et al.: Circulation 1994;89:2552–2561.)

underestimation of viability occurred in inferior segments (16 of 20 patients) and may be related to the known attenuation of Tc-99m activity in this region. The PET images are correcrted for attenuation.

In contrast, Udelson et al.[93] found that Tl-201 uptake and Tc-99m–sestamibi uptake were comparable in akinetic or dyskinetic myocardial regions when both tracers were administered at rest to patients with CAD and a mean LVEF of 35% ± 11% (Fig. 9–31). Among segments demonstrating significant reversibility of left ventricular dysfunction after revascularization, mean redistribution activity was 72% ± 11%. Tc-99m sestamibi activity was 75% ± 9% in these segments. Preliminary observations in 20 patients with chronic CAD and LV dysfunction who underwent both resting Tl-201 and sestamibi SPECT imaging in our laboratory suggests that Tc-99m–sestamibi uptake is comparable to delayed Tl-201 uptake in asynergic myocardium, confirming the findings of Udelson et al.[93] Figure 9–32 shows rest and delayed Tl-201 images and a resting Tc-99m sestamibi image obtained in the same patient. Note that tracer uptake on the resting delayed Tl-201 tomograms and the rest Tc-99m sestamibi tomograms is similar in the anterior, apical, and inferior defects. In fact, greater Tc-99m sestamibi uptake can be appreciated in the inferior wall. The issue of whether or not Tc-99m sestamibi is as accurate as Tl-201 for distinguishing between ischemia and infarction is not entirely resolved. Despite less redistribution over time than Tl-201, substantial uptake of Tc-99m sestamibi appears to occur in regions of hibernating myocardium that are viable. Our own experience using quantitative planar imaging indicates that the detection rate of reversible defects on exercise stress imaging is similar for Tl-201 and Tc-99m sestamibi in a given patient population.[94]

Tc-99m–sestamibi imaging has been performed in con-

junction with iodine-123 phenylpentadecanoic acid imaging[94a] or FDG PET imaging[94b] for determination of viability. Zones of diminished Tc-99m–sestamibi uptake were associated with increased uptake of these metabolic tracers correlated with functional variables indicative of viability.

Technetium-99m Sestamibi Imaging for Assessment of Viability After Thrombolytic Therapy

Since Tc-99m sestamibi demonstrates little redistribution, separate injections of the radionuclide are administered during stress and rest. This separate injection technique may be particularly useful in assessing the efficacy

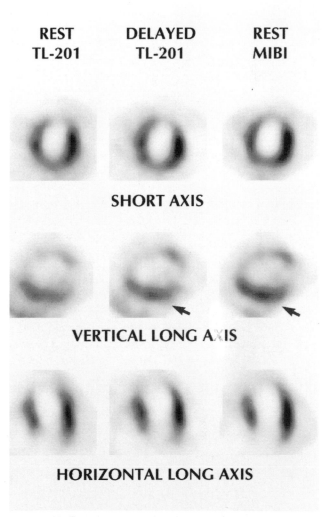

Figure 9–32. Early (first column) and delayed (second column) resting Tl-201 SPECT images and a Tc-99m sestamibi (MIBI) rest image acquired immediately after the delayed Tl-201 image in a patient with CAD and left ventricular dysfunction. Note the comparability in tracer uptake between the delayed Tl-201 image and the Tc-99m sestamibi image in the anterior and apical defects. Greater inferior wall Tc-99m sestamibi uptake than Tl-201 uptake is observed *(arrows).*

of thrombolytic therapy (see Chap. 6). The first dose of Tc-99m sestamibi is administered just before thrombolytic therapy, but imaging can be postponed until several hours later, following the complete infusion of a thrombolytic agent. In this way, institution of thrombolysis during the acute phase of infection is not delayed. A "snapshot" of the perfusion pattern at the time of admission before reperfusion is obtained with this first injection of Tc-99m sestamibi. Even if one waits 4 to 6 hours after injection for obtaining the prethrombolysis images, one can still observe clearly the perfusion pattern that existed at the time of presentation during acute coronary occlusion. A second injection of Tc-99m sestamibi is administered sometime after the first images are acquired, which will delineate the degree of improvement in regional flow and extent of salvage.

Several experimental and clinical studies have been completed that validate the approach described above.[87,88] These are reviewed in some detail in Chapter 6. Wackers et al.[95] and Gibbons et al.[96] with the assistance of several collaborating institutions, successfully applied serial Tc-99m–sestamibi imaging in patients with acute MI who received thrombolytic therapy. Patients with a patent infarct vessel had a significantly greater decrease in defect size on repeat images 18 to 48 hours after thrombolytic therapy than patients with persistently occluded vessels. A relative decrease of more than 30% in the size of Tc-99m–sestamibi perfusion defects on planar images predicted patency of the infarct-related vessel. Final Tc-99m defect size correlated well with the predischarge LVEF in these infarct patients. Christian et al.[95a] reported that infarct size by Tc-99m sestamibi had a closer correlation with LV ejection fraction at 6 weeks than did infarct size determined by reinjection Tl-201 imaging. In this study, a significant association between resting infarct size with Tc-99m sestamibi and reinjection Tl-201 was observed, although the estimates by Tl-201 were consistently larger.

The above observations are clinically significant, since presently there are few reliable nonangiographic methods that predict successful reperfusion. Tc-99m–sestamibi imaging could become a useful technique to incorporate into future clinical research trials aimed at evaluating the efficacy of pharmacologic or mechanical approaches to reperfusion in the setting of acute MI. Figure 9–33 shows the dipyridamole and rest Tc-99m–sestamibi images obtained before hospital discharge in a patient who received intravenous streptokinase on admission for an acute inferior MI. Mild inferoapical and inferior perfusion defects are apparent.

Simultaneous Evaluation of Flow and Function

One feature of Tc-99m–sestamibi imaging for viability assessment is the capability to simultaneously assess regional blood flow and regional myocardial wall motion (see Chap. 2). This may be a unique feature applicable to assessment of myocardial viability in chronic CAD or in acute ischemic syndromes. Regional wall motion is assessed by gating either planar or SPECT perfusion images and viewing the end-systolic and end-diastolic images derived from the scans (see Chap. 2). Regions that show preserved Tc-99m–sestamibi uptake as well as preserved systolic thickening are judged to represent viable myocardium. Regions that demonstrate abnormal systolic thickening but preserved Tc-99m–sestamibi uptake suggest viable but stunned or hibernating myocardium. A marked reduction in Tc-99m

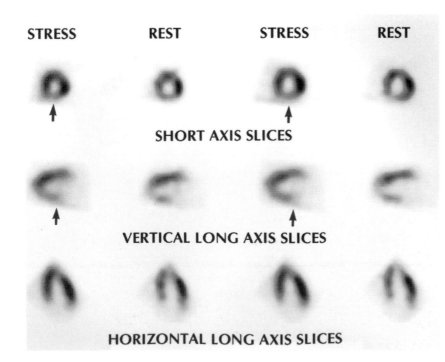

STRESS   REST   STRESS   REST

SHORT AXIS SLICES

VERTICAL LONG AXIS SLICES

HORIZONTAL LONG AXIS SLICES

Figure 9–33. Dipyridamole stress (STRESS) and resting (REST) Tc-99m–sestamibi SPECT images in a 41-year-old man with an inferior MI treated with intravenous streptokinase. Representative short-axis, vertical long-axis, and vertical long-axis slices demonstrate mild, irreversible inferoapical and inferior defects *(arrows).*

sestamibi activity with total absence of systolic thickening would indicate a zone of predominantly irreversible myocardial injury.

Iodine-123 Phenylpentadecanoic Acid for Viability Assessment

Iodine-123 phenylpentadecanoic acid (IPPA) is a synthetic fatty acid that holds considerable promise as an imaging agent for the assessment of myocardial viability in patients with CAD and LV dysfunction.[96a–96f] The basic radiopharmacologic properties of the iodinated radiolabeled fatty acids are discussed in Chapter 2. The initial uptake of IPPA is dictated mainly by regional myocardial blood flow. As with other tracers, there is a plateau of uptake at high flows. IPPA metabolism results in a biexponential myocardial washout pattern with a rapid first phase reflecting beta oxidation and a slower second phase representing turnover in the remaining lipid pools (e.g., triglycerides). Myocardial ischemia causes a reduction in beta oxidation of fatty acids with a relative increase in the proportion of fatty acids in the slowly metabolizing intracardiac lipid pool. Ischemia thus diminishes the myocardial washout rate of radiolabeled fatty acids. Nonviable and irreversibly injured myocardium would show significantly reduced IPPA uptake after a resting injection without much change in relative activity in the defect zone over time. The absence of change in activity implies no metabolic activity. With resting hypoperfusion resulting in hibernation, IPPA uptake is initially decreased early after tracer administration.[96c–96f] Subsequently, there is filling in of the defect over time because of reduced washout. The reduced washout compared to the faster normal washout results in IPPA "redistribution" and relative defect normalization. Preliminary data from our laboratory suggest that IPPA redistribution is more rapid than Tl-201 redistribution when both tracers were administered to dogs with a sustained reduction in resting coronary blood flow.

To assess viability in patients with CAD and LV dysfunction using IPPA, a serial SPECT imaging protocol is utilized. Imaging is performed 4, 12, 20, 28, and 36 minutes after IPPA administration.[96d] Preliminary clinical studies have indicated that quantitative assessment of IPPA uptake and clearance on serial SPECT IPPA images can differentiate viable from nonviable myocardium and predict improvement in LV function after revascularization.[96b–96g] Figure 9–34 shows the relative IPPA activity versus time in ischemic and nonischemic myocardial regions in a patient who presented with unstable angina and multivessel disease.[96c] Decreased activity on initial images was seen in the inferolateral wall. On subsequent images, the $T_{1/2}$ for IPPA clearance using a fit to the monoexponential decay was 36 minutes in the normal region and 50 minutes in the ischemic region. This represents differences in metabolism between the two regions and corresponded to relative improvement in defect contrast over time.

Murray et al.[96e] reported 92% sensitivity and 86% specificity of IPPA metabolic imaging for viability detection using myocardial biopsy findings at the time of revascularization for establishing the criteria for viability. IPPA washout was 17.8% ± 2.3% in biopsy-viable segments as compared with 21.2% ± 5.0% in healthy volunteers and was 13.4% ± 2.4% in biopsy nonviable segments ($P < 0.001$ vs. biopsy-viable segments). Eighty percent of IPPA-viable dysfunctional segments demonstrated improved regional wall motion postoperatively. Hansen et al.[96d] reported findings of a study in which IPPA clearance slopes derived from linear regression of the log of activity in bull's-eye plots on serial SPECT IPPA images were predictive of improvement of left ventricular function after revascularization. Further studies comparing the accuracy of IPPA imaging with serial resting SPECT Tl-201 imaging and PET imaging appear warranted.

INFARCT-AVID IMAGING WITH RADIOLABELED MYOSIN-SPECIFIC ANTIBODY

Infarct-avid imaging has been available for many years to identify zones of myocardial necrosis in patients with

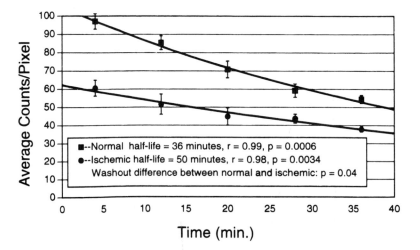

Figure 9–34. Washout of I-123 IPPA from ischemic and normal myocardium in a patient with unstable angina and multivessel CAD. The difference in clearance ratio is significant and represents altered metabolism of IPPA in underperfused myocardium. (Reprinted by permission of the Society of Nuclear Medicine from Hansen CL, et al.: J Nucl Med 1994;35(Suppl):385–425.)

acute MI (see Chap. 6). With this nuclear cardiology technique, the radiopharmaceutical that is administered is selectively bound in myocardial regions of recent necrosis, yielding a ''hot spot'' of radioactivity that can be detected and localized on myocardial scintigraphy. Tc-99m stannous pyrophosphate was the agent most commonly utilized in this approach. More recently, a new infarct-avid imaging technique has emerged involving the scintigraphic detection and quantification of myocardial necrosis after intravenous administration of radiolabeled myosin-specific antibody (see Chap. 6).[97] This approach is based on the principle that antibody specific for cardiac myosin will bind to the intracellular protein when sarcolemmal membrane integrity has been altered by ischemic myocardial injury (see Chap. 2). Experimental studies have shown that the location of antimyosin antibody uptake correlates with the region of necrosis as determined by histologic techniques.[98]

As with Tc-99m pyrophosphate, a delay of 16 to 24 hours after administration of radiolabeled antimyosin antibody is required before imaging can be performed. This delay permits clearance of the agent from the blood pool. To detect myocardial necrosis, a discrete ''hot spot'' of antimyosin uptake should be demonstrated. As discussed in Chapter 6, indium-111 (In-111) antimyosin antibody imaging has 90% specificity and equally high sensitivity for identifying regions of myocardial necrosis after acute MI. For viability assessment after infarction, the greater the area of In-111 antimyosin uptake, the greater the degree of irreversible cellular injury. Dual imaging with Tl-201 and In-111 antimyosin after infarction can delineate the total area of hypoperfusion, either during stress or at rest using the Tl-201 defect area, and extent of necrosis by measuring the In-111 antimyosin zone of increased uptake.[99] A large perfusion defect associated with a small zone of antimyosin uptake (mismatch) is suggestive of a large extent of jeopardized but viable myocardium with a small infarct. When the Tl-201 defect size matches the In-111 antimyosin defect size, the extent of viable myocardium is considered minimal. Thus, determination of myocardial viability can be undertaken with a dual imaging technique where both In-111 antimyosin antibody and Tl-201 are administered to patients with acute infarction and severe myocardial asynergy. Zones of preserved Tl-201 uptake contiguous to regions of antimyosin uptake would suggest viable myocardium despite persistence of severe systolic dysfunction. The identification of reversible perfusion abnormalities on stress Tl-201 imaging in myocardial zones outside an area of infarction showing intense antimyosin uptake reflects ischemia in addition to irreversible cellular injury. This pattern indicates that areas of ischemic and jeopardized myocardium are present in addition to the zone of myocardium that was rendered necrotic and suggests underlying multivessel CAD.

There are limitations of antimyosin antibody imaging that deserve mention. The actual role that this imaging technique will have in the clinical setting has not yet been ascertained. Myocardial viability can be determined after MI solely with the use of Tl-201 rest scintigraphy and assessment of regional wall motion.

POSITRON EMISSION TOMOGRAPHY TO ASSESS MYOCARDIAL VIABILITY

More sophisticated imaging techniques such as metabolic imaging with PET may be even more sensitive for identifying zones of myocardial viability than conventional single-photon imaging approaches.[99a–99c] Table 9–4 lists the various PET approaches that have been used to assess myocardial viability by assessment of flow and metabolism. Under basal normal physiologic conditions, myocardial metabolic activity is predominantly aerobic. The working heart meets its energy requirements chiefly by oxidative metabolism of fatty acids and glucose. Under fasting conditions, nonesterified fatty acids are still the preferred energy fuel. When ischemia develops, oxidation of fatty acids is impaired and anaerobic metabolism of glucose becomes proportionally more dominant. Fluorine-18-labeled deoxyglucose (FDG) is a glucose analog that mimics the initial steps of the glucose metabolic flux by the heart, including transport across the cell membrane and hexokinase-mediated phosphorylation (see Chap. 2). The phosphorylated FDG is trapped within the myocardial cell because the myocyte is relatively impermeable to it and because it is not a good substrate for subsequent metabolism by either glycolytic or glycogen synthetic pathways. Dephosphorylation of FDG-6-phosphate appears to be quite slow. Increased regional uptake and phosphorylation of FDG in a zone of myocardial asynergy, representing sustained or enhanced glycolytic activity, identifies myocardial tissue that is metabolically active and, thus, is viable.

Presence of FDG in regions with depressed systolic function and reduced blood flow has been shown accurately to distinguish reversible from irreversible myocardial injury.[6,7] The imaging technique involves intravenous administration of FDG and then allowing 30 to 40 minutes for metabolic trapping of the tracer. Images are then recorded for 20 to 30 minutes. Regional myocardial perfusion is simultaneously assessed using a PET agent capable of measuring blood flow (e.g., N-13 ammonia, rubidium-82 [Rb-82]). For assessment of myocardial hibernation, imaging of FDG uptake should be undertaken after oral glucose loading. This

Table 9–4. Assessment of Myocardial Viability by PET

1. Enhanced uptake of ^{18}F-labeled FDG in myocardial zones of reduced perfusion
2. Preserved regional oxidative metabolism assessed by quantitative analysis of ^{11}C-acetate kinetics
3. Preserved uptake and retention of Rb-82
4. Quantitation of water-perfusable tissue index (PTI) with oxygen-15–labeled water

will enhance the contrast between viable and nonviable myocardium. Supplemental glucose should not, however, be given to diabetic patients. Extra insulin might be given to such diabetic patients prior to FDG imaging. Both perfusion and FDG images are analyzed qualitatively and quantitatively. Three possible patterns are identified. The first is normal uniform blood flow associated with normal uniform glucose utilization, which indicates viable and normal myocardium. The second pattern is characterized by a regional reduction in blood flow paralleled by a proportional reduction in glucose utilization referred to as *perfusion-metabolism match*. This pattern is indicative of myocardial necrosis and nonviability. The third scintigraphic pattern is characterized by a regional decrease in blood flow associated with a relative or absolute increase in FDG, which is called a *perfusion-metabolism mismatch*. Figure 9–35 is an example of this mismatch pattern, which is suggestive of myocardial viability. Patients with a mismatch pattern and regional left ventricular dysfunction have less myocardial fibrosis as determined from myocardial biopsies obtained during coronary bypass surgery compared with patients exhibiting a watch pattern preoperatively.[99d]

A relative increase in FDG is defined as an increase relative to the reduction of blood flow. An absolute increase in FDG means that FDG uptake is increased relative to FDG activity in normal myocardium. A perfusion-metabolism match would be indicative of infarcted myocardium, whereas a mismatch implies preserved metabolic integrity and, thus, viability. The extent and severity of myocardial perfusion abnormalities and metabolic alternations are best evaluated by inspection of reoriented, short-axis tomographic images from the PET scans. The short-axis images can be displayed semiquantitatively into polar maps employing color codes to depict extent and severity of regionally abnormal blood flow and metabolism matches and mismatches.

Clinical Positron Emission Tomography Imaging of Metabolism of Fluorine-18 2,Deoxyglucose and Perfusion

PET with N-13 ammonia and FDG was used to assess regional myocardial perfusion and viability, respectively, in patients with chronic CAD and ECG Q waves.[100] Infarcted regions were identified by a matched reduction in regional N-13 ammonia activity and FDG utilization, whereas viable regions were identified by enhanced FDG uptake in regions of diminished N-13 ammonia activity. Figure 9–36 shows the ECG and representative tomographic PET images from a patient with a Q-wave infarction in this study. Glucose metabolism was well preserved in severely hypokinetic regions, corresponding to Q waves and decreased N-13 ammonia perfusion. In this study, PET with FDG revealed evidence of persistent glucose metabolism in a large proportion of myocardial regions, correlating with chronic ECG Q waves and wall motion abnormalities, thereby identifying viable myocardium not easily detected by conven-

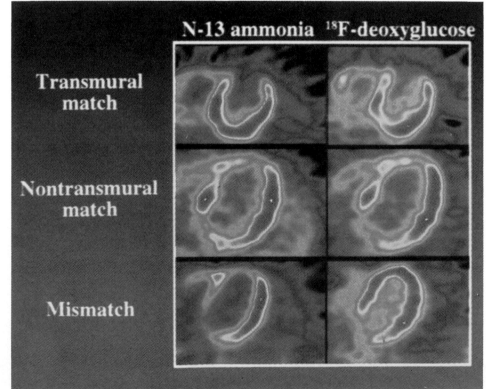

Figure 9–35. Example of a mismatch pattern between myocardial blood flow (*left,* N-13 ammonia images) and myocardial metabolism (*right,* images FDG). Note the increase in FDG uptake in the zone of hypoperfusion indicating preserved viability. Also shown are "transmural match" and "nontransmural match" patterns. The former suggests nonviability, as in a transmural infarction, whereas the latter suggests a mixture of viable and nonviable myocardial tissue. (Reprinted by permission of the Society of Nuclear Medicine from Maddahi J, et al.: J Nucl Med 1994; 35: 707–715.)

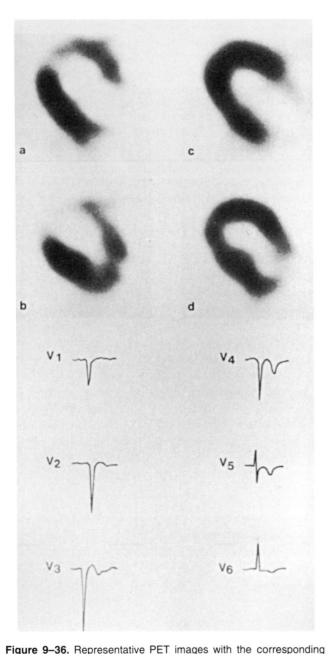

Figure 9–36. Representative PET images with the corresponding resting ECG in a patient with a MI and pathologic Q waves in ECG leads V_1 to V_4. The left ventricular ejection fraction on radionuclide angiography—26%—was associated with severe hypokinesis of the anterior wall and akinesis of the intraventricular septum. Perfusion defects are noted on the N-13 ammonia study in the anterior and septal segments (**a, b**). Preserved glucose metabolism (**c, d**) with substantial uptake of FDG in the defect regions. (Brunken R, et al.: Circulation 1986;73:951–963.)

tional evaluation. Schwaiger et al.[100a] performed FDG imaging studies in postinfarction patients within 72 hours of onset of symptoms. Decreased metabolic activity in the infarct zone was predictive of no subsequent improvement in regional systolic function. FDG uptake was higher in patients with patent infarct vessels than in those with an occluded infarct-related artery. Pierard et al.[101] compared FDG uptake patterns after acute infarction with dobutamine echocardiography at 9 days and again at 9 months after

hospital admission. Absence of metabolic activity in PET scans was associated with no further enhancement of function with dobutamine. However, in patients with preserved FDG uptake, the functional response was quite variable. Only one of six patients with a mismatch pattern (high glucose-perfusion ratio) demonstrated late functional recovery. FDG uptake patterns do not correlate with presence or absence of visualized angiographic collaterals.[102a] The extent of mismatch (perfusion defect with enhanced FDG) was unrelated to either presence or magnitude of collateral vessels in 42 patients with 78 completely occluded arteries subtending asynergic myocardial zones. Figure 9–37 shows the extent of PET patterns of viability in individual coro-

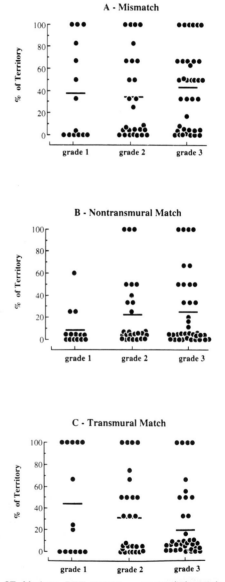

Figure 9–37. Various PET viability patterns (mismatch, nontransmural match, and transmural match) versus angiographic collateral grade in individual coronary territories. The extent of PET mismatch (Panel A) as a percentage of a territory was unrelated to collateral grade. (Grade 1 = absent; Grade 2 = faint opacification of distal vessel via collateral channels; Grade 3 = well-developed collaterals and entire distal vessel densely opacified.) (Reprinted with permission from the American College of Cardiology (Journal of the American College of Cardiology, 1994, Vol. 23, pp. 860–868).)

nary territories versus the angiographic collateral grade. The relationship was highly variable.

In some patients with left ventricular dysfunction, FDG may be reduced in some myocardial zones, despite normal flow. Perrone-Filardi et al.[101a] found that 26% of myocardial regions with flow of at least 0.7 ml/g/minute had moderately reduced FDG uptake. Of these, 32% had absent systolic thickening at rest; 63% had corresponding reversible Tl-201 scan defects. The authors concluded that such segments represent an admixture of fibrotic and reversibly ischemic myocardium.

There are some potential limitations to the use of FDG imaging in the subacute phase of acute infarction for evaluation of viability in the infarct zone.[102–103b] Intravenous heparin administered to most infarct patients in the early course of hospitalization can raise plasma free fatty acid levels, which may suppress FDG uptake by myocardial tissue.[102] Elevated serum catecholamines consequent to the acute infarction process can also suppress myocardial glucose uptake.[103] The very early performance of PET imaging with FDG in the first hours of infarction to assess myocardium at jeopardy is not feasible since it would unduly delay institution of thrombolytic therapy.

Brunken et al.[57] showed evidence of preserved glucose uptake by PET in many segments that demonstrated only partial Tl-201 redistribution or in zones corresponding to fixed Tl-201 defects. In that study, 58% of segments that showed no Tl-201 redistribution at 4 hours demonstrated some preservation of regional FDG uptake. These authors concluded that markers of perfusion alone would underestimate the extent of viable myocardium, particularly in regions supplied by severely stenotic vessels. Reinjection of a second dose of Tl-201 at 4 hours on quantitative image analysis to enhance the sensitivity of Tl-201 scintigraphy for distinguishing viable from nonviable myocardium was not undertaken in this study.

Perrone-Filardi et al.[104] found that FDG uptake was observed in 97% of hypokinetic and normal regions and in 74% of akinetic regions in patients with ischemic LV dysfunction (mean LVEF, 27% ± 10%). Perfusion was assessed by oxygen-15 (O-15)–labeled water. End-diastolic wall thickness was greater in akinetic regions that demonstrated FDG uptake than in those that did not. Figure 9–38 relates FDG uptake to systolic function for segments analyzed in this study. Thus, a large percentage of asynergic regions remain viable in patients with chronic CAD and LV dysfunction. The percentage of akinetic or dyskinetic segments showing FDG uptake in this study (74%) is almost identical to the percentage of severely asynergic segments demonstrating viability by resting Tl-201 criteria (73%) in the study by Ragosta et al.[52] in a similar patient population. Gewirtz et al.[104a] reported that assessment of flow alone by quantitative N-13 ammonia PET imaging was valuable in assessing myocardial viability in zones of asynergy resulting from acute MI. In 26 patients mismatch between blood flow and FDG uptake, with a single exception, was not seen in any segment with flow less than 0.25 ml/minute/g. Also, all dyskinetic segments had flow less than 0.25 ml/minute/g. In contrast, 43 of 45 myocardial segments with normal or hypokinetic contraction had flow at least 0.39 ml/minute/g. Average flow in these segments was 0.78 ± .35 ml/minute/g.

Predicting Response to Revascularization by Positron Emission Tomography

PET imaging with FDG can be used to predict which asynergic myocardial segments will improve systolic function after coronary revascularization.[105–108e] Tillisch et al.[105] monitored the functional outcome of segmental wall motion abnormalities after bypass surgery relative to the preoperative FDG findings on PET. Systolic function was enhanced in 85% of myocardial segments that showed mismatch be-

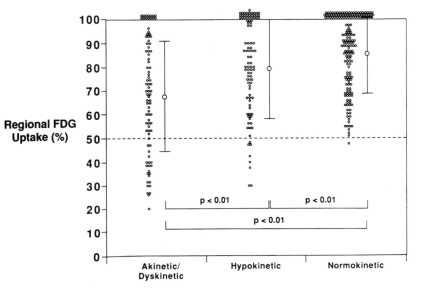

Figure 9–38. Relationship between FDG uptake and systolic wall motion patterns in patients with ischemic LV dysfunction. FDG uptake was observed in 97% of hypokinetic and normal regions and in 74% of akinetic regions demonstrating substantial viability in regions with abnormal wall motion. (Reprinted with permission from the American College of Cardiology (Journal of the American College of Cardiology, 1992, Vol. 20, pp. 161–168).)

tween blood flow and FDG uptake, whereas no improvement was noted in 92% of patients who had a matched diminution in blood flow and metabolism. Tamaki et al.[106] found that 78% of segments that showed preserved FDG uptake had improvement in regional function after bypass surgery, compared to improvement in only 22% of segments without FDG uptake. Schwaiger et al.[107] found in 29 patients who underwent revascularization that improvement in regional systolic function occurred in 75% of segments with akinesis or dyskinesis and relatively increased FDG uptake preoperatively. Lack of FDG uptake in zones of akinesis or dyskinesis had 90% predictive accuracy for failure to recover contractile function after bypass surgery.

After coronary revascularization, most hibernating myocardial segments show a reduction of FDG activity that corresponds to the improvement in perfusion and function.[108] This reduction reflects a shift back to using fatty acids as the predominant substrate for metabolism. However, some myocardial regions continue to show abnormal elevation of FDG uptake as late as 5 months after revascularization. Marwick et al.[108] found that these segments were characterized before intervention by more severe malperfusion. Figure 9–39 shows PET images from a patient in this study who after surgery exhibited normalization of perfusion but not of metabolism. Persistent elevation of FDG activity can be discerned in the inferior wall, despite improvement in RB-82 uptake.

Thus, PET imaging of blood flow and metabolism appears to be useful for preoperative evaluation of patients with markedly depressed LV function. Many patients with chronic CAD have severe regional wall motion abnormalities, and myocardial viability is an important factor with respect to consideration and outcome of bypass surgery. The positive predictive accuracy of a perfusion-metabolism mismatch for improvement of segmental function after coronary bypass surgery is in the range of 80% to 85%. The accuracy of a match of perfusion and metabolism for predicting that function will not improve following revascularization ranges from 80% to 90%.[7, 108a–108d] Table 9–5 summarizes the predictive accuracy of perfusion-FDG PET imaging of metabolism for recovery of regional LV dysfunction after myocardial revascularization.[108a] The presence of a mismatch pattern also has prognostic significance.[108b] Survival was shown to be poorer among patients with a mismatch than among those with a match pattern if treated medically (92% vs. 50%). Patients with mismatch who underwent revascularization had a higher survival rate than those treated medically (88% vs. 50%; $P = 0.03$). Figure 9–40 summarizes these findings. This study emphasizes that patients with marked LV dysfunction who have a significant extent of hibernating myocardium have a poor prognosis when treated medically.

Improvement in exercise capacity after revascularization can be predicted by a postexercise increase in FDG uptake. Marwick et al.[108e] reported that patients with multiple FDG-avid regions demonstrated a significantly greater improvement in peak rate-pressure product and maximal peak heart rate during exercise stress after revascularization compared to remaining patients with a lesser amount of postexercise FDG uptake.

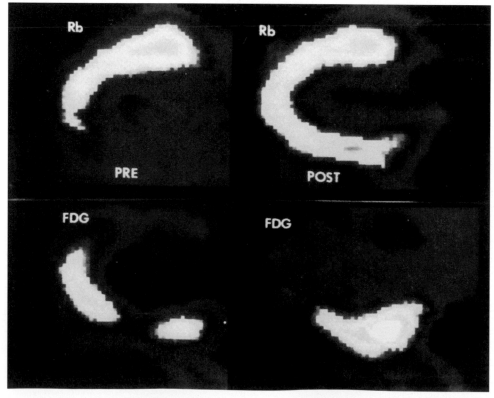

Figure 9–39. Sagittal PET images with apex oriented to the left, which demonstrate improvement in Rb-82 uptake in the inferior wall after revascularization *(upper panels)* with persistent elevation of FDG activity in the inferior wall after surgery *(lower right panel).* (See Color Figure 9–39.) (Marwick TH et al.: Circulation 1992;85:1347–1353.)

See Color Figure 9–39.

Table 9–5. Predictive Accuracy of Perfusion-FDG Metabolism PET Imaging for Recovery of Regional Left Ventricular Dyssynergy After Myocardial Revascularization

Investigator, Year	Number of Patients (segs)	Predictive Accuracy	
		Positive	*Negative*
Tillisch, 1986[105]	17 (67)	35/41 (85%)	24/26 (92%)
Tamaki, 1989[106]	20 (46)	18/23 (78%)	18/23 (78%)
Tamaki, 1991[64]	11 (56)	40/50 (80%)	6/6 (100%)
Lucignani, 1992[94b]	14 (54)	37/39 (95%)	12/15 (80%)
Carrel, 1992[108c]	23 (23)	16/19 (84%)	3/4 (75%)
Gropler, 1992[122]	16 (53)	19/24 (79%)	24/29 (83%)
Marwick, 1992[108]	16 (85)	25/37 (68%)	38/48 (79%)
Gropler, 1993[108d]	34 (57)	21/29 (72%)	23/28 (82%)
Total	154 (441)	211/262 (80%)	148/179 (83%)

(Adapted from Maddahi J, et al.: J Nucl Med 1994;35:707–715.[108a])

CARBON-11 PALMITATE IMAGING

Carbon-11 (C-11) palmitate, a tracer of fatty acid metabolism, clears from the myocardium in a biexponential manner with an early rapid and a late slow clearance phase (see Chap. 2). It was originally thought that by quantitating the early rapid phase, oxidative metabolism could be noninvasively assessed. With oxidation, it is the efflux of C-11 carbon dioxide that is being monitored. However, subsequent studies at Washington University in St. Louis showed that, with ischemia, the correlation between the $T_{1/2}$ of early palmitate clearance after administration of C-11 palmitate and myocardial oxygen consumption is not close. Nearly 50% of tracer efflux is accounted for by clearance of nonmetabolized palmitate, referred to as *back-diffusion.*[109] Rosamond et al.[110] found that, in normal hearts of open-chest dogs, 10% of initially extracted radiolabeled palmitate is retained in tissue as triglycerides, phospholipids, or other lipids, 74% was oxidized, and 16% back-diffused unaltered.

With ischemia, 28% was retained, 27% oxidized, and 44% back-diffused. With prolonged ischemia, triglycerides, diglycerides, and nonesterified fatty acids comprise a greater fraction of initially extracted radioactivity. These authors concluded that, during ischemia, externally detected C-11 palmitate clearance rates cannot be used as a direct measure of fatty-acid metabolism because of the effect on efflux of nonmetabolized radiolabeled palmitate and the distribution of tracer retained in tissue.

Despite these limitations, C-11 palmitate imaging has shown to be useful in certain clinical studies.[110a] Grover-McKay et al.[111] showed attenuation in the increase in fatty acid oxidation in myocardium distal to a coronary stenosis with atrial pacing in patients with CAD. Segments with altered C-11 palmitate kinetics showed new wall motion abnormalities on echocardiography in 50% of the patients studied. Regional C-11 palmitate imaging has been utilized to assess metabolic activity in reperfused myocardium following thrombolysis.[112] The earlier the initiation of reper-

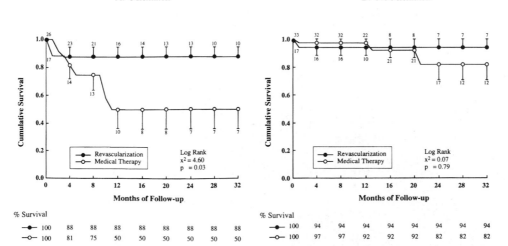

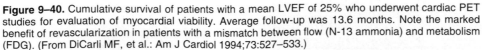

Figure 9–40. Cumulative survival of patients with a mean LVEF of 25% who underwent cardiac PET studies for evaluation of myocardial viability. Average follow-up was 13.6 months. Note the marked benefit of revascularization in patients with a mismatch between flow (N-13 ammonia) and metabolism (FDG). (From DiCarli MF, et al.: Am J Cardiol 1994;73:527–533.)

fusion, the greater the intensity and extent of C-11 palmitate uptake in the infarct zone.[113] Recovery of metabolic function after reperfusion could be predicted by the ability soon after reflow to accumulate C-11 palmitate.[114] Efficacy of adjunctive therapy to enhance myocardial salvage with reperfusion could also be assessed by PET imaging of C-11 palmitate.[115] C-11 palmitate kinetics may remain abnormal for a prolonged period after reperfusion following transient ischemia, and metabolic recovery occurs in parallel with recovery of regional function.[116]

CARBON-11 ACETATE IMAGING

More recently, PET imaging of C-11 acetate has been evaluated to assess myocardial oxygen consumption. The kinetics of C-11 acetate in the myocardium are reviewed in Chapter 2. Measurement of the oxidation of acetate could provide an indirect noninvasive measure of regional oxygen utilization. The regional uptake and clearance of C-11 acetate have been used as a noninvasive approach to calculating myocardial oxygen consumption and oxidative myocardial reserve.[116a] Henes et al.[117] quantitated the metabolic response of normal myocardium to increased work by measuring clearance of myocardial C-11 activity after C-11 acetate administration to normal subjects at rest and during dobutamine infusion. At rest, clearance of C-11 was monoexponential and homogeneous. With an increased rate-pressure product (RPP) with dobutamine infusion, C-11 clearance became biexponential with a significant change in the k_1 (rate constant of first phase of C-11 clearance). However, the slope of the k_1/RPP relation remained consistent, which indicated that oxidative metabolic reserve can be adequately evaluated by this technique. Since increases in the rate of clearance of C-11 acetate are proportional to in-creases in cardiac work, this approach may be used to assess oxidative metabolic reserve in patients with cardiovascular diseases.

Armbrecht et al.[118] validated the use of C-11 acetate as a tracer of oxidative myocardial metabolism for use with PET in the open-chest dog model. They found that the rate constant k_1 for the first rapid clearance phase of C-11 correlated closely with myocardial oxygen consumption ($r = 0.94$) during control, ischemic, reperfusion, and dipyridamole-induced experimental conditions. Experiments performed with carbon-14 (C-14) acetate demonstrated that the rapid acetate clearance phase represents nearly exclusively TCA cycle turnover of the tracer. The clearance of radioactivity from myocardium after injection of labeled acetate was almost exclusively in the form of labeled carbon dioxide. Once extracted, acetate is rapidly converted to acetyl coenzyme A, which enters the citric acid cycle in the mitochondria.

In patients with reperfused anterior MI studied between 2 weeks and 3 months after the acute event, regional oxidative metabolism as assessed by PET imaging of C-11 acetate is reduced in proportion to residual blood flow.[119] Infarct segments that exhibit increased FDG uptake relative to flow had faster acetate clearance than segments without flow-metabolism mismatch; though, at similar levels of hypoperfusion, this study showed no significant difference in acetate clearance among segments with and those without flow-metabolism (by FDG) mismatch. Figure 9–41 shows the scatterplot of the correlation between the acetate clearance slope and myocardial blood flow. Walsh et al.[120] imaged patients with C-11 acetate in the acute stage of infarction. They found a marked reduction in C-11 acetate clearance rates at the center of the infarct with a mild decrease in the hypoperfused periinfarction zone. The recovery of oxidative metabolism after reperfusion in acute

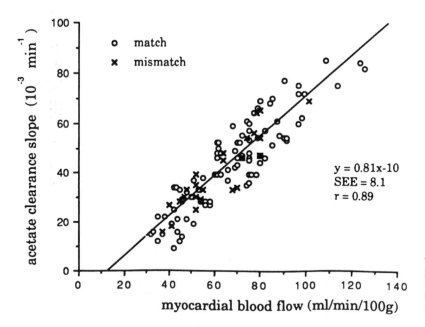

$$y = 0.81x - 10$$
$$SEE = 8.1$$
$$r = 0.89$$

Figure 9–41. Scatter plots of correlation between acetate clearance slope and myocardial blood flow in hypoperfused regions with a matched pattern between regional glucose uptake and blood flow (o) or a mismatch pattern between flow and glucose uptake (x). (Vanoverschelde JL, et al.: Circulation 1992;85:9–21.)

MI may lag behind the recovery of blood flow.[120] In the study by Henes et al.,[121] flow was nearly normal as assessed by O-15 water after thrombolytic therapy, but oxidative metabolism as assessed by C-11 acetate remained at 45% ± 22% of normal. C-11 acetate kinetics progressively improved during hospitalization. Early recovery of wall motion was predicted by improved oxidative metabolism. In a subsequent study from the same group, Gropler et al.[122] demonstrated that dysfunctional but viable myocardium after infarction exhibited oxidative metabolism equivalent to 74% of that of normal myocardium. Preservation of oxidative metabolism was found to be a necessary condition for recovery of function after revascularization, and C-11 acetate imaging was superior to FDG imaging for identification of viable but asynergic segments. This group also reported that the combination of O-15 water perfusion imaging and C-11 acetate imaging could be successfully employed to predict recovery of function in asynergic myocardium after revascularization.[122a] Figure 9–42 shows wall motion scores in viable and nonviable myocardium before and after revascularization in this study. A significant improvement in wall motion was seen only in segments judged viable by C-11 acetate imaging. The wall motion score fell from 2.61 ± 0.77 to 1.38 ± 0.58.

The clinical utility of this PET metabolic imaging technique still is not well-defined. Certainly, residual oxidative metabolism in zones of myocardial jeopardy in CAD patients with ischemic dysfunction and in patients with a recent MI can be assessed. This may assist in decision making about therapeutic strategies aimed at enhancing regional flow and function.

RUBIDIUM-82 IMAGING OF MYOCARDIAL VIABILITY

PET imaging of blood flow using Rb-82 may prove to be a useful approach to identifying viable myocardium. Myocardial viability is predicated on the fact that metabolically active myocardium must have some flow preservation. Estimates of myocardial membrane integrity based upon Rb-82 tissue kinetics compare favorably with myocardial uptake of FDG.[123] The rationale for the use of Rb-82 imaging for assessing myocardial viability is based on the concept that transiently ischemic but viable myocardium can retain extracted Rb-82 whereas nonviable myocardium exhibits back-diffusion of the tracer.[124, 125] Upon delivery by coronary blood flow to the myocardium, Rb-82 is extracted by normal cells, where it equilibrates with the intracellular potassium pool. If these cells are necrotic and cannot retain the tracer, it washes out rapidly after initial distribution. The rate of Rb-82 washout can be measured by rapid sequential PET imaging.

In a study reported by Gould et al.[126] 43 patients with evolving MI had PET imaging using FDG and Rb-82. The goal of the study was to determine whether cell membrane dysfunction as evidenced by abnormal kinetics of Rb-82 paralleled the abnormal cellular metabolism of FDG. Infarct size based on Rb-82 kinetics correlated closely with size and location on FDG images ($r = 0.93$), suggesting that loss of cellular function for sequestering Rb-82 parallels the loss of metabolic integrity of cellular glucose metabolism. Figure 9–43 shows the relation of infarct size by Rb-82 compared to FDG in this study. In a subsequent report from

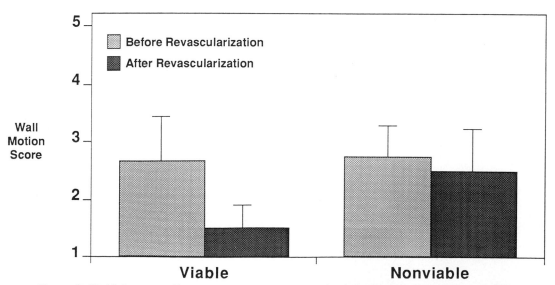

Figure 9–42. Histograms with average wall motion scores (and standard deviations) for segments containing viable and nonviable myocardium, before and after revascularization. Viability was determined by C-11 acetate imaging for identifying zones of preserved oxidative metabolism. Although before revascularization, viable and nonviable segments showed similar degrees of severity of mechanical dysfunction, after revascularization only viable regions demonstrated significantly improved function. (Reprinted with permission from the American College of Cardiology (Journal of the American College of Cardiology, 1992, Vol. 20, pp. 569–577).)

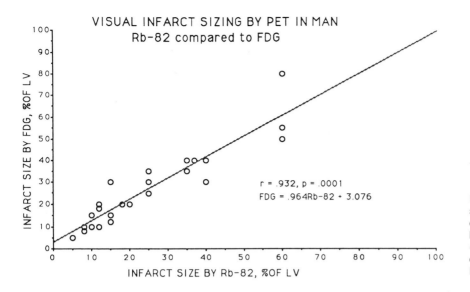

Figure 9–43. Relationship between infarct size by Rb-82 imaging expressed as a percentage of left ventricle (LV) and infarct size by FDG, also expressed as percentage of LV. (Reprinted by permission of the Society of Nuclear Medicine from Gould KL, et al.: J Nucl Med 1991;32:1–9.)

this group, size of scar and viable myocardium by PET using Rb-82, was highly predictive of 3-year mortality in patients who had a previous infarction.[126a] MI or scar on 23% or more of the left ventricle was associated with a 3-year mortality rate of 43% versus 5% for those with scar comprising less than 23% of the left ventricle. Also in this study, patients with viable myocardium had a significantly lower mortality rate than patients with nonviable myocardium in risk zones (Fig. 9–44). This may be attributed to the fact that 75% of these patients underwent revascularization.

OXYGEN-15 WATER AND ASSESSMENT OF MYOCARDIAL VIABILITY

Quantification of absolute blood flow with PET imaging of O-15–labeled water (see Chap. 2) could prove feasible for the determination of myocardial viability without the necessity of concomitant metabolic imaging with FDG or C-11 acetate. Yamamoto investigated the use of the water-perfusable tissue index (PTI), defined as the proportion of the total anatomic tissue within a given region of interest that is capable of rapidly exchanging water.[127] This variable is obtained from analysis of transmission, blood volume (O-15 carbon monoxide), and myocardial blood flow (O-15 water) PET images. These investigators showed that PTI was a better index of recovery of function than measurement of blood flow alone. PTI values also correlated well with FDG-flow ratios. Thus, PTI, which measures the proportion of myocardium functionally exchanging water, provides a quantitative index of myocardial viability that appears to provide similar predictive information as measurement of FDG-flow ratios.

CLINICAL DECISION MAKING IN RADIONUCLIDE ASSESSMENT OF MYOCARDIAL VIABILITY

There is no doubt that radionuclide imaging of myocardial perfusion, function, and metabolism for assessment of

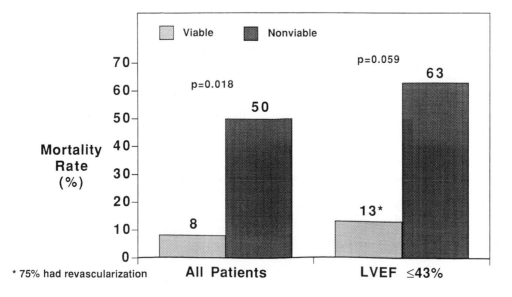

Figure 9–44. Myocardial viability by PET utilizing Rb-82 imaging in risk zones versus mortality during follow-up in all patients and in patients with a resting LV ejection fraction of 43% or less. Note that patients who demonstrate viable myocardium had a significantly lower mortality rate in these groups compared to patients with nonviable myocardium. Seventy-five percent of the patients underwent revascularization. (Reprinted with permission from the American College of Cardiology (Journal of the American College of Cardiology, 1993, Vol. 22, pp. 984–997).)

myocardial viability can assist in clinical decision making in certain subsets of patients with CAD. As described in this chapter, measurement of regional myocardial systolic function alone may not be adequate to distinguish viable from irreversibly injured myocardium in patients who have recently undergone coronary reperfusion or who have severe CAD and manifest "stunned" or "hibernating" myocardium as the cause of LV dysfunction. In these clinical situations, stress-redistribution or solely resting Tl-201 imaging, or resting Tc-99m sestamibi or Tc-99m tetrofosmin imaging, will help distinguish ischemic from necrotic myocardium. With SPECT exercise Tl-201 imaging, it is preferable to administer a second dose of Tl-201 following the "reinjection" protocol to best differentiate reversible ischemia from myocardial scar. With quantitative planar imaging, reinjection of a second dose of Tl-201 may not be necessary.

In patients who are unable to exercise, resting Tl-201 scintigraphy alone, preferably employing quantitation, should be highly accurate in identifying asynergic regions that are still viable. Demonstration of preserved Tl-201 uptake, even if it is reduced, suggests that following revascularization regional function should improve. Patients with severe CAD and depressed function who are most likely to benefit from revascularization exhibit Tl-201 uptake with standard stress and 4-hour redistribution imaging, by stress and delayed 18- to 24-hour imaging, or by enhanced Tl-201 uptake with reinjection. Tl-201 uptake in the resting state, alone, even if mildly diminished (less than 50% reduced compared to normal uptake) with no delayed redistribution, indicates viability and also predicts improvement in function after revascularization. Patients with no evidence of viable myocardium in the distribution of severely obstructed vessels by Tl-201 scan criteria (severe defect with no enhanced uptake after reinjection) would be spared the risk of surgery and a probable suboptimal long-term outcome if revascularization surgery or angioplasty were technically successful. Most of these patients exhibit end-diastolic thinning of the myocardium by 2-D echocardiography or magnetic resonance imaging (MRI) and manifest Q waves on ECG. Similarly, greater than 50% uptake of Tc-99m sestamibi in zones of myocardial asynergy is predictive of viability as reflected by a subsequent improvement in function in these zones after revascularization.

It is somewhat premature to predict whether or not Tc-99m–sestamibi imaging will prove more beneficial than Tl-201 scintigraphy for identifying viable myocardium after coronary reperfusion. Certainly, the results of clinical studies in which regional function and perfusion are simultaneously assessed by gated Tc-99m–sestamibi imaging will be of interest. It is quite likely that Tc-99m–sestamibi imaging in acute MI patients undergoing thrombolytic therapy will prove more useful than Tl-201 imaging in this patient population for the early assessment of success of reflow and extent of myocardial salvage. The clinical studies reported to date are certainly encouraging in this regard. Acute infarction patients who do not exhibit a significant reduction in Tc-99m–sestamibi defect on serial imaging after thrombolysis might be candidates for "rescue angioplasty." No defect reduction would suggest failure to reperfuse with pharmacologic therapy.

Dual-isotope imaging with Tl-201 injected at rest and Tc-99m sestamibi injected during exercise is presently under investigation to determine if defect reversibility is better detected than by imaging with either radionuclide alone. The concept is that the resting Tl-201 images provide information relevant to viability, whereas the exercise Tc-99m–sestamibi images are acquired for detection of stress-induced ischemia.

Infarct-avid imaging with In-111 antimyosin antibody may not gain extensive use in clinical practice for evaluation of viability after acute infarction. Perhaps a limited diagnostic role for this imaging approach will emerge in patients with suspected infarction who have uninterpretable ECG findings (e.g., bundle branch blocks) or whose creatine kinase enzyme values are nondiagnostic (e.g., those admitted more than 48 hours after onset of symptoms).

The cost effectiveness of the more expensive PET imaging techniques for assessment of viability have not yet been adequately ascertained. The superiority to conventional imaging techniques of PET imaging of myocardial metabolism with FDG or C-11 acetate or other tracers for detection of CAD and determination of myocardial viability has not clearly been ascertained. The studies cited in this chapter seem to indicate almost comparable sensitivity for SPECT Tl-201 imaging using the reinjection protocol and PET imaging with FDG for distinguishing viable from nonviable myocardium. However, further comparative studies between PET and SPECT studies in a larger number of patients, in which the gold standard for viability is enhanced regional function after revascularization, should be conducted. Certainly, the PET studies with FDG and with C-11 acetate appear promising with respect to quantitating alterations in regional myocardial metabolism in patients in acute infarction and in patients with chronic CAD and depressed LV function.

DOBUTAMINE ECHOCARDIOGRAPHY AND VIABILITY ASSESSMENT

Low-dose dobutamine in conjunction with echocardiography may have value for the assessment of myocardial viability.[128, 128a] An increase in wall thickening or wall motion in asynergic segments correlates with viable myocardium as judged by PET imaging of FDG uptake.[102] Dobutamine echocardiography involves recording 2-D echocardiograms at baseline and after doses of 5 or 10 μg/kg/minute of dobutamine. Augmented LV systolic thickening or endocardial motion constitutes a positive response for viability. Smart et al.[129] infused dobutamine in 63 patients recovering from an acute MI, all of whom had received thrombolytic therapy. The low-dose dobutamine protocol was associated with 86% sensitivity and 90% specificity for reversible dysfunction as assessed by serial echocardiography. Dobutamine echocardiography may not be as useful for detecting viability in hibernating myocardium in patients with severe multivessel CAD. In that situation, even low-dose dobutamine infusion could cause ischemia due to an increase in oxygen demand that cannot be met with an increase in regional myocardial blood flow. Low-dose dobutamine (2.5 mg/minute) in pigs with a chronic reduction in CAD flow caused a further reduction in creatine phosphate and ATP after only 5 minutes of drug infusion.[130] This was associated with an increase in regional myocardial work. In the study of Sansoy et al.[89] small doses of dobutamine (5 mg/kg/minute) in dogs with a severe LAD stenosis failed to increase systolic thickening in zones of asynergy that were viable by rest Tl-201 uptake criteria. Thus, unless some flow enhancement occurs commensurate with the inotropic effect of dobutamine, enhanced systolic contraction will not be detected in the supply zone of a severely stenotic artery. In contrast, dobutamine echocardiography should be very sensitive for detecting viability in stunned myocardium as observed with coronary reperfusion. This is because flow has been restored, permitting a further increase in regional blood flow consequent to dobutamine-induced inotropy. Nevertheless, substantial Tl-201, Tc-99m–sestamibi, or Tc-99m–tetrofosmin uptake should also be seen in myocardium rendered asynergic by stunning.

REFERENCES

1. Alderman EL, Bourassa MG, Cohen LS, Davis KB, Kaiser GG, Killip T, Mock MB, Pettinger M, Robertson TL: Ten-year follow-up of survival and myocardial infarction in the randomized Coronary Artery Surgery Study. Circulation 1990;82:1629–1646.
2. Varnauskas E: Twelve-year follow-up of survival in the randomized European Coronary Surgery Study. N Engl J Med 1988;319:332–337.
3. Veterans Administration Coronary Artery Bypass Surgery Cooperative Study Group: Eleven-Year Survival in the Veterans Administration Randomized Trial of Coronary Bypass Surgery for Stable Angina. N Engl J Med 1984;311:1333–1339.
4. Bolli R: Myocardial 'stunning' in man. Circulation 1992;86:1671–1691.
5. Rahimtoola SH: The hibernating myocardium. Am Heart J 1989;117:211–221.
6. Schelbert HR: Current status and prospects of new radionuclides and radiopharmaceuticals for cardiovascular nuclear medicine. Semin Nucl Med 1987;17:145–181.
7. Schwaiger M, Hicks R: The clinical role of metabolic imaging of the heart by positron emission tomography. J Nucl Med 1991;32:565–578.
8. Bonow RO, Dilsizian V: Thallium 201 for assessment of myocardial viability. Semin Nucl Med 1991;21:230–241.
9. Beller GA, Ragosta M, Watson DD, Gimple LW: Myocardial thallium-201 scintigraphy for assessment of viability in patients with severe left ventricular dysfunction. Am J Cardiol 1992;70:18E–22E.
10. Lemlek J, Heo J, Iskandrian AS: The clinical relevance of myocardial viability in patient management. Am Heart J 1992;124:1327–1331.
10a. Schelbert HR: Metabolic imaging to assess myocardial viability. J Nucl Med 1994;35(Suppl):85–145.
11. Braunwald E, Kloner RA: The stunned myocardium: Prolonged, postischemic ventricular dysfunction. Circulation 1982;66:1146–1149.
12. Ross J Jr: Myocardial perfusion-contraction matching. Implications for coronary heart disease and hibernation. Circulation 1991;83:1076–1083.
13. Moore CA, Cannon J, Watson DD, Kaul S, Beller GA: Thallium 201 kinetics in stunned myocardium characterized by severe postischemic systolic dysfunction. Circulation 1990;81:1622–1632.
14. Nicklas JM, Becker LC, Bulkley BH: Effects of repeated brief coronary occlusion on regional left ventricular function and dimension in dogs. Am J Cardiol 1985;56:473–478.
15. Swain JL, Sabina RL, McHale PA, Greenfield JC Jr, Holmes EW: Prolonged myocardial nucleotide depletion after brief ischemia in the open-chest dog. Am J Physiol 1982;242:H818–H826.
16. Greenfield RA, Swain JL: Disruption of myofibrillar energy use: Dual mechanisms that may contribute to postischemic dysfunction in stunned myocardium. Circulation Res 1987;60:283–289.
17. Stahl LD, Weiss HR, Becker LC: Myocardial oxygen consumption, oxygen supply/demand heterogeneity, and microvascular patency in regionally stunned myocardium. Circulation 1988;77:865–872.
18. Ciuffo AA, Ouyang P, Becker LC, Levin L, Weisfeldt ML: Reduction of sympathetic inotropic response after ischemia in dogs. Contributor to stunned myocardium. J Clin Invest 1985;75:1504–1509.
19. Kusuoka H, Porterfield JK, Weisman HF, Weisfeldt ML, Marban E: Pathophysiology and pathogenesis of stunned myocardium. Depressed Ca²⁺ activation of contraction as a consequence of reperfusion-induced cellular calcium overload in ferret hearts. J Clin Invest 1987;79:950–961.
20. Zimmerman AN, Hulsmann WC: Paradoxical influence of calcium ions on the permeability of the cell membranes of the isolated rat heart. Nature 1966;211:646–647.
21. Grinwald PM, Brosnahan C: Sodium imbalance as a cause of calcium overload in post-hypoxic reoxygenation injury. J Molec Cell Cardiol 1987;19:487–495.
22. Engler RL: Free radical and granulocyte-mediated injury during myocardial ischemia and reperfusion. Am J Cardiol 1989;63:19E–23E.
23. Zhao MJ, Zhang H, Robinson TF, Factor SM, Sonnenblick EH, Eng C: Profound structural alterations of the extracellular collagen matrix in postischemic dysfunctional (''stunned'') but viable myocardium. J Am Coll Cardiol 1987;10:1322–1334.
24. Bolli R: Oxygen-derived free radicals and postischemic myocardial dysfunction (''stunned myocardium''). J Am Coll Cardiol 1988;12:239–249.
25. Buxton DB, Nienaber CA, Luxen A, Ratib O, Hansen H, Phelps ME, Schelbert HR: Noninvasive quantitation of regional myocardial oxygen consumption in vivo with [1-11C] acetate and dynamic positron emission tomography. Circulation 1989;79:134–142.
26. Topol EJ, Weiss JL, Brinker JA, Brin KP, Gottlieb SO, Becker LC, Bulkley BH, Chandra N, Flaherty JT, Gerstenblith G, et al.: Regional wall motion improvement after coronary thrombolysis with recombinant tissue plasminogen activator: Importance of coronary angioplasty. J Am Coll Cardiol 1985;6:426–433.
27. Anderson JL, Marshall HW, Bray BE, Lutz JR, Frederick PR, Yanowitz FG, Datz FL, Klausner SC, Hagan AD: A randomized trial of intracoronary streptokinase in the treatment of acute myocardial infarction. N Engl J Med 1983;308:1312–1318.
28. Defeyter P, Suryapranta H, Serreys P, Beatt K, Vandenbrand M, Hugenholtz G: Effects of successful PTCA on global and regional left ventricular function in unstable angina pectoris. Am J Cardiol 1987;60:993.
29. de Zwaan C, Cheriex EC, Braat SH, Stappers JL, Wellens HJ: Improvement of systolic and diastolic left ventricular wall motion by serial echocardiograms in selected patients treated for unstable angina. Am Heart J 1991;121:789–797.
30. Stack RS, Phillips HR, Grierson DS, Behar VS, Kong Y, Peter RH, Swain JL, Greenfield JC Jr: Functional improvement of jeopardized myocardium following intracoronary streptokinase infusion in acute myocardial infarction. J Clin Invest 1983;72:84–95.
31. Touchstone DA, Beller GA, Nygaard TW, Tedesco C, Kaul S: Effects of successful intravenous reperfusion therapy on regional myocardial function and geometry in humans: A tomographic assessment using two-dimensional echocardiography. J Am Coll Cardiol 1989;13:1506–1513.
32. Edwards NC, Sinusas AJ, Bergin JD, Watson DD, Ruiz M, Beller GA: Influence of subendocardial ischemia on transmural myocardial function. Am J Physiol 1992;262:H568–H576.

33. Lewis SJ, Sawada SG, Ryan T, Segar DS, Armstrong WF, Feigenbaum H: Segmental wall motion abnormalities in the absence of clinically documented myocardial infarction: Clinical significance and evidence of hibernating myocardium. Am Heart J 1991; 121:1088–1094.

34. Brundage BH, Massie BM, Botvinick EH: Improved regional ventricular function after successful surgical revascularization. J Am Coll Cardiol 1984;3:902–908.

35. Topol EJ, Weiss JL, Guzman PA, Dorsey-Lima S, Blanck TJ, Humphrey LS, Baumgartner WA, Flaherty JT, Reitz BA: Immediate improvement of dysfunctional myocardial segments after coronary revascularization: Detection by intraoperative transesophageal echocardiography. J Am Coll Cardiol 1984;4:1123–1134.

36. Nienaber CA, Brunken RC, Sherman CT, Yeatman LA, Gambhir SS, Krivokapich J, Demer LL, Ratib O, Child JS, Phelps ME, et al.: Metabolic and functional recovery of ischemic human myocardium after coronary angioplasty. J Am Coll Cardiol 1991;18:966–978.

37. van den Berg EK Jr, Popma JJ, Dehmer GJ, Snow FR, Lewis SA, Vetrovec GW, Nixon JV: Reversible segmental left ventricular dysfunction after coronary angioplasty. Circulation 1990;81:1210–1216.

38. Linderer T, Guhl B, Spielberg C, Wunderlich W, Schnitzer L, Schroder R: Effect on global and regional left ventricular functions by percutaneous transluminal coronary angioplasty in the chronic stage after myocardial infarction. Am J Cardiol 1992;69:997–1002.

39. Montalescot G, Faraggi M, Drobinski G, Messian O, Evans J, Grosgogeat Y, Thomas D: Myocardial viability in patients with Q wave myocardial infarction and no residual ischemia. Circulation 1992;86:47–55.

40. Smucker ML, Beller GA, Watson DD, Kaul S: Left ventricular dysfunction in excess of the size of infarction: A possible management strategy. Am Heart J 1988;115:749–753.

40a. Galli M, Marcassa C, Balli R, Giannuzzi P, Temporelli PL, Imparato A, Orrego PLS, Giubbini R, Giordano A, Tavazzi L: Spontaneous delayed recovery of perfusion and contraction after the first 5 weeks after anterior infarction. Evidence for hibernating myocardium in the infarcted area. Circulation 1994;90:1386–1397.

41. Sinusas AJ, Watson DD, Cannon JM Jr, Beller GA: Effect of ischemia and postischemic dysfunction on myocardial uptake of technetium-99m–labeled methoxyisobutyl isonitrile and thallium-201. J Am Coll Cardiol 1989;14:1785–1793.

42. Goldhaber SZ, Newell JB, Alpert NM, Andrews E, Pohost GM, Ingwall JS: Effects of ischemic-like insult on myocardial thallium-201 accumulation. Circulation 1983;67:778–786.

43. Granato JE, Watson DD, Flanagan TL, Beller GA: Myocardial thallium-201 kinetics and regional flow alterations with 3 hours of coronary occlusion and either rapid reperfusion through a totally patent vessel or slow reperfusion through a critical stenosis. J Am Coll Cardiol 1987;9:109–118.

44. Pohost GM, Zir LM, Moore RH, McKusick KA, Guiney TE, Beller GA: Differentiation of transiently ischemic from infarcted myocardium by serial imaging after a single dose of thallium-201. Circulation 1977;55:294–302.

45. Grunwald AM, Watson DD, Holzgrefe HH Jr, Irving JF, Beller GA: Myocardial thallium-201 kinetics in normal and ischemic myocardium. Circulation 1981;64:610–618.

46. Pohost GM, Okada RD, O'Keefe DD, Gewirtz H, Beller G, Strauss HW, Chaffin JS, Leppo J, Daggett WM: Thallium redistribution in dogs with severe coronary artery stenosis of fixed caliber. Circulation Res 1981;48:439–446.

47. Watson DD, Campbell NP, Read EK, Gibson RS, Teates CD, Beller GA: Spatial and temporal quantitation of plane thallium myocardial images. J Nucl Med 1981;22:577–584.

48. Nielsen AP, Morris KG, Murdock R, Bruno FP, Cobb FR: Linear relationship between the distribution of thallium-201 and blood flow in ischemic and nonischemic myocardium during exercise. Circulation 1980;61:797–801.

49. Gibson RS, Watson DD, Taylor GJ, Crosby IK, Wellons HL, Holt ND, Beller GA: Prospective assessment of regional myocardial perfusion before and after coronary revascularization surgery by quantitative thallium-201 scintigraphy. J Am Coll Cardiol 1983;1:804–815.

50. Gewirtz H, Beller GA, Strauss HW, Dinsmore RE, Zir LM, McKusick KA, Pohost GM: Transient defects of resting thallium scans in patients with coronary artery disease. Circulation 1979;59:707–713.

51. Berger BC, Watson DD, Burwell LR, Crosby IK, Wellons HA, Teates CD, Beller GA: Redistribution of thallium at rest in patients with stable and unstable angina and the effect of coronary artery bypass surgery. Circulation 1979;60:1114–1125.

52. Ragosta M, Beller G, Watson D, Kaul S, Gimple L: Quantitative planar rest-redistribution Tl-201 imaging in detection of myocardial viability and prediction of improvement in left ventricular function after coronary bypass surgery in patients with severely depressed left ventricular function. Circulation 1993;87:1630–1641.

53. Berger BC, Watson DD, Taylor GJ, Craddock GB, Martin RP, Teates CD, Beller GA: Quantitative thallium-201 exercise scintigraphy for detection of coronary artery disease. J Nucl Med 1981;22:585–593.

53a. Yamamoto K, Asada S, Masuyama T, et al.: Myocardial hibernation in the infarcted region cannot be assessed from the presence of stress-induced ischemia. Usefulness of delayed image of exercise thallium-201 scintigraphy. Am Heart J 1993;125:33–40.

54. Liu P, Kiess MC, Okada RD, Block PC, Strauss HW, Pohost GM, Boucher CA: The persistent defect on exercise thallium imaging and its fate after myocardial revascularization: Does it represent scar or ischemia? Am Heart J 1985;110:996–1001.

55. Ohtani H, Tamaki N, Yonekura Y, Mohiuddin IH, Hirata K, Ban T, Konishi J: Value of thallium-201 reinjection after delayed SPECT imaging for predicting reversible ischemia after coronary artery bypass grafting. Am J Cardiol 1990;66:394–399.

56. Cloninger KG, DePuey EG, Garcia EV, Roubin GS, Robbins WL, Nody A, DePasquale EE, Berger HJ: Incomplete redistribution in delayed thallium-201 single photon emission computed tomographic (SPECT) images: An overestimation of myocardial scarring. J Am Coll Cardiol 1988;12:955–963.

57. Brunken R, Schwaiger M, Grover-McKay M, Phelps ME, Tillisch J, Schelbert HR: Positron emission tomography detects tissue metabolic activity in myocardial segments with persistent thallium perfusion defects. J Am Coll Cardiol 1987;10:557–567.

58. Kiat H, Berman DS, Maddahi J, De Yang L, Van Train K, Rozanski A, Friedman J: Late reversibility of tomographic myocardial thallium-201 defects: An accurate marker of myocardial viability. J Am Coll Cardiol 1988;12:1456–1463.

59. Yang LD, Berman DS, Kiat H, Resser KJ, Friedman JD, Rozanski A, Maddahi J: The frequency of late reversibility in SPECT thallium-201 stress-redistribution studies. J Am Coll Cardiol 1990;15:334–340.

60. Gutman J, Berman DS, Freeman M, Rozanski A, Maddahi J, Waxman A, Swan HJ: Time to completed redistribution of thallium-201 in exercise myocardial scintigrpahy: Relationship to the degree of coronary artery stenosis. Am Heart J 1983;106:989–995.

61. Watson D: Quantitative analysis of Tl-201 redistribution at 24 hours compared to 2 and 4 hours post-injection (Abstract). J Nucl Med 1990;31:763.

62. Dilsizian V, Rocco TP, Freedman NM, Leon MB, Bonow RO: Enhanced detection of ischemic but viable myocardium by the reinjection of thallium after stress-redistribution imaging. N Engl J Med 1990;323:141–146.

63. Rocco TP, Dilsizian V, McKusick KA, Fischman AJ, Boucher CA, Strauss HW: Comparison of thallium redistribution with rest "reinjection" imaging for the detection of viable myocardium. Am J Cardiol 1990;66:158–163.

64. Tamaki N, Ohtani H, Yamashita K, Magata Y, Yonekura Y, Nohara R, Kambara H, Kawai C, Hirata K, Ban T, et al.: Metabolic activity in the areas of new fill-in after thallium-201 reinjection: Comparison with positron emission tomography using fluorine-18-deoxyglucose. J Nucl Med 1991;32:673–683.

65. Dilsizian V, Freedman NM, Bacharach SL, Perrone–Filardi P, Bonow RO: Regional thallium uptake in irreversible defects. Magnitude of change in thallium activity after reinjection distinguishes viable from nonviable myocardium. Circulation 1992;85:627–634.

66. Kiat H, Friedman JD, Wang FP, Van Train KF, Maddahi J, Takemoto K, Berman DS: Frequency of late reversibility in stress-redistribution thallium-201 SPECT using an early reinjection protocol. Am Heart J 1991;122:613–619.

67. Dilsizian V, Bonow RO: Differential uptake and apparent 201Tl washout after thallium reinjection. Options regarding early redistribution imaging before reinjection or late redistribution imaging after reinjection. Circulation 1992;85:1032–1038.

68. Melin JA, Wijns W, Keyeux A, Gurne O, Cogneau M, Michel C,

Bol A, Robert A, Charlier A, Pouleur H: Assessment of thallium-201 redistribution versus glucose uptake as predictors of viability after coronary occlusion and reperfusion. Circulation 1988;77:927–934.

69. Bonow RO, Dilsizian V, Cuocolo A, Bacharach SL: Identification of viable myocardium in patients with chronic coronary artery disease and left ventricular dysfunction. Comparison of thallium scintigraphy with reinjection and PET imaging with 18F-fluorodeoxyglucose. Circulation 1991;83:26–37.

70. Perrone-Filardi P, Bacharach SL, Dilsizian V, Maurea S, Frank JA, Bonow RO: Regional left ventricular wall thickening. Related to regional uptake of 18-fluorodeoxyglucose and 201Tl in patients with chronic coronary artery disease and left ventricular dysfunction. Circulation 1992;86:1125–1137.

71. Dilsizian V, Smeltzer WR, Freedman NM, Dextras R, Bonow RO: Thallium reinjection after stress-redistribution imaging. Does 24-hour delayed imaging after reinjection enhance detection of viable myocardium? Circulation 1991;83:1247–1255.

72. Kayden DS, Sigal S, Soufer R, Mattera J, Zaret BL, Wackers FJ: Thallium-201 for assessment of myocardial viability: Quantitative comparison of 24-hour redistribution imaging with imaging after reinjection at rest [published erratum appears in J Am Coll Cardiol 1991 Apr; 19(5):1121]. J Am Coll Cardiol 1991;18:1480–1486.

73. Watson DD, Smith W, Vinson E, Kaul S, Blackburn T, Beller G: Quantitative analysis of rest reinjection compared to redistribution (Abstract). J Am Coll Cardiol 1992;19(3):129A.

74. Glover D, Ruiz M, Simanis J, Smith W, Watson D, Beller G: Thallium-201 reinjection does improve detection of defect reversibility compared with quantitative Tl-201 redistribution in a canine ischemia model. Circulation 1992;86:I-418.

74a. Maublant JC, Lipiecki J, Citron B, Karsenty B, Mestas D, Boire JY, Veyre A, Ponsonnaille J: Reinjection as an alternative to rest imaging for detection of exercise-induced ischemia with thallium-201 emission tomography. Am Heart J 1993;125:330–335.

74b. Galli M, Marcassa C: Thallium-201 redistribution after early reinjection in patients with severe stress defects and ventricular dysfunction. Am Heart J 1994;128:41–52.

75. Leppo J, Boucher CA, Okada RD, Newell JB, Strauss HW, Pohost GM: Serial thallium-201 myocardial imaging after dipyridamole infusion: Diagnostic utility in detecting coronary stenoses and relationship to regional wall motion. Circulation 1982;66:649–657.

76. Okada RD, Dai YH, Boucher CA, Pohost GM: Serial thallium-201 imaging after dipyridamole for coronary disease detection: Quantitative analysis using myocardial clearance. Am Heart J 1984;107:475–481.

77. Eichorn E, Kosinski E, Lewis S, et al.: Usefulness of dipyridamole-thallium-201 perfusion scanning for distinguishing ischemic from nonischemic cardiomyopathy. Am J Cardiol 1988;62:985–951.

77a. Gimple LW, Beller GA: Myocardial viability. Assessment by cardiac scintigraphy. Cardiology Clinics 1994;12:317–332.

77b. Iskandrian AS, Heo J, Stanberry C: When is myocardial viability an important clinical issue? J Nucl Med 1994;35(Suppl):4S–7S.

78. Hakki AH, Iskandrian AS, Kane SA, Amenta A: Thallium-201 myocardial scintigraphy and left ventricular function at rest in patients with rest angina pectoris. Am Heart J 1984;108:326–332.

79. Mori T, Minamiji K, Kurogane H, Ogawa K, Yoshida Y: Rest-injected thallium-201 imaging for assessing viability of severe asynergic regions. J Nucl Med 1991;32:1718–1724.

79a. Dilsizian V, Perrone-Filardi P, Arrighi JA, Bacharach SL, Quyyumi AA, Freedman MT, Bonow RO: Concordance and discordance between rest-redistribution-reinjection thallium imaging for assessing viable myocardium: Comparison with metabolic activity by positron emission tomography. Circulation 1993;88:941–952.

80. Reduto LA, Freund GC, Gaeta JM, Smalling RW, Lewis B, Gould KL: Coronary artery reperfusion in acute myocardial infarction: Beneficial effects of intracoronary streptokinase on left ventricular salvage and performance. Am Heart J 1981;102:1168–1177.

81. De Coster PM, Melin JA, Detry JM, Brasseur LA, Beckers C, Col J: Coronary artery reperfusion in acute myocardial infarction: Assessment by pre- and postintervention thallium-201 myocardial perfusion imaging. Am J Cardiol 1985;55:889–895.

82. Schwarz F, Hofmann M, Schuler G, von Olshausen K, Zimmermann R, Kubler W: Thrombolysis in acute myocardial infarction: Effect of intravenous followed by intracoronary streptokinase application on estimates of infarct size. Am J Cardiol 1984;53:1505–1510.

83. Granato JE, Watson DD, Flanagan TL, Gascho JA, Beller GA: Myocardial thallium-201 kinetics during coronary occlusion and reperfusion: Influence of method of reflow and timing of thallium-201 administration. Circulation 1986;73:150–160.

84. Ritchie JL, Cerqueira M, Maynard C, Davis K, Kennedy JW: Ventricular function and infarct size: The Western Washington Intravenous Streptokinase in Myocardial Infarction Trial. J Am Coll Cardiol 1988;11:689–697.

85. Okada RD, Glover D, Gaffney T, Williams S: Myocardial kinetics of technetium-99m-hexakis-2-methoxy-2-methylpropyl-isonitrile. Circulation 1988;77:491–498.

86. Meerdink DJ, Leppo JA: Comparsion of hypoxia and ouabain effects on the myocardial uptake kinetics of technetium-99m hexakis 2-methoxyisobutyl isonitrile and thallium-201. J Nucl Med 1989;30:1500–1506.

87. Verani MS, Jeroudi MO, Mahmarian JJ, Boyce TM, Borges-Neto S, Patel B, Bolli R: Quantification of myocardial infarction during coronary occlusion and myocardial salvage after reperfusion using cardiac imaging with technetium-99m hexakis 2-methoxyisobutyl isonitrile. J Am Coll Cardiol 1988;12:1573–1581.

88. Sinusas AJ, Trautman KA, Bergin JD, Watson DD, Ruiz M, Smith WH, Beller GA: Quantification of area at risk during coronary occlusion and degree of myocardial salvage after reperfusion with technetium-99m methoxyisobutyl isonitrile. Circulation 1990;82:1424–1437.

88a. Beller GA, Glover DK, Edwards NC, Ruiz M, Simanis JP, Watson DD: 99mTc-sestamibi uptake and retention during myocardial ischemia and reperfusion. Circulation 1993;87:2033–2042.

89. Sansoy V, Glover D, Watson D, Ruiz M, Smith W: Comparison of thallium-201 rest redistribution, technetium-99m sestamibi uptake and functional response to dobutamine for assessment of myocardial viability. Circulation, in press.

90. Leon AR, Eisner RL, Martin SE, Schmarkey LS, Aaron AM, Boyers AS, Burnham KM, Oh DJ, Patterson RE: Comparison of single-photon emission computed tomographic (SPECT) myocardial perfusion imaging with thallium-201 and technetium-99m sestamibi in dogs. J Am Coll Cardiol 1992;20:1612–1625.

91. Melon PG, Beanlands RS, DeGrado TR, Nguyen N, Petry NA, Schwaiger M: Comparison of technetium-99m sestamibi and thallium-201 retention characteristics in canine myocardium. J Am Coll Cardiol 1992;20:1277–1283.

91a. Dahlberg ST, Meerdink DJ, Gilmore MP, Leppo JA: Myocardial extraction of technetium-99m-[2-(1-methoxybutyl) isonitrile] in the isolated rabbit heart: A myocardial perfusion agent with high extraction and stable retention. J Nucl Med 1993;34:927–931.

91b. Li QS, Solot G, Frank TL, Wagner HN Jr, Becker LC: Myocardial redistribution of technetium-99m-methoxyisobutyl isonitrile. J Nucl Med 1990;31:1069–1076.

91c. Glover DK, Okada RD: Myocardial technetium-99m sestamibi kinetics after reperfusion in a canine model. Am Heart J 1993;125:657–666.

91d. Taillefer R, Primeau M, Costi P, Lambert R, Leveille J, Latour Y: Technetium-99m-sestamibi myocardial perfusion imaging in detection of coronary artery disease: Comparison between initial (1-hour) and delayed (3-hour) postexercise images. J Nucl Med 1991;32:1961–1965.

91e. Villanueva-Meyer J, Mena I, Diggles L, Narahara KA: Assessment of myocardial perfusion defect size after early and delayed SPECT imaging with technetium-99m-hexakis 2-methoxyisobutyl isonitrile after stress. J Nucl Med 1993;34:187–192.

92. Cuocolo A, Pace L, Ricciardelli B, Chiariello M, Trimarco B, Salvatore M: Identification of viable myocardium in patients with chronic coronary artery disease: Comparison of thallium-201 scintigraphy with reinjection and technetium-99m-methoxyisobutyl isonitrile. J Nucl Med 1992;33:505–511.

92a. Marzullo P, Sambuceti G, Parodi O: The role of sestamibi scintigraphy in the radioisotopic assessment of myocardial viability. J Nucl Med 1992;33:1925–1930.

92b. Marzullo P, Parodi O, Reisenhofer B, Sambuceti G, Picano E, Distante A, Gimelli A, L'Abbate A: Value of rest thallium-201/technetium-99m sestamibi scans and dobutamine echocardiography for detecting myocardial viability. Am J Cardiol 1993;71:166–172.

92c. Maurea S, et al.: Rest-injected thallium-201 redistribution and resting technetium-99m methoxyisobutylisonitrile uptake in coronary artery disease: Relation to the severity of coronary artery stenosis. Eur J Nucl Med 1993;20:502–510.

92d. Rocco TP, Dilsizian V, Strauss HW, Boucher CA: Technetium-99m isonitrile myocardial uptake at rest. Relation to clinical markers of potential viability. J Am Coll Cardiol 1989;14:1678–1684.

92e. Dilsizian V, Arrighi J, Diodati JG, et al: Myocardial viability in patients with chronic coronary artery disease. Comparison of 99mTc-sestamibi with thallium reinjection and [^{18}F]-fluorodeoxyglucose. Circulation 1994;89:578–587.

92f. Sawada SG, Allman KC, Muzik O, Beanlands RSB, Wolfe ER, Gross M, Lorraine F, Schwaiger M: Positron emission tomography detects evidence of viability in rest technetium-99m sestamibi defects. J Am Coll Cardiol 1994;23:92–98.

93. Udelson JE, Coleman PS, Metherall J, Pandian NG, Gomez AR, Griffith JL, Shea NL, Oates E, Konstam MA: Predicting recovery of severe regional ventricular dysfunction. Comparison of resting scintigraphy with 201Tl and 99mTc-sestamibi. Circulation 1994; 89:2552–2561.

94. Sinusas AJ, Beller GA, Smith WH, Vinson EL, Brookeman V, Watson DD: Quantitative planar imaging with technetium-99m methoxyisobutyl isonitrile: Comparison of uptake patterns with thallium-201. J Nucl Med 1989;30:1456–1463.

94a. Kuikka JT, Mussalo H, Hietakorpi S, Vanninen E, Lansimies E: Evaluation of myocardial viability with technetium-99m hexakis-2-methoxyisobutyl isonitrile and iodine-123 phenylpentadecanoic acid and single-photon emission tomography. Eur J Nucl Med 1992;19:882–889.

94b. Lucignani G, Paolini G, Landoni C, Zuccari M, Paganelli G, Galli L, Di Credico G, Vanoli G, Rossetti C, Mariani MA, et al.: Presurgical identification of hibernating myocardium by combined use of technetium-99m hexakis 2-methoxyisobutylisonitrile single photon emission tomography and fluorine-18-fluoro-2-deoxy-D-glucose positron emission tomography in patients with coronary artery disease. Eur J Nucl Med 1992;19:874–881.

94c. Bisi G, Sciagrà R, Santoro GM, Fazzini PF: Rest technetium-99m sestamibi tomography in combination with short-term administration of nitrates: Feasibility and reliability for prediction of postrevascularization outcome of asynergic territories. J Am Coll Cardiol 1994;24:1282–1289.

94d. Baer FM, Smolarz K, Theissen P, Voth E, Schicha H, Sechtem U: Regional 99mTc-methoxyisobutyl-isonitrile uptake at rest in patients with myocardial infarcts: Comparison with morphological and functional parameters obtained from gradient-echo magnetic resonance imaging. Eur Heart J 1994;15:97–107.

95. Wackers FJ, Gibbons RJ, Verani MS, Kayden DS, Pellikka PA, Behrenbeck T, Mahmarian JJ, Zaret BL: Serial quantitative planar technetium-99m isonitrile imaging in acute myocardial infarction: Efficacy for noninvasive assessment of thrombolytic therapy. J Am Coll Cardiol 1989;14:861–873.

95a. Christian TF, O'Connor MK, Hopfenspirger MR, Gibbons RJ: Comparison of reinjection thallium-201 and resting technetium-99m sestamibi tomographic images for the quantification of infarct size after acute myocardial infarction. J Nucl Cardiol 1994;1:17–28.

96. Gibbons RJ, Verani MS, Behrenbeck T, Pellikka PA, O'Connor MK, Mahmarian JJ, Chesebro JH, Wackers FJ: Feasibility of tomographic 99mTc-hexakis-2-methoxy-2-methylpropyl-isonitrile imaging for the assessment of myocardial area at risk and the effect of treatment in acute myocardial infarction. Circulation 1989;80:1277–1286.

96a. Reske SN: Experimental and clinical experience with iodine 123–labeled iodophenylpentadecanoic acid in cardiology. J Nucl Cardiol 1994;1:S58–S64.

96b. Corbett J: Clinical experience with iodine-123-iodophenylpentadecanoic acid. J Nucl Med 1994;35(suppl):32S–37S.

96c. Hansen CL: Preliminary report of an ongoing phaseI/II dose range, safety and efficacy study of iodine-123-phenylpentadecanoic acid for the identification of viable myocardium. J Nucl Med 1994;35(Suppl):38S–42S.

96d. Hansen CL, Heo J, Iskandrian AS: Prediction of improvement of left ventricular function after coronary revascularization from alterations in myocardial metabolic activity detected with I-123-phenylpentadecanoic acid dynamic SPECT imaging (Abstract). J Am Coll Cardiol 1994; March:344A.

96e. Murray GL, Schad NC, Magill HL, Vander Zwaag R: Myocardial viability assessment with dynamic low-dose iodine-123-iodophenyl-pentadecanoic acid metabolic imaging: Comparison with myocardial biopsy and reinjection SPECT thallium after myocardial infarction. J Nucl Med 1994;35(suppl):43S–48S.

96f. Powers J, Cave V, Wasserliben V, Cassel D, Heo J, Iskandrian AS: Mechanisms and implications of redistribution during dynamic rest SPECT I-123 IPPA imaging. J Am Coll Cardiol 1994; March:423A.

96g. Tamaki N, Kawamoto M: The use of iodinated free fatty acids for assessing fatty acid metabolism. J Nucl Cardiol 1994;1:S72–S78.

97. Corbett J, Quaife R, Parkey R: Current state of infarct avid imaging—advantages of SPECT evaluations: Promise of antimyosin antibodies. Am J Cardiac Imaging 1992;6:59.

98. Takeda K, LaFrance ND, Weisman HF, Wagner HN Jr, Becker LC: Comparison of indium-111 antimyosin antibody and technetium-99m pyrophosphate localization in reperfused and nonreperfused myocardial infarction. J Am Coll Cardiol 1991;17:519–526.

99. Johnson LL, Seldin DW, Keller AM, Wall RM, Bhatia K, Bingham CO, Tresgallo ME: Dual isotope thallium and indium antimyosin SPECT imaging to identify acute infarct patients at further ischemic risk. Circulation 1990;81:37–45.

99a. Schelbert HR: Merits and limitations of radionuclide approaches to viability and future developments. J Nucl Cardiol 1994;1:S86–S96.

99b. Tamaki N: Current status of viability assessment with positron tomography. J Nucl Cardiol 1994;1:S40–S47.

99c. Bergmann SR: Use and limitations of metabolic tracers labeled with positron-emitting radionuclides in the identification of viable myocardium. J Nucl Med 1994;35(Suppl):15S–22S.

99d. Maes A, Flameng W, Nugts J, et al.: Histological alterations in chronically hypoperfused myocardium. Correlation with PET findings. Circulation 1994;90:735–745.

100. Brunken R, Tillisch J, Schwaiger M, Child JS, Marshall R, Mandelkern M, Phelps ME, Schelbert HR: Regional perfusion, glucose metabolism, and wall motion in patients with chronic electrocardiographic Q wave infarctions: Evidence for persistence of viable tissue in some infarct regions by positron emission tomography. Circulation 1986;73:951–963.

100a. Schwaiger M, Brunken R, Grover-McKay M, Krivokapich J, Child J, Tillisch JH, Phelps ME, Schelbert HR: Regional myocardial metabolism in patients with acute myocardial infarction assessed by positron emission tomography. J Am Coll Cardiol 1986;8:800–808.

101. Pierard LA, De Landsheere CM, Berthe C, Rigo P, Kulbertus HE: Identification of viable myocardium by echocardiography during dobutamine infusion in patients with myocardial infarction after thrombolytic therapy: Comparison with positron emission tomography. J Am Coll Cardiol 1990;15:1021–1031.

101a. Perrone-Filardi P, Bachrach SL, Dilsizian V, Marin-Neto JA, Maurea S, Arrighi JA, Bonow RO: Clinical significance of reduced regional myocardial glucose uptake in regions with normal blood flow in patients with chronic coronary artery disease. J Am Coll Cardiol 1994;23:608–616.

102. Wyns W, Schwaiger M, Huang SC, Buxton DB, Hansen H, Selin C, Keen R, Phelps ME, Schelbert HR: Effects of inhibition of fatty acid oxidation on myocardial kinetics of 11C-labeled palmitate. Circulation Res 1989;65:1787–1797.

102a. Di Carli M, Sherman T, Khanna S, et al.: Myocardial viability in asynergic regions subtended by occluded coronary arteries: Relation to the status of collateral flow in patients with chronic coronary artery disease. J Am Coll Cardiol 1994;23:860–868.

103. Merhige ME, Ekas R, Mossberg K, Taegtmeyer H, Gould KL: Catecholamine stimulation, substrate competition, and myocardial glucose uptake in conscious dogs assessed with positron emission tomography. Circulation Res 1987;61:II124–II129.

103a. Bergmann S: Use and limitations of metabolic tracers labeled with positron-emitting radionuclides in the identification of viable myocardium. J Nucl Med 1994;35(suppl):15S–22S.

103b. Gropler RJ: Methodology governing the assessment of myocardial glucose metabolism by positron emission tomography and fluorine 18-labeled fluorodeoxyglucose. J Nucl Cardiol 1994;1:S4–S14.

104. Perrone-Filardi P, Bacharach SL, Dilsizian V, Maurea S, Marin-Neto JA, Arrighi JA, Frank JA, Bonow RO: Metabolic evidence of viable myocardium in regions with reduced wall thickness and absent wall thickening in patients with chronic ischemic left ventricular dysfunction. J Am Coll Cardiol 1992;20:161–168.

104a. Gewirtz H, Fischman AJ, Abraham S, Gilson M, Strauss HW, Alpert NM: Positron emission tomographic measurements of absolute regional myocardial blood flow permits identification of nonviable myocardium in patients with chronic myocardial infarction. J Am Coll Cardiol 1994;23:851–859.

105. Tillisch J, Brunken R, Marshall R, Schwaiger M, Mandelkern M, Phelps M, Schelbert H: Reversibility of cardiac wall-motion abnormalities predicted by positron tomography. N Engl J Med 1986;314:884–888.

106. Tamaki N, Yonekura Y, Yamashita K, Saji H, Magata Y, Senda M, Konishi Y, Hirata K, Ban T, Konishi J: Positron emission tomography using fluorine-18 deoxyglucose in evaluation of coronary artery bypass grafting. Am J Cardiol 1989;64:860–865.

107. Schwaiger M, Hicks R: The clinical role of metabolic imaging of the heart by positron emission tomography. J Nucl Med 1991;32:565–578.

107a. vom Dahl J, Eitzman DT, Al-Aovar ZR, Kanter HL, Hicks RJ, Deeb M, Kirsh MM, Schwaiger M: Relation of regional function, perfusion, and metabolism in patients with advanced coronary artery disease undergoing surgical revascularization. Circulation 1994;90:2356–2366.

108. Marwick TH, MacIntyre WJ, Lafont A, Nemec JJ, Salcedo EE: Metabolic responses of hibernating and infarcted myocardium to revascularization. A follow-up study of regional perfusion, function, and metabolism. Circulation 1992;85:1347–1353.

108a. Maddahi J, Schelbert H, Brunken R, Di Carli M: Role of thallium-201 and PET imaging in evaluation of myocardial viability and management of patients with coronary artery disease and left ventricular dysfunction. J Nucl Med 1994;35:707–715.

108b. Di Carli MF, Davidson M, Little R, et al.: Value of metabolic imaging with positron emission tomography for evaluating prognosis in patients with coronary artery disease and left ventricular dysfunction. Am J Cardiol 1994;73:527–533.

108c. Carrel T, Jenni R, Haubold-Reuter S, Von Schulthess G, Pasic M, Turina M: Improvement of severely reduced left ventricular function after surgical revascularization in patients with preoperative myocardial infarction. Eur J Cardiothorac Surg 1992;6:479–484.

108d. Gropler RJ, Geltman EM, Sampathkumaran K, et al.: Comparison of carbon-11 acetate with fluorine-18-fluorodeoxyglucose for delineating viable myocardium by positron emission tomography. J Am Coll Cardiol 1993;22:1587–1597.

108e. Marwick TH, Nemec JJ, Lafont A, Salcedo EE, MacIntyre WJ: Prediction by postexercise fluoro-18 deoxyglucose positron emission tomography of improvement in exercise capacity after revascularization. Am J Cardiol 1992;69:854–859.

109. Fox KA, Abendschein DR, Ambos HD, Sobel BE, Bergmann SR: Efflux of metabolized and nonmetabolized fatty acid from canine myocardium. Implications for quantifying myocardial metabolism tomographically. Circulation Res 1985;57:232–243.

110. Rosamond TL, Abendschein DR, Ambos HD, Sobel BE, Bergmann SR, Fox KA: Metabolic fate of radiolabeled palmitate in ischemic canine myocardium: Implications for positron emission tomography. J Nucl Med 1987;28:1322–1329.

110a. Geltman EM: Assessment of myocardial fatty acid metabolism with 1-¹¹C-palmitate. J Nucl Cardiol 1994;1:S15–S22.

111. Grover-McKay M, Schelbert HR, Schwaiger M, Sochor H, Guzy PM, Krivokapich J, Child JS, Phelps ME: Identification of impaired metabolic reserve by atrial pacing in patients with significant coronary artery stenosis. Circulation 1986;74:281–292.

112. Sobel BE, Geltman EM, Tiefenbrunn AJ, Jaffe AS, Spadaro JJ Jr, Ter-Pogossian MM, Collen D, Ludbrook PA: Improvement of regional myocardial metabolism after coronary thrombolysis induced with tissue-type plasminogen activator or streptokinase. Circulation 1984;69:983–990.

113. Bergmann SR, Lerch RA, Fox KA, Ludbrook PA, Welch MJ, Ter-Pogossian MM, Sobel BE: Temporal dependence of beneficial effects of coronary thrombolysis characterized by positron tomography. Am J Med 1982;73:573–581.

114. Knabb RM, Bergmann SR, Fox KA, Sobel BE: The temporal pattern of recovery of myocardial perfusion and metabolism delineated by positron emission tomography after coronary thrombolysis. J Nucl Med 1987;28:1563–1570.

115. Knabb RM, Rosamond TL, Fox KA, Sobel BE, Bergmann SR: Enhancement of salvage of reperfused ischemic myocardium by diltiazem. J Am Coll Cardiol 1986;8:861–871.

116. Schwaiger M, Schelbert HR, Keen R, Vinten-Johansen J, Hansen H, Selin C, Barrio J, Huang SC, Phelps ME: Retention and clearance of C-11 palmitic acid in ischemic and reperfused canine myocardium. J Am Coll Cardiol 1985;6:311–320.

116a. Melin JA, Vanoverschelde J-L, Boe A, Heyndrickx G, Wijns W: The use of carbon 11-labeled acetate for assessment of aerobic metabolism. J Nucl Cardiol 1994;1:S48–S57.

117. Henes CG, Bergmann SR, Walsh MN, Sobel BE, Geltman EM: Assessment of myocardial oxidative metabolic reserve with positron emission tomography and carbon-11 acetate. J Nucl Med 1989;30:1489–1499.

118. Armbrecht JJ, Buxton DB, Schelbert HR: Validation of [1-¹¹C] acetate as a tracer for noninvasive assessment of oxidative metabolism with positron emission tomography in normal, ischemic, postischemic, and hyperemic canine myocardium. Circulation 1990; 81:1594–1605.

119. Vanoverschelde JL, Melin JA, Bol A, Vanbutsele R, Cogneau M, Labar D, Robert A, Michel C, Wijns W: Regional oxidative metabolism in patients after recovery from reperfused anterior myocardial infarction. Relation to regional blood flow and glucose uptake. Circulation 1992;85:9–21.

120. Walsh MN, Bergmann SR, Steele RL, Kenzora JL, Ter-Pogossian MM, Sobel BE, Geltman EM: Delineation of impaired regional myocardial perfusion by positron emission tomography with H₂¹⁵O. Circulation 1988;78:612–620.

121. Hanes C, Bergman S, Perez J, Sobel B, Geltman A: The time course of restoration of nutritive perfusion, myocardial oxygen consumption, and regional function after coronary thrombosis. Coronary Artery Dis 1990;1:687–696.

122. Gropler RJ, Siegel BA, Sampathkumaran K, Perez JE, Sobel BE, Bergmann SR, Geltman EM: Dependence of recovery of contractile function on maintenance of oxidative metabolism after myocardial infarction. J Am Coll Cardiol 1992;19:989–997.

122a. Gropler RJ, Geltman EM, Sampathkumaran K, Perez JE, Moerlein SM, Sobel BE, Bergmann SR, Siegel BA: Functional recovery after coronary revascularization for chronic coronary artery disease is dependent on maintenance of oxidative metabolism. J Am Coll Cardiol 1992;20:569–577.

123. Gould KL, Yoshida K, Hess MJ, Haynie M, Mullani N, Smalling RW: Myocardial metabolism of fluorodeoxyglucose compared to cell membrane integrity for the potassium analogue rubidium-82 for assessing infarct size in man by PET. J Nucl Med 1991;32:1–9.

124. Goldstein RA: Kinetics of rubidium-82 after coronary occlusion and reperfusion. Assessment of patency and viability in open-chested dogs. J Clin Invest 1985;75:1131–1137.

125. Goldstein RA: Rubidium-82 kinetics after coronary occlusion: Temporal relation of net myocardial accumulation and viability in open-chested dogs. J Nucl Med 1986;27:1456–1461.

126. Gould KL, Yoshida K, Hess MJ, Haynie M, Mullani N, Smalling RW: Myocardial metabolism of fluorodeoxyglucose compared to cell membrane integrity for the potassium analogue rubidium-82 for assessing infarct size in man by PET. J Nucl Med 1991;32:1–9.

126a. Yoshida K, Gould K: Quantitative relation of myocardial infarct size and myocardial viability by positron emission tomography to left ventricular ejection fraction and 3-year mortality with an without revascularization. J Am Coll Cardiol 1993;22:984–997.

127. Yamamoto Y, de Silva R, Rhodes CG, Araujo LI, Iida H, Rechavia E, Nihoyannopoulos P, Hackett D, Galassi AR, Taylor CJ, et al.: A new strategy for the assessment of viable myocardium and regional myocardial blood flow using ¹⁵O-water and dynamic positron emission tomography. Circulation 1992;86:167–178.

128. Marcovitz P, Armstrong W: Assessing myocardial viability with dobutamine stress echocardiagraphy. Am J Cardiac Imaging 1992; 6:214.

128a. Smart SC: The clinical utility of echocardiography in the assessment of myocardial viability. J Nucl Med 1994;35(Suppl):49S–58S.

129. Smart S, Sawada S, Ryan T, Sega D, Atherton L, Berkovitz K, Bourdillion P, Fcigenbaum H: Low dose dobutamine echocardiography detects reversible dysfunction after thrombolytic therapy of acute myocardial infarction. Circulation 1993;88:405–415.

130. Schultz R, Rose J, Martin C, Broddle O, Hensch G: Development of short-term myocardial hibernation. Circulation 1993;88:684–695.

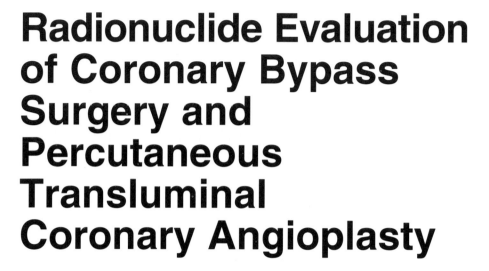

Chapter 10

Radionuclide Evaluation of Coronary Bypass Surgery and Percutaneous Transluminal Coronary Angioplasty

EXERCISE THALLIUM-201 SCINTIGRAPHY FOR ASSESSMENT OF CORONARY BYPASS SURGERY

Exercise thallium-201 (Tl-201) scintigraphy has been utilized successfully for preoperative and postoperative assessment of regional myocardial blood flow and regional myocardial viability in patients with coronary artery disease (CAD). Table 10–1 summarizes the potential clinical applications of stress perfusion imaging for the preoperative and postoperative assessment of patients with CAD. As I discussed extensively in Chapter 4, exercise stress Tl-201 imaging performed preoperatively in patients with CAD can identify high-risk subgroups who enjoy a greater survival benefit from revascularization than from medical therapy. Patients at high risk demonstrate multiple myocardial perfusion abnormalities, often spanning more than one coronary supply region, or increased pulmonary Tl-201 uptake.[1-5] The greater the number of redistribution defects observed on serial planar or single-photon emission computed tomography (SPECT) scintigraphy, the higher is the subsequent cardiac event rate during follow-up and the greater the likelihood of underlying multivessel or left main

CAD (see Chap. 4). Patients with increased lung Tl-201 uptake and transient left ventricular (LV) cavity dilatation on serial postexercise images also have a higher cardiac event rate when treated medically and demonstrate a high incidence of underlying multivessel CAD as determined by angiography.[6-8] Exercise Tl-201 scintigraphy can be utilized even after coronary anatomic findings are known following cardiac catheterization to determine potential benefit for

Table 10–1. **Clinical Applications of Stress Perfusion Imaging for Preoperative and Postoperative Assessment of Patients with Coronary Artery Disease**

Preoperative assessment
  Determination of presence and extent of inducible ischemia
  Identification of which high-risk patients are most likely to benefit
    from revascularization
  Determination of viability in asynergic myocardium
  Prediction of postoperative functional response
Postoperative assessment
  Determination of extent of enhanced perfusion
  Detection of graft stenosis or occlusion
  Differential diagnosis of chest pain
  Diagnosis of perioperative MI
  Following progression of native CAD

bypass surgery. Specifically, patients with multivessel disease and depressed LV function who exhibit large areas of residual jeopardized myocardium are more likely to benefit from revascularization than patients with a similar degree of LV dysfunction and coronary anatomic disease but scant evidence of residual jeopardized myocardium. The latter subgroup of patients with LV dysfunction from previous myocardial infarction (MI) exhibit predominantly persistent defects in the distribution of the coronary narrowings but not additional reversibility with Tl-201 reinjection.

Prediction of Operative Response

Preoperative exercise Tl-201 scintigraphy may be clinically useful for predicting the subsequent response to revascularization in patients with CAD.[9] Myocardial zones that demonstrate redistribution-type defects before surgery usually show improved Tl-201 uptake and washout after revascularization.[10] This improvement in perfusion should be accompanied by an improvement in resting regional and global LV function.[10] In contrast, persistent defects showing severe reduction in Tl-201 uptake (more than 50% compared with normal zones) demonstrate little improvement in perfusion and function as assessed on postoperative noninvasive studies. Figure 10–1 shows preoperative and postoperative planar Tl-201 scans showing marked improvement in myocardial tracer uptake in a region that corresponds to a preoperative persistent defect. Rozanski et al.[11] reported improvement in function in 54% of preoperative asynergic segments after bypass surgery in 25 patients studied. Preoperative Tl-201 exercise scintigraphy was very predictive of the pattern of postoperative asynergy. Redistribution was observed in 90% of segments with reversible asynergy and absent in 76% of segments with irreversible asynergy. Tl-201 imaging was superior to the presence or absence of pathologic Q waves in this differentiation.

The use of preoperative Tl-201 scintigraphy for assessing myocardial viability is discussed in more detail in Chapter 9. Preoperative Tl-201 imaging in conjunction with contrast ventriculography, radionuclide angiography, or two-dimensional (2-D) echocardiography is helpful for determining myocardial viability in regions of severe asynergy. Segments that exhibit akinetic wall motion on the functional study that are associated with severe persistent Tl-201 defects in the same region on the perfusion study are less likely to show improvement in regional wall motion after revascularization. These regions are predominantly composed of fibrous scar. On echocardiography, such segments appear thinned during diastole and demonstrate lack of thickening during systole and lack of enhancement of systolic thickening during intravenous dobutamine infusion (see Chap. 9). In contrast, the majority of patients with akinetic or dyskinetic segments that on serial imaging show total or partial redistribution or mild persistent defects often

show improvement in both perfusion and function after successful revascularization.[12] These abnormally contracting regions of preserved Tl-201 uptake in the presence of akinesis most likely represent "hibernating myocardium" and have the potential for enhanced systolic performance when flow, oxygen, and substrate availability are increased with revascularization. The global left ventricular ejection fraction (LVEF) also improves after successful bypass surgery in patients with "ischemic cardiomyopathy" attributable at least in part to hibernating myocardium.[12] Mild persistent Tl-201 defects that demonstrate improvement after revascularization also show increased fluorine-18 2-deoxyglucose (FDG) uptake on positron emission scintigrams.[13] Persistent Tl-201 defects that are more severe and exhibit more than a 50% reduction in Tl-201 uptake usually do not show enhanced FDG uptake preoperatively.

In patients who are unable to exercise adequately because of heart failure or marked limitation in exercise capacity, rest Tl-201 scintigraphy can provide useful information on the potential benefit of coronary revascularization.[12, 14] In the study by Iskandrian et al., normal resting Tl-201 uptake or rest redistribution correctly identified 86% of patients who showed improved LV function postoperatively. Twelve of fourteen patients with normal resting Tl-201 uptake or a reversible defect on serial rest images showed improved EF after coronary bypass surgery. Only two patients with normal Tl-201 uptake or a reversible defect on resting images showed no improvement in LVEF after revascularization. In contrast, of nine patients who showed persistent Tl-201 defects on preoperative rest images, only two showed improved EF after revascularization. Figure 10–2 shows the changes in LVEF after bypass surgery in relation to the preoperative Tl-201 scan results in this study.

Data by Ragosta et al.[12] showed that Tl-201 uptake on resting scintigrams was useful in predicting improvement or lack of improvement in regional and global function after bypass surgery. The greater the number of severe persistent defects (more than 50% reduction in regional Tl-201 uptake) on rest Tl-201 scintigrams, the less the improvement in regional wall motion score or LVEF after revascularization (see Chap. 9). Thus, in patients who are unable to exercise because of significant myocardial dysfunction or clinical symptoms or signs of heart failure, rest Tl-201 scintigraphy can be used preoperatively to identify a subgroup who stand to benefit most, with respect to improvement in cardiac function and amelioration of heart failure symptoms, with bypass surgery.

Postoperative Use of Thallium-201 Scintigraphy

In addition to utilizing exercise or rest Tl-201 scintigraphy to identify patients with CAD who are adequate candidates for bypass surgery, stress or rest myocardial perfusion imaging can be performed after revascularization to deter-

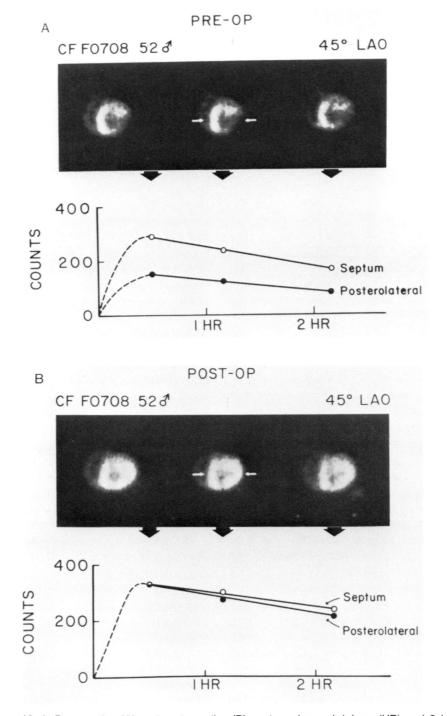

Figure 10–1. Preoperative **(A)** and postoperative **(B)** postexercise and 1 hour (HR) and 2 hour redistribution planar 45° left anterior oblique Tl-201 scintigrams showing marked improvement in myocardial perfusion in a region corresponding to a preoperative persistent posterolateral Tl-201 defect (see *arrows*). Below each set of images are the quantitative myocardial Tl-201 time–activity curves showing a significant reduction in Tl-201 counts in the posterolateral wall on the preoperative images. (Reprinted with permission from the American College of Cardiology (Journal of the American College of Cardiology, 1983, Vol. 1, pp. 804–815).)

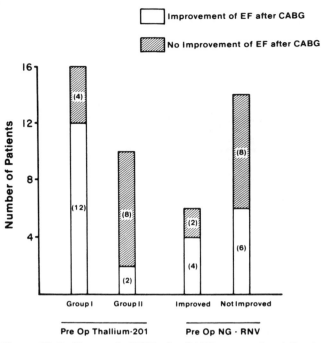

Figure 10-2. Changes in LVEF after CABG surgery in relation to the results of preoperative (preop) Tl-201 images and nitroglycerin (NG) interventional radionuclide ventriculograms (RNV). Group I patients had normal perfusion scans or redistribution defects; group II patients had persistent defects. (Iskandrian AS, et al.: Am J Cardiol 1983;51:1312–1316.)

mine if intraoperative myocardial injury occurred and for evaluation of internal mammary or saphenous vein bypass graft flow. Patients with patent grafts should demonstrate improved regional myocardial perfusion at faster exercise heart rates or workload when tested after surgery (Fig. 10–3). Hirzel et al.[15] found that 81% of patients who showed normal perfusion after revascularization surgery had patent coronary bypass grafts. Figure 10–4 shows the bypass graft patency rate relative to the scintigraphic findings in this study. The patency rate was 81% for patients whose perfusion within the preoperative ischemic regions returned to normal after exercise and at rest. At the other extreme, the patency rate was 15% for patients who postoperatively had enlarged perfusion defects or new ones. Thus, patients with patent grafts who have not suffered an intraoperative MI should show normal or significantly improved regional Tl-201 uptake after surgery.

Detection of Graft Occlusion

Patients who present with atypical chest pain after seemingly successful revascularization surgery benefit from postoperative stress Tl-201 scintigraphy rather than immediate referral for coronary angiography. Those who have stenotic or occluded grafts usually show persistence of Tl-201 scan abnormalities—or new ones—after surgery. Perioperative MI is characterized by a new persistent defect

on postoperative scintigraphy as compared with the preoperative scan, in which only a redistribution defect or normal Tl-201 uptake was observed. Perioperative infarction is also accompanied by a new regional wall motion abnormality on a resting functional study, seen on either radionuclide ventriculography or 2-D echocardiography.

Quantitative imaging should be superior to visual scan analysis alone for evaluation of graft patency. The determination of myocardial Tl-201 washout rates was useful for establishing graft patency after coronary artery bypass graft (CABG) surgery.[16] Zimmermann et al.[16] found that, postoperatively, 50 of 57 segments supplied by a patent graft showed normal Tl-201 washout rates, whereas in 9 of 11 segments occlusion of the graft was indicated by a decreased washout rate. By comparing preoperative and postoperative myocardial scintigrams, the postoperative assessment of washout rates increased both sensitivity (82% vs. 64%) and specificity (88% vs. 77%) for the evaluation of bypass graft patency. Thus, these authors concluded that quantitative assessment of regional Tl-201 washout rates improves the diagnostic accuracy of the noninvasive detection of myocardial ischemia with respect to the evaluation of coronary revascularization surgery.

Quantitative planar Tl-201 scintigraphy was used to assess postoperative flow reserve in internal mammary bypass grafts by Johnson et al.[17] In a group of 24 consecutive patients with proximal left anterior descending (LAD) coronary stenosis who underwent internal mammary grafting, the ratio of anteroseptal activity to posterolateral wall activity 8 weeks after surgery was 0.97 ± 0.15. This compared to a ratio of 1.0 ± 0.15 for a group of control patients with angiographically normal coronary arteries. Of interest, the anteroseptal-posterolateral wall Tl-201 activity ratio was not significantly different for a group of 28 saphenous vein graft recipients who also underwent postoperative stress Tl-201 scintigraphy (0.96 ± 0.19).

The efficacy of CABG surgery with a gastroepiploic artery has also been evaluated with exercise Tl-201 myocardial scintigraphy.[18] The scintigraphic studies showed that myocardial blood flow improved significantly after operations using the gastroepiploic artery as a graft conduit. This correlated with postoperative angiography showing patency of grafts.

It is unusual to see complete normalization of stress-induced defects after coronary revascularization. In a study reported by Verani et al.,[19] postoperative improvement in Tl-201 uptake was observed in 19 of 23 patients, but in only 9 patients did myocardial perfusion distribution return entirely to normal. Figure 10–5 shows images made before and after revascularization and the coronary angiographic findings from one of the patients who postoperatively showed complete normalization of perfusion. Interestingly, failure of regional myocardial perfusion to improve postoperatively in that study did not preclude marked alleviation of angina and improved exercise tolerance after surgery. The amelioration of angina symptoms may be related

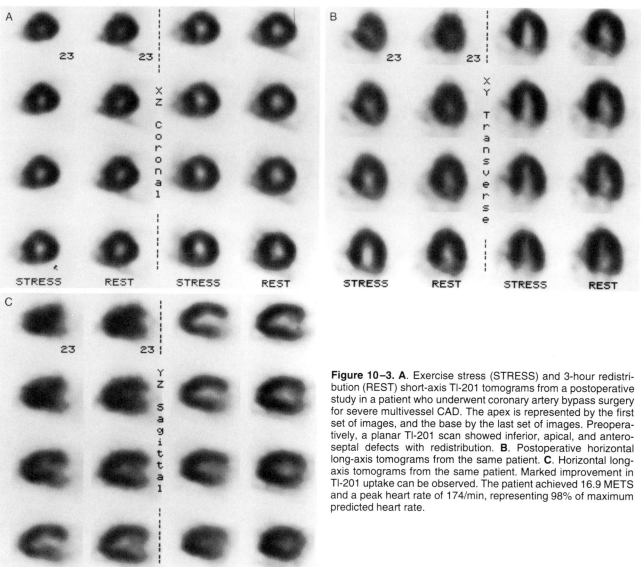

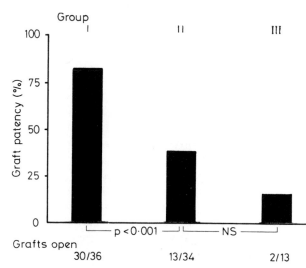

Figure 10–3. A. Exercise stress (STRESS) and 3-hour redistribution (REST) short-axis TI-201 tomograms from a postoperative study in a patient who underwent coronary artery bypass surgery for severe multivessel CAD. The apex is represented by the first set of images, and the base by the last set of images. Preoperatively, a planar TI-201 scan showed inferior, apical, and anteroseptal defects with redistribution. **B**. Postoperative horizontal long-axis tomograms from the same patient. **C**. Horizontal long-axis tomograms from the same patient. Marked improvement in TI-201 uptake can be observed. The patient achieved 16.9 METS and a peak heart rate of 174/min, representing 98% of maximum predicted heart rate.

Figure 10–4. Bypass graft patency rate (%) relative to TI-201 scintigraphic findings. Patency rate was higher in group I patients, whose perfusion scan normalized postoperatively as compared with group II, whose postoperative perfusion was unchanged, and group III, whose postoperative perfusion was worse by TI-201 criteria. (Hirzel HO, et al.: Br Heart J 1980;43:426–435.)

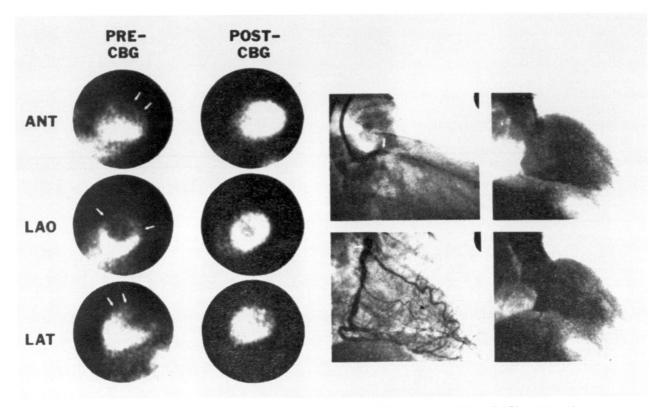

Figure 10–5. Pre- and post-CABG images in the anterior (ANT), left anterior oblique (LAO), and lateral (LAT) projections in a patient with multivessel CAD. The left ventriculogram shows marked anterior wall hypokinesis. The preoperative scintigrams (column 1) show perfusion defects in the anterolateral wall, the upper septum, and high posterolateral wall. The postoperative scintigram shows improved perfusion in these defects following three bypass grafts. (Reprinted by permission of the Society of Nuclear Medicine from Verani MS, et al.: J Nucl Med 1978;19:765–772.)

to significant enhancement of regional blood flow to the zone of jeopardized myocardium supplied by the physiologically most severe stenosis as determined preoperatively on coronary angiography. That is, as long as the "culprit lesion"—the one likely responsible for angina at a low level of exertion—is successfully revascularized, symptoms may diminish. Residual defects remote from the culprit lesion on postoperative Tl-201 imaging may not be functionally significant. Nevertheless, the greater the improvement in total myocardial perfusion postoperatively, the greater should be the improvement in exercise tolerance and amelioration of anginal symptoms.

Greenberg et al.[20] found that, as an indicator of postoperative coronary lesions, chest pain lacked sensitivity (60%) and was nonspecific (20%). The stress electrocardiogram (ECG) had poor sensitivity (60%) but good specificity (86%), but it was not helpful for patients with equivocal exercise ECGs or suboptimal stress tests. In contrast, the exercise Tl-201 scintigram had good sensitivity (77%) and was highly specific (100%) for the diagnosis of a postoperative coronary stenosis. It was significantly more specific than chest pain ($P < 0.01$) and rendered excellent localizing information. The exercise Tl-201 scintigram added to the accuracy of both conclusive and inconclusive ECG stress tests.

Exercise Tl-201 scintigraphy performed postoperatively has a rather low predictive value for graft patency in infarct zones that have been revascularized. Wainwright et al.[21] detected 79% of patent grafts but only 50% of occluded ones in 48 patients who underwent exercise scintigraphy and coronary angiography at a mean interval of 15 months after bypass surgery. For grafts that supply noninfarcted myocardium, however, the predictive accuracy of graft patency and graft occlusion was 85% and 81%, respectively. In that study, stress ECG alone failed to detect 15 of 21 patients who showed scintigraphic evidence of regional myocardial ischemia by Tl-201 scintigraphy criteria. These authors also showed the benefit of complete revascularization for patients undergoing bypass surgery for CAD. Additional residual ischemia attributed to ungrafted CAD was detected by stress Tl-201 scintigraphy in 67% of patients. Most commonly it occurred in the distribution of the diagonal branch of the LAD coronary artery, particularly when the distal LAD graft was patent. The results of that study showed that independent grafts to the diagonal branch of the LAD artery are recommended at the time of bypass surgery. Iskandrian et al.[22] point out that some patients with incomplete revascularization have normal postoperative Tl-201 scintigrams. Generally, they have at least one patent graft, and the ungrafted or incompletely regrafted lesion is generally limited to the right coronary artery or to diagonal vessels. Postoperative exercise-induced perfusion abnormalities on Tl-201 scintigrams denoted either graft occlusion or disease in nongrafted vessels.

If intraoperative transapical venting of the left ventricle is performed during bypass surgery, postoperative apical Tl-201 defects are observed in approximately two-thirds of cases.[23] In this study, serial Tl-201 imaging was 80% sensitive, 88% specific, and 86% accurate overall in detecting or excluding graft occlusion, which was predicted by redistribution defects as well as new persistent defects. Occluded grafts were correctly localized by Tl-201 scintigraphy in 61% of patients. Table 10–2 summarizes the results of this study pertaining to the accuracy of Tl-201 imaging to detect bypass graft occlusion. Reduced capacity for physical work correlated with detection of new perfusion defects postoperatively.

Technetium-99m (Tc-99m)–labeled perfusion agents can be substituted for Tl-201 for either preoperative or postoperative evaluation of coronary bypass patients.[22a] The published literature is predominantly confined to studies using Tl-201, but sensitivity and specificity of Tc-99m–sestamibi and Tl-201 imaging are comparable. Figure 10–6 shows postoperative exercise and rest Tc-99m sestamibi short axis SPECT images in a patient who underwent a "redo" coronary bypass 8 weeks previously with an internal mammary graft anastamosed to his LAD. He developed postoperative angina, and the sestamibi study showed a reversible anteroapical defect and a partially reversible anterior wall defect.

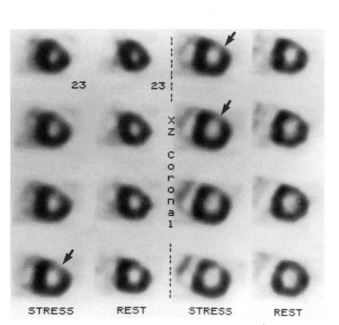

Figure 10–6. Postoperative exercise (STRESS) and resting (REST) short-axis Tc-99m sestamibi tomograms in a patient with postoperative angina after a "redo" coronary bypass operation. A partially reversible anterior defect *(arrow)* can be seen. The sequence begins with the apex in the first pair of images in the first two rows and ends with the base in the last pair of images in the third and fourth rows.

Table 10–2. Sensitivity, Specificity, and Accuracy of Tl-201 Imaging for Detecting Patients with Bypass Graft Occlusion at 1-Year Follow-Up

Finding	Patients	
	No.	**%**
Patients with at least one occluded graft (15)		
Ischemia	8	53
New scar	6	40
Ischemia/new scar	12	80 (Sensitivity)
Patients with all grafts patent (34)		
Ischemia	3/34	
New scar	2/34	
No new defects	30/34	88 (Specificity)
True Tl-201 results (42)		
Total tests (49)		86 (Accuracy)

(Pfisterer M, et al.: Circulation 1982; 66:1017–1024.)

EXERCISE THALLIUM-201 SCINTIGRAPHY FOR EVALUATING PERCUTANEOUS TRANSLUMINAL CORONARY ANGIOPLASTY

Postprocedure Assessment of Myocardial Perfusion

Exercise myocardial perfusion imaging can be undertaken to predict the efficacy of percutaneous transluminal coronary angioplasty (PTCA).[23a–23c] Patients who are the most suitable candidates for angioplasty are those who suffer exertional angina and before the procedure demonstrate significant stress-induced reversible perfusion defects or only mild persistent defects. Following successive balloon dilation of a stenotic vessel, substantial improvement in regional myocardial perfusion during exercise scintigraphy performed after the procedure can be expected (Fig. 10–7).[23b] Okada et al.[24] performed exercise Tl-201 scintigraphy before and 1 week after PTCA. Tl-201 scintigrams were analyzed using a computer method that quantitated regional Tl-201 uptake, redistribution, and washout. Significant improvement in Tl-201 uptake was observed in myocardial segments perfused by the LAD 1 week after successful PTCA. This increase in stress-induced perfusion was associated with a significant reduction in the degree of delayed Tl-201 redistribution in these same segments. Tl-201 clearance rate in myocardial scan segments supplied by the dilated vessel also improved after PTCA. Of the 17 patients who demonstrated abnormal lung Tl-201 uptake before PTCA, only four demonstrated this high-risk scintigraphic variable after balloon dilation. The improvement in myocardial Tl-201 uptake and washout was associated with an improvement in the exercise LVEF. Relief of angina symptoms and improved exercise tolerance are associated with

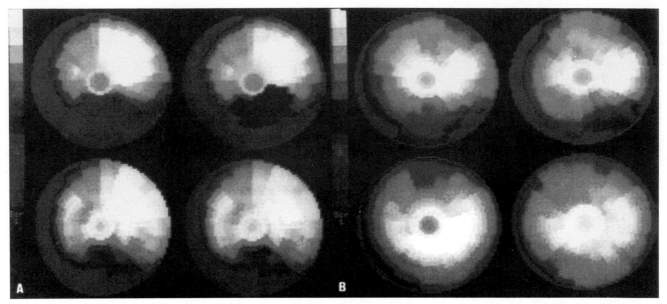

See Color Figure 10–7.

Figure 10–7. Bull's-eye polar maps from SPECT images obtained after exercise *(top row)* and 4 hours after tracer injection *(bottom row)*. The preangioplasty bull's-eye maps are shown in the left panel, **A,** and the postangioplasty bull's-eye maps are shown in the right panel, **B.** Note that, following successful right coronary artery angioplasty, both the immediate and 4-hour delayed bull's-eye plots are normal. In the preangioplasty study, a significant diminution in tracer uptake is seen in the inferior wall, with partial redistribution at 4 hours (see Color Figure 10–7). (DePuey E: Circulation 1991;84:I-59–I-65.)

the disappearance of Tl-201 redistribution after PTCA. Approximately 90% of preprocedure ischemic-type Tl-201 defects improve significantly or normalize after balloon dilation.

Verani et al.[25] studied 61 patients before and after PTCA utilizing quantitative analysis of Tl-201 uptake and washout. Tl-201 uptake in defect areas increased from 49% ± 1.3% to 71.3% ± 1.9% after PTCA ($P < 0.0001$), and 68 (65%) of the areas that before PTCA showed abnormal uptake returned to normal. There was a concomitant improvement in Tl-201 washout. Of eight patients with exclusively a "pre-PTCA" Tl-201 washout abnormality, six showed normalization of washout after PTCA. Residual Tl-201 scan abnormalities were observed in approximately 50% of patients, most often in regions of previous MI, in the region of an undilated stenotic vessel.

Several studies compared the diagnostic value of exercise Tl-201 scintigraphy and stress ECG for evaluating the results of PTCA. Scholl et al.[26] found that, of 36 asymptomatic patients studied 1 month after PTCA, the number of patients with an abnormal exercise ECG decreased from 20 to 7 ($P < 0.01$), and with an abnormal Tl-201 scintigram, from 21 to 6 ($P < 0.001$). Of the 10 patients with a persistently positive exercise ECG or abnormal Tl-201 scintigram, two had residual stenoses of 50% to 70% severity, two had significant lesions in a nondilated vessel, and three had an abnormal scintigram 1 month after PTCA that subsequently became negative at 6 months. Manyari et al.[27] reported that additional improvement in myocardial perfusion could oc-

cur until 6 months after PTCA as assessed by serial Tl-201 scintigraphy. Figure 10–8 shows continued improvement in myocardial Tl-201 uptake in one of the representative patients in this study. Similarly, abnormal flow reserve continues to improve in reperfused ischemic myocardium after successful angioplasty in patients with acute MI. Pharmacologically inducible flow reserve was improved at the time of hospital discharge compared with that at day 1 postinfarction in this study.[27a] Thus, abnormal perfusion scans on studies obtained soon after PTCA do not necessarily reflect suboptimal dilation or early restenosis. Abnormal flow reserve in the distribution of the dilated vessel may last long in patients who have what initially appears to be a successful angiographic result.

Lim et al.[28] reported a new computer method designed to quantitate improvement in myocardial perfusion after PTCA. Computer-derived functional images were used to demonstrate the extent of redistribution and the extent of change in regional perfusion before and after PTCA. Tl-201 activity, expressed as a percentage of maximal myocardial activity, increased from 72% to 82% in anterior segments and from 67% to 75% a week after PTCA in patients with a proximal LAD lesion who were serially evaluated. The increase in Tl-201 uptake was associated with a reduction in the amount of Tl-201 redistribution between initial and postexercise images and with enhancement of myocardial Tl-201 clearance. By this quantitative analysis approach, improvement in Tl-201 scintigrams following PTCA was seen in 14 of 20 patients.

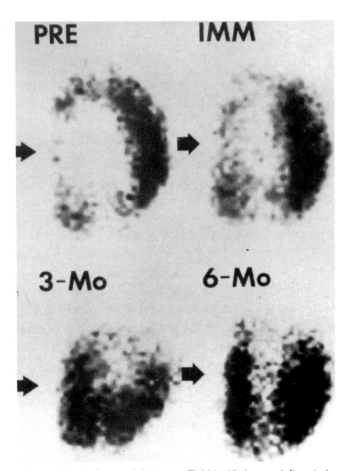

Figure 10–8. Sequential stress Tl-201 45-degree left anterior oblique images in a patient with proximal LAD coronary artery stenosis who underwent successful coronary angioplasty. Note the progressive improvement in septal Tl-201 uptake over 3 months following the procedure. Regional septal Tl-201 uptake was quantitated at 52% before angioplasty (pre), 72% at 5 days after angioplasty (1mm), 101% at 3 months after angioplasty (3-mo), and 98% at 6 months after angioplasty (6-mo). (Manyari DE, et al.: Circulation 1988;77:86–95.)

Kanemoto et al.[29] showed that PTCA improved Tl-201 uptake in the distribution of a dilated region and improved resting and exercise LVEF, as long as the luminal diameter was dilated more than 20%. Improvement in Tl-201 uptake in the previously ischemic region correlated directly with the improvement in exercise EF. DePuey et al.[30] showed that the greatest improvement in Tl-201 uptake after PTCA was demonstrated when dilatation was attempted in areas of severe coronary stenosis, and when luminal diameter was most markedly increased. Improvement in Tl-201 uptake was directly related to the change in luminal diameter achieved by PTCA, although the correlation between the change in percentage of stenosis and the improvement in the Tl-201 defect score was weak ($r = 0.41$).

A radionuclide imaging agent can be injected intravenously in the cardiac catheterization laboratory during balloon occlusion performed for angioplasty to assess the area at risk distal to the coronary narrowing. The imaging can

be repeated after conclusion of the procedure, to determine the degree in improvement in blood flow or viability. Heller et al.[30a] found that the number of defects on Tc-99m–teboroxime images decreased significantly from 4.13 ± 1.01 during balloon occlusion to 0.27 ± 0.44 after reperfusion ($P = 0.0006$). There was a 30% decrease in the defect–normal zone count–pixel ratios for these 15 patients during balloon occlusion, which normalized after successful dilation. Similar findings were reported by Haronian et al.,[30b] who used Tc-99m–sestamibi imaging. In that study, angiographic risk scores correlated only moderately with Tc-99m–sestamibi risk area ($r = 0.54$). As expected, the LAD risk area (scored from 0 to 60) was larger than that observed for the other vessels (22 ± 15 vs. 7 ± 11; $P = 0.002$). Figure 10–9 depicts the Tc-99m–sestamibi defect size on planar angioplasty images relative to LAD and extra-LAD angioplasty sites. There was a wide range of risk area for similar angiographic sites of balloon occlusion. Borges-Neto et al.[30c] found that perfusion defect size determined after Tc-99m–sestamibi injection during balloon occlusion was larger (28% ± 3%) than the Tc-99m–sestamibi defect size with exercise imaging (13% ± 2%; $P < 0.01$). This discrepancy is most likely due to the fact that with exercise scintigraphy, the coronary stenosis may permit some antegrade flow, whereas with balloon dilatation, the lumen of the vessel is totally occluded.

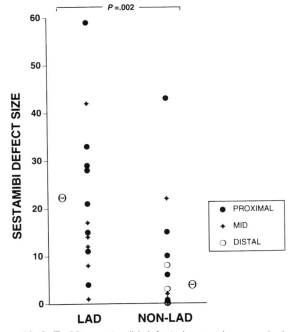

Figure 10–9. Tc-99m–sestamibi defect size on planar angioplasty images in relation to the angioplasty site. The risk area for patients undergoing LAD artery angioplasty was larger than that for those who underwent angioplasty of other vessels. Note, however, the wide range of risk area for similar locations of coronary occlusion as well as the overlap between LAD and non-LAD angioplasty sites. (Reprinted with permission from the American College of Cardiology (Journal of the American College of Cardiology, 1993, Vol. 22, pp. 1033–1043).)

Detection of Restenosis

Restenosis, one of the major limitations of PTCA, occurs in approximately 30% to 40% of patients who initially experience a successful angiographic and clinical result after balloon dilation. Exercise- or dipyridamole Tl-201 scintigraphy can be utilized to detect restenosis after PTCA.[30d] Table 10–3 list the causes of perfusion defects seen on post-PTCA perfusion scans. Evidence of persistence of Tl-201 redistribution defects on post-PTCA stress scintigraphy in asymptomatic patients is predictive of early recurrence of angina and implies that there was either incomplete dilatation, early restenosis, or a functionally important stenosis that was not dilated at the time of pre-PTCA. This stenosis might be more distal to the proximally dilated lesion or in one or more of the other major coronary vessels that was not considered significant at the time of preprocedure coronary angiography. Thus, some patients with residual defects have multivessel disease and coronary narrowing in a nondilated vessel. When, after the initial dilation, the patient exercises more vigorously, ischemia can be induced in the myocardial supply region of such a nondilated stenosis.

Data published by Stuckey et al.[31] demonstrated that exercise Tl-201 scintigraphy performed soon after PTCA in patients who had a clinically successful result was predictive of recurrence of angina. Patients who exhibited asymptomatic Tl-201 redistribution on post-PTCA exercise scintigraphy performed 2 weeks after the procedure had a high probability of developing recurrent angina in the ensuing 6 months (Fig. 10–10); however, although the predictive specificity of Tl-201 redistribution for recurrent angina was high in this study (91%), overall sensitivity was only 39%. Nevertheless, Tl-201 redistribution on post-PTCA exercise scintigraphy was the only significant independent predictor of recurrent angina by logistic regression analysis. After repeat angiography was performed in 17 of the 23 patients who had recurrent angina, 14 (82%) demonstrated resteno-

sis and three (18%) had progressive narrowing distal to or remote from the site of dilation. The presence of exercise-induced Tl-201 redistribution had a positive predictive value of 69% for recurrent angina, which was higher than the 41% value for exercise ST-segment depression. The negative predictive value of Tl-201 redistribution was 75%, slightly higher than the 69% for ST-segment depression.

In contrast to the protocol employed by Stuckey et al.,[31] Wijns et al.[32] performed post-PTCA Tl-201 scintigraphy 4 weeks—rather than 2 weeks—after the procedure. Patients were followed for an average of 6 months for recurrence of angina, and all underwent repeat coronary angiography at 6 months, or earlier if symptoms recurred. Restenosis was defined as an increase of the stenosis to more than 50% luminal diameter. For the 89 patients in their study, Tl-201 scintigraphy was superior to exercise ECG stress testing alone for predicting recurrence of angina after PTCA (66% vs. 38%). Restenosis was predicted in 74% of patients by Tl-201 scintigraphy, but in only 50% by the exercise ECG. Figure 10–11 shows the predictive value for angiographic restenosis for the possible combinations of noninvasive test results in this study. These authors concluded that significant but asymptomatic restenosis must have occurred by 4 weeks after PTCA in most patients in whom subsequently it was observed. In a subsequent study by the same group,[33] multivariate analysis was performed in 111 patients who were studied prospectively with repeat coronary angiography and exercise Tl-201 scintigraphy at an interval of 6 ±

Table 10–3. Causes of Myocardial Perfusion Defects on Postangioplasty Stress Perfusion Scans

Restenosis of dilated lesion
Ischemia in distribution of nondilated lesion
Myocardial scar, though lesion was successfully dilated
Abnormal flow reserve without evidence of restenosis
Progression of native CAD
False-positive defect secondary to artifact

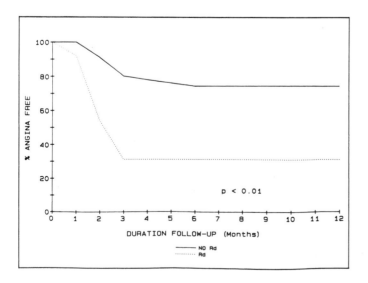

Figure 10–10. Percentage of patients who remained angina free among those who did *(dotted line)* or did not *(solid line)* exhibit Tl-201 redistribution (Rd) on exercise scintigraphy after coronary angioplasty. (Reprinted with permission from the American College of Cardiology (Journal of the American College of Cardiology, 1989, Vol. 63, pp. 517–521).)

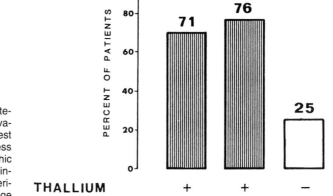

Figure 10–11. The predictive value for angiographic restenosis after angioplasty for possible combinations of noninvasive test results: (+), abnormal test; and (−), normal test result. (Key: Ex Test, exercise electrocardiographic stress test; shaded columns, patients with abnormal scintigraphic responses; open columns, patients with negative Tl-201 scintigraphic results.) (Reprinted with permission from the American College of Cardiology (Journal of the American College of Cardiology, 1985, Vol. 55, pp. 357–361).)

2 months after complete revascularization by PTCA. Four factors were found to relate independently to the increased risk of restenosis. In order of importance they were: (1) recurrence of angina ($P < 0.0001$), (2) an abnormal finding on exercise Tl-201 scintigraphy ($P < 0.001$), (3) absolute postangioplasty stenosis diameter ($P < 0.002$), and (4) exercise ST-segment depression ($P < 0.01$). Using a logistic model, these predictors of restenosis were combined into a restenosis probability score classified as high, intermediate, or low. The predictive value for restenosis in the high-risk group (probability greater than 80%) was 100%, and the predictive value for no restenosis in the low-risk group (probability less than 20%) was 94%.

The predictive value of exercise Tl-201 scintigraphy for detecting restenosis is greater in the studies reported by Wijns et al. and Renkin et al.,[32, 33] as compared to the results reported by Stuckey et al.[31] This may be attributable to the fact that, in the Belgian studies, post-PTCA exercise Tl-201 scintigraphy was performed later (after 4 weeks) following dilation. Since angiographic restenosis is a progressive process and is time related, it is not surprising that the sensitivity of perfusion imaging for predicting recurrent angina due to restenosis is higher the longer the interval between the procedure and the noninvasive evaluation after initially successful balloon dilatation.

Breisblatt et al.[34] evaluated the predictive accuracy of exercise Tl-201 scintigraphy for detection of restenosis after PTCA in 121 patients who had a successful angiographic result after the procedure. Of 104 asymptomatic patients evaluated 4 to 6 weeks after PTCA, 25% had persistent Tl-201 redistribution on scintigraphy. Restenosis, as judged by angiography, was confirmed by 6 months in 85% of these patients and by 1 year in 96%. These investigators also confirmed that myocardial perfusion imaging was superior to exercise ECG stress testing alone for detecting restenosis. Miller et al.[35] assessed the prognostic value of quantitative exercise Tl-201 scintigraphy performed after PTCA for re-

stenosis prediction using stepwise logistic regression analysis. They reported that a combination of an abnormal exercise scintigram, showing redistribution defects, together with a post-PTCA gradient of 20 mm Hg or greater identified patients who showed a fourfold greater risk for restenosis and recurrent angina or MI during 12 months' follow-up. The number of segments that exhibited delayed Tl-201 clearance was also predictive of restenosis.

SPECT Thallium-201 Imaging and Detection of Restenosis

Investigators at Emory University evaluated SPECT Tl-201 scintigraphy as a possible predictor of restenosis after 6 months. In a series of 158 patients, scintigraphic evidence of a perfusion defect in the territory of a dilated vessel was associated with poor sensitivity (44%) and specificity (67%).[36] The low specificity of an abnormal scan after early PTCA in predicting restenosis in that study is probably attributable to early postprocedure evaluation. Abnormal flow reserve in the distribution of a successfully dilated vessel causing Tl-201 perfusion abnormalities on exercise scintigraphy can be seen up to 6 months after technically successful PTCA.[27] Perfusion defects seen on early post-PTCA Tl-201 scintigraphy do not necessarily imply restenosis but can reflect reversible functional flow reserve abnormalities.

Hecht et al.[37] evaluated the utility of SPECT Tl-201 scintigraphy for detection of restenosis after PTCA. The study group comprised 116 consecutive patients referred for evaluation of possible restenosis where, for 65% of them, the indication for angiographic reevaluation was recurrent chest pain. This population differs from previous ones in that 47% of the patients underwent multivessel PTCA. A total of 185 vessels were dilated in 116 patients. Complete revascularization was achieved in 77%, and partial revascularization in 33% of patients. SPECT Tl-201 imaging demonstrated superior sensitivity (93%) for detection of restenosis over exercise ECG stress testing (52%). Similarly, specificity was also superior (77% vs. 64%). This yielded accuracies of 86% and 57% for SPECT Tl-201 scintigraphy and exercise ECG testing, respectively ($P <$ 0.001). Table 10–4 summarizes the results of these analyses. SPECT Tl-201 scintigraphy was 86% sensitive, specific, and accurate for restenosis detection in specific vessels and results were comparable for one-vessel and for multivessel PTCA, and for complete versus partial revascularization. Exercise Tl-201 scintigraphy can be utilized to determine the significance of 40% to 70% diameter narrowing at the site of previous stenting or directional atherectomy at 6 months postprocedure.[37a] Cardiac events were low in patients in this study who had "intermediate" restenosis but no inducible ischemia and were similar to the event rate in patients with less than 40% diameter narrowing.

SPECT Tl-201 scintigraphy appears to be as sensitive for detecting restenosis in asymptomatic patients as it is in patients with recurrent angina. Hecht et al.[38] found that sensitivity, specificity, and accuracy for detection of restenosis by SPECT were 96%, 75%, and 86% in asymptomatic patients, as compared with 91%, 77%, and 85% in symptomatic patients (Table 10–4). In patients with silent and asymptomatic ischemia, restenosis was associated with comparable amounts and degrees of severity of ischemic defects in the two groups. Pfisterer et al.[38a] found a 60% prevalence of silent ischemia on exercise Tl-201 scintigraphic testing 6 months after PTCA. Exercise electrocardiography results were negative in 74% of patients with scintigraphic ischemia and angiographic restenosis, and the degree of restenosis was similar in patients with symptomatic or silent ischemia (80% ± 16% vs. 81% ± 21%). Prognosis was comparable in silent and symptomatic ischemia groups. Figure 10–12 shows the cardiac event rate with and without chest pain included as an event in this study. Repeat PTCA in patients manifesting ischemia reduced the subsequent cardiac event rate.

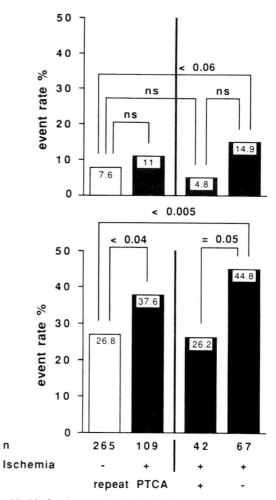

Figure 10–12. Cardiac event rate (excluding repeat coronary angioplasty at 6 months as an event) in relation to presence *(black bars)* or absence *(white bars)* of ischemia by Tl-201 imaging and in relation to repeat angioplasty. In the lower panel, exercise-induced chest pain is included as an event. Patients undergoing repeat angioplasty for ischemia had one-third of the critical event rate (cardiac death, myocardial infarction, revascularization for recurrent symptoms, and hospital admission for chest pain) of patients with ischemia but no repeat intervention (5% vs. 15%). (Reprinted with permission of the American College of Cardiology (Journal of the American College of Cardiology, 1993, Vol. 22, pp. 1446–1554).)

Exercise Tl-201 scintigraphy can be employed for identification of the culprit lesion in patients with multivessel CAD and symptomatic angina. Breisblatt et al.[39] reported that approximately half of the patients who underwent successful dilation of a culprit lesion and who had multivessel CAD exhibited scintigraphic evidence of ischemia in a second vascular redistribution on repeat exercise Tl-201 perfusion imaging. Of the subgroup who had no evidence of ischemia on repeat evaluation, only 13% required repeat PTCA of a second vessel at 1-year follow-up. This study points out the importance of complete revascularization in patients with multivessel CAD for elimination of stress-induced ischemia.

Thus, exercise perfusion imaging, when performed at the earliest 4 to 6 weeks after angioplasty, provides useful information pertaining to symptomatic or asymptomatic re-

Table 10–4. Detection of Restenosis After Angioplasty by SPECT Thallium Imaging and Exercise ECG: Silent Versus Symptomatic Ischemia

	Sensitivity (%)	Specificity (%)	Accuracy (%)
Silent ischemia			
SPECT	96*	75	88*
Exercise ECG	40	50	44†
Symptomatic ischemia			
SPECT	91*	77	85*
Exercise ECG	59	71	64

*$P < 0.001$ vs. exercise ECG.
†$P < 0.05$ vs. symptomatic ischemia.
(Reprinted with permission of the American College of Cardiology (Journal of the American College of Cardiology, 1991, Vol. 17, pp. 670–677).)

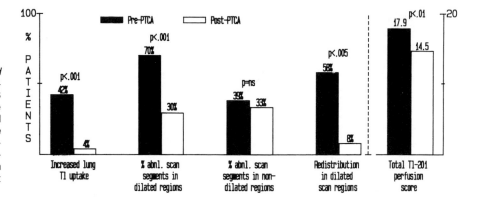

Figure 10–13. Changes in exercise Tl-201 scan variables from preangioplasty *(solid bars)* to postangioplasty *(open bars)* in 24 patients undergoing angioplasty after CAB surgery for recurrent angina. Note the marked decrease in prevalence of increased lung Tl-201 (Tl) uptake and the percentage of abnormal (abnl) scan segments in the distribution of the dilated lesion. The percentage of scan segments with redistribution was also markedly reduced. (Reed DC, et al.: Am Heart J 1989;117:60–71.)

stenosis. Waiting at least 4 to 6 weeks postprocedure for stress imaging can enhance both sensitivity and specificity of Tl-201 or Tc-99m sestamibi for detection of restenosis. Perfusion imaging is more sensitive than exercise electrocardiographic testing alone for detection of ischemia due to restenosis after PTCA.[39a] Specificity of the ST segment response for ischemia detection after PTCA is also suboptimal. In fact, ST depression can be observed in absence of ischemia in patients with preprocedure regional ventricular dysfunction.[39b]

Assessment of Percutaneous Transluminal Coronary Angioplasty in Bypass Grafts

Exercise Tl-201 scintigraphy has also been used to assess efficacy of coronary angioplasty in patients who undergo PTCA bypass grafts for recurrent angina after CABG. Reed et al.[40] showed that, after PTCA of stenotic bypass grafts, abnormal lung Tl-201 uptake, the number of abnormal scan segments, and the magnitude of redistribution in dilated lesions were significantly reduced (Fig. 10–13). Redistribution defects seen in 38% of patients on post-PTCA scans indicated a substantial degree of residual ischemia after angiographically successful dilation of diseased grafts. All patients with post-PTCA redistribution defects subsequently developed angina. Of the various clinical, angiographic, exercise ECG stress test, and Tl-201 scan variables, only delayed redistribution was found to be an independent predictor of recurrent angina. Restenosis was the most common underlying cause for this exercise-induced perfusion abnormality. Thus, as stress Tl-201 scintigraphy can be used to detect restenosis with native CAD, this study is applicable to coronary bypass grafts.

Summary

In conclusion, there is no doubt that, after successful dilatation as judged by coronary angiography after PTCA, an improvement in regional myocardial Tl-201 uptake and washout in the supply region of the dilated vessel can be

expected on postprocedure exercise scintigraphy. Pre-PTCA ischemic-type transient Tl-201 defects should improve or normalize when a stress perfusion study is performed at least 4 weeks after the dilation procedure. Early post-PTCA stress Tl-201 scintigraphy may reveal residual Tl-201 perfusion abnormalities that can be attributed to abnormal flow reserve rather than early restenosis.[40a] Uren et al.[40] reported abnormal coronary vasodilator response after angioplasty 7 days after vasodilation. By 3 months, the coronary vasodilator response had returned to normal. Figure 10–14 summarizes these data. The precise mechanism for this early flow-reserve abnormality in the distribution of a recently dilated vessel is unclear. When symptoms reappear, restenosis is often the cause, and Tl-201 scintigraphic results become abnormal again. Asymptomatic restenosis can be detected by stress Tl-201 scintigraphy, and such scan abnormalities are similar in magnitude and extent to those seen in patients with the current angina who then submit to post-PTCA scintigraphy. Exercise Tl-201 scintigraphy may also be valuable in determining the functional significance of coronary stenoses, in addition to

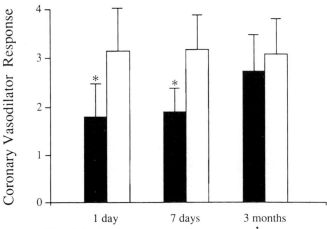

Figure 10–14. Bar graph showing the coronary vasodilator response in the angioplasty *(solid bars)* and the remote *(open bars)* regions at 1 day, 7 days, and 3 months after successful angioplasty. Note the depressed coronary vasodilator response in the angioplasty region at 1 day and 7 days, compared with the 3-month value (*, *P* < 0.05). (Reprinted with permission from the American College of Cardiology (Journal of the American College of Cardiology, 1993, Vol. 21, pp. 612–621).)

the one dilated in patients with multivessel disease in whom only the presumed culprit lesion is dilated. At higher exercise heart rates, new perfusion abnormalities in the distribution of nondilated stenoses in the substrate of multivessel disease may become evident. Finally, Tl-201 scintigraphy performed in patients with atypical chest pain after PTCA may obviate coronary angiography. A normal exercise Tl-201 perfusion scan under such circumstances suggests that the chest pain is not due to restenosis, progression of distal disease, or a significant stenosis in a nondilated vessel.

RADIONUCLIDE ANGIOGRAPHY IN THE ASSESSMENT OF PATIENTS BEFORE AND AFTER CORONARY ARTERY BYPASS GRAFT SURGERY

Exercise radionuclide angiography has been utilized to identify patients at high risk who may expect to benefit from CABG surgery. As discussed in Chapter 4, patients who demonstrate a subnormal LVEF in response to exercise are those who tend to have more extensive angiographic CAD and are at a higher risk for subsequent cardiac mortality than are patients who exhibit a normal global functional response to exercise. In a nonrandomized study performed at Duke University, patients who demonstrated the greatest amount of exercise-induced LV dysfunction preoperatively had the most favorable outcome with coronary artery bypass surgery, as judged by mortality statistics and pain relief.[41] Patients who underwent bypass surgery and who preoperatively had a normal LVEF on exercise enjoyed no better survival or long-term pain relief than those treated medically. Patients with an abnormal response to exercise preoperatively survived longer and enjoyed more effective pain relief with surgery compared to those patients with an abnormal response who received medical therapy alone.

Kronenberg et al.[42] found that the preoperative EF response predicted the degree of improvement in exercise performance after bypass surgery. Patients who showed the greatest improvement were those who had the most signifi-

cant drop in EF before revascularization. These data from nonrandomized studies suggest that exercise radionuclide angiography, like Tl-201 scintigraphy, may be useful in selecting the CAD patients at high risk who are most likely to benefit from bypass surgery. Patients who preoperatively exhibit a significant drop in LVEF from rest to exercise might benefit more from coronary bypass surgery than patients who exhibit little evidence during stress-induced ischemia.

Exercise radionuclide angiographic assessment can identify patients who have occluded or stenosed bypass grafts after revascularization. Lim et al.[43] found that the resting LVEF was unchanged after CABG surgery, as assessed by both first-pass and equilibrium-gated radionuclide angiography in 20 patients with chronic stable angina who were studied. At the maximum workload, the mean LVEF was significantly greater postoperatively than preoperatively (63% ± 17% vs. 53% ± 17%), indicating reversal of stress-induced ischemia. Of five patients whose mean LVEF decreased significantly during exercise postoperatively, all had one or more occluded or stenosed grafts. Figure 10–15 shows the LVEF response of the left ventricle in response to graded supine bicycle exercise before and after coronary bypass surgery.

Kent and colleagues also determined the effect of coronary bypass surgery on exercise EF and exercise regional wall motion.[44] After revascularization the average resting LVEF remained unchanged, but 17 of the 20 patients demonstrated an improvement in exercise LVEF. All patients whose LVEF improved during exercise after bypass surgery improved "symptomatically." Regional function also showed improvement during exercise. These authors concluded that both EF during exercise and exercise-induced wall motion abnormalities improve after surgery in most patients who demonstrate symptomatic improvement after coronary revascularization. An abnormal LVEF response to exercise postoperatively would indicate either intraoperative myocardial damage, incomplete revascularization, or graft occlusion or stenosis. A new wall motion abnormality on resting radionuclide angiography would suggest intraoperative myocardial infarction or resting ischemia.

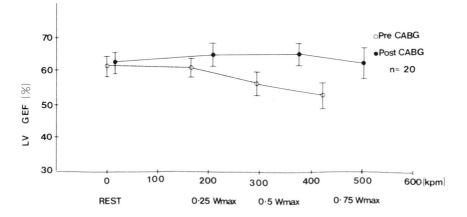

Figure 10–15. Mean global LVEF (GEF) during graded bicycle exercise (Wmax) before (pre) and after (post) CABG surgery. (Lim YL, et al.: Circulation 1982;66:972–979.)

EXERCISE RADIONUCLIDE ANGIOGRAPHY FOR ASSESSMENT OF PERCUTANEOUS TRANSLUMINAL CORONARY ANGIOPLASTY

Like exercise perfusion imaging, exercise radionuclide angiography has been used to evaluate the results of PTCA. Successful PTCA should be associated with a reversal of exercise-induced wall motion abnormalities and an improvement in the exercise LVEF response. Restenosis can also be detected by exercise radionuclide angiography. DePuey et al.[45] found that patients with less than a 5% increase in LVEF or who had wall motion deterioration early after PTCA on testing eventually were found to have a greater degree of restenosis than did patients with normal post-PTCA findings. The accuracy of abnormal radionuclide angiographic findings in predicting a 50% or greater restenosis of the dilated vessel was 73% immediately after PTCA and 77% at the time of follow-up angiography at 4 to 12 months. Patients with residual stenoses of 20% or less had only a 5% incidence of abnormal EF responses after PTCA. In contrast, 75% of patients whose restenosis achieved luminal diameter reduction of 50% or greater had an abnormal exercise radionuclide EF result. Figure 10–16 shows the change in LVEF from rest to peak exercise before and after PTCA grouped according to the degree of restenosis on angiography. Patients with no more than 20% residual stenosis had the most marked improvement in exercise LVEF after PTCA. These authors concluded that radionuclide angiography was useful in predicting coronary restenosis after angioplasty. Kanemoto et al.[46] also showed that LV function during exercise was enhanced if the luminal diameter was dilated by more than 20% by PTCA. Patients who had a successful angiographic result increased their EF during exercise from 39.9% ± 10.5% to 49.4% ± 10.9% ($P < 0.001$) after the procedure.

An alternative to exercise RNA for detection of restenosis is exercise echocardiography (see Chap. 3). Mertes et al.[46a] reported 83% sensitivity and 85% specificity for de-

tection of recurrent ischemia after coronary angioplasty using bicycle stress echocardiography in 86 patients studied 6.5 ± 1.3 months after nonsurgical coronary artery revascularization. Hecht et al.,[46b] who also used bicycle exercise, found 87% sensitivity and 95% specificity for detection of restenosis, values superior to those obtained for exercise ECG testing, which were 55% and 79%, respectively.

PHARMACOLOGIC STRESS THALLIUM-201 SCINTIGRAPHY FOR ASSESSMENT OF MYOCARDIAL REVASCULARIZATION

The clinical applications of pharmacologic stress Tl-201 perfusion imaging employing intravenous infusion of dipyridamole or adenosine are discussed in detail in Chapter 8. Pharmacologic stress perfusion imaging techniques can be employed as a substitute for exercise scintigraphy for detection of graft stenosis or occlusion after coronary bypass surgery or detection of restenosis after initially successful PTCA. Studies have shown comparable stenosis detection rates for (1) dipyridamole scintigraphy and exercise scintigraphy, and (2) adenosine scintigraphy and exercise Tl-201 scintigraphy. Patients who benefit most from pharmacologic stress imaging for detection of restenosis are those who had diminished exercise capacity or have noncardiac factors that prevent them from attaining a diagnostic exercise heart rate or workload. Eichhorn et al.[47] performed dipyridamole Tl-201 SPECT imaging at a mean interval of 1.5 days before, and 6.3 days after, PTCA. Angiographic success was achieved in 23 of 24 patients. Before PTCA, 3 of 24 scans were interpreted as normal, and there was no change following PTCA. Of the 19 patients who showed redistribution defects before PTCA, 17 showed improvement on postprocedure dipyridamole Tl-201 scintigraphy. Quantitative scan analysis showed significant improvement in Tl-201 uptake in myocardial regions supplied by successfully dilated regions, but not in remote regions. Jain et al.[48] reported the value of dipyridamole Tl-201 imaging for

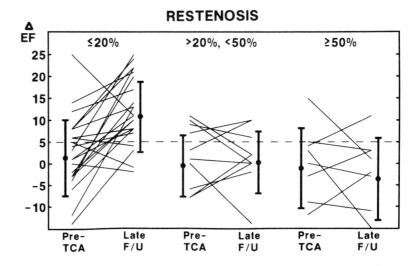

Figure 10–16. Change in EF from rest to peak exercise before transluminal coronary angioplasty (pre-TCA) and at 4- to 12-month follow-up (late F/U). Patients are grouped according to degree of angiographic restenosis. Data are depicted as mean ± 1 standard deviation. A normal change in EF is ≥5 points, which would lie above the horizontal dashed line. (DePuey E, et al.: J Am Coll Cardiol 1984;4:1103–1113.)

predicting restenosis. Restenosis developed in 71% of patients with an ischemic Tl-201 defect after PTCA, as compared with 11.5% for patients who had no ischemic defect. Dipyridamole echocardiography and exercise planar Tl-201 scintigraphy showed similar sensitivity (75% vs. 83%) and specificity (90% vs. 84%) for detection of restenosis.[47a] In this study, all patients had ST-segment depression on exercise testing, were asymptomatic, and received a large dose of dipyridamole (0.84 mg/kg over 10 minutes). Dobutamine echocardiography can be utilized to evaluate the efficacy of PTCA in reversing stress-induced ischemia. Akosah et al.[49] found that before PTCA, dobutamine infusion induced wall motion abnormalities in 88% of 35 patients. Wall motion improved in 90% of these patients when dobutamine was infused 24 to 48 hours after successful PTCA.

A host of new techniques are emerging in the field of interventional cardiology that are supplementary or alternative to balloon dilation. These include coronary atherectomy, laser angioplasty, and stent placement. Results of stress myocardial perfusion–imaging techniques can be used as endpoints in assessing the efficacy of these techniques for enhancing myocardial blood flow. Nuclear cardiology stress testing could certainly be incorporated into clinical trials to determine the rate of restenosis with these new devices.

REFERENCES

1. Brown KA, Boucher CA, Okada RD, Guiney TE, Newell JB, Strauss HW, Pohost GM: Prognostic value of exercise thallium-201 imaging in patients presenting for evaluation of chest pain. J Am Coll Cardiol 1983;1:994–1001.
2. Ladenheim ML, Pollock BH, Rozanski A, Berman DS, Staniloff HM, Forrester JS, Diamond GA: Extent and severity of myocardial hypoperfusion as predictors of prognosis in patients with suspected coronary artery disease. J Am Coll Cardiol 1986;7:464–471.
3. Iskandrian AS, Hakki AH, Kane-Marsch S: Prognostic implications of exercise thallium-201 scintigraphy in patients with suspected or known coronary artery disease. Am Heart J 1985;110:135–143.
4. Kaul S, Lilly DR, Gascho JA, Watson DD, Gibson RS, Oliner CA, Ryan JM, Beller GA: Prognostic utility of the exercise thallium-201 test in ambulatory patients with chest pain: Comparison with cardiac catheterization. Circulation 1988;77:745–758.
5. Pollock SG, Abbott RD, Boucher CA, Beller GA, Kaul S: Independent and incremental prognostic value of tests performed in hierarchical order to evaluate patients with suspected coronary artery disease. Validation of models based on these tests. Circulation 1992;85:237–248.
6. Gill JB, Ruddy TD, Newell JB, Finkelstein DM, Strauss HW, Boucher CA: Prognostic importance of thallium uptake by the lungs during exercise in coronary artery disease. N Engl J Med 1987;317:1486–1489.
7. Kaul S, Finkelstein DM, Homma S, Leavitt M, Okada RD, Boucher CA: Superiority of quantitative exercise thallium-201 variables in determining long-term prognosis in ambulatory patients with chest pain: A comparison with cardiac catheterization. J Am Coll Cardiol 1988;12:25–34.
8. Weiss AT, Berman DS, Lew AS, Nielsen J, Potkin B, Swan HJ, Waxman A, Maddahi J: Transient ischemic dilation of the left ventricle on stress thallium-201 scintigraphy: A marker of severe and extensive coronary artery disease. J Am Coll Cardiol 1987;9:752–759.
9. Beller GA, Gibson RS, Watson DD: Radionuclide methods of identifying patients who may require coronary artery bypass surgery. Circulation 1985;72:V9–22.
10. Gibson RS, Watson DD, Taylor GJ, Crosby IK, Wellons HL, Holt ND, Beller GA: Prospective assessment of regional myocardial perfusion before and after coronary revascularization surgery by quantitative thallium-201 scintigraphy. J Am Coll Cardiol 1983;1:804–815.
11. Rozanski A, Berman DS, Gray R, Levy R, Raymond M, Maddahi J, Pantaleo N, Waxman AD, Swan HJ, Matloff J: Use of thallium-201 redistribution scintigraphy in the preoperative differentiation of reversible and nonreversible myocardial asynergy. Circulation 1981;64:936–944.
12. Ragosta M, Gimple W, Kron I, Beller G: Preoperative assessment of myocardial viability by rest-thallium-201 imaging in patients with reduced ventricular function. Circulation 1990;82:III-294–III-294.
13. Bonow RO, Dilsizian V, Cuocolo A, Bacharach SL: Identification of viable myocardium in patients with chronic coronary artery disease and left ventricular dysfunction. Comparison of thallium scintigraphy with reinjection and PET imaging with ^{18}F-fluorodeoxyglucose. Circulation 1991;83:26–37.
14. Iskandrian AS, Hakki AH, Kane SA, Goel IP, Mundth ED, Segal BL: Rest and redistribution thallium-201 myocardial scintigraphy to predict improvement in left ventricular function after coronary arterial bypass grafting. Am J Cardiol 1983;51:1312–1316.
15. Hirzel HO, Nuesch K, Sialer G, Horst W, Krayenbuehl HP: Thallium-201 exercise myocardial imaging to evaluate myocardial perfusion after coronary artery bypass surgery. Br Heart J 1980;43:426–435.
16. Zimmermann R, Tillmanns H, Knapp WH, Neumann FJ, Saggau W, Kubler W: Noninvasive assessment of coronary artery bypass patency: Determination of myocardial thallium-201 washout rates. Eur Heart J 1988;9:319–327.
17. Johnson AM, Kron IL, Watson DD, Gibson RS, Nolan SP: Evaluation of postoperative flow reserve in internal mammary artery bypass grafts. J Thorac Cardiovasc Surg 1986;92:822–826.
18. Kusukawa J, Hirota Y, Kawamura K, Suma H, Takeuchi A, Adachi I, Akagi H: Efficacy of coronary artery bypass surgery with gastroepiploic artery. Assessment with thallium-201 myocardial scintigraphy. Circulation 1989;80:I135–140.
19. Verani MS, Marcus ML, Spoto G, Rossi NP, Ehrhardt JC, Razzak MA: Thallium-201 myocardial perfusion scintigrams in the evaluation of aorto-coronary saphenous bypass surgery. J Nucl Med 1978;19:765–772.
20. Greenberg BH, Hart R, Botvinick EH, Werner JA, Brundage BH, Shames DM, Chatterjee K, Parmley WW: Thallium-201 myocardial perfusion scintigraphy to evaluate patients after coronary bypass surgery. Am J Cardiol 1978;42:167–176.
21. Wainwright RJ, Brennand-Roper DA, Maisey MN, Sowton E: Exercise thallium-201 myocardial scintigraphy in the follow-up of aorto-coronary bypass graft surgery. Br Heart J 1980;43:56–66.
22. Iskandrian AS, Haaz W, Segal BL, Kane SA: Exercise thallium-201 scintigraphy in evaluating aortocoronary bypass surgery. Chest 1981;80:11–15.
22a. Iskandrian AE, Kegel JG, Tecce MA, Wasserleben V, Cave V, Heo J: Simultaneous assessment of left ventricular perfusion and function with technetium-99m sestamibi after coronary artery bypass grafting. Am Heart J 1993;126:1199–1203.
23. Pfisterer M, Emmenegger H, Schmitt HE, Muller-Brand J, Hasse J, Gradel E, Laver MB, Burckhardt D, Burkart F: Accuracy of serial myocardial perfusion scintigraphy with thallium-201 for prediction of graft patency early and late after coronary artery bypass surgery. A controlled prospective study. Circulation 1982;66:1017–1024.
23a. Kuijper A, Van Eck-Smit L, Neimeyer M, et al.: The role of scintigraphic techniques in the evaluation of functional results of coronary bypass grafting and percutaneous transluminal coronary angioplasty. Int J Cardiac Imaging 1993;9:49–58.
23b. DePuey EG: Myocardial perfusion imaging with thallium-201 to evaluate patients before and after transluminal coronary angioplasty. Circulation 1991;84:I-59–I-65.
23c. Haronian HL, Cabin HS: Nuclear cardiology: The inverventionalists' perspective. J Nucl Cardiol 1994;1:415–419.
24. Okada RD, Lim YL, Boucher CA, Pohost GM, Chesler DA, Block PC: Clinical, angiographic, hemodynamic, perfusional and functional changes after one-vessel left anterior descending coronary angioplasty. Am J Cardiol 1985;55:347–356.
25. Verani MS, Tadros S, Raizner AE, Phillips R, Matcek G, Lewis JM, Roberts R: Quantitative analysis of thallium-201 uptake and washout before and after transluminal coronary angioplasty. Int J Cardiol 1986;13:109–124.
26. Scholl JM, Chaitman BR, David PR, Dupras G, Brevers G, Val PG, Crepeau J, Lesperance J, Bourassa MG: Exercise electrocardiography

and myocardial scintigraphy in the serial evaluation of the results of percutaneous transluminal coronary angioplasty. Circulation 1982;66:380–390.

27. Manyari DE, Knudtson M, Kloiber R, Roth D: Sequential thallium-201 myocardial perfusion studies after successful percutaneous transluminal coronary artery angioplasty: Delayed resolution of exercise-induced scintigraphic abnormalities. Circulation 1988;77:86–95.

27a. Suryapranata H, Zijlstra F, MacLeod DC, van den Brand M, de Feyter PJ, Surruys PW: Predictive value of reactive hyperemic response on reperfusion on recovery of regional myocardial function after coronary angioplasty in acute myocardial infarction. Circulation 1994;89:1109–1117.

28. Lim YL, Okada RD, Chesler DA, Block PC, Boucher CA, Pohost GM: A new approach to quantitation of exercise thallium-201 scintigraphy before and after an intervention: Application to define the impact of coronary angioplasty on regional myocardial perfusion. Am Heart J 1984;108:917–925.

29. Kanemoto N, Hor G: Improvement of regional myocardial perfusion following percutaneous transluminal coronary angioplasty in patients with coronary artery disease. Jpn Heart J 1985;26:495–508.

30. Depuey E, Roubin G, Cloninger K, et al.: Correlation of transluminal coronary angioplasty parameters and quantification thallium-201 tomography. J Invasive Cardiol 1988;1:40–49.

30a. Heller L, Villegas B, Weiner B, McSherry B, Dahlberg S, Leppo J: Sequential teboroxime imaging during and after balloon occlusion of a coronary artery. J Am Coll Cardiol 1993;21:1319–1327.

30b. Haronian H, Remetz M, Sinusas A, Baron J, Miller H, Cleman M, Zaret B, Wackers B: Myocardial risk area defined by technetium-99m sestamibi imaging during percutaneous transluminal coronary angiography. J Am Coll Cardiol 1993;22:1033–1043.

30c. Borges-Neta S, Puma J, Jones RH, Sketch MH, Stack R, Hanson MW, Coleman RE: Myocardial perfusion and ventricular function measurements during total coronary artery occlusion in humans: A comparison with rest and exercise radionuclide studies. Circulation 1994;89:278–284.

30d. Miller DD, Verani MS: Current status of myocardial perfusion imaging after percutaneous transluminal coronary angioplasty. J Am Coll Cardiol 1994;24:260–266.

31. Stuckey TD, Burwell LR, Nygaard TW, Gibson RS, Watson DD, Beller GA: Quantitative exercise thallium-201 scintigraphy for predicting angina recurrence after percutaneous transluminal coronary angioplasty. Am J Cardiol 1989;63:517–521.

32. Wijns W, Serruys PW, Reiber JH, de Feyter PJ, van den Brand M, Simoons ML, Hugenholtz PG: Early detection of restenosis after successful percutaneous transluminal coronary angioplasty by exercise-redistribution thallium scintigraphy. Am J Cardiol 1985;55:357–361.

33. Renkin J, Melin J, Robert A, Richelle F, Bachy JL, Col J, Detry JM, Wijns W: Detection of restenosis after successful coronary angioplasty: Improved clinical decision making with use of a logistic model combining procedural and follow-up variables. J Am Coll Cardiol 1990;16:1333–1340.

34. Breisblatt WM, Barnes JV, Weiland F, Spaccavento LJ: Incomplete revascularization in multivessel percutaneous transluminal coronary angioplasty: The role for stress thallium-201 imaging. J Am Coll Cardiol 1988;11:1183–1190.

35. Miller DD, Liu P, Strauss HW, Block PC, Okada RD, Boucher CA: Prognostic value of computer-quantitated exercise thallium imaging early after percutaneous transluminal coronary angioplasty. J Am Coll Cardiol 1987;10:275–283.

36. Cloninger KG, DePuey EG, Garcia EV, Roubin GS, Robbins WL, Nody A, DePasquale EE, Berger HJ: Incomplete redistribution in delayed thallium-201 single photon emission computed tomographic (SPECT) images: An overestimation of myocardial scarring. J Am Coll Cardiol 1988;12:955–963.

37. Hecht HS, Shaw RE, Bruce TR, Ryan C, Stertzer SH, Myler RK: Usefulness of tomographic thallium-201 imaging for detection of restenosis after percutaneous transluminal coronary angioplasty. Am J Cardiol 1990;66:1314–1318.

37a. Gordon PC, Friedrich SP, Piana RN, et al.: Is 40% to 70% diameter narrowing at the site of previous stenting or directional coronary atherectomy clinically significant? Am J Cardiol 1994;74:26–32.

38. Hecht HS, Shaw RE, Chin HL, Ryan C, Stertzer SH, Myler RK: Silent ischemia after coronary angioplasty: Evaluation of restenosis and extent of ischemia in asymptomatic patients by tomographic thallium-201 exercise imaging and comparison with symptomatic patients. J Am Coll Cardiol 1991;17:670–677.

38a. Pfisterer M, Rickenbacher P, Kiowski W, Müller-Brand J, Burkart F: Silent ischemia after percutaneous transluminal coronary angioplasty: Incidence and prognostic significance. J Am Coll Cardiol 1993; 22:1446–1454.

39. Breisblatt WM, Barnes JV, Weiland F, Spaccavento LJ: Incomplete revascularization in multivessel percutaneous transluminal coronary angioplasty: The role for stress thallium-201 imaging. J Am Coll Cardiol 1988;11:1183–1190.

39a. Marie PY, Danchin N, Karcher G, Grentzinger A, Juillière Y, Olivier P, Buffet P, Anconina J, Beurrier D, Cherrier F, Bertrand A: Usefulness of exercise SPECT-thallium to detect asymptomatic restenosis in patients who had angina before coronary angioplasty. Am Heart J 1993;126:571–577.

39b. Beregi J-P, Bauters C, McFadden EP, Quandalle P, Bertrand ME, Lablanche J-M: Exercise-induced ST-segment depression in patients without restenosis after coronary angioplasty: Relation to preprocedural impaired left ventricular function. Circulation 1994;90:148–155.

40. Reed DC, Beller GA, Nygaard TW, Tedesco C, Watson DD, Burwell LR: The clinical efficacy and scintigraphic evaluation of post–coronary bypass patients undergoing percutaneous transluminal coronary angioplasty for recurrent angina pectoris. Am Heart J 1989;117:60–71.

40a. Uren NG, Crake T, Lefroy DC, de Silva R, Davies GJ, Maseri A: Delayed recovery of coronary resistive vessel function after coronary angioplasty. J Am Coll Cardiol 1993;21:612–621.

41. Jones EL, Craver JM, Hurst JW, Bradford JA, Bone DK, Robinson PH, Cobbs BW, Thompkins TR, Hatcher CR Jr: Influence of left ventricular aneurysm on survival following the coronary bypass operation. Ann Surg 1981;193:733–742.

42. Kronenberg MW, Pederson RW, Harston WE, Born ML, Bender HW Jr, Friesinger GC: Left ventricular performance after coronary artery bypass surgery. Prediction of functional benefit. Ann Intern Med 1983;99:305–313.

43. Lim YL, Kalff V, Kelly MJ, Mason PJ, Currie PJ, Harper RW, Anderson ST, Federman J, Stirling GR, Pitt A: Radionuclide angiographic assessment of global and segmental left ventricular function at rest and during exercise after coronary artery bypass graft surgery. Circulation 1982;66:972–979.

44. Kent KM, Borer JS, Green MV, Bacharach SL, McIntosh CL, Conkle DM, Epstein SE: Effects of coronary-artery bypass on global and regional left ventricular function during exercise. N Engl J Med 1978;298:1434–1439.

45. DePuey EG, Leatherman LL, Leachman RD, Dear WE, Massin EK, Mathur VS, Burdine JA: Restenosis after transluminal coronary angioplasty detected with exercise-gated radionuclide ventriculography. J Am Coll Cardiol 1984;4:1103–1113.

46. Kanemoto N, Hor G, Kober G, Maul FD, Klepzig H Jr, Standke R, Kaltenbach M: Noninvasive assessment of left ventricular performance following transluminal coronary angioplasty. Int J Cardiol 1983;3:281–294.

46a. Mertes H, Erbel R, Nixdorff U, Mohr-Kahaly S, Kruger S, Meyer J: Exercise echocardiography for the evaluation of patients after nonsurgical coronary artery revascularization. J Am Coll Cardiol 1993;21:1087–1093.

46b. Hecht HS, DeBord L, Shaw R, Dunlap R, Ryan C, Stertzer SH, Myler RK: Usefulness of supine bicycle stress echocardiography for detection of restenosis after percutaneous transluminal coronary angioplasty. Am J Cardiol 1993;71:293–296.

47. Eichhorn EJ, Konstam MA, Salem DN, Isner JM, Deckelbaum L, Stransky NB, Metherall JA, Toltzis HI: Dipyridamole thallium-201 imaging pre- and post-coronary angioplasty for assessment of regional myocardial ischemia in humans. Am Heart J 1989;117:1203–1209.

47a. Pirelli S, Danzi GB, Massa D, Piccalo G, Faletra F, Cannizzaro G, Sarullo F, Picano E, De Vita C, Campolo L: Exercise thallium scintigraphy versus high-dose dipyridamole echocardiography testing for detection of asymptomatic restenosis in patients with positive exercise tests after coronary angioplasty. Am J Cardiol 1993;71:1052–1056.

48. Jain A, Mahmarian JJ, Borges-Neto S, Johnston DL, Cashion WR, Lewis JM, Raizner AE, Verani MS: Clinical significance of perfusion defects by thallium-201 single photon emission tomography following oral dipyridamole early after coronary angioplasty. J Am Coll Cardiol 1988;11:970–976.

49. Akosah KO, Porter TR, Simon R, Funai JT, Minisi AJ, Mohanty PK: Ischemia-induced regional wall motion abnormality is improved after coronary angioplasty: Demonstration by dobutamine stress echocardiography. J Am Coll Cardiol 1993;21:584–589.

Chapter 11

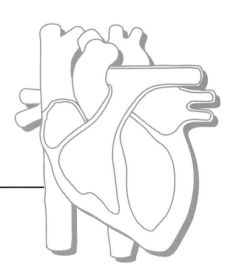

Radionuclide Imaging in Noncoronary and Congenital Heart Disease

MYOCARDIAL PERFUSION ABNORMALITIES IN NONCORONARY HEART DISEASE

Myocardial perfusion abnormalities associated with noncoronary cardiovascular disorders may lead to a misdiagnosis of coronary artery disease (CAD). Table 11–1 lists some of the noncoronary conditions in which thallium-201 (Tl-201) scintigraphy revealed perfusion abnormalities.

Hypertrophic Cardiomyopathy

Tl-201 scintigraphy can occasionally assist in the detection of septal hypertrophy in patients with presumed idiopathic hypertrophic subaortic stenosis.[1] A ratio of septum to left ventricular (LV) free wall thickness of 1.7 has been observed in patients with asymmetric septal hypertrophy. In normal volunteers and in patients with concentric LV hypertrophy, this ratio is approximately 1.0. A significant percentage of patients with hypertrophic cardiomyopathy demonstrate focal stress-induced perfusion abnormalities on Tl-201 scintigraphy.[2–5] Perfusion abnormalities were observed in all regions of the left ventricle, though persistent Tl-201 defects were predominantly observed in segments of the LV wall that were normal or showed mildly increased thickness.[2] In contrast, a great proportion of the redistribution defects in patients with hypertrophic cardio-

myopathy were detected in areas of moderate-to-marked wall thickness. Patients with perfusion defects showing complete redistribution had normal or hyperdynamic LV systolic function, whereas the majority of patients with persistent defects or partial redistribution had a subnormal LV ejection fraction (LVEF).

Cannon et al.[3] found that reversible Tl-201 abnormalities during stress are markers of myocardial ischemia in patients

Table 11–1. Abnormal Tl-201 Scintigrams in Noncoronary Cardiac Disease

Hypertrophic cardiomyopathy with normal epicardial coronary arteries
Progressive systemic sclerosis with diffuse scleroderma
Hypertensive heart disease
Diabetic heart disease with normal coronary arteries
Duchenne-type muscular dystrophy
Myocarditis
Nonischemic dilated cardiomyopathy
Left bundle branch block with normal coronary arteries
Anomalous left coronary artery arising from the pulmonary artery
Myocardial sarcoidosis
Cardiac lymphoma
Sickle cell anemia
Coarctation of the aorta
Thickened interventricular septum on 45-degree left anterior oblique view in hypertrophic subaortic stenosis
Increased right ventricular Tl-201 activity in pulmonary hypertension

(Beller GA: Myocardial perfusion imaging with thallium-201. *In* Marcus M, et al (eds): Cardiac Imaging, ed 3. Philadelphia, WB Saunders, 1991, pp 1047–1073.)

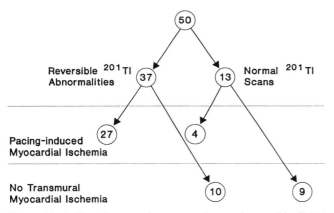

Figure 11–1. Flow diagram shows prevalence of reversible Tl-201 defects in association with myocardial ischemia determined by great cardiac vein lactate levels during pacing stress in 50 patients with hypertrophic cardiomyopathy. (Cannon RO, et al.: Circulation 1991;83:1660–1667.)

with hypertrophic cardiomyopathy. Of 50 patients with hypertrophic cardiomyopathy undergoing exercise scintigraphy, 74% had inducible defects that normalized after 3 hours of rest. Twenty-six patients had apparent LV cavity dilatation with exercise. Of the 37 patients with reversible Tl-201 defects, 73% had metabolic evidence of myocardial ischemia during rapid atrial pacing as determined by measurement of coronary sinus lactate levels. Patients with an ischemic ST-segment response to exercise had an 80% prevalence of reversible Tl-201 defects and a 70% prevalence of pacing-induced lactate abnormalities. Figure 11–1 shows the prevalence of reversible Tl-201 defects and association with lactate criteria for pacing-induced ischemia in the 50 patients with hypertrophic cardiomyopathy who constituted this study cohort. Patients with hypertrophic cardiomyopathy and exertional chest pain were found to

have less total 3-hour washout of Tl-201 after dipyridamole scintigraphy than did those without chest pain. Patients with chest pain also showed greater maximal LV wall thickness than those without chest pain (27 ± 7 vs 23 ± 7mm; $P = 0.03$), and there was a weak inverse correlation between regional Tl-201 washout and wall thickness. This finding may reflect altered coronary flow dynamics in hypertrophic myocardium in this patient population in the absence of stenosis in the large coronary vessels. Dilsizian et al.[3a] studied the relationship between ischemia on electrocardiographic (ECG) monitoring and Tl-201 scintigraphy and the incidence of ventricular tachycardia, cardiac arrest, or syncope in patients with hypertrophic cardiomyopathy. They found that sudden cardiac arrest or syncope is frequently related to ischemia rather than to "primary arrhythmogenic substrate" as determined by inducibility of ventricular tachycardia on programmed electrical stimulation in the electrophysiology laboratory. In this study, anti-ischemia therapy improved regional Tl-201 uptake in seven of eight patients (88%), three of whom showed reversion to normal Tl-201 studies. Figure 11–2 shows Tl-201 tomograms before and after verapamil therapy in a patient from this study; a marked diminution in exercise-induced Tl-201 perfusion defects was observed after verapamil therapy. Udelson et al.[5a] showed a marked reduction in redistribution defects with verapamil therapy in 10 of 14 patients with hypertrophic cardiomyopathy, as compared with the pretreatment exercise Tl-201 scintigrams.[5a]

Surgical relief of ventricular outflow obstruction in patients with obstructive hypertrophic cardiomyopathy can result in normalization or improvement of myocardial perfusion in the majority of patients with reversible and fixed Tl-201 defects.[4] Figure 11–3 shows an example of normalization of exercise-induced perfusion defects after septal myectomy in a patient in this study.

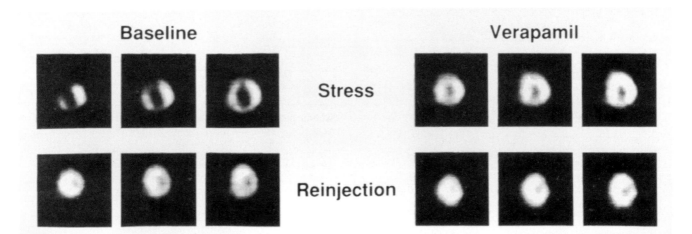

Figure 11–2. Tl-201 SPECT tomograms at baseline and after verapamil therapy in a patient with hypertrophic cardiomyopathy. Before verapamil, the left panel shows exercise-induced perfusion defects in the anterior, septal, and inferior regions that normalize after Tl-201 reinjection. After verapamil therapy, perfusion during stress and after reinjection improved. (Reprinted with permission from the American College of Cardiology (Journal of the American College of Cardiology, 1993, Vol. 22, pp. 796–804).)

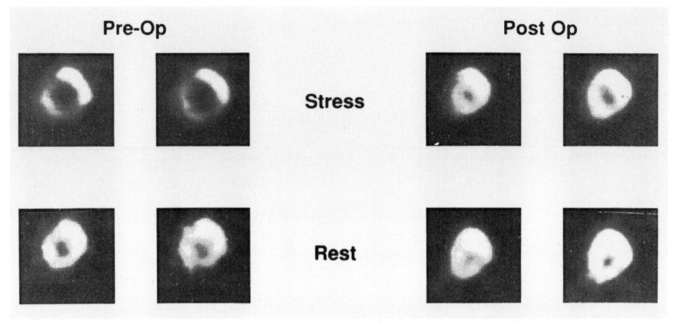

Figure 11–3. Preoperative (pre-op) and postoperative (post-op) SPECT short-axis images with stress and after rest in a patient with hypertrophic cardiomyopathy who demonstrated a 100-mm Hg basal gradient across the aortic outflow track. After septal myectomy and relief of this gradient, perfusion defects after exercise resolved. (Cannon RO, et al.: Circulation 1992;85:1039–1045.)

The configuration of the hypertrophic myocardium has also been assessed by single-photon emission computed tomography (SPECT) Tl-201 imaging. Ventricular septal wall thickness has been observed to increase with an increased septum-to–posterior wall Tl-201 activity ratio of 1.45.[6] Abnormalities of ventricular systolic and diastolic function in hypertrophic cardiomyopathy can be detected by gated radionuclide angiography.[6a–6e] The peak filling rate and time to peak filling, indices of diastolic function, are reduced in hypertrophic cardiomyopathy, and they improve in response to verapamil therapy. Iodine-123–metaiodobenzylguanidine (MIBG) imaging of cardiac sympathetic nerve terminals (see Chap. 2) has been used to evaluate patients with hypertrophic cardiomyopathy.[6f, 6g] Nakajima et al.[6f] found enhanced MIBG clearance in zones of increased myocardial thickness (more than 20 mm), which was attributed to damage to the sympathetic nervous system. I-123 MIBG is diffusely reduced in patients with idiopathic dilated cardiomyopathy, and this correlates with the diminution in LVEF.[6h] When patients enter the dilated phase of hypertrophic cardiomyopathy, evidence for cellular necrosis is observed on In-111 antimyosin imagery.[6i] Fatty acid utilization as assessed by Iodine-123–labeled beta-methyl–branched fatty acid (I-123-BMIPP) imaging was shown to be impaired in patients with hypertrophic cardiomyopathy.[6j]

Progressive Systemic Sclerosis and Scleroderma

Myocardial perfusion abnormalities have been observed in progressive systemic sclerosis and diffuse scleroderma.[7–11]

Approximately half of scleroderma patients have Tl-201 redistribution defects, and more show persistent defects.[8] Findings with coronary angiography in such patients usually are within normal limits. A disturbance of the myocardial microcirculation has been hypothesized to be the underlying pathophysiologic cause of myocardial perfusion abnormalities in progressive systemic sclerosis with diffuse scleroderma.[11] Nitenberg et al.,[11] who assessed maximal coronary vasodilation capacity after intravenous dipyridamole in seven patients with scleroderma, found that coronary reserve, measured as the dipyridamole–basal coronary sinus flow ratio, was 2.54 ± 1.37 in the scleroderma group, as compared with 4.01 ± 0.56 ($P < 0.05$) in the control subjects. This decrease in coronary flow reserve was not explained by an alteration of LV function. Both right ventricular (RV) and LV dysfunction have been observed in this disease, suggesting ischemia-induced injury. Figure 11–4 shows the resting LVEF plotted against Tl-201 defect size in patients with diffuse scleroderma in studies by Follansbee et al.[8] The group with Tl-201 defect scores above the median had a significantly lower mean LVEF than did the group with a lesser amount of hypoperfusion by Tl-201 scan criteria. Some patients with systemic sclerosis and scleroderma show cold-induced redistribution defects and reversible systolic function abnormalities.[7] Cold exposure could cause reflex coronary constriction, resulting in reversible ischemia.

Hypertension

Hypertensive patients who have a low pretest likelihood of CAD are more likely to have abnormal Tl-201 test re-

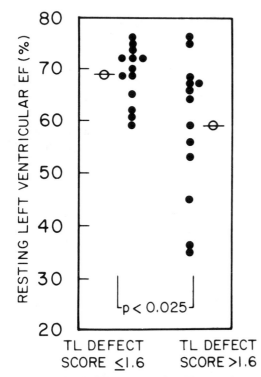

Figure 11–4. Resting LVEF plotted against Tl-201 defect size in 26 patients with progressive systemic sclerosis with diffuse scleroderma. (Reprinted by permission of *The New England Journal of Medicine* from Follansbee WP, et al.: N Engl J Med 1984;310:142–148. Copyright 1984, Massachusetts Medical Society.)

sults than their normotensive counterparts.[12] Schulman et al.[12] showed that 29% of hypertensive patients who had little likelihood of CAD had abnormal Tl-201 scans whereas 7% of their normotensive counterparts did. Hypertension may independently produce myocardial changes and changes in perfusion that are detected on myocardial perfusion imaging. Abnormal coronary vascular reserve in hypertension patients may play a role in the scan abnormalities observed. Results of a study by Tubeau et al.[13] showed that Tl-201 scintigraphic perfusion defects were observed in 20% of symptomatic patients with hypertension and LV hypertrophy. Seventy-five percent of the patients with an abnormal scan or abnormal computerized treadmill exercise score developed typical angina pectoris during follow-up. Thus, there are some asymptomatic patients with hypertension and LV hypertrophy whose stress-induced Tl-201 scan abnormalities do not represent a false-positive result but perhaps represent abnormal flow reserve in the presence of mild to moderate stenoses. Wasserman et al.[14] found that hypertensive patients without CAD did not exhibit a significant increase in LVEF from resting values during exercise, and slightly less than a third developed a stress-induced regional wall motion abnormality (Fig. 11–5). These findings are consistent with those described above for abnormal flow reserve in hypertensive patients during exercise stress.

Our own experience has not borne out a significant false-positive rate for exercise perfusion imaging in patients with hypertension. More often, such patients have false-positive ischemic ST-segment responses with normal myocardial perfusion scans.

Diabetes

Certain diabetes patients may demonstrate abnormal myocardial perfusion on Tl-201 scintigrams who do not have significant large-vessel CAD.[15–19] Microcirculatory dysfunction or noncoronary pathologic abnormalities may be the explanation for abnormal Tl-201 scintigrams in this group of diabetics.[15] Diabetes patients with CAD have a higher prevalence of painless abnormal Tl-201 scintigrams consistent with ischemia than do nondiabetics.[16] Koistinen et al.[17] performed exercise SPECT Tl-201 imaging in 136 diabetes patients who had no symptoms of heart disease. Of these, 33 had stress perfusion defects and 19 had ST-segment depression of at least 1.0 mm. For 13 patients both test results were positive. Of the patients undergoing catheterization, many had angiographically normal coronary arteries, yielding a positive predictive value of the Tl-201 scan of only 48%. The authors speculated that some of these "false-positive" scans for CAD might have been due to disease of the small intramyocardial arteries.

Left Bundle Branch Block

Certain patients with left bundle branch block (LBBB) are evaluated by stress Tl-201 scintigraphy for possible CAD. The exercise ECG cannot be diagnostic in such patients. A substantial number of patients with LBBB and angiographically normal coronary arteries can demonstrate ab-

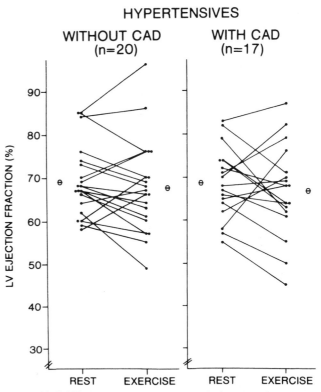

Figure 11–5. EF at rest and with exercise in hypertensive patients with and without CAD. (Reprinted by permission of *The New England Journal of Medicine* from Wasserman AG, et al.: N Engl J Med 1984;311: 1276–1280. Copyright 1984, Massachusetts Medical Society.)

normal myocardial perfusion on exercise scintigraphy.[20–29a] Most often, these perfusion defects are localized to the intraventricular septum and do not show delayed redistribution.

Rothbart et al.[23] evaluated the diagnostic and prognostic value of exercise Tl-201 scintigraphy in 74 consecutive patients with LBBB who were being evaluated for possible CAD. Only 18 (24%) had a normal quantitative planar perfusion scan by quantitative criteria. Catheterization was performed in 22 patients for clinical indications, and abnormal scans were observed in 91%, 19 of whom had defects in the territory of the left anterior descending (LAD) coronary artery. Only 10 of these 22 patients who underwent catheterization had significant CAD. All had abnormal scintigrams. Six catheterized patients had nonischemic cardiomyopathy with angiographically normal coronary arteries. Of major interest, though, were the six totally normal patients, four of whom demonstrated redistribution defects in the LAD scan segments despite normal coronary angiograms. Figure 11–6 shows the quantitative planar scintigraphic data from a patient with LBBB and angiographically normal coronary arteries from this study by Rothbart et al.[23] A septal redistribution defect is observed.

The entire cohort of 74 patients were separated on the basis of presence (group I) or the absence (group II) of clinical or catheterization evidence of heart disease (Table 11–2). Abnormal scintigrams were seen in 95% of group I patients and in 56% of group II patients. Group I patients had a higher prevalence of multivessel scan abnormalities, LV dilatation, and increased lung Tl-201 uptake than group II patients. During 22 ± 16 months' follow-up, 11 patients from group I, but none from group II, experienced sudden death or myocardial infarction (MI) or underwent coronary bypass surgery. When all Tl-201 scintigraphic variables and the presence versus the absence of overt heart disease were entered into a stepwise discriminate function analysis, the only significant predictors of adverse outcome were clinically overt heart disease and increased lung Tl-201 uptake.

In another study by Matzer et al.,[29] the accuracy for detection of LAD disease in patients with LBBB was significantly better when an apical defect was used as a criterion for the disease rather than septal or anterior defects. In this SPECT Tl-201 study, anterior and septal defects were common in patients with LBBB without CAD. Larcos et al.[25] sought to validate whether abnormal apical or anterior perfusion abnormalities on exercise Tl-201 scintigraphy could increase the diagnostic accuracy for detection of LAD disease in patients with LBBB. By receiver-operating characteristics analysis, a fixed or reversible defect in the apex was the best criterion for detection of LAD disease. Although an apical defect was highly sensitive, it was neither specific nor accurate. Perfusion abnormalities in the anterior wall and septum were also of limited diagnostic accuracy. By quantitative criteria, although the sensitivity of an apical defect was 93% for CAD detection in patients with LBBB, specificity was only 19% and accuracy 55%. Tawahara et

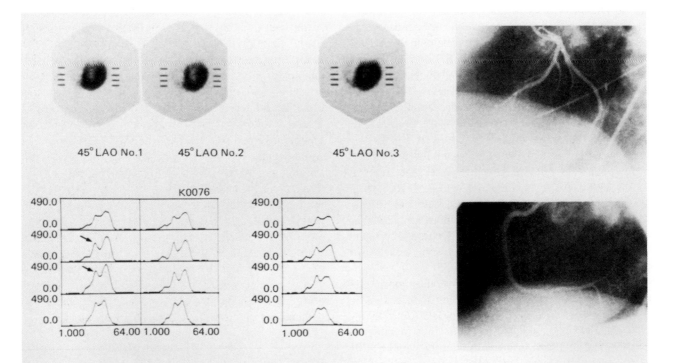

Figure 11–6. Forty-five–degree left anterior oblique (LAO) Tl-201 scintigrams at 10 minutes (no. 1), 1 hour (no. 2), and 2½ hours (no. 3) after exercise showing a septal redistribution defect. The horizontal quantitative count profiles are shown beneath each image, the arrow pointing to the decrease in Tl-201 counts in the midseptum. The patient had left bundle branch block and angiographically normal coronary arteries *(right)*. (Rothbart R, et al.: Am J Noninvas Cardiol 1987;1:197–205.)

Table 11–2. Frequency of Tl-201 Scintigraphic Findings Based on Presence or Absence of Clinically Overt Cardiovascular Disease in Patients with Left Bundle Branch Block

	Clinical Disease		
	Present (N = 38) Group I (No.) (%)	Absent (N = 36) Group II (No.) (%)	P Value*
Any Tl-201 defect	36 (95)	20 (56)	<0.001
LV dilatation	12 (32)	0 (0)	<0.001
Abnormal lung uptake of Tl-201	10 (26)	1 (3)	<0.007
Multivessel scintigraphic pattern	15 (39)	3 (8)	<0.02
Redistribution	27 (71)	17 (47)	<0.06

*Fisher's exact test.
(Rothbart R, et al.: Am J Noninvas Cardiol 1987;1:197–205.)

al.[27] assessed the specificity of SPECT imaging for CAD detection in patients with LBBB. Specificity was 30% compared to 94% in patients with normal intraventricular conduction. In contrast, no significant difference in specificity was observed in patients with right bundle branch block (RBBB) or Wolff-Parkinson-White syndrome and in those with normal conduction. As expected, defects were seen in anterior, septal, and inferior segments in patients with LBBB and in the septal and inferior segments in patients with RBBB and left-axis deviation despite absence of coronary stenoses.

Dipyridamole Tl-201 scintigraphy may be more specific than exercise scintigraphy for detection of CAD.[29a–29e] Burns et al.[29a] reported 100% sensitivity and 90% specificity for dipyridamole SPECT Tl-201 imaging for CAD detection and 83% and 20%, respectively, for exercise imaging. Rockett et al.[29b] found normal dipyridamole SPECT Tl-201 scans in 14 of 19 patients with LBBB. Morais et al.[29c] found fewer false-positive Tl-201 scans in patients with LBBB employing dipyridamole stress than exercise stress. O'Keefe and coworkers studied 173 consecutive LBBB patients who underwent either exercise (N = 56) or adenosine (N = 117) Tl-201 scintigraphy.[29d] The overall predictive accuracy was 93% in the adenosine group and 68% in the exercise group (P = 0.01). Specificity for septal defects was 42% with exercise as compared with 82% for adenosine stress imaging (P < 0.0002). Thus, these studies suggest that vasodilator stress imaging is more accurate than exercise imaging in patients with LBBB because of better specificity for detecting coronary stenosis in vessels that supply the interventricular septum.

The mechanism for myocardial perfusion abnormalities in the interventricular septum in patients with LBBB in angiographically normal coronary arteries is unclear. In one study,[21] electrical induction of LBBB in dogs in most instances resulted in a comparable reduction in septal Tl-201 uptake. The investigators suggested that these septal defects in the presence of LBBB may reflect functional ischemia caused by asynchronous septal contraction. Ono et al.[28] showed diminished Tl-201 activity in the septum in open-chest dogs undergoing RV pacing. In that study, fluorine-18–labeled 2-fluoro-2-deoxyglucose was reduced in the septum, as compared with the free wall of the left ventricle. Regional flow was 0.53 ml/min/g in the septum and 0.84 ml/min/g in the free wall. These findings were associated with diminished systolic septal thickening. Thus, LBBB, by itself, may reduce regional perfusion and metabolism in the septum because of impaired systolic contraction.

Coronary Artery Anomalies

Perfusion abnormalities can be found in the anterolateral wall in patients with anomalous origin of the left coronary artery arising from the pulmonary artery.[30–35a] After surgery, there may be improvement in anterior wall myocardial perfusion, but most often persistent defects remain postoperatively, since myocardial fibrosis is usually present. Manier et al.[35] reported a case of a 3½-month-old patient with an anomalous left coronary artery arising from the pulmonary artery who presented with ECG and scintigraphic evidence of an anterolateral wall infarction, which almost completely resolved following surgical revision. Figure 11–7 shows preoperative and postoperative SPECT Tl-201 images in an adult patient, reported by Anguenot et al.,[32] who had an anomalous left coronary artery arising from the pulmonary trunk. This patient was treated with reimplantation of the left coronary artery to the aorta. Postoperatively, a marked improvement in Tl-201 uptake was noted in anterior regions where persistent defects were seen on preoperative scans. Kawakami et al.[36] found transient perfusion defects on Tl-201 scans in 40% of patients with multiple arteriovenous connections. Postoperative Tl-201 imaging may be useful in assessing the results of surgical repair of hemodynamically significant coronary artery anomalies.[37]

Right Ventricular Thallium-201 Imaging

Imaging of the RV myocardium can be accomplished with Tl-201 scintigraphy. Several groups have shown exercise-induced transient defects in the right ventricle on serial

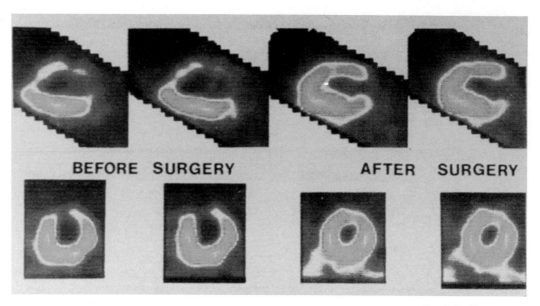

See Color Figure 11–7.

Figure 11–7. Pre- and postoperative Tl-201 SPECT images in a patient with an anomalous left coronary artery arising from the pulmonary trunk. The vertical long-axis slices *(upper row)* and the short-axis slices *(bottom row)* demonstrate reduced tracer uptake in the septum and the anterior wall before surgery. The postoperative images show resolution of these defects. (See Color Figure 11–7.) (Reprinted by permission of the Society of Nuclear Medicine from Anguenot TJ, et al.: J Nucl Med 1991;32:1788–1790.)

redistribution imaging. This is most often associated with a high-grade right coronary artery stenosis.[38, 39] RV overloading has been successfully detected by Tl-201 scintigraphy (Fig. 11–8). With pressure overload, the degree of RV Tl-201 visualization correlates with elevation of RV systolic pressure.[40] Normally, in the absence of heart failure or RV overload, the RV free wall is not visualized at rest with Tl-201 imaging. When pulmonary hypertension develops, the RV free wall becomes visualized on resting perfusion images. Figure 11–8 shows prominent RV Tl-201 uptake in a

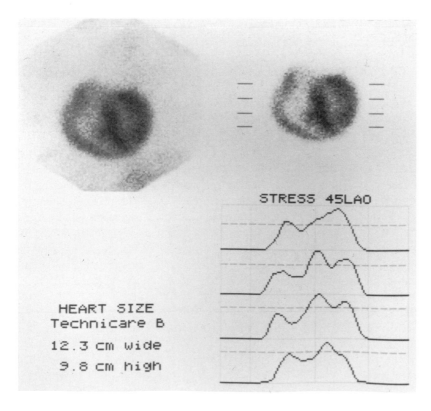

STRESS 45LAO

HEART SIZE
Technicare B
12.3 cm wide
9.8 cm high

Figure 11–8. A stress 45-degree left anterior oblique (LAO) Tl-201 scintigram in a patient with an atrial septal defect. Note the enlarged right ventricle and prominent tracer uptake in the right ventricular myocardium. The quantitative horizontal count profiles are shown below the background-subtracted image.

patient with an atrial septal defect and a left-to-right shunt who underwent exercise scintigraphy. RV Tl-201 uptake is prominently identified after MI complicated by congestive heart failure.[41]

The RV-LV average count ratio is a good predictor of RV-LV pressure ratio ($r = 0.91$) in patients with either an atrial septal defect, ventricular septal defect, tetralogy of Fallot, or a double outlet right ventricle.[42] The data from this study are summarized in Figure 11–9. Wackers et al.[43] found that RV visualization at rest on Tl-201 images does not necessarily indicate RV hypertrophy but may be due to an acute increase in RV workload.

Dilated Cardiomyopathy

Tl-201 imaging has been undertaken in conjunction with resting radionuclide angiography or echocardiography in the assessment of patients with cardiomegaly and severe

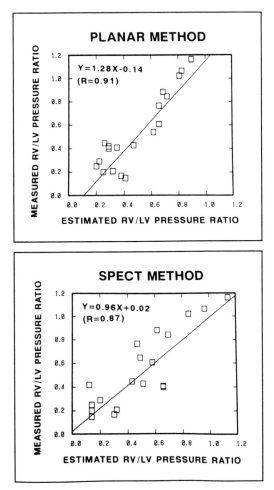

Figure 11–9. Predictability of the right ventricular (RV) and left ventricular (LV) count ratio (horizontal axis) for estimating the RV-LV pressure ratio (vertical axis) in children with congenital heart disease. The planar method results are shown in the upper panel, and the SPECT method is shown in the lower panel. (Reprinted by permission of the Society of Nuclear Medicine from Nakajima K, et al.: J Nucl Med 1991;32:2215–2220.)

congestive heart failure.[44–48] The combined approach may be useful for distinguishing ischemic cardiomyopathy from idiopathic dilated cardiomyopathy. Figure 11–10 shows end-diastolic and end-systolic images in a patient with a nonischemic cardiomyopathy. There is symmetrical decrease in LV function with global hypokinesis. Tl-201 scintigrams in patients with ischemic cardiomyopathy most often have defects involving more than 40% of the circumference of the LV image, which corresponds well to the segmental wall motion abnormalities observed on radionuclide angiography or echocardiography. Patients with dilated congestive cardiomyopathy usually show relatively homogeneous, albeit reduced, Tl-201 uptake in a thin-walled ventricle or have defects less than 20% of the image circumference. Some patients with dilated cardiomyopathy have more focal-type defects, particularly involving the apex, despite having normal coronary arterics (Fig. 11–11). Patients with the greatest extent of hypoperfusion with dilated cardiomyopathy have the lowest survival rate.[48] Death from progressive heart failure tended to occur in patients with extensive perfusion defects. Tauberg et al. found that increased lung Tl-201 uptake occurs more frequently in ischemic than in idiopathic dilated cardiomyopathy.[47] Ninety percent of patients with ischemic cardiomyopathy had a large defect with severe reduction in Tl-201 uptake compared with 5% of idiopathic cardiomyopathy patients having a large, severe defect (Fig. 11–12).

In vivo PET imaging of myocardial concentration of beta receptors can be undertaken using the ligand carbon-11 (C-11) CGP-12177.[48a] In this study of 10 patients with idiopathic cardiomyopathy and heart failure, a 53% decrease in C-11 CGP was observed, as compared with imaging data obtained in 8 normal subjects. Beta-receptor concentration obtained by PET correlated well with receptor density determined from binding studies on myocardial biopsy samples. Decreased beta-receptor concentration by PET also correlated with contractile responsiveness to intracoronary dobutamine. The use of iodine-123–labeled metaiodobenzylguanidine (I-123 MIBG) to image adrenergic neurodensity in the myocardium is reviewed in Chapter 2. Reduced MIBG uptake has been observed in patients with heart failure and correlates with reduction in indices of left ventricular function.[48b]

Other Disorders

Resting Tl-201 defects have been reported in patients with myocardial sarcoidosis.[49] Patients with Duchenne's-type muscular dystrophy have been reported to demonstrate abnormalities in SPECT Tl-201 scintigrams. In one study,[50] SPECT Tl-201 scintigrams showed hypoperfusion in 90% of boys with Duchenne's-type dystrophy and in 61% of patients with either facioscapulohumeral, limb-girdle, or myotonic dystrophy. Multifocal Tl-201 defects have been observed in patients who present with clinically docu-

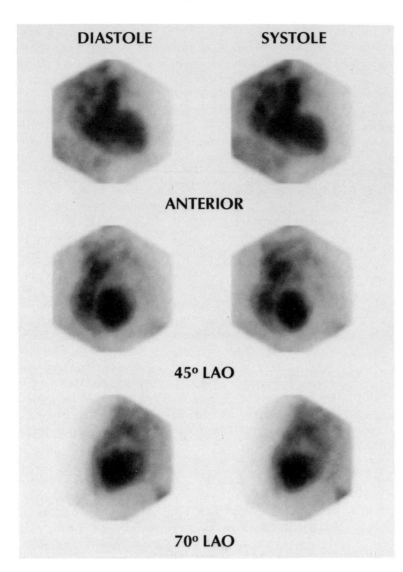

DIASTOLE SYSTOLE

ANTERIOR

45° LAO

70° LAO

Figure 11–10. End-diastolic *(left)* and end-systolic *(right)* equilibrium-gated cardiac blood pool scans in anterior, 45-degree left anterior oblique (LAO) and 70-degree LAO projections showing global hypokinesis of the left ventricle.

mented myocarditis, characterized by ECG abnormalities and elevation of cardiac enzymes.[51] These defects were observed at rest in the presence of angiographically normal coronary arteries. Many patients with Chagas' disease have chest pain as a prominent symptom. Reversible defects have been observed in myocardial zones demonstrating hypokinesis in patients with Chagas' heart disease[52]; however, the majority of perfusion defects are persistent and correspond to regions of severe asynergy where myocardial fibrosis is present. In a retrospective study by Hagar and Rahimtoola[53] in patients with Chagas' heart disease and no evidence for CAD, seven had exercise Tl-201 scan abnormalities and six showed reversible defects, suggesting ischemia. An LV aneurysm was found in 14 of the 25 pa-

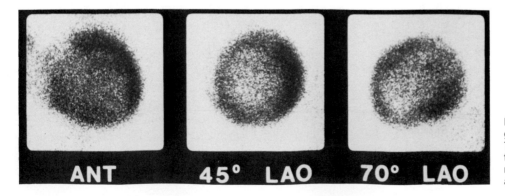

ANT 45° LAO 70° LAO

Figure 11–11. Anterior (ANT), 45-degree left anterior oblique (LAO), and 70-degree LAO Tl-201 images in a patient with a dilated nonischemic cardiomyopathy. Note the thinning of the apex and the interventricular septum.

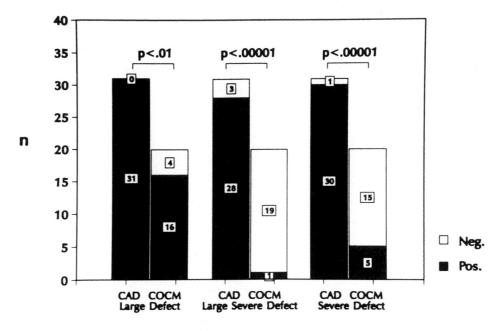

Figure 11–12. Distribution of defect size and varying defect severity in patients with either ischemic cardiomyopathy (CAD) or idiopathic cardiomyopathy (COCM). The height of each bar represents the number *(n)* of patients in that group. All patients with CAD had large defects, and in 90% these defects were also severe. Only 5% of patients with COCM had severe reduction in Tl-201 uptake *(center bars)*. (Key: Neg., negative test; Pos., positive test.) (Tauberg SG, et al.: Am J Cardiol 1993;71: 674–680.)

tients reviewed. Abnormal Tl-201 perfusion scans have also been reported in sickle-cell anemia,[54] Takayasu's arteritis,[55] blunt chest trauma,[56] Kawasaki's disease,[57] postoperative coarctation of the aorta,[58] and cardiac lymphoma.[59] Patients with mitral valve prolapse usually do not have focal perfusion abnormalities unless CAD is also present.[60, 61] Perfusion abnormalities have also been seen on SPECT Tc-99m sestamibi images obtained after anatomic correction (arterial switch procedure) for transposition of the great vessels.[61a] This procedure involves coronary artery mobilization and reimplantation, which may cause some myocardial flow alterations. Interestingly, these perfusion defects lessen with exercise,[61b] and exercise tolerance is not impaired.

RADIONUCLIDE ANGIOGRAPHY FOR ASSESSMENT OF ADULT CONGENITAL DISEASE AND RIGHT VENTRICULAR FUNCTION

Radionuclide Quantitation of Left-to-Right Cardiac Shunts

The quantitative determination of intracardiac shunts by radionuclide angiography was first introduced by Maltz and Treves.[62, 63a] The method involves determining the ratio of pulmonary to systemic blood flow (QP/QS) calculated from $A_1/(A_1 - A_2)$, where A_1 is defined as the integral of a gamma variate function fitted to the first-pass portion of the pulmonary time-activity curve and A_2 is the integral of a gamma variate fitted to the early recirculation peak. The recirculation peak is derived by subtracting the gamma variate fit from the observed pulmonary time-activity curve. This technique is based on the observation that intracardiac shunts greater than 30% of systemic blood flow can be

recognized on serial first-pass images by rapid normal transit of the technetium-99m (Tc-99m) tracer through the lungs and early reappearance of the tracer in right heart chambers distal to the site of the shunt. The tracer activity that is shunted deforms the exponential decline of counts, resulting in this second recirculation curve. The approach to quantitation of the left-to-right shunt using the tracer curves requires separation of the initial circulation of tracer from its subsequent transit through the lungs. The way the bolus of radioactivity is injected is very important, since a biphasic injection would be detrimental to shunt quantitation because the counts that reflect the initial transit must be separated from those that result from left-to-right shunt flow. Thus, bolus dispersion should be avoided. If the bolus disperses, either because of the technique of injection or because of hemodynamic abnormalities such as heart failure, the technique overestimates the shunt fraction. Deconvolution techniques for quantitative evaluation of QP/QS have been recommended.[64–66] Figure 11–13 shows a normal pulmonary time-activity curve and a pulmonary curve in a left-to-right shunt. Early pulmonary recirculation due to premature recirculation of radioactivity to the lungs via the shunt can be appreciated.

Madsen et al.[66] reported a new technique for quantifying QP/QS in left-to-right shunts. In this method, the gamma variate, which is fitted to the first-pass portion of the pulmonary curve, is used to generate a curve, which simulates the response curve of a normal lung with systemic recirculation. The difference between this curve and the observed lung curve is then used to calculate QP/QS. This method yielded QP/QS values in 30 patients referred for cardiac shunt studies that were more accurate and had less intraobserver variation than those obtained from the method of Maltz and Treves (Fig. 11–14). The authors state that their method is preferable, since in the Maltz and Treves method

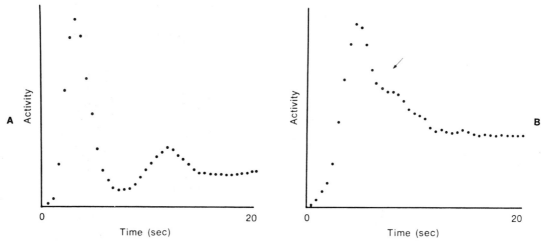

Figure 11–13. Pulmonary time-activity curves taken at 2 frames/second. **A.** Normal curve. **B.** Pulmonary curve and a left-to-right shunt. Note the early pulmonary recirculation *(arrow)* due to radiolabeled blood returning prematurely to the lungs. (Treves S, Parker A: Cardiovascular Nuclear Medicine, ed 2. St. Louis, CV Mosby, 1979, pp 148–161.)

there is often no clear demarcation to guide the selection of points for the second gamma variate fit. In the method of Madsen et al.,[66] only one gamma variate fit is required, and the accuracy of the QP/QS calculation depends on how well normal lung recirculation can be estimated.

An occasional patient with an undiagnosed left-to-right shunt is referred to the nuclear cardiology laboratory for symptoms of dyspnea and diminished exercise tolerance. A radionuclide angiogram in such a patient would demonstrate RV volume overload and a premature and discrete recirculation curve seen on the pulmonary time-activity downslope.

Right-to-Left Shunt Detection

Right-to-left shunts can also be recognized on radionuclide angiograms.[67, 68] Radioactive counts are detected in the aorta soon after tracer appears in the right side of the heart when a right-to-left shunt is present. Data to quantitate the shunt fraction are recorded from a site distant to the heart, such as the carotid arteries. This is because counts recorded from sites such as the ascending aorta may include counts scattered from the adjacent pulmonary artery. The systemic radionuclide curves measured in the carotid artery of patients with right-to-left shunts have configurations similar to those obtained with dye indicator dilution methods. In 20 children reported by Peter et al.,[67] right-to-left shunts determined by radionuclide angiographic data correlated well with the shunt measurements determined from the Fick data.

Jones[68] points out that the definition of the path of blood flow through the central circulation represents an important use of radionuclide angiography in congenital heart disease patients. Examples given are the demonstration of a persistent left superior vena cava in a patient with an atrial septal defect, evaluation of vena cava flow after Mustard repair of transposition of the great vessels, and definitions of relative flow to each lung after Fontan correction of tricuspid atresia.

Postoperative Evaluation

Postoperative studies may also provide valuable information on the adequacy of complete closure of septal de-

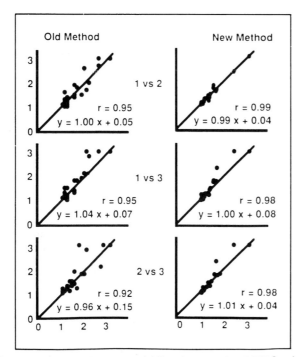

Figure 11–14. Interobserver variability plots showing QP/QS values obtained by three operators for the conventional old method *(left)* and the new method *(right)* for quantitation of left-to-right shunts. The top plot shows results of operator 1 vs. operator 2; the middle plot shows operator 1 vs. operator 3, and the bottom plot is operator 2 vs. operator 3. (Reprinted by permission of the Society of Nuclear Medicine from Madsen MT, et al.: J Nucl Med 1991;32:1808–1812.)

fects. Perhaps the most appropriate application of radionuclide angiography in congenital heart disease is in the long-term follow-up of patients with complex congenital heart disease who have undergone corrective surgery. Many of these patients now survive into adulthood. Some patients may have normal LV and RV function after operations for correcting complex congenital lesions but may still manifest subnormal responses to exercise stress. In some patients, the documentation of a deterioration in LV or RV function with exercise can explain symptoms of diminished exercise tolerance and dyspnea.[68a] Jones[68] points out that measurements of ventricular function during exercise may provide valuable insight into myocardial reserve capacity in children who have undergone surgically correction of a congenital heart disorder.

Assessment of Resting Right Ventricular Performance

Right Ventricular Infarction

Imaging the size and contraction pattern of the right ventricle is particularly useful for evaluating patients with acute inferior wall MI who exhibit signs of peripheral hypoperfusion.[69, 70] Patients with hemodynamically significant RV infarction show a depressed RVEF and RV dilatation, although the LVEF may be normal or only mildly reduced. The recognition of RV infarction as a cause of hypotension following an acute inferior MI has important therapeutic implications because in such instances rapid intravenous fluid administration, with or without dobutamine infusion, may be lifesaving, whereas diuretic therapy could be dangerous and life threatening.

Pulmonary Disease

Impairment of ventilatory function as a consequence of chronic obstructive pulmonary disease may result in respiratory symptoms that are indistinguishable from those seen in congestive heart failure. In chronic pulmonary disease without associated coronary valve or hypertensive disease, the LVEF is often normal and the dominant abnormality is seen with right-sided function.[71, 72] Figure 11–15 shows the RVEF and LVEF at rest and with submaximal exercise for 30 patients with chronic obstructive lung disease from the study of Berger et al.[71] RVEF failed to increase normally with exercise, although the LVEF response was unaltered. RV dysfunction is frequently seen at rest in patients with chronic obstructive lung disease, even without clinical or chest X-ray evidence of cor pulmonale. An abnormal RVEF appears to be predictive of the subsequent development of cor pulmonale and RV failure in chronic pulmonary disease patients. Thus, in a patient with primary impairment of ventilatory function, a normal LVEF and normal diastolic filling parameters on radionuclide angiography lead to the conclusion that the cause of dyspnea is most likely pulmo-

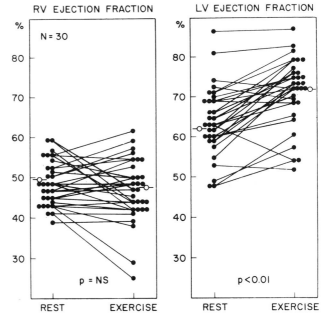

Figure 11–15. Right ventricular (RV) and left ventricular (LV) ejection fractions at rest and with submaximal exercise in 30 patients with chronic obstructive pulmonary disease. Mean values are shown at the sides of each panel. For the overall group, RV ejection fraction was unchanged with exercise, whereas LV ejection fraction increased normally. (Berger HJ, Matthay RA: Am J Cardiol 1981;47: 950–962.)

nary disease. Therapeutic measures aimed at reducing pulmonary vascular resistance would be indicated.

Radionuclide measurements of RVEF have been correlated by Koor et al. with hemodynamics on the right side of the heart as determined during catheterization.[73] These investigators found a significant linear correlation between RVEF and mean pulmonary artery pressure ($r = -0.82$; Fig. 11–16) and between RVEF and RV end-diastolic pressure ($r = -0.67$). Patients with elevated RV end-diastolic *and* mean pulmonary artery pressures had a more severely depressed RVEF than patients with elevated mean pulmonary artery pressure alone. Thus, these investigators concluded that an abnormal RVEF by radionuclide angiography in the absence of primary RV volume overload suggests abnormal right heart pressures, whereas a normal value excludes severe pulmonary artery hypertension or an elevated RV end-diastolic pressure.

Postoperative Assessment

RV performance during supine bicycle exercise was evaluated by gated equilibrium radionuclide angiography in 19 clinically well children with D-transposition of the great arteries an average of 6.4 years after Mustard's operation.[74] The mean resting EF was 44% $\pm$ 12% and was unchanged at peak exercise. Eight children had a normal EF response, whereas 11 had either no increase or a decrease in EF (Fig. 11–17). Patients with an abnormal EF response exhibited a decline in the relative end-diastolic volume. The data de-

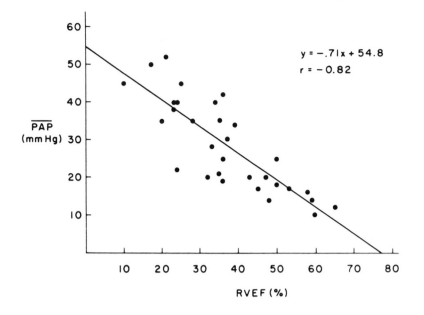

$$y = -.71x + 54.8$$
$$r = -0.82$$

Figure 11–16. Relation between mean pulmonary arterial pressure (PAP) and right ventricular ejection fraction (RVEF) for 31 patients who underwent right-side heart catheterization. Data are included from patients with CAD and normal LV function, from patients who had an elevated mean pulmonary arterial pressure but normal RV end-diastolic pressure, and from patients with an elevated RV end-diastolic pressure. (Korr KS, et al.: Am J Cardiol 1982;49:71–78.)

scribed in this report indicated that, after Mustard's procedure, clinically well children may have abnormal RV function under stress.

Right Ventricular Function During Stress

Berger et al.[75] showed that the normal response of the right ventricle to exercise was at least a 5% absolute increase in the RVEF. By multivariate analysis, the RVEF during exercise is inversely related to total pulmonary vascular resistance.[75a] In patients with CAD, the RVEF either decreased or remained the same during exercise in 19 of 32 patients studied.[75] Patients with an abnormal RVEF most often had a concomitant abnormal exercise LVEF. In that study there was a significant linear relationship between the direction and magnitude of change from rest to exercise of LVEF and RVEF ($r = 0.77$; Fig. 11–18). The RV response to exercise was not primarily dependent on the presence or absence of a proximal right coronary stenosis. The data from this study suggested that the major determinant of an abnormal exercise RV reserve response on exercise testing was the concomitant LV dysfunction with exercise. Airway obstruction and arterial hypoxemia are significantly more severe in patients exhibiting abnormal compared to normal right ventricular functional responses to exercise.[75b]

Comparison to Echocardiography

Two-dimensional (2-D) echocardiography provides very useful noninvasive information on RV function and pulmonary hypertension. Although the RVEF is more accurately determined by radionuclide angiography than by echocardiography because of limitations of a geometric— as opposed to a count-based—approach for EF quantitation, echocardiography provides important information for qualitative assessment of RV dynamics. It may be easier and

less costly to use echocardiography for detection of acute RV infarction in the CCU setting than to employ radionuclide angiography for this purpose. Bellamy et al.[76] reported that, of 50 patients with acute inferior MI, 20 had regional wall motion abnormalities detected by 2-D echo-

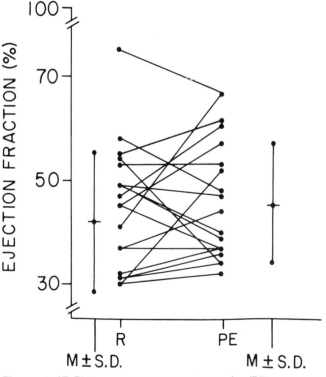

Figure 11–17. RVEF at rest (R) and peak exercise (PE) in children with D-transposition of the great arteries 6.4 ± 2.7 years after Mustard's operation. Mean EF was 44 ± 12% at rest and 46 ± 11% at peak exercise. Eleven of the 19 children had an abnormal EF response to stress. (Benson LN, et al.: Circulation 1982;65:1052–1059.)

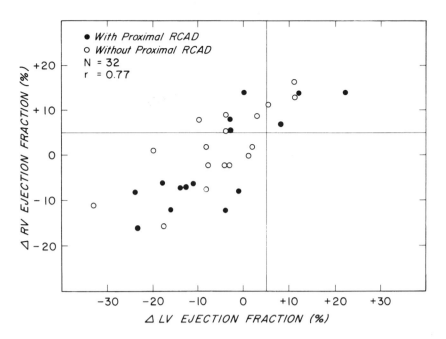

Figure 11–18. Linear relationship of changes in RV and LV responses to exercise. The RV response to exercise was not primarily dependent on the presence or absence of a proximal right coronary stenosis (RCAD). The normal responses are indicated by the horizontal and vertical lines at +5%. (Berger BC, et al.: Circulation 1979;60:1292–1300.)

cardiography, as compared with 22 in whom MI was detected by gated equilibrium blood pool scanning. The sensitivity and specificity for the detection of RV infarction were 82% and 93%, respectively, for 2-D echocardiography and 50% and 71% for ST-segment elevation in lead AVR of the 12-lead ECG. Arditti et al.[77] reported the detection of RV dysfunction in 60 of 104 patients with acute inferior MI by 2-D echocardiography and equilibrium radionuclide angiography. In that study, eight patients presented with regional wall motion abnormalities by 2-D echocardiography, and a normal EF was found on the radionuclide imaging study. Conversely, five patients without regional wall motion abnormalities demonstrated a subnormal RVEF.

Doppler echocardiographic techniques used to assess LV systolic function can be utilized to assess global RV systolic function. Both pulse-wave and continuous-wave Doppler can be employed to measure ejection velocities in the outflow tract of the right ventricle and in the pulmonary artery trunk. Measurement of peak ejection velocity may be useful in noninvasively estimating pulmonary artery pressure. With development of pulmonary hypertension, peak ejection velocity appears earlier in systole and has a characteristic systolic "spike" on the velocity curve.[78] Normally, the peak ejection velocity of the right ventricle occurs in midsystole and the systolic velocity curve has a smooth appearance at its peak. If pulmonary acceleration time is 60 milliseconds or shorter, significant pulmonary hypertension most likely is present. There is an inverse relationship between acceleration time and mean pulmonary artery pressure.[79] Such information cannot readily be obtained from radionuclide angiography, though the higher the pulmonary artery pressure the worse the RV systolic EF.

Assessment of Pharmacologic Therapy

Determination of RVEF by radionuclide angiography may provide useful information for gauging the results of pharmacologic therapy for congestive heart failure. Konstam et al.[80] found that the greatest improvement in RV systolic performance with vasodilators could be expected in patients with the largest RV end-systolic volume at baseline. They reported a significant negative correlation between RV end-systolic pressure-volume slope and the end-systolic volume. Exercise capacity in persons who have congestive heart failure may be predicted by the degree of impairment of the RVEF. Baker et al.[81] showed a good correlation between RVEF determined in the resting state and exercise capacity measured by maximal oxygen uptake. Interestingly, they found no correlation between the LV resting EF and exercise capacity.

Right Ventricular Function in Patients with Aortic or Mitral Stenosis

Often, elderly patients present with significant congestive heart failure and a systolic ejection murmur consistent with aortic stenosis. It is most unusual for patients with aortic stenosis and congestive failure symptoms to demonstrate significant RV dysfunction. If biventricular dilatation and systolic dysfunction are observed on radionuclide angiography in a patient with a systolic ejection murmur, the primary cause of the heart failure state probably is not the aortic stenosis. This is important, since some patients with severe aortic stenosis can have gradients below 35 mm Hg. An occasional patient with occult mitral stenosis may be referred to the nuclear cardiology laboratory for the evaluation of dyspnea. In a patient with hemodynamically significant mitral stenosis, a normal LVEF with diminished LV volume would be observed in the presence of RV enlargement. If pulmonary hypertension were significant, RV systolic dysfunction would be apparent.

Right Ventricular Dynamics in Other Congenital Heart Diseases

Radionuclide angiography of RV dynamics yields some useful clinical information in patients with pulmonic stenosis, in patients with Ebstein's anomaly of the tricuspid valve, and in patients with ventricular septal defects. In patients with congenital pulmonic stenosis, the RV chamber is enlarged. In Ebstein's anomaly, the radionuclide angiogram provides information on the size and performance of the dysplastic functional right ventricle that may help in the selection of patients for repair and in determining the need for tricuspid valve replacement. The first-pass portion of the study would confirm the presence of a right-to-left shunt. The presence and degree of tricuspid regurgitation can also be assessed by radionuclide angiography, though Doppler echocardiography is superior for this purpose. In certain patients with tricuspid atresia who have a suboptimal echocardiographic window, radionuclide angiography may yield some useful information. The right ventricle would not be visualized with cavitary presence of the radioisotopic label.

Detection of Doxorubicin Cardiotoxicity

Radionuclide angiography at rest or during exercise is useful for monitoring LV function in patients receiving cardiotoxic chemotherapeutic agents.[82-84] In a study by Alexander et al.,[82] all patients who demonstrated signs of congestive heart failure due to doxorubicin cardiotoxicity had a resting LVEF below 30% and showed a decline in EF by at least 15%, to a final value of not more than 45%

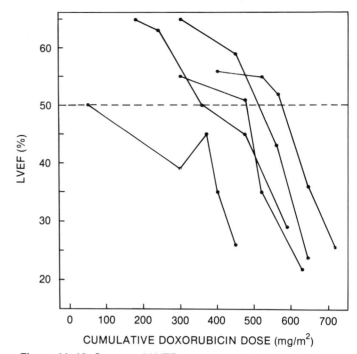

Figure 11–19. Segmental LVEF measurements related to the cumulative dose of doxorubicin in patients who developed congestive heart failure. Each patient passed through a phase of moderate cardiotoxicity defined by an absolute fall in LVEF of at least 15%. (Reprinted by permission of *The New England Journal of Medicine* from Alexander J, et al.: N Engl J Med 1979;30:278–283. Copyright 1979, Massachusetts Medical Society.)

before clinical manifestations were observed. When the drug was discontinued because of a decline in LVEF, a further drop was not seen during follow-up and heart failure did not develop. Figure 11–19 shows sequential measurements of LVEF in five patients who developed severe congestive heart failure in response to cumulative increases in doxorubicin dose. Iodine-labeled MIBG imaging may show diminished accumulation of MIBG in the heart in early adriamycin-induced cardiomyopathy.[85] The decrease

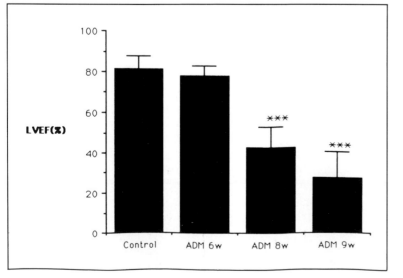

Figure 11–20. Progression of LV dysfunction with adriamycin (ADM) treatment. Rats were treated with 2 mg/kg of ADM once a week for 6, 8, 9, and 10 weeks (W). Note that the LVEF abruptly decreased in the 8-week group and decreased farther in the 9-week group (***, *P* < 0.001 compared with controls). (Reprinted by permission of the Society of Nuclear Medicine from Wakasugi S, et al.: J Nucl Med 1993;34:1529–1535.)

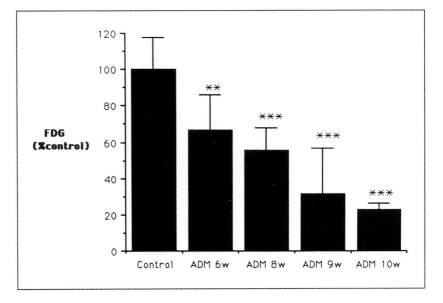

Figure 11–21. Progression of decrease in F-18 deoxyglucose (FDG) accumulation in the myocardium in adriamycin-treated animals. Decrease in FDG accumulation occurred earlier than deterioration in LVEF and progressed more linearly. (Key: **, $P < 0.01$; ***, $P < 0.001$; compared with controls.) (Reprinted by permission of the Society of Nuclear Medicine from Wakasugi S, et al.: J Nucl Med 1993;34:1529–1535.)

appears to be dose dependent and greater in the left ventricle than in the right ventricle; the decrease also correlates with the diminution in LVEF. This same group reported progressive decreases in F-18-FDG and I-125-BMIPP uptake in a rat model of adriamycin toxicity, reflecting diminished myocardial utilization of glucose and fatty acids, respectively.[86] Decrease in F-18-FDG uptake appeared earlier than deterioration in LVEF (Figs. 11–20, 11–21). These metabolic changes developed without evidence for a reduction in regional myocardial blood flow as assessed by Tc-99m–sestamibi uptake. Finally, increased In-111 antimyosin uptake can be observed in patients with doxorubicin toxicity, reflecting severe cell injury.[87] The uptake of this tracer may be seen before LVEF deteriorates.

SUMMARY

The content of this chapter, as well as the review of imaging agents in Chapter 2, indicates that noninvasive imaging of myocardial perfusion, function, metabolism, viability, and adrenergic function provides clinically relevant information on the status of patients with noncoronary disease. Often, perfusion abnormalities may be observed in the absence of significant narrowing on coronary angiography, which may not represent a "false-positive" test result but suggest abnormal nutrient blood flow of another cause. Similarly, global and regional systolic dysfunction of the left ventricle or right ventricle can be seen in a variety of extracoronary disease states, and radionuclide angiography can help detect and quantify the extent of dysfunction.

REFERENCES

1. Bulkley BH, Hutchins GM, Bailey I, Strauss HW, Pitt B: Thallium-201 imaging and gated cardiac blood pool scans in patients with ischemic and idiopathic congestive cardiomyopathy. A clinical and pathologic study. Circulation 1977;55:753–760.
2. O'Gara PT, Bonow RO, Maron BJ, Damske BA, van Lingen A, Bacharach SL, Larson SM, Epstein SE: Myocardial perfusion abnormalities in patients with hypertrophic cardiomyopathy: Assessment with thallium-201 emission computed tomography. Circulation 1987;76:1214–1223.
3. Cannon RO, Dilsizian V, O'Gara PT, Udelson JE, Schenke WH, Quyyumi A, Fananapazir L, Bonow RO: Myocardial metabolic, hemodynamic, and electrocardiographic significance of reversible thallium-201 abnormalities in hypertrophic cardiomyopathy. Circulation 1991;83:1660–1667.
3a. Dilsizian V, Bonow RO, Epstein SE, Fananapazir L: Myocardial ischemia detected by thallium scintigraphy is frequently related to cardiac arrest and syncope in young patients with hypertrophic cardiomyopathy. J Am Coll Cardiol 1993;22:796–804.
4. Cannon RO, Dilsizian V, O'Gara PT, Udelson JE, Tucker E, Panza JA, Fananapazir L, McIntosh CL, Wallace RB, Bonow RO: Impact of surgical relief of outflow obstruction on thallium perfusion abnormalities in hypertrophic cardiomyopathy. Circulation 1992;85:1039–1045.
5. von Dohlen TW, Prisant LM, Frank MJ: Significance of positive or negative thallium-201 scintigraphy in hypertrophic cardiomyopathy. Am J Cardiol 1989;64:498–503.
5a. Udelson JE, Bonow RO, O'Gara PT, Maron BJ, van Lingen A, Bachrach SE, Epstein SE: Verapamil prevents silent myocardial perfusion abnormalities during exercise in patients with hypertrophic cardiomyopathy. Circulation 1989;79:1052–1060.
6. Suzuki Y, Kadota K, Nohara R, Tamaki S, Kambara H, Yoshida A, Murakami T, Osakada G, Kawai C, Tamaki N, et al.: Recognition of regional hypertrophy in hypertrophic cardiomyopathy using thallium-201 emission-computed tomography: Comparison with two-dimensional echocardiography. Am J Cardiol 1984;53:1095–1098.
6a. Nishimura T: Approaches to identify and characterize hypertrophic myocardium. J Nucl Med 1993;34:1013–1019.
6b. Bonow R, Frederick T, Bacharach S, Green M, Goose P, Maron B, Rosing D: Atrial systole and left ventricular filling in hypertrophic cardiomyopathy: Effect of verapamil. Am J Cardiol 1983;51:1386–1391.
6c. Bonow RO, Rosing DR, Bacharach SL, Green MV, Kent KM, Lipson LC, Maron BJ, Leon MB, Epstein SE: Effects of verapamil on left ventricular systolic function and diastolic filling in patients with hypertrophic cardiomyopathy. Circulation 1981;64:787–796.
6d. Bonow RO, Dilsizian V, Rosing DR, Maron BJ, Bacharach SL, Green MV: Verapamil-induced improvement in left ventricular diastolic filling and increased exercise tolerance in patients with hypertrophic cardiomyopathy: Short- and long-term effects. Circulation 1985;72:853–864.

6e. Pandis I, Nestico P, Hakki A, Mintz G, Segal B, Iskandrian A: Systolic and diastolic left ventricular performance at rest and during exercise in apical hypertrophic cardiomyopathy. Am J Cardiol 1986;57:356–358.

6f. Nakajima K, Bunko H, Taki J, Shimizu M, Muramori A, Hisada K: Quantitative analysis of 123I-meta-iodobenzylguanidine (MIBG) uptake in hypertrophic cardiomyopathy. Am Heart J 1990;119:1329–1337.

6g. Taki J, Nakajima K, Bunko H, Simizu M, Muramori A, Hisada K: Whole-body distribution of iodine 123 metaiodobenzylguanidine in hypertrophic cardiomyopathy: Significance of its washout from the heart. Eur J Nucl Med 1990;17:264–268.

6h. Schofer J, Spielmann R, Schuchert A, Weber K, Schluter M: Iodine-123 *meta*-iodobenzylguanidine scintigraphy: A noninvasive method to demonstrate myocardial adrenergic nervous system disintegrity in patients with idiopathic dilated cardiomyopathy. J Am Coll Cardiol 1988;12:1252–1258.

6i. Nishimura T, Nagata S, Uehara T, Hayashida K, Mitani I, Kumita S: Assessment of myocardial damage in dilated-phase hypertrophic cardiomyopathy by using indium-111-antimyosin Fab myocardial scintigraphy. J Nucl Med 1991;32:1333–1337.

6j. Kurata C, Tawarahara K, Taguchi T, Aoshima S, Kobayashi A, Yamazaki N, Kawai H, Kaneko M: Myocardial emission computed tomography with iodine-123–labeled beta-methyl-branched fatty acid in patients with hypertrophic cardiomyopathy. J Nucl Med 1992;33:6–13.

7. Alexander EL, Firestein GS, Weiss JL, Heuser RR, Leitl G, Wagner HN Jr, Brinker JA, Ciuffo AA, Becker LC: Reversible cold-induced abnormalities in myocardial perfusion and function in systemic sclerosis. Ann Intern Med 1986;105:661–668.

8. Follansbee WP, Curtiss EI, Medsger TA Jr, Steen VD, Uretsky BF, Owens GR, Rodnan GP: Physiologic abnormalities of cardiac function in progressive systemic sclerosis with diffuse scleroderma. N Engl J Med 1984;310:142–148.

9. Kahan A, Devaux JY, Amor B, Menkes CJ, Weber S, Nitenberg A, Venot A, Guerin F, Degeorges M, Roucayrol JC: Nifedipine and thallium-201 myocardial perfusion in progressive systemic sclerosis. N Engl J Med 1986;314:1397–1402.

10. Corbett JR, Dehmer GJ, Lewis SE, Woodward W, Henderson E, Parkey RW, Blomqvist CG, Willerson JT: The prognostic value of submaximal exercise testing with radionuclide ventriculography before hospital discharge in patients with recent myocardial infarction. Circulation 1981;64:535–544.

11. Nitenberg A, Foult JM, Kahan A, Perennec J, Devaux JY, Menkes CJ, Amor B: Reduced coronary flow and resistance reserve in primary scleroderma myocardial disease. Am Heart J 1986;112:309–315.

12. Schulman DS, Francis CK, Black HR, Wackers FJ: Thallium-201 stress imaging in hypertensive patients. Hypertension 1987;10:16–21.

13. Tubau JF, Szlachcic J, Hollenberg M, Massie BM: Usefulness of thallium-201 scintigraphy in predicting the development of angina pectoris in hypertensive patients with left ventricular hypertrophy. Am J Cardiol 1989;64:45–49.

14. Wasserman AG, Katz RJ, Varghese PJ, Leiboff RH, Bren GG, Schlesselman S, Varma VM, Reba RC, Ross AM: Exercise radionuclide ventriculographic responses in hypertensive patients with chest pain. N Engl J Med 1984;311:1276–1280.

15. Genda A, Mizuno S, Nunoda S, Nakayama A, Igarashi Y, Sugihara N, Namura M, Takeda R, Bunko H, Hisada K: Clinical studies on diabetic myocardial disease using exercise testing with myocardial scintigraphy and endomyocardial biopsy. Clin Cardiol 1986;9:375–382.

16. Nesto RW, Phillips RT, Kett KG, Hill T, Perper E, Young E, Leland OS Jr: Angina and exertional myocardial ischemia in diabetic and nondiabetic patients: Assessment by exercise thallium scintigraphy [published erratum appears in Ann Intern Med 1988 Apr;108:646]. Ann Intern Med 1988;108:170–175.

17. Koistinen MJ, Huikuri HV, Pirttiaho H, Linnaluoto MK, Takkunen JT: Evaluation of exercise electrocardiography and thallium tomographic imaging in detecting asymptomatic coronary artery disease in diabetic patients. Br Heart J 1990;63:7–11.

18. Koistinen MJ: Prevalence of asymptomatic myocardial ischaemia in diabetic subjects. Br Med J 1990;301:92–95.

19. Abenavoli T, Rubler S, Fisher VJ, Axelrod HI, Zuckerman KP: Exercise testing with myocardial scintigraphy in asymptomatic diabetic males. Circulation 1981;63:54–64.

20. DePuey EG, Guertler-Krawczynska E, Robbins WL: Thallium-201 SPECT in coronary artery disease patients with left bundle branch block. J Nucl Med 1988;29:1479–1485.

21. Hirzel HO, Senn M, Nuesch K, Buettner C, Pfeiffer A, Hess OM, Krayenbuehl HP: Thallium-201 scintigraphy in complete left bundle branch block. Am J Cardiol 1984;53:764–769.

22. Huerta EM, Rodriguez Padial L, Castro Beiras JM, Illera JP, Asin Cardiel E: Thallium-201 exercise scintigraphy in patients having complete left bundle branch block with normal coronary arteries. Int J Cardiol 1987;16:43–46.

23. Rothbart R, Beller G, Watson D, et al.: Diagnostic accuracy and prognostic significance of quantitative thallium-201 scintigraphy in patients with left bundle branch block. Am J Noninv Cardiol 1987;1:197–205.

24. Braat SH, Brugada P, Bar FW, Gorgels AP, Wellens HJ: Thallium-201 exercise scintigraphy and left bundle branch block. Am J Cardiol 1985;55:224–226.

25. Larcos G, Gibbons RJ, Brown ML: Diagnostic accuracy of exercise thallium-201 single-photon emission computed tomography in patients with left bundle branch block. Am J Cardiol 1991;68:756–760.

26. Civelek AC, Gozukara I, Durski K, Ozguven MA, Brinker JA, Links JM, Camargo EE, Wagner HN Jr, Flaherty JT: Detection of left anterior descending coronary artery disease in patients with left bundle branch block. Am J Cardiol 1992;70:1565–1570.

27. Tawarahara K, Kurata C, Taguchi T, Kobayashi A, Yamazaki N: Exercise testing and thallium-201 emission computed tomography in patients with intraventricular conduction disturbances. Am J Cardiol 1992;69:97–102.

28. Ono S, Nohara R, Kambara H, Okuda K, Kawai C: Regional myocardial perfusion and glucose metabolism in experimental left bundle branch block. Circulation 1992;85:1125–1131.

29. Matzer L, Kiat H, Friedman JD, Van Train K, Maddahi J, Berman DS: A new approach to the assessment of tomographic thallium-201 scintigraphy in patients with left bundle branch block. J Am Coll Cardiol 1991;17:1309–1317.

29a. Burns RJ, Galligan L, Wright LM, Lawand S, Burke RJ, Gladstone PJ: Improved specificity of myocardial thallium-201 single-photon emission computed tomography in patients with left bundle branch block by dipyridamole. Am J Cardiol 1991;68:504–508.

29b. Rockett JF, Wood WC, Moinuddin M, Loveless V, Parrish B: Intravenous dipyridamole thallium-201 SPECT imaging in patients with left bundle branch block. Clin Nucl Med 1990;15:401–407.

29c. Morais J, Soucy JP, Sestier F, Lamoureux F, Lamoureux J, Danais S: Dipyridamole testing compared to exercise stress for thallium-201 imaging in patients with left bundle branch block. Can J Cardiol 1990;6:5–8.

29d. O'Keefe JH Jr, Bateman TM, Barnhart CS: Adenosine thallium-201 is superior to exercise thallium-201 for detecting coronary artery disease in patients with left bundle branch block. J Am Coll Cardiol 1993;21:1332–1338.

29e. Krishnan R, Lu J, Zhu Y, Dae MW, Botvinick EH: Myocardial perfusion scintigraphy in left bundle branch block: A perspective on the issue from image analysis in a clinical context. Am Heart J 1993;126:578–586.

30. Gutgesell HP, Pinsky WW, DePuey EG: Thallium-201 myocardial perfusion imaging in infants and children. Value in distinguishing anomalous left coronary artery from congestive cardiomyopathy. Circulation 1980;61:596–599.

31. Moodie DS, Cook SA, Gill CC, Napoli CA: Thallium-201 myocardial imaging in young adults with anomalous left coronary artery arising from the pulmonary artery. J Nucl Med 1980;21:1076–1079.

32. Anguenot TJ, Bernard YF, Cardot JC, Boumal D, Bassand JP, Maurat JP: Isotopic findings in anomalous origin of the left coronary artery from the pulmonary artery: Report of an adult case. J Nucl Med 1991;32:1788–1790.

33. Finley JP, Howman-Giles R, Gilday DL, Olley PM, Rowe RD: Thallium-201 myocardial imaging in anomalous left coronary artery arising from the pulmonary artery. Applications before and after medical and surgical treatment. Am J Cardiol 1978;42:675–680.

34. Rabinovitch M, Rowland TW, Castaneda AR, Treves S: Thallium 201 scintigraphy in patients with anomalous origin of the left coronary artery from the main pulmonary artery. J Pediatrics 1979;94:244–247.

35. Manier S, Blue P, Abreu S, Nostrand D, Eggli D, Ghaed N: Thallium-201 scintigraphy in anomalous origin of the coronary artery from the pulmonary artery: Ischemia masquerading as infarction. Am J Cardiac Imaging 1987;1:267.

35a. Katsuragi M, Yamamoto K, Tashiro T, Nishihara H, Toudou K: Thallium-201 myocardial SPECT in Bland-White-Garland syndrome: Two adult patients with inferoposterior perfusion defect. J Nucl Med 1993;34:2182–2184.

36. Kawakami K, Shimada T, Yamada S, Murakami R, Morioka S, Moriyama K: The detection of myocardial ischemia by thallium-201 myocardial scintigraphy in patients with multiple coronary arterioventricular connections. Clin Cardiol 1991;14:975–980.

37. Rajfer SI, Oetgen WJ, Weeks KD Jr, Kaminski RJ, Rocchini AP: Thallium-201 scintigraphy after surgical repair of hemodynamically significant primary coronary artery anomalies. Chest 1982;81:687–692.

38. Brown KA, Boucher CA, Okada RD, Strauss HW, McKusick KA, Pohost GM: Serial right ventricle thallium-201 imaging after exercise: Relation to anatomy of the right coronary artery. Am J Cardiol 1982;50:1217–1222.

39. Lahiri A, Carboni GP, Crawley JW, Raftery EB: Reversible ischaemia of right ventricle detected by exercise thallium-201 scintigraphy. Br Heart J 1982;48:260–264.

40. Ohsuzu F, Handa S, Kondo M, Yamazaki H, Tsugu T, Kubo A, Takagi Y, Nakamura Y: Thallium-201 myocardial imaging to evaluate right ventricular overloading. Circulation 1980;61:620–625.

41. Cohen HA, Baird MG, Rouleau JR, Fuhrmann CF, Bailey IK, Summer WR, Strauss HW, Pitt B: Thallium-201 myocardial imaging in patients with pulmonary hypertension. Circulation 1976;54:790–795.

42. Nakajima K, Taki J, Ohno T, Taniguchi M, Bunko H, Hisada K: Assessment of right ventricular overload by a thallium-201 SPECT study in children with congenital heart disease. J Nucl Med 1991;32:2215–2220.

43. Wackers FJ, Klay JW, Laks H, Schnitzer J, Zaret BL, Geha AS: Pathophysiologic correlates of right ventricular thallium-201 uptake in a canine model. Circulation 1981;64:1256–1264.

44. Bulkley BH, Hutchins GM, Bailey I, Strauss HW, Pitt B: Thallium 201 imaging and gated cardiac blood pool scans in patients with ischemic and idiopathic congestive cardiomyopathy. A clinical and pathologic study. Circulation 1977;55:753–760.

45. Dunn RF, Uren RF, Sadick N, Bautovich G, McLaughlin A, Hiroe M, Kelly DT: Comparison of thallium-201 scanning in idiopathic dilated cardiomyopathy and severe coronary artery disease. Circulation 1982;66:804–810.

46. Yamaguchi S, Tsuiki K, Hayasaka M, Yasui S: Segmental wall motion abnormalities in dilated cardiomyopathy: Hemodynamic characteristics and comparison with thallium-201 myocardial scintigraphy. Am Heart J 1987;113:1123–1128.

47. Tauberg SG, Orie JE, Bartlett BE, Cottington EM, Flores AR: Usefulness of thallium-201 for distinction of ischemic from idiopathic dilated cardiomyopathy. Am J Cardiol 1993;71:674–680.

48. Tamai J, Nagata S, Nishimura T, Yutani C, Miyatake K, Sakakibara H, Nimura Y: Hemodynamic and prognostic value of thallium-201 myocardial imaging in patients with dilated cardiomyopathy. Int J Cardiol 1989;24:219–224.

48a. Merlet P, Delforge J, Syrota A, Angevin E, Maziere B, Crouzel C, Valette H, Loisance D, Castaigne A, Rande JL: Positron emission tomography with ^{11}C CGP-12177 to assess beta-adrenergic receptor concentration in idiopathic dilated cardiomyopathy. Circulation 1993;87:1169–1178.

48b. Merlet P, Valetti H, Dubois-Randé JL, et al.: Iodine-123-labeled metaiodobenzylguanidine imaging in heart disease. J Nucl Cardiol 1994;1:S79–S85.

49. Makler PT, Lavine SJ, Denenberg BS, Bove AA, Idell S: Redistribution on the thallium scan in myocardial sarcoidosis: Concise communication. J Nucl Med 1981;22:428–432.

50. Yamamoto S, Matsushima H, Suzuki A, Sotobata I, Indo T, Matsuoka Y: A comparative study of thallium-201 single-photon emission computed tomography and electrocardiography in Duchenne and other types of muscular dystrophy. Am J Cardiol 1988;61:836–843.

51. Tamaki N, Yonekura Y, Kadota K, Kambara H, Torizuka K: Thallium-201 myocardial perfusion imaging in myocarditis. Clin Nucl Med 1985;10:562–566.

52. Marin-Neto JA, Marzullo P, Marcassa C, Gallo Junior L, Maciel BC, Bellina CR, L'Abbate A: Myocardial perfusion abnormalities in chronic Chagas' disease as detected by thallium-201 scintigraphy. Am J Cardiol 1992;69:780–784.

53. Hagar JM, Rahimtoola SH: Chagas' heart disease in the United States. N Engl J Med 1991;325:763–768.

54. Manno BV, Burka ER, Hakki AH, Manno CS, Iskandrian AS, Noone AM: Biventricular function in sickle-cell anemia: Radionuclide angiographic and thallium-201 scintigraphic evaluation. Am J Cardiol 1983;52:584–587.

55. Hashimoto Y, Numano F, Maruyama Y, Oniki T, Kasuya K, Kakuta T, Wada T, Yajima M, Maezawa H: Thallium-201 stress scintigraphy in Takayasu arteritis. Am J Cardiol 1991;67:879–882.

56. Bodin L, Rouby JJ, Viars P: Myocardial contusion in patients with blunt chest trauma as evaluated by thallium 201 myocardial scintigraphy. Chest 1988;94:72–76.

57. Kondo C, Hiroe M, Nakanishi T, Takao A: Detection of coronary artery stenosis in children with Kawasaki disease. Usefulness of pharmacologic stress 201Tl myocardial tomography. Circulation 1989;80:615–624.

58. Kimball BP, Shurvell BL, Mildenberger RR, Houle S, McLaughlin PR: Abnormal thallium kinetics in postoperative coarctation of the aorta: Evidence for diffuse hypertension-induced vascular pathology. J Am Coll Cardiol 1986;7:538–545.

59. McDonnell PJ, Becker LC, Bulkley BH: Thallium imaging in cardiac lymphoma. Am Heart J 1981;101:809–814.

60. Klein GJ, Kostuk WJ, Boughner DR, Chamberlain MJ: Stress myocardial imaging in mitral leaflet prolapse syndrome. Am J Cardiol 1978;42:746–750.

61. Gaffney FA, Wohl AJ, Blomqvist CG, Parkey RW, Willerson JT: Thallium-201 myocardial perfusion studies in patients with the mitral valve prolapse syndrome. Am J Med 1978;64:21–26.

61a. Hayes AM, Baker EJ, Kakadeker A, Parsons JM, Martin RP, Radley-Smith R, Qureshi SA, Yacoub M, Maisey MN, Tyman M: Influence of anatomic correction for transposition of the great arteries on myocardial perfusion: Radionuclide imaging with technetium-99m 2-methoxy isobutyl isonitrile. J Am Coll Cardiol 1994;24:769–777.

61b. Weindling SN, Wernovsky G, Colan SD, Parker JA, Boutin C, Mone SM, Costello J, Castañeda AR, Treves T: Myocardial perfusion, function and exercise tolerance after the arterial switch operation. J Am Coll Cardiol 1994;23:424–433.

62. Maltz DL, Treves S: Quantitative radionuclide angiocardiography: Determination of Qp:Qs in children. Circulation 1973;47:1049–1056.

63. Treves S: Detection and quantitation of cardiovascular shunts with commonly available radionuclides. Semin Nucl Med 1980;10:16–26.

63a. Treves S, Parlar A: Detection and quantification of intracardiac shunts. *In* Strauss HW, Pitt B (eds): Cardiovascular Nuclear Medicine, 2nd Ed. St. Louis, CV Mosby, 1979, pp 148–161.

64. Ham HR, Dobbeleir A, Virat P, Piepsz A, Lenaers A: Radionuclide quantitation of left-to-right cardiac shunts using deconvolution analysis: Concise communication. J Nucl Med 1981;22:688–692.

65. Bourguignon MH, Links JM, Douglass KH, Alderson PO, Roland JM, Wagner HN Jr: Quantification of left to right cardiac shunts by multiple deconvolution analysis. Am J Cardiol 1981;48:1086–1090.

66. Madsen MT, Argenyi E, Preslar J, Grover-McKay M, Kirchner PT: An improved method for the quantification of left-to-right cardiac shunts. J Nucl Med 1991;32:1808–1812.

67. Peter CA, Armstrong BE, Jones RH: Radionuclide quantitation of right-to-left intracardiac shunts in children. Circulation 1981;64:572–577.

68. Jones R: Radionuclide angiography. *In* Marcus M, Schelbert H, Skorton D, Wolff G (eds): Cardiac Imaging, ed 3. Philadelphia, WB Saunders, 1991, pp 1006–1026.

68a. Imbriaco M, Cuocolo A, Pace L, Nicolai E, Nappi A, Celentano L, Palma G, Vosa C: Technetium-99m methoxy isobutyl isonitrile simultaneous evaluation of ventricular function and myocardial perfusion in patients with congenital heart disease. Clin Nucl Med 1994;19:28–32.

69. Tobinick E, Schelbert HR, Henning H, LeWinter M, Taylor A, Ashburn WL, Karliner JS: Right ventricular ejection fraction in patients with acute anterior and inferior myocardial infarction assessed by radionuclide angiography. Circulation 1978;57:1078–1084.

70. Rigo P, Murray M, Taylor DR, Weisfeldt ML, Kelly DT, Strauss HW, Pitt B: Right ventricular dysfunction detected by gated scintiphotography in patients with acute inferior myocardial infarction. Circulation 1975;52:268–274.

71. Berger HJ, Matthay RA: Noninvasive radiographic assessment of cardiovascular function in acute and chronic respiratory failure. Am J Cardiol 1981;47:950–962.

72. Berger HJ, Matthay RA, Pytlik LM, Gottschalk A, Zaret BL: First-pass radionuclide assessment of right and left ventricular performance

in patients with cardiac and pulmonary disease. Semin Nucl Med 1979;9:275–295.

73. Korr KS, Gandsman EJ, Winkler ML, Shulman RS, Bough EW: Hemodynamic correlates of right ventricular ejection fraction measured with gated radionuclide angiography. Am J Cardiol 1982;49:71–77.

74. Benson LN, Bonet J, McLaughlin P, Olley PM, Feiglin D, Druck M, Trusler G, Rowe RD, Morch J: Assessment of right ventricular function during supine bicycle exercise after Mustard's operation. Circulation 1982;65:1052–1059.

75. Berger BC, Watson DD, Burwell LR, Crosby IK, Wellons HA, Teates CD, Beller GA: Redistribution of thallium at rest in patients with stable and unstable angina and the effect of coronary artery bypass surgery. Circulation 1979;60:1114–1125.

75a. Morrison D, Sorensen S, Caldwell J, Wright AL, Ritchie J, Kennedy JW, Hamilton G: The normal right ventricular response to supine exercise. Chest 1982;82:686–691.

75b. Matthay RA, Berger HJ, Davies RA, Loke J, Mahler DA, Gottschalk A, Zaret BL: Right and left ventricular exercise performance in chronic obstructive pulmonary disease: Radionuclide assessment. Ann Intern Med 1980;93:234–239.

76. Bellamy GR, Rasmussen HH, Nasser FN, Wiseman JC, Cooper RA: Value of two-dimensional echocardiography, electrocardiography, and clinical signs in detecting right ventricular infarction. Am Heart J 1986;112:304–309.

77. Arditti A, Lewin RF, Hellman C, Sclarovsky S, Strasberg B, Agmon J: Right ventricular dysfunction in acute inferoposterior myocardial infarction. An echocardiographic and isotopic study. Chest 1985;87:307–314.

78. Dabestani A, Mahan G, Gardin JM, Takenaka K, Burn C, Allfie A, Henry WL: Evaluation of pulmonary artery pressure and resistance by pulsed Doppler echocardiography. Am J Cardiol 1987;59:662–668.

79. Isobe M, Yazaki Y, Takaku F, Koizumi K, Hara K, Tsuneyoshi H, Yamaguchi T, Machii K: Prediction of pulmonary arterial pressure in adults by pulsed Doppler echocardiography. Am J Cardiol 1986;57:316–321.

80. Konstam MA, Cohen SR, Salem DN, Conlon TP, Isner JM, Das D, Zile MR, Levine HJ, Kahn PC: Comparison of left and right ventricular end-systolic pressure-volume relations in congestive heart failure. J Am Coll Cardiol 1985;5:1326–1334.

81. Baker BJ, Wilen MM, Boyd CM, Dinh H, Franciosa JA: Relation of right ventricular ejection fraction to exercise capacity in chronic left ventricular failure. Am J Cardiol 1984;54:596–599.

82. Alexander J, Dainiak N, Berger HJ, Goldman L, Johnstone D, Reduto L, Duffy T, Schwartz P, Gottschalk A, Zaret BL: Serial assessment of doxorubicin cardiotoxicity with quantitative radionuclide angiocardiography. N Engl J Med 1979;300:278–283.

83. Schwartz RG, McKenzie WB, Alexander J, Sager P, D'Souza A, Manatunga A, Schwartz PE, Berger HJ, Setaro J, Surkin L, et al.: Congestive heart failure and left ventricular dysfunction complicating doxorubicin therapy. Seven-year experience using serial radionuclide angiocardiography. Am J Med 1987;82:1109–1118.

84. Palmeri S, Bonow R, Myers C, Seipp C, Jenkins J, Green M, Bacharach S, Rosenberg S: Prospective evaluation of doxorubicin cardiotoxicity by rest and exercise radionuclide angiography. Am J Cardiol 1985;58:607–613.

85. Wakasugi S, Fischman AJ, Babich JW, Aretz HT, Callahan RJ, Nakaki M, Wilkinson R, Strauss HW: Meta-iodobenzylguanidine: Evaluation of its potential as a tracer for monitoring doxorubicin cardiomyopathy. J Nucl Med 1993;34:1283–1286.

86. Wakasugi S, Fischman A, Babich J, Callahan R, Elmaleh D, Wilkinson R, Strauss H: Myocardial substrate utilization and left ventricular function in adriamycin cardiomyopathy. J Nucl Med 1993;34:1529–1535.

87. Carrio I, Lopez-Pousa A, Estroch M, Duncker D, Berma L, Torres G, Andres L: Detection of doxorubicin cardiotoxicity in patients with sarcomas by indium-111-antimyosin myoclonal antibody. J Nucl Med 1993;34:1503–1507.

Chapter 12

Radionuclide Imaging in Valvular Heart Disease

INTRODUCTION

Either first-pass or equilibrium radionuclide angiography (RNA) may provide clinically relevant information for the assessment of patients with valvular heart disease. Isolated mitral valvular stenosis is perhaps the only disorder in which radionuclide imaging plays a very minor role. Echocardiography is the technique of choice for the noninvasive determination of the hemodynamic severity of mitral stenosis. A highly accurate estimation of valve area as well as the diastolic gradient across the valve can be made, permitting the clinician to determine the appropriate timing of mitral surgery to alleviate the obstruction to left ventricular (LV) filling and reduce the symptoms and signs of congestive heart failure. RNA techniques performed in the resting state or during exercise are more appropriate for evaluating valvular regurgitant lesions than for assessing stenotic lesions. RNA can be an important noninvasive procedure in the quantitation of left ventricular ejection fraction (LVEF) in patients with aortic valvular stenosis. The technique for quantitating the LVEF from first-pass or equilibrium-gated RNA is discussed in Chapter 1. In some instances, contrast ventriculography may be hazardous for patients with suspected severe aortic stenosis with symptoms of congestive heart failure and echocardiographic demonstration of diminished LV systolic performance. RNA in such patients with aortic stenosis can provide an accurate measurement of the LVEF, thus eliminating the need for the ventriculographic determination of LVEF at catheterization.

In certain patients with mild aortic stenosis and angina, stress myocardial perfusion imaging may be useful in determining whether the ischemic symptoms are due to physiologically important concomitant coronary artery disease (CAD) rather than to aortic stenosis alone. If focal perfusion defects are observed showing delayed redistribution in a patient with mild to moderate aortic stenosis, the angina symptoms may be due more to CAD or the combination of a coronary stenosis and aortic stenosis.

In this chapter, the focus is directed to the clinical utility of RNA in the noninvasive work-up or follow-up of patients with aortic or mitral regurgitation or mixed valvular disease in which the regurgitant lesion is thought to be dominant.

AORTIC REGURGITATION

Rest Radionuclide Angiography

Rest RNA can be used to distinguish between acute and chronic aortic regurgitation in a patient who presents with congestive heart failure and an aortic regurgitation murmur but who previously had no known cardiac disease. Perhaps the most common cause of acute aortic regurgitation in a patient without a history of cardiac disease is infective endocarditis. Rest RNA in acute regurgitation shows no significant dilatation or hypertrophy of the left ventricle. With acute regurgitation there is no time for adaptive dilatation of the left ventricle to occur with increased compliance. LV systolic performance is normal or hyperkinetic with acute aortic regurgitation in association with signs of pulmonary congestion.

As described in Chapter 1, a semiquantitative measurement of left-sided regurgitation can be achieved with RNA techniques.[1, 2] The most common technique for making this measurement is the ratio of the LV stroke volume to the right ventricular (RV) stroke volume. In patients with no valvular regurgitation, this ratio is usually in the range of 1.15. In patients with aortic or mitral regurgitation, the ratio increases to more than 1.30. Although this technique results in significant overlap between patients who have mild regurgitation and those with none, it can be utilized to distinguish between significant regurgitation and none at all. Certainly, overlap of atrial technetium-99m (Tc-99m) activity may interfere with the accurate measurement of ventricular stroke counts. Right atrial activity can be excluded by using a caudal tilt of the collimator or by subtracting right atrial activity.[3]

With chronic aortic regurgitation, the LV end-diastolic volume is increased and systolic performance is either normal or depressed. The measurements of LVEF by RNA in patients with aortic regurgitation are quite accurate and reflect the consequences of the regurgitant lesion on LV muscle function. In patients with chronic aortic insufficiency, useful information may also be gained from serial measurements of relative LV volume changes in aortic regurgitation, and volume measurement can be employed to assess responses to either medical or surgical therapy in addition to monitoring changes in LVEF.[2, 4]

RNA performed in the resting state may assist in the timing of aortic valve surgery in patients with aortic insufficiency. Aortic valve surgery is indicated in patients with aortic insufficiency who present with moderate or severe symptoms, the most dominant being progressive dyspnea with exertion and reduction in exercise tolerance. Aortic valve replacement in patients with significant symptoms lessens their severity and enhances survival, as compared with medical therapy.[5, 6] In symptomatic patients, RNA may be useful in predicting the short- and long-term outcomes after aortic replacement. The worse the preoperative LV function, the less the chance of postoperative improvement in EF, and perhaps the less impact on reducing mortality long-term. In symptomatic patients undergoing aortic valve surgery, the resting radionuclide EF is an important variable for determination of postoperative LV dysfunction.[4] Postoperative morbidity and mortality increase as the preoperative EF—as measured by any technique—decreases.[7–9]

Rest RNA plays a more important role in the determination of timing of aortic valve replacement in patients who have asymptomatic aortic regurgitation.[4] Certain asymptomatic patient groups may benefit from early operation for aortic insufficiency, before symptoms develop. Many clinicians now feel that early operation is beneficial for patients with minimal or no symptoms who exhibit evidence of diminished LV systolic performance. Despite substantial regurgitation and LV volume overload, patients with aortic regurgitation can remain free of symptoms for many years, and even decades. The critical issue is that when symptoms

do occur, clinical deterioration will most certainly progress rapidly with acceleration of LV dysfunction. Therefore, many clinicians now desire to intervene earlier in the natural history of aortic regurgitation, affording the patient enhanced survival and quality of life after a valve replacement. The goal of early surgery is to obviate irreversible LV dysfunction that results from progressive dilatation and eccentric hypertrophy in this valvular lesion.

The National Institutes of Health (NIH) group has published the results of several important studies dealing with the RNA assessment of asymptomatic patients with aortic insufficiency and its role in determining more optimal timing of valvular surgery. Figure 12–1 shows the preoperative and 6-month postoperative LVEF measurements obtained by rest RNA in a group of 93 patients undergoing valve replacement for chronic aortic regurgitation at the NIH.[4] As shown, many aortic insufficiency patients who had EFs less than 40% demonstrated persistence or deterioration of LV dysfunction after surgery. Patients whose preoperative EF was more than 50% almost always had normal or improved postoperative LV function. Bonow et al.[9] have further shown that the 6-month postoperative EF is predictive of long-term functional results. When impaired LV systolic

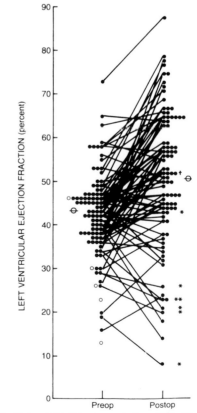

Figure 12–1. Plots of LVEF at rest before (preop) and 6 months after (postop) aortic valve replacement in 93 consecutive patients with chronic aortic regurgitation. Open circles indicate patients who died before 6-month follow-up. Asterisks indicate patients who died of CHF after the 6-month study, and a cross indicates a single patient who died suddenly after the 6-month study. (Bonow RO: Circulation 1991;84:I-296–I-302.)

function was seen 6 months after surgery, late postoperative improvement (up to 8 years) was unlikely.

Measurement of systolic function by RNA can provide prognostic information on survival after valve surgery.[8, 10–12] As shown in Figure 12–2 from the work of Bonow,[11a] patients with preoperative LV dysfunction are at relatively high risk for postoperative death. These data were obtained in 80 consecutive patients undergoing aortic valve replacement. Depression of LVEF at rest was defined as a value below 45%. Patients with normal preoperative LV function who have undergone aortic valve replacement have an excellent long-term postoperative prognosis. The survival rate was 96% for patients with normal systolic function preoperatively, as compared to 63% for patients with a preoperative EF of less than 45%.[11] Preoperative exercise tolerance and duration of LV dysfunction were additional variables that contributed to mortality risk in patients whose EF was abnormal preoperatively. Patients with a short duration of LV dysfunction showed a greater diminution in LV volume and enhancement in LVEF after aortic valve replacement than patients whose LV dysfunction was allowed to go on longer before surgical intervention. In the NIH study,[11] survival after surgery was suboptimal for patients who exhibited poor exercise tolerance or a resting depression of LVEF known to have been present 18 months or longer. When resting LV function was diminished for less than 14 months and exercise tolerance was preserved, postoperative survival was far better.

These observations support the notion that asymptomatic patients with aortic regurgitation can be followed at regular intervals with determinations of resting LVEF. If a deterioration in LV function is observed, even in the absence of symptoms, aortic valve replacement should be seriously considered. If exercise tolerance is also determined to have deteriorated, then the recommendation for early valve replacement is supported with even greater confidence. The decision to recommend surgery to an asymptomatic patient must always be weighed against operative risk. With cur-

rent approaches to intraoperative myocardial preservation and operative monitoring, the mortality rate and morbidity following aortic valve replacement have decreased. When this watchful waiting approach is employed in asymptomatic patients with aortic insufficiency and normal LV function, approximately 4% require operative intervention each year.[13] Patients who are followed in this manner should, of course, be referred for aortic valve replacement if cardiac symptoms develop between office visits and between resting functional determinations. Most patients who develop symptoms manifest a concomitant deterioration of LV function. Asymptomatic patients who continue to exhibit normal systolic function at rest do not require prophylactic aortic valve replacement to prevent deterioration of LV function. The annual mortality rate for asymptomatic patients with aortic insufficiency and normal EF is less than 0.5%.[13, 14]

Other noninvasive variables have been proposed as being useful in the decision-making process for determining the optimal time for surgical intervention in patients with aortic regurgitation. Preoperative echocardiographic measurements have been examined to determine their ability to predict outcome after aortic valve surgery. Some studies suggested that an LV end-systolic dimension on M-mode echocardiography of at least 15 mm and fractional shortening of no more than 30% predicted a poor postoperative outcome.[10] Subsequent data reported in the literature cast doubt on the utilization of these criteria for operative intervention in asymptomatic patients with aortic regurgitation. Postoperative mortality did not correlate well with the LV end-systolic dimension or fractional shortening in these subsequent studies.[15, 16] Severe aortic regurgitation can result in premature closure of the mitral valve at end-diastole as shown by echocardiography. This early mitral valve closure is due to a rapid early rise of the LV diastolic pressure attributed to the volume overload. Patients who exhibit this echocardiographic finding are usually symptomatic and have symptoms consistent with marked left-sided heart fail-

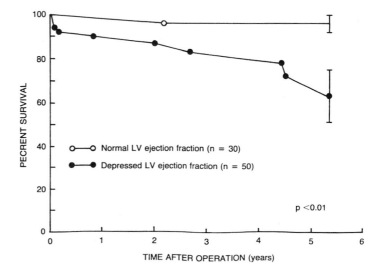

Figure 12–2. Survival curves in patients who underwent aortic valve replacement for aortic regurgitation separated by those with a normal LVEF preoperatively or an abnormal LVEF before surgery. (Bonow RO: Circulation 1991;84:I-296–I-302.)

ure. It is not often seen in patients with asymptomatic regurgitation.

Exercise Radionuclide Angiography

As discussed in the previous section, the patient with aortic regurgitation may experience irreversible myocardial dysfunction before clinical symptoms appear. Some investigators have suggested that the myocardial reserve capacity in patients with aortic insufficiency might be as stressed during stress conditions so that early intrinsic myocardial dysfunction could be detected.[17, 18] Figure 12–3 shows the effect of exercise on LVEF in symptomatic and asymptomatic patients with aortic regurgitation in this study. The clinical utility of the LVEF response to exercise in decision-making concerning timing of valve surgery in asymptomatic aortic regurgitation is controversial. The early studies of the utility of exercise RNA for identifying subclinical LV dysfunction with aortic regurgitation suggested that patients with an exercise LVEF below 0.55 had LV dysfunction that was unmasked by exercise. A significant number of asymptomatic aortic regurgitation patients had an abnormal LVEF response to exercise, which suggested that this index might be overly sensitive.

Boucher et al.[19] compared the LVEF with filling pres-

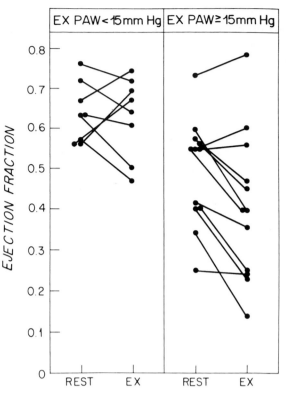

Figure 12–4. Rest and exercise (Ex) EF values for patients with aortic regurgitation who demonstrated an exercise pulmonary artery wedge pressure (PAW) of 15 mm Hg or more *(right panel)* or less than 15 mm Hg. Note that the exercise EF values were higher in those whose PAW was less than 15 mm Hg. (Boucher CA, et al.: Circulation 1983;67:1091–1100.)

sures during supine exercise in asymptomatic or minimally symptomatic patients with aortic regurgitation. The exercise LVEF was higher in patients with a peak exercise pulmonary capillary wedge pressure below 15 mm Hg than in patients with a peak pulmonary wedge pressure during exercise of 15 mm Hg or more (Fig. 12–4). However, there was significant overlap in values between the two groups. These investigators, using multiple regression analysis, found that the best correlate of the peak exercise pulmonary capillary wedge pressure was the peak oxygen uptake. The rest and exercise LVEF values demonstrated a correlation with peak exercise pulmonary capillary wedge pressure, but the change in LVEF with exercise did not. Bonow[4] points out that, although in some patients an abnormal LVEF to maximal exercise may represent early evidence of myocardial dysfunction in aortic regurgitation, an abnormal functional response to exercise in the volume-overloaded left ventricle is a nonspecific finding because the LVEF may be influenced by loading changes that occur during exercise. The hemodynamic effects of both pressure and volume overload are complex. Because the volume of regurgitation decreases with each beat as exercise increases, and because of a shorter diastolic filling time and a decrease in systemic vascular resistance, the total stroke volume and end-diastolic volume can actually fall during exercise, but forward

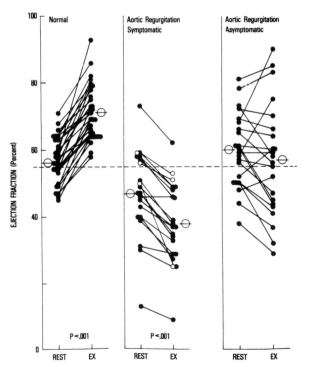

Figure 12–3. Effect of exercise (Ex) and LVEF in normal patients *(left panel)*, patients with symptomatic aortic regurgitation *(middle panel)*, and patients with asymptomatic aortic regurgitation *(right panel)*. Open circles represent values from patients with minimal symptoms. The dashed line at the ejection value of 55% represents the lower limit of normal during exercise. (Borer JS, et al.: Am J Cardiol 1978;42:351–356.)

stroke volume increases. Since the LVEF reflects the total stroke volume and does not separate the regurgitant volume from forward volume, it is possible for such patients to have both a falling EF and an increasing forward stroke volume during exercise. The fall in the exercise EF is directly proportional to the severity of resting LV dilatation and wall stress, and to the degree of aortic regurgitation.[20–23]

Another factor that influences exercise radionuclide studies in aortic regurgitation is the position of the patient during exercise. When upright bicycle exercise was utilized with first-pass RNA, no difference was noted in rest or exercise EF or in volumes between class I or II and class III or IV patients.[24] Other studies have also shown that, in contrast to the data acquired during supine exercise, most asymptomatic patients appear to have an increase in EF with upright exercise.[25, 26] Marks et al.[26] compared supine and upright exercise functional responses in the same patients. In that study, only 2 of 12 patients had a fall in LVEF of 0.05 or greater during upright exercise, as compared with 8 of 12 patients during supine exercise. This points out that one cannot apply EF criteria based on one technique to another technique in which the exercise protocol is different. To date, no study has convincingly demonstrated the independent prognostic value of the exercise LVEF response in patients with aortic regurgitation. There are no definitive data to indicate that asymptomatic patients should be referred for valve replacement solely on the basis of an abnormal LVEF response to exercise RNA, particularly when performed in the supine position.

Bonow et al.[13] found that a third of aortic insufficiency patients who increased their LVEF by 5% or more ended up requiring aortic valve replacement within 4 years. This, again, casts doubt on the value of the exercise EF variable in identifying patients who might need prophylactic valve replacement before symptoms occur.

Borer et al.[18] found that, though the exercise LVEF improved after aortic valve replacement in patients with aortic insufficiency, it was still subnormal relative to that seen in normal patients without valve disease (Fig. 12–5). This suggests that LV dysfunction is only partially reversible with valve replacement, even when timing of surgery is thought to be appropriate. Postoperatively, patients with aortic valve replacement for aortic regurgitation can demonstrate a transient diminution in the LV resting EF postoperatively. Boucher et al.[27] reported that the LVEF fell from 55% preoperatively to 40% postoperatively at 2 to 4 weeks in 20 patients undergoing aortic valve replacement for aortic insufficiency. Several years later, when the LVEF was remeasured, it had increased to a level comparable to that seen preoperatively. It was proposed that the early decline in LVEF may be due to the sudden decrease in end-diastolic volume that occurs immediately after valve replacement.

MITRAL REGURGITATION

Rest Radionuclide Angiography

Volume overload patterns resulting from mitral regurgitation as the cause of congestive heart failure can be identified by resting RNA. Figure 12–6 illustrates how RNA might differentiate aortic from mitral regurgitation.[27a] Patients with mitral valve regurgitation have an enlarged end-diastolic volume but a normal or nearly normal LVEF as long as irreversible myocardial damage has not occurred. The first-pass transit time is also normal or shortened. In patients with a murmur of mitral insufficiency, a markedly depressed LVEF with global hypokinesis on RNA leads to the impression that the murmur is due to "secondary" mitral regurgitation. Although systolic impairment of the papillary muscles plays a role in secondary mitral regurgitation in cardiomyopathy, LV chamber dilation with secondary dilation of the mitral annulus also plays a major role. It is important to identify patients with secondary mitral regurgitation since vasodilator therapy tends to redirect secondary mitral regurgitation in a forward direction, thus increasing forward LVEF and stroke volume.

In contrast, patients with preserved LV function as assessed by RNA and mitral insufficiency will benefit from valve replacement, since regurgitation is of primary pathophysiologic importance in the demonstration of heart failure symptoms. Some of these patients demonstrate abnormal

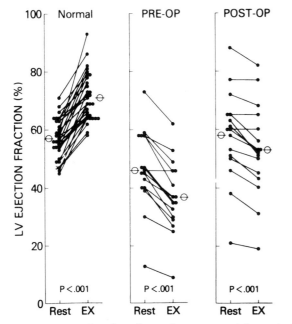

Figure 12–5. Effect of aortic valve replacement on left ventricular function at rest and after exercise (Ex) as assessed by radionuclide angiography. The preoperative values (pre-op) are shown in the center panel for 16 asymptomatic patients with aortic regurgitation. The right panel represents values obtained with repeat study 6 months after surgery (post-op) in the same patients. The open circles represent mean values for ejection fraction. (Borer JS, et al.: Am J Cardiol 1979;44:1297–1305.)

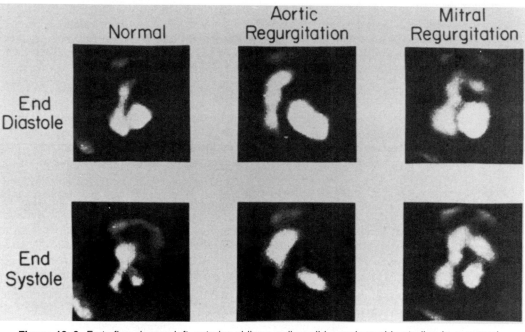

Figure 12–6. Forty-five–degree left anterior oblique radionuclide angiographic studies in a normal subject *(left panel),* a patient with aortic regurgitation *(middle panel),* and a patient with mitral regurgitation *(right panel).* The upper row shows end-diastolic images and the bottom row, end-systolic images. In aortic regurgitation, the left ventricle is shown to be displaced laterally and downward and well separated from the right ventricle. In mitral regurgitation, the right and left ventricles are not separated, and there is greater right ventricular enlargement than seen with aortic regurgitation. (Sorenson S, et al.: Circulation 1980;62:1089–1098.)

RV dynamics on RNA. From the first-pass portion of the gated equilibrium radionuclide study, tricuspid regurgitation may be evidenced by systolic reflux of the tracer into the inferior vena cava. If pulmonary hypertension is present, the right and left pulmonary arteries appear dilated.

The operative results of mitral valve replacement for mitral regurgitation are directly related to the degree of irreversible myocardial damage that developed in the natural course of the disease; however, because of the unloading of LV pressure into the left atrium early during systole, the resting LVEF may remain within "normal limits" despite primary irreversible myocardial damage. The resting LVEF is still important in the assessment of patients with mitral regurgitation, since an EF that begins to fall even if it remains in the normal range would indicate progression of myocardial dysfunction. Phillips et al.[28] demonstrated that the preoperative rest EF was related to prognosis following mitral valve replacement for mitral regurgitation. Of 105 consecutive patients undergoing mitral valve replacement for mitral regurgitation, those who had an EF of 0.50 or greater had an 89% 5-year survival rate. This contrasted to a 71% survival rate for patients with a preoperative EF of 0.40 to 0.49 and 38% for those whose preoperative EF was below 0.40 (Fig. 12–7).

Resting M-mode and 2-D echocardiography and Doppler are more valuable than RNA in the assessment of patients at rest with mitral regurgitation. Echocardiography permits the detailed analysis of the morphology of the mitral valve, which provides information on the etiology of the regurgitation. Entities such as rheumatic mitral regurgitation, mitral valve prolapse, ruptured chordae with or without a flail leaflet, papillary muscle dysfunction, calcified mitral annulus, and vegetations or valvular erosion from infective endocarditis can all be identified on echocardiography. This morphologic examination of the mitral valve apparatus can help the surgeon determine whether or not mitral valve repair or mitral valve replacement is the surgical procedure of choice.

Another important variable that contributes to long-term prognosis in patients with mitral regurgitation is the size of the left atrium.[29] This can be measured more precisely with echocardiography than by RNA. The left atrium is sometimes massively enlarged in patients with mitral regurgitation. The dimensions of the left ventricle can also be measured with echocardiographic techniques. When mitral regurgitation is severe, there is a progressive increase in the end-diastolic dimension, the end-systolic dimension, and stroke volume. Fractional shortening is often increased in patients without heart failure but is decreased when myocardial dysfunction develops. Another important role of echocardiography and RNA in mitral regurgitation patients is the identification of regional wall motion abnormalities, which may be secondary to a previous infarction. In this instance, mitral regurgitation could be secondary to papillary muscle functional abnormalities consequent to the development of myocardial and papillary muscle scar.

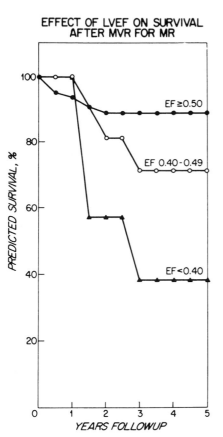

Figure 12–7. Survival curves showing the predicted survival rates of the study population stratified according to the left ventricular ejection fraction. Patients with an ejection fraction below 0.40 had a significantly reduced survival rate. The study population consisted of 105 consecutive patients undergoing mitral valve replacement for isolated mitral regurgitation. (Phillips HR, et al.: Am J Cardiol 1981;48:647–654.)

Doppler echocardiography has been utilized increasingly for the detection of mitral regurgitation and for "semiquantitating" its severity.[30] Color Doppler can display the regurgitant jet, and the distance attained by the jet in the LV chamber correlates with the degree of regurgitation. Echocardiography can also be valuable intraoperatively to determine the efficacy of mitral valve repair and is the approach of choice for intraoperative assessment of mitral regurgitation.

Exercise Radionuclide Angiography

The clinical application of exercise RNA in mitral regurgitation is somewhat more limited than in aortic insufficiency because the hemodynamic response of the left ventricle to exercise is markedly influenced by the unloading effect of early regurgitation into the left atrium during systole. This reduces afterload stress during systole. Evaluation of RVEF during exercise may be more useful than evaluation of the exercise LVEF. A fall in RVEF should correlate with severity of pulmonary hypertension. The LVEF response to exercise stress may deteriorate after surgery[31];

however, RVEF should increase toward the normal range after successful valve surgery.

As mentioned above with respect to patients with aortic regurgitation, patients with mitral regurgitation who become symptomatic should be evaluated immediately for valve repair or replacement. Asymptomatic patients with mitral regurgitation should be strongly considered for surgery if there is evidence of impaired LV function at rest. Even an LVEF that is in the 50% to 55% range may be "abnormal" in patients with mitral regurgitation. The early unloading effect of regurgitation during systole should produce a resting EF in excess of 60% if underlying myocardial contractility is not impaired.

TRICUSPID REGURGITATION

Tricuspid regurgitation is best evaluated with echocardiographic techniques. Nevertheless, first-pass RNA permits the detection of systemic venous reflux, which strongly suggests tricuspid regurgitation.[32] In addition to observing systemic reflux in the venae cavae with tricuspid regurgitation, intraventricular septal wall motion abnormalities and an abnormal RV-LV stroke volume index would be useful parameters for determining severity of tricuspid regurgitation.

If tricuspid regurgitation is a primary disorder due to rheumatic heart disease, RV systolic function on RNA should be normal because of the unloading of the RV pressure into the right atrium. If tricuspid regurgitation is secondary to RV dysfunction, the radionuclide angiogram would demonstrate diffusely hypokinetic RV wall motion. If there is severe pulmonary hypertension, the right ventricle is enlarged and demonstrates diminished systolic function. In that instance, the pulmonary artery and the outflow tract may appear enlarged.

SUMMARY

Clearly, in valvular heart disease patients RNA is most useful for serially assessing resting LV function to determine the most appropriate timing for valve repair or replacement in patients with minimal or no symptoms. For patients with symptoms that appear consequent to the hemodynamic effects of the valve lesion, surgery should be recommended regardless of RNA findings. Exercise RNA now is rarely performed as a means for determining whether or not valve surgery is required. Finally, echocardiography plays a more important role than nuclear cardiology techniques for evaluating patients with valvular heart disease.

REFERENCES

1. Rigo P, Alderson PO, Robertson RM, Becker LC, Wagner HN Jr: Measurement of aortic and mitral regurgitation by gated cardiac blood pool scans. Circulation 1979;60:306–312.

2. Iskandrian AS, Heo J: Radionuclide angiographic evaluation of left ventricular performance at rest and during exercise in patients with aortic regurgitation. Am Heart J 1986;111:1143–1149.

3. Henze E, Schelbert HR, Wisenberg G, Ratib O, Schon H: Assessment of regurgitant fraction and right and left ventricular function at rest and during exercise: A new technique for determination of right ventricular stroke counts from gated equilibrium blood pool studies. Am Heart J 1982;104:953–962.

4. Bonow RO: Radionuclide angiography in the management of asymptomatic aortic regurgitation. Circulation 1991;84:I296–I302.

5. Roberts DL, DeWeese JA, Mahoney EB, Yu PN: Long-term survival following aortic valve replacement. Am Heart J 1976;91:311–317.

6. Copeland JG, Griepp RB, Stinson EB, Shumway NE: Long-term follow-up after isolated aortic valve replacement. J Thoracic Cardiovasc Surg 1977;74:875–889.

7. Cohn PF, Gorlin R, Cohn LH, Collins JJ Jr: Left ventricular ejection fraction as a prognostic guide in surgical treatment of coronary and valvular heart disease. Am J Cardiol 1974;34:136–141.

8. Forman R, Firth BG, Barnard MS: Prognostic significance of preoperative left ventricular ejection fraction and valve lesion in patients with aortic valve replacement. Am J Cardiol 1980;45:1120–1125.

9. Bonow RO, Dodd JT, Maron BJ, O'Gara PT, White GG, McIntosh CL, Clark RE, Epstein SE: Long-term serial changes in left ventricular function and reversal of ventricular dilatation after valve replacement for chronic aortic regurgitation. Circulation 1988;78:1108–1120.

10. Henry WL, Bonow RO, Borer JS, Ware JH, Kent KM, Redwood DR, McIntosh CL, Morrow AG, Epstein SE: Observations on the optimum time for operative intervention for aortic regurgitation. I. Evaluation of the results of aortic valve replacement in symptomatic patients. Circulation 1980;61:471–483.

11. Bonow RO, Picone AL, McIntosh CL, Jones M, Rosing DR, Maron BJ, Lakatos E, Clark RE, Epstein SE: Survival and functional results after valve replacement for aortic regurgitation from 1976 to 1983: Impact of preoperative left ventricular function. Circulation 1985;72:1244–1256.

11a. Bonow RO: Radionuclide angiography in the management of asymptomatic aortic regurgitation. Circulation 1991;84:1296–1302.

12. Greves J, Rahimtoola SH, McAnulty JH, DeMots H, Clark DG, Greenberg B, Starr A: Preoperative criteria predictive of late survival following valve replacement for severe aortic regurgitation. Am Heart J 1981;101:300–308.

13. Bonow RO, Rosing DR, McIntosh CL, Jones M, Maron BJ, Lan KK, Lakatos E, Bacharach SL, Green MV, Epstein SE: The natural history of asymptomatic patients with aortic regurgitation and normal left ventricular function. Circulation 1983;68:509–517.

14. Siemienczuk D, Greenberg B, Morris C, Massie B, Wilson RA, Topic N, Bristow JD, Cheitlin M: Chronic aortic insufficiency: Factors associated with progression to aortic valve replacement. Ann Intern Med 1989;110:587–592.

15. Fioretti P, Roelandt J, Bos RJ, Meltzer RS, van Hoogenhuijze D, Serruys PW, Nauta J, Hugenholtz PG: Echocardiography in chronic aortic insufficiency. Is valve replacement too late when left ventricular end-systolic dimension reaches 55 mm? Circulation 1983;67:216–221.

16. Daniel WG, Hood WP Jr, Siart A, Hausmann D, Nellessen U, Oelert H, Lichtlen PR: Chronic aortic regurgitation: Reassessment of the prognostic value of preoperative left ventricular end-systolic dimension and fractional shortening. Circulation 1985;71:669–680.

17. Borer JS, Bacharach SL, Green MV, Kent KM, Henry WL, Rosing DR, Seides SF, Johnston GS, Epstein SE: Exercise-induced left ventricular dysfunction in symptomatic and asymptomatic patients with aortic regurgitation: Assessment with radionuclide cineangiography. Am J Cardiol 1978;42:351–357.

18. Borer JS, Rosing DR, Kent KM, Bacharach SL, Green MV, McIntosh CJ, Morrow AG, Epstein SE: Left ventricular function at rest and during exercise after aortic valve replacement in patients with aortic regurgitation. Am J Cardiol 1979;44:1297–1305.

19. Boucher CA, Wilson RA, Kanarek DJ, Hutter AM Jr, Okada RD, Liberthson RR, Strauss HW, Pohost GM: Exercise testing in asymptomatic or minimally symptomatic aortic regurgitation: Relationship of left ventricular ejection fraction to left ventricular filling pressure during exercise. Circulation 1983;67:1091–1100.

20. Lewis S, Riba A, Berger H, Davis R, Wackers F, Alexander J, Sands M, Cohen L, Zaret B: Radionuclide angiographic exercise left ventricular performance in chronic aortic regurgitation: Relationship to resting echocardiographic ventricular dimensions and systolic wall stress. Am Heart J 1982;103:498.

21. Gerson MC, Engel PJ, Mantil JC, Bucher PD, Hertzberg VS, Adolph RJ: Effects of dynamic and isometric exercise on the radionuclide-determined regurgitant fraction in aortic insufficiency. J Am Coll Cardiol 1984;3:98–106.

22. Goldman ME, Packer M, Horowitz SF, Meller J, Patterson RE, Kukin M, Teichholz LE, Gorlin R: Relation between exercise-induced changes in ejection fraction and systolic loading conditions at rest in aortic regurgitation. J Am Coll Cardiol 1984;3:924–929.

23. Bonow RO, Picone AL, McIntosh CL, Jones M, Rosing DR, Maron BJ, Lakatos E, Clark RE, Epstein SE: Survival and functional results after valve replacement for aortic regurgitation from 1976 to 1983: Impact of preoperative left ventricular function. Circulation 1985;72:1244–1256.

24. Peter CA, Jones RH: Cardiac response to exercise in patients with chronic aortic regurgitation. Am Heart J 1982;104:85–91.

25. Iskandrian AS, Hakki AH, Kane SA, Segal BL: Quantitative radionuclide angiography in assessment of hemodynamic changes during upright exercise: Observations in normal subjects, patient with coronary artery disease and patients with aortic regurgitation. Am J Cardiol 1981;48:239–246.

26. Marks A, Borkowski H, Sands M, Wolfson S, Berger H, Zaret B: Exercise left ventricular performance in aortic regurgitation: Dissimilar responses in supine and upright positions (Abstract). Circulation 1982;66:II–354.

27. Boucher CA, Bingham JB, Osbakken MD, Okada RD, Strauss HW, Block PC, Levine FH, Phillips HR, Pohost GM: Early changes in left ventricular size and function after correction of left ventricular volume overload. Am J Cardiol 1981;47:991–1004.

27a. Sorensen S, O'Rourke RA, Chaudhuri TK: Noninvasive quantitation of valvular regurgitation by gated equilibrium radionuclide angiography. Circulation 1980;62:1089–1098.

28. Phillips HR, Levine FH, Carter JE, Boucher CA, Osbakken MD, Okada RD, Akins CW, Daggett WM, Buckley MJ, Pohost GM: Mitral valve replacement for isolated mitral regurgitation: Analysis of clinical course and late postoperative left ventricular ejection fraction. Am J Cardiol 1981;48:647–654.

29. Reed D, Abbott RD, Smucker ML, Kaul S: Prediction of outcome after mitral valve replacement in patients with symptomatic chronic mitral regurgitation. The importance of left atrial size. Circulation 1991;84:23–34.

30. Abbasi AS, Allen MW, DeCristofaro D, Ungar I: Detection and estimation of the degree of mitral regurgitation by range-gated pulsed Doppler echocardiography. Circulation 1980;61:143–147.

31. Johnston DL, Lesoway R, Kostuk WJ: Ventricular function following mitral valve surgery: Assessment using radionuclide ventriculography. Can J Surg 1984;27:349–353.

32. Winzelberg GG, Boucher CA, Pohost GM, McKusick KA, Bingham JB, Okada RD, Strauss HW: Right ventricular function in aortic and mitral valve disease. Chest 1981;79:520–528.

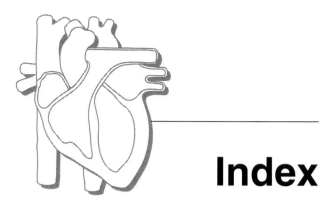

Index

Note: Page numbers in *italics* refer to illustrations; page numbers followed by t refer to tables.

ISBN 0-7216-3335-3